NUTRITION

NUTRITION
THE CHALLENGE OF BEING WELL NOURISHED

Dorothy A. Wenck
Martin Baren, M.D.
Sat Paul Dewan, Ph.D.

Reston Publishing Company, Inc.
A Prentice-Hall Company
Reston, Virginia

Library of Congress Cataloging in Publication Data
Wenck, Dorothy A
   Nutrition.

   Bibliography: p. 577
   Includes index.
   1. Nutrition.   I. Baren, Martin, joint author.
II. Dewan, Sat Paul, joint author.   III. Title.
TX354.W42   641.1   79-23425
ISBN 0-8359-5061-1

© 1980 by Reston Publishing Company, Inc.
A Prentice-Hall Company
Reston, Virginia 22090

10   9   8   7   6   5   4   3   2   1

Printed in the United States of America

CONTENTS

PREFACE   vii

Part I   FOODS, NUTRITION, AND CONSUMER CHOICES   1
            1   What Is Nutrition?   3
            2   Why We Eat What We Eat   23
            3   The Confused Consumer   57

Part II   ENERGY AND BODY WEIGHT   75
            4   Our Need for Energy   77
            5   The Challenge of Maintaining Ideal Weight   89
            6   Underweight   109

Part III   THE NUTRIENTS AND THE FOODS THAT SUPPLY
            THEM   115
            7   Carbohydrates and Fiber   117
                Supermarket Nutrition: Choosing Foods in the Bread
                                        and Cereal Group, 133
                                        Choosing Sugars and
                                        Sweeteners, 145
            8   Fats   151
                Supermarket Nutrition: Choosing Fats and Oils, 162
            9   Proteins   169
                Supermarket Nutrition: Choosing Foods in the Meat
                                        Group, 186
                                        Choosing a No-Meat Diet, 202

v

10   Our Need For Water   209
11   Mineral Elements   215
       Supermarket Nutrition: Choosing Foods in the Milk
                                Group, 237
12   Vitamins   247
       Supermarket Nutrition: Choosing Foods in the Vegetable
                                and Fruit Group, 269

Part IV   NUTRITION THROUGHOUT THE LIFE CYCLE   285
13   Nutrition During Pregnancy and Lactation   287
14   Infant Nutrition   303
15   Nutrition During Childhood   327
16   Nutrition During Adolescence   351
17   Nutrition in Adulthood   371

Part V   CONTEMPORARY ISSUES IN DIET AND HEALTH   383
18   Dietary Goals for the United States   385
19   Diet and Disease   389
20   Diet and Drugs   417
       Supermarket Nutrition: Buying Nutrient Supplements,
                                433

Part VI   NUTRIENTS: ARE THEY THERE WHEN WE EAT THE
     FOOD?   437
21   Variables Affecting Nutrients in Food   439
22   Loss and Retention of Nutrients in Food   447
       Supermarket Nutrition: Fresh Versus Processed
                                Foods, 458

Part VII   WHAT'S IN FOODS BESIDES NUTRIENTS?   463
23   Natural Toxicants   465
24   Intentional Additives   471
25   Contaminants   485
26   Who Protects Your Food?   501
       Supermarket Nutrition: "Natural," "Organic," and
                                "Health" Foods, 502

Part VIII   MEETING THE NUTRITION CHALLENGE   507
27   Food Management to Reach Nutrition Goals   509
28   Nutrition Challenges: Yesterday, Today, and
     Tomorrow   527

Appendix   NUTRITIVE VALUE OF FOODS   533

            RECOMMENDED DIETARY ALLOWANCES   572

            RELIABLE NUTRITION INFORMATION SOURCES   577

            INDEX   591

PREFACE

Survival is man's most basic nutrition challenge. Most of early man's efforts were spent getting enough to eat in order to survive. It was only after man developed efficient methods of obtaining food that he had time and energy left to begin developing other aspects of civilized life. In underdeveloped parts of the world, getting enough to eat is still the most pressing nutrition challenge.

But in affluent societies, such as the United States, where one farmer can produce enough to feed 50 or more people, our nutrition challenge is to be *well nourished* in the midst of plenty. The majority of people in the United States face the problem of eating too much—especially too much of the wrong kinds of food. Our challenge is to choose from among the many foods available to us those that will provide optimum nutrition.

For help in this decision making process, we turn to nutrition scientists who study the biochemistry of food and the reactions of the components of food inside the body. Through their research, we learn about the nutrients we need and how we can get them from our food.

The purpose of this book is to give you a sound basis for making decisions—based on current nutrition knowledge—about the foods you eat. Many people, even with a thorough knowledge of the basic facts, do not eat very well. Therefore, our emphasis is on the practical aspects of choosing foods—the translation of nutrition knowledge into food choices—and on the factors that affect our nutrient needs, our eating habits, and the nutritional value of our everyday foods. This endeavor becomes somewhat difficult at times because of the many controversies in the field of nutrition. These controversies tend to make our challenge that much more stimulating.

Only a simplified version of the chemistry and physiology of nutrition is presented here, as background to enable the reader to understand some of the reasons behind the "rules." If this introduction to applied nutrition whets your appetite, you may want to study subjects such as organic chemistry, biochemistry, and physiology in preparation for a more in-depth study of nutrition science. The reference section at the end of the book lists resources that provide more information on the scientific aspects of nutrition.

As you study nutrition, remember that it is a relatively young science and that nutrition scientists don't know all the answers. The body of nutrition knowledge is expanding rapidly with the development of new research techniques. Many facts are yet to be learned. And on some questions, nutrition scientists are not in agreement among themselves!

For this reason, you must recognize that educating yourself about nutrition is an ongoing process. You need to update your knowledge continually with current readings in reliable publications. And you need to read popular nutrition books and articles with a questioning mind, for much nutrition information put forth as "fact" is merely theory or speculation unsubstantiated by valid research. The reference list includes periodicals that can be relied upon to give you up-to-date, scientifically based information.

The primary focus of this book is, therefore, on the practical, everyday application of nutrition principles to food choices. The main thrust deals with the day-to-day issues that affect food choices and subsequently the health of the individual.

The goals of *Nutrition* include the following:

1. To make the reader aware of the basic chemical and physiological concepts of nutrition.

2. To examine the concepts of under- and overnutrition, and to study the various nutrients and learn how they apply to our daily lives.

3. To acquaint the reader with the necessity of different food choices for the various age groups and for people with special requirements due to medical conditions.

4. To address some of the controversial and newer issues in nutrition and to help the reader make some sense out of the often puzzling array of information.

5. To enable the reader to translate knowledge into food choice—to understand just what he or she is putting on the table.

6. To stimulate the student of nutrition to educate himself continually and to try to evaluate the information supplied in a meaningful,

nonbiased, and inquisitive manner in order to arrive at a meaningful conclusion.

Finally, we must remember that even "nutrition experts" may disagree among themselves. Thus, it is important not to become too dogmatic about what you *know* about this subject. It is often necessary to say "based upon what we know" or "let's wait until we have more facts." An open mind is healthy for growth!

We feel that *Nutrition* will be helpful and useful as a guide to informed and practical nutrition. If it is true that "we are what we eat," we should certainly understand exactly what it is that we *are* eating. It is our hope that this book will be just the beginning of a lifelong interest in a subject that is so vital to our health.

The authors gratefully acknowledge the aid and close support of Mrs. Janice Parks, nutrition educator at Santa Ana (California) Community College. Her expert advice, from the inception of this book through its organization and final review, is immensely appreciated. We also wish to thank Mrs. Parks for supplying chapter objectives, chapter summaries, and essential information about the needs of the students for whom this book is intended.

Because food selection is such a vital part of your nutrition challenge, chapters on the nutrients (Chapters 7, 8, 9, 11, 12, 20, 22, and 26) contain sections on "supermarket nutrition." These sections will help you make a connection between the nutrients discussed and choosing the foods that contain them.

Part I

FOODS, NUTRITION, AND CONSUMER CHOICES

WHAT
IS
NUTRITION? 1

Highlights

Components of nutrition

Recommended Dietary Allowances (RDA) and U.S. RDA

Pros and cons of food guides with emphasis on the Basic Four
  system

Malnutrition

Nutritional status

What is nutrition? Better yet, what is good nutrition?

The person who wants to find the answers to these questions might easily become lost in the mysterious maze of informational corridors, confused by the wealth of technical information provided by scientists or misled by simplistic answers provided by those who may have products to sell. Somewhere in between is some reasonable, common sense information that we can use to guide us in our quest for sound nutrition knowledge.

NUTRITION AND FOOD: DEFINITIONS

The word *nutrition* is often paired with the word *food* because the two go together. They are interdependent, but not interchangeable.

Food might be defined as any edible substance that provides nourishment when consumed. Food contains ingredients known as *nutrients*, which we must have to have energy for activities, to grow, and to maintain health. (See Exhibit 1.1.) These essential nutrients are categorized as carbohydrates (which are sugars, starches and fibers), fats, proteins, minerals, vitamins, and water.

Exhibit 1.1   The Three Functions of Foods and Nutrients

Provide energy for activities
Build and maintain body tissue
Regulate body processes

Food also contains many other substances that are not nutrients but that may have other functions such as providing flavor or color.

Nutrition might be defined as the *process* whereby we obtain the essential nutrients and use them to make many other substances our bodies need. This process would include eating and digesting food and absorbing and using, or metabolizing, the nutrients it contains.

We can obtain all of the essential nutrients from food. However, it is possible to obtain nourishment without eating and digesting food—if, for example, the nutrients are injected directly into our veins as in intravenous feeding.

Thus it is the nutrients that are essential, and the food that normally provides them. Since food is vital, we need to know the nutritive content of foods, which ones are the best sources of the various nutrients, and how to combine them into a healthful diet.

The term *good nutrition* implies that we are obtaining from our food all of the essential nutrients in the amounts needed to keep our bodies functioning and to maintain optimum health. A very simplified definition of good nutrition might be "eating the right foods in the right amounts."

The work of nutrition scientists involves finding the answers to questions about the nutrients—their function in the body, the amount of each that we need, what happens when we receive too much or too little—and about food and diet—what foods we should eat and in what amount.

Yet nutrition science in its broadest sense has many more facets: the influence of sensory factors of flavor, color, and texture of food on eating behavior; the psychological, cultural, emotional, and social aspects of food intake; and even the economics of food availability and consumer behavior in the purchase of food have an impact on nutrition. Some of these considerations will be discussed in the next chapter.

THE NUTRIENTS

To date nutrition scientists have identified some 40 to 45 substances as essential nutrients. But the list is growing as new nutrients continue to be identified. The history of nutrition science contains fascinating stories about the ways food substances have been identified as essential nutrients. In some instances, medical researchers seeking the cause of a particular disease found that the problem was due to a deficiency of a single substance, and that when this substance was added to the diet, the symptoms of the disease disappeared. A number of vitamins were discovered in this way.

Nutrients might be divided into two general categories based on the amount that we need. These are the *macronutrients* (carbohydrates, fats, proteins, and water), which we need in relatively large amounts, and the *micronutrients* (mineral elements and vitamins), which we need in relatively small amounts. All of the nutrients except for mineral elements and water are classified as organic substances because they contain the element carbon. Mineral elements and water are inorganic substances because they do not contain carbon.

Exhibit 1.2 gives an overview of the most common nutrients. Fats, carbohydrates, and proteins will be discussed in Chapters 7 through 9; water, mineral elements, and vitamins in Chapters 10 through 12.

The vitamins are divided into two general categories based on their solubility in either water or fat. The fat-soluble vitamins are vitamins A, D, E, and K; the water-soluble vitamins include vitamin C (ascorbic acid), niacin, thiamin, riboflavin, folic acid (also called folacin), pantothenic acid, pyridoxine, vitamin B_{12}, and biotin.

The mineral elements are divided into two categories based on the quantity of them that we need. Macroelements are those needed in relatively large amounts while microelements are those needed in very

Exhibit 1.2   Classification of Nutrients

MACRONUTRIENTS		

Carbohydrates (sugar and starch; also fiber)
Proteins
Fats
Water

MICRONUTRIENTS	WATER SOLUBLE	FAT SOLUBLE
Vitamins	C (ascorbic acid)	A
	Niacin	D
	Thiamin	E
	Riboflavin	K
	Folic Acid (or Folacin)	
	Pantothenic Acid	
	Pyridoxine (B_6)	
	B_{12}	
	Biotin	

	MACROELEMENTS	MICROELEMENTS
Mineral Elements	Calcium	Iron
	Phosphorus	Manganese
	Sodium	Copper
	Potassium	Iodine
	Chlorine	Fluorine
	Sulfur	Zinc
	Magnesium	Cobalt
		Molybdenum
		Selenium

small amounts. Some examples of macroelements are sodium, potassium, calcium, and phosphorous. Some examples of microelements are iron, iodine, manganese, zinc, and fluorine.

RECOMMENDED DIETARY ALLOWANCES

Once a nutrient is identified, one of the principal research efforts of nutrition scientists is to determine how much of it is needed by people at various ages and stages of life. Initial studies usually are conducted with laboratory animals, but the information developed in these studies cannot be applied directly to humans since people's needs often are quite different from animals' needs. Human nutrition studies, on the other hand, are time-consuming, costly, and difficult to conduct, especially because of the problems of controlling variables and possibly causing harm to the individuals involved. Because of the obstacles to collecting accurate data, our present knowledge of nutrient needs is incomplete, and the requirements of humans for many nutrients have not been established.

However, the data on human and animal needs currently available are used by nutrition scientists to establish estimates of the amounts of essential nutrients per day that will meet the needs of most healthy persons. In the United States, the most widely used nutrient guidelines are the Recommended Dietary Allowances (RDA), which are issued by the National Academy of Sciences, National Research Council, Food and Nutrition Board. They are updated every four to six years, and the 1979 RDA are used in this book (see Appendix A).

The RDA serve as dietary or nutritional standards for a wide range of age–weight–sex groups such as infants, children, adolescents, pregnant and lactating women, and younger and older adults. They are recommendations, not average requirements, for satisfactory levels of intake of essential nutrients for population groups of average, healthy people. They do not take account of special needs certain individuals may have due to genetic makeup, metabolic disorders, chronic infections, and other abnormalities, which may result in their needing different levels of nutrients.

To allow for individual differences, the RDA usually are set with a generous margin of safety. Thus they are thought to meet the needs of 95 to 97 percent of the people within each age-sex group. In other words, the RDA exceed the requirements of most individuals to ensure that the needs of nearly all are met. For this reason, a person who consumes a diet that provides less than the RDA for one or more essential nutrients is not necessarily getting a diet that is nutritionally inadequate. What can be concluded, however, is that the farther the intake of an essential nutrient falls below the RDA, the greater the probability of nutritional inadequacy. On the other hand, if an individual is getting all the essential nutrients at or above the RDA level of his or her age, chances are good that the diet is nutritionally adequate.

An exception is the RDA for energy, or calories, which are not designed as guides for individual calorie needs. Other variables not included in the RDA, such as body size and physical activity, are involved in an individual's calorie requirements.

Another factor considered when the RDA are established is the availability of the nutrient and the factors that affect how efficiently it is used in the body. For some nutrients, such as iron, absorption or use in the body may be incomplete; so the RDA needs to be set high enough to allow for this. And because in the case of certain other nutrients, substances in foods, called *precursors*, may be converted into the nutrient in the body, the RDA needs to allow for this. An example is *carotene*, the orange-colored substance found in carrots and other vegetables and fruits, which our bodies convert to vitamin A.

On the other side of the coin, receiving too much of certain nutrients, amounts significantly above the RDA, can be just as harmful as not obtaining enough. Certain vitamins (such as A and D) and minerals can be highly toxic if high doses are used over a period of time. Thus the RDA can serve as guidelines for optimal nutrient intake from the standpoint of both maximum and minimum levels.

The most appropriate use of the RDA, the one for which they were originally established, is as guides in the planning and procurement of food supplies for population groups such as the armed services and residents of schools, hospitals, mental, and penal institutions. Another major use is for standards against which to evaluate diet of population groups in a study of their nutritional status. However, when the results of dietary surveys are compared with the RDA, caution should be exercised in drawing conclusions.

An adaptation of the RDA is now being used as part of the nutrition-labeling program. The Food and Drug Administration (FDA) has adopted the U.S. Recommended Daily Allowances (U.S. RDA) as a standard for giving information about the nutrient value of foods on labels. The U.S. RDA consist of single values for each nutrient, usually the highest RDA value for any age group. The nutrition labels show the nutrient content of each food as a percentage of the U.S. RDA. For example, a label may tell you that one cup of milk provides 20 percent of the U.S. RDA for protein, 6 percent of the U.S. RDA for vitamin A, 30 percent of the U.S. RDA for calcium, and so on.

Since the U.S. RDA for adults are based on the needs of the age group (usually teenage boys) having the highest need for each nutrient, most people do not need to obtain 100 percent of the U.S. RDA for every nutrient. In some cases the differences between an individual's need for a nutrient and the U.S. RDA may be as high as 50 percent. Thus, nutrition label information must be used with caution.

Another way foods are compared is on the basis of their *nutrient density*, that is, the relative proportion of nutrients to calories (calories measure the energy value of foods). Foods high in calories and relatively low in other nutrients are said to have low nutrient density while foods low in calories and high in other nutrients have a high nutrient density.

FOODS AS SOURCES OF NUTRIENTS

All of the nutrients needed by the body are available from the food we eat. So in addition to establishing the amounts of the individual nutrients that humans need, nutrition scientists also are concerned with finding out where we get the nutrients, that is, in learning what foods contain what nutrients and in what amounts.

This information is needed for developing recommendations for foods and diets that will provide good nutrition. The "balanced diet" concept in which there is a good combination of all the foods needed for good health derives from this knowledge.

As we will learn in Chapter 21, the nutrient level of foods can be highly variable and depend on many factors including genetics, growing conditions, and the way the food is handled from the time it is harvested until it is eaten.

The information compiled by researchers over the years about the nutritive value of foods is assembled in food composition tables. Appendix B provides an abbreviated listing of the estimated nutrient values of many of our common foods.

The average consumer, however, is not interested in using food composition tables to plan meals and choose foods that provide good nutrition. Realizing this, nutrition educators have attempted to bridge the gap between the scientist and the consumer with simplified guides to food selection. In most food guides everyday foods are classified into basic groups according to similarity of nutrient content, and suggestions are made for the amounts of each group of food that should be eaten daily. The assumption is that if foods from each group are eaten every day in the recommended amounts, the consumer will have a reasonably balanced diet.

The basic purpose of food guides is nutrition education. They are used in many nations throughout the world and differ considerably from one country to another since they tend to reflect the food customs of the people as well as the availability of food.

In the United States the first food guide was developed during World War I and was based on five groups: (1) vegetables and fruits; (2) meat, fish, and milk; (3) cereals; (4) sugar; and (5) fat. During World War II the grouping was revised and became the *Basic Seven*: (1) citrus fruits; (2) leafy green vegetables; (3) other vegetables and fruits; (4) meat, fish, poultry, eggs, dried beans, peas, and nuts; (5) milk and cheese; (6) breads and cereals; and (7) fats.

After using this guide for some 10 years, nutrition educators decided that the number of groups was too high and the system was too complicated for the average person to remember and use.

Finally, the system widely used today was introduced. Called the *Basic Four*, or the *Four Food Groups*, it consists of four groups: (1) milk and cheese; (2) vegetables and fruits; (3) breads and cereals; and (4) meat, poultry, eggs, fish, dried beans and peas, and nuts. Exhibit 1.3 shows the kinds of foods and nutrients prominent in each group. Typical nutrition education flyers, showing the foods and servings suggested in this food guide are pictured in Exhibits 1.4 and 1.5.

In the Four Food Groups, fat and sugar are excluded altogether to deemphasize their use and prevent their being considered necessary additons to the diet. (We can get plenty of sugar and fat as natural or added ingredients of the foods in the four groups.)

Exhibit 1.3   The Four Food Groups

	NUTRIENTS	
	GOOD SOURCE OF:	POOR SOURCE OF:

I. Milk Group

| Milk, cheese, yogurt, cottage cheese, ice cream | Calcium Vitamins A and D Riboflavin Protein | Iron Vitamin C |

* Servings: Adults: 2 each day, 8 oz or equivalent
     Teenagers: 4 each day   Children: 2–3 each day
     Pregnancy and lactation: 4–5 each day

II. Meat Group

| All meats, fish, poultry eggs Dry beans and dry peas (legumes), nuts, peanut butter | Protein B Vitamins Iron Fats | Vitamins A and D Vitamin C |

Servings: 2 each day, 2–3 oz servings

III. Vegetable - Fruit Group

| All vegetables *Deep yellow*—carrots, squash *Dark Green*—green peppers, broccoli, spinach, kale, endive, asparagus *Other*—tomato, lettuce, peas, onion, corn, lima beans, beets, potato, cabbage, cauliflower, celery Citrus Fruits: orange, grapefruit Other Fruits: apple, banana, peach, pear, plum, apricot, grapes, berries, prunes | Vitamin C Vitamin A Carbohydrate and fiber Iron | Fat |

Servings: 4 each day, ½ cup serving

IV. Bread-Cereal Group

| (These should be whole grain or enriched.) Bread Cereal (ready to eat) Cereal (cooked) Noodles Macaroni Spaghetti Rice Grits Crackers | Carbohydrate (starch, fiber) B Vitamins Iron | Vitamin C |

Servings: 4 each day, 1 slice or 1 oz

DAILY FOOD GUIDE
some choices for thrifty families

MILK GROUP
some for everyone

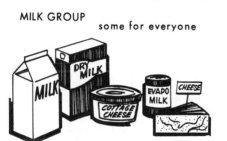

MEAT GROUP
2 or more servings

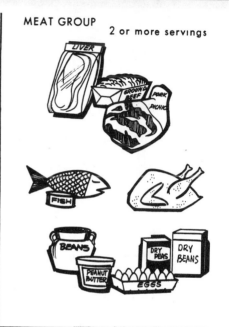

VEGETABLE - FRUIT GROUP
4 or more servings

Dark Green

Deep Yellow

Citrus and Tomatoes

others

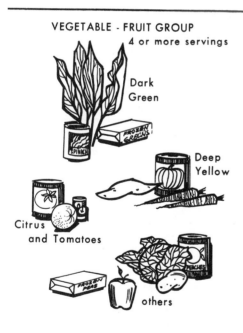

BREAD - CEREAL GROUP
4 or more servings

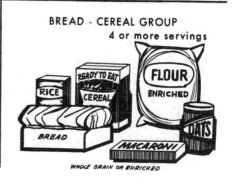

WHOLE GRAIN OR ENRICHED

everyday eat foods from each group
EAT OTHER FOODS AS NEEDED TO ROUND OUT MEALS

Exhibit 1.4.

Follow the Food Guide
Every Day

SOME
for
EVERYONE

MILK GROUP
COUNT AS A SERVING 1 CUP OF MILK

Children under 9 — to	Adults — or more
Children 9-12 — or more	Pregnant Women — or more
Teenagers — or more	Nursing Mothers — or more

Cheese can be used for part of the MILK

2
or more
SERVINGS

MEAT GROUP
COUNT AS A SERVING 2 OR 3 OUNCES OF COOKED LEAN MEAT, POULTRY OR FISH — — SUCH AS

A HAMBURGER   OR A CHICKEN LEG   OR A FISH

ALSO-2 EGGS

OR 1 CUP COOKED DRY BEANS OR PEAS

OR 4 TABLESPOONS PEANUT BUTTER

4
or more
SERVINGS

VEGETABLE-FRUIT GROUP
COUNT AS A SERVING ½ CUP (RAW OR COOKED)

OR 1 PORTION SUCH AS

OR   OR

4
or more
SERVINGS

BREAD-CEREAL GROUP (WHOLE GRAIN OR ENRICHED)
COUNT AS A SERVING   1 TORTILLA — — —

1 SLICE OF BREAD OR 1 BISCUIT

OR 1 OUNCE READY-TO-EAT CEREAL — — — —

OR ½ CUP TO ¾ CUP COOKED CEREAL,

CORNMEAL, GRITS, MACARONI, RICE, OR SPAGHETTI

EAT OTHER FOODS AS NEEDED TO ROUND OUT THE MEALS

U.S. DEPARTMENT OF AGRICULTURE • Consumer and Marketing Service • Agricultural Research Service • July 1966

ADAPTED BY UNIVERSITY OF CALIFORNIA AGRICULTURAL EXTENSION SERVICE

Co-operative Extension work in Agriculture and Home Economics, United States Department of Agriculture and University of California co-operating

Exhibit 1.5.

The Four Food Group system is easy to understand and provides a simple method for consumers to follow when planning and evaluating their diets. However, in recent years, the system has been criticized by nutrition scientists as being both oversimplified and outdated because of the many changes in foods and food habits that have taken place since the system was developed.

Some of their specific criticisms include:

1. When consumed in recommended amounts, the Four Food Groups provide only 1,200-1,300 calories (too few for almost everyone except dieters), and they also are low in iron, for women, and thiamin, for men.

2. Other nutrients such as folacin, vitamin E, Vitamin B_6, zinc, and magnesium, whose importance has been realized only in recent years, are not provided for in the Four Food Groups.

3. Many highly processed, fabricated, and convenience foods are not nutritionally equivalent to the less processed foods that they replace. A sugared fruit-flavored drink fortified with vitamin C is nowhere near the equivalent of orange juice, for example, and enriched white flour lacks the trace minerals found in whole grain flour.

4. All foods in each group are not equally nutritious and interchangeable. In the meat group, for example, when beans or peas or nuts are substituted for animal protein, no vitamin B_{12} is supplied. Some fruits, for example, pears, have few nutrients compared to other fruits, such as citrus.

5. Individuals may choose the least nutritious foods in each group or not have serving sizes sufficiently large and as a result not meet their nutritional requirements. A study by California nutrition scientists showed that improper choices from the Four Food Groups can result in a diet providing less than two-thirds of the RDA for magnesium, iron, zinc, vitamin B_6 and vitamin C.[1] This may be especially true in periods of increased needs such as pregnancy and lactation.

However, the Four Food Groups can be useful for planning a foundation diet with some modifications. You can make up for some of its potential deficiencies if you:

1. Choose a wide variety of foods in each group. The more narrow your choices, the more likely you are to miss some important nutrients.

2. Include as many unprocessed or lightly processed foods as practical and not depend on highly processed convenience foods exclusively. Whole grains are preferred over enriched cereals because of their content of magnesium, zinc, folacin, iron, and vitamin B_6.

[1]J. King, S. Cohenour, C. Corruccini, P. Schneeman, "Evaluation and Modification of the Basic Four Food Guide." *Journal of Nutrition Education* , Vol. 10, No. 1, Jan-March, 1978, p. 27.

3. Use plenty of dark green leafy vegetables as a good source of folacin, calcium, and riboflavin.

4. Increase serving sizes or add a third serving from the meat or milk group. For example, use nuts as a snack food for a good source of thiamin. Use liver or other organ meats regularly. Legumes contain more vitamin B_6, folacin, iron, zinc, and magnesium than does animal protein.

5. Use some margarine or other type of vegetable oil, for example, in cooking or salad dressing, as a source of vitamin E.

6. Add extra foods to meet your calorie needs from other foods in the Four Food Groups as much as possible rather than using low-nutrient-density foods that are high in sugar, fat, or alcohol.

To sum up, while the Four Food Group system has its faults, no alternative system has been developed that is as simple and practical. But if you use it, use it wisely.

EVALUATING NUTRITIONAL STATUS

The nutritional status of an individual or group of people and how to measure it are other questions that concern both the nutrition scientist and the health professional. We know that nutrition plays a major role in the maintenance of good health for people of all ages. Thus, deviations from good nutrition are likely to be associated with lack of optimal health or performance.

Since good nutrition implies the presence of a diet that contains all the nutrients in proportions that are necessary for the proper functioning of the body, it follows that in malnutrition (*mal* meaning bad) there is a deviation in the optimum amount of one or more of the nutrients, which may lead to the impairment of health. In malnutrition there could be a lack, excess, or imbalance of nutrients.

The continuum of nutritional status that could result under various levels of nutrient intake is illustrated in Exhibit 1.6. Overnutrition is associated with an excess of one or more of the nutrients. Undernutrition may be caused by a deficiency of any of the essential nutrients or by a generalized insufficient intake of foods and all or nearly all of the nutrients. Undernutrition also may result when an adequate diet is eaten, but the body is not able to utilize the food due to some disorder or disease. This type of nutritional disorder may include conditions such as:

1. Lack of ingestion—vomiting, gastrointestinal blockage

2. Difficulty in absorption and transportation of food in gastrointestinal tract due to liver, pancreas, and intestinal enzyme disorders

3. Lack of utilization—metabolic disorders such as diabetes mellitus

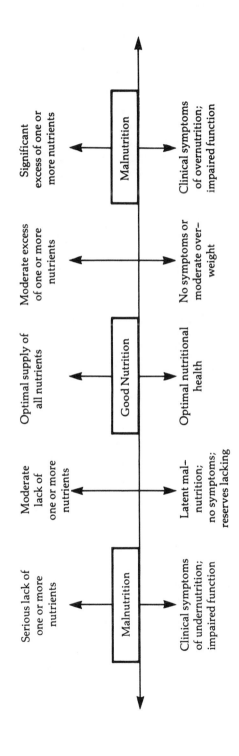

Exhibit 1.6. Continuum of Nutritional Status

15

4. Increased metabolism due to fever, injury

5. Excessive excretion—diarrhea, bowel, and kidney diseases

The main concern of this book is with the type of nutritional disorder associated with diet rather than physiological malfunctioning. Some nutritional disorders which are directly caused by a lack of nutrients are anemia (iron), marasmus (calories), kwashiorkor (protein), beri-beri and pellagra (B vitamins), scurvy (vitamin C), and rickets (vitamin D, calcium). The results of an overabundance of nutrients might cause an easily observed symptom such as obesity or a serious reaction to toxic doses of vitamin or mineral supplements. An imbalance of nutrients, especially too much sugar, might be a contributing cause of dental caries.

Scientists study the nutritional status of population groups in several ways. They may survey available food supplies and draw inferences about the quality of the diet of the population from the disappearance of foods from the marketplace. Annual food consumption statistics from the U.S. Department of Agriculture (USDA) are actually "disappearance" statistics that may be used for this type of study.

Another study method is to conduct a food purchasing or consumption survey of a random sample of people in a population group and compare the diets consumed with a nutrition standard such as the RDA. Once every decade the U.S. Department of Agriculture has conducted this type of survey among a cross section of people in the United States and from the information gathered has reported some general conclusions about the nutritional quality of the American diet.

In neither of these types of surveys is the actual food consumed or the nutritional health of individuals measured. To collect this type of data scientists employ diet diaries or dietary recalls, clinical evaluations, and biochemical analyses of individuals being studied.

In a diet diary, the individual records all foods eaten, usually as they are eaten, over a period of time, while in a diet recall, the person is asked to remember what was eaten for a time period such as 24 hours. Food intake may then be compared to a norm, such as a food guide, or it may be analyzed for nutrients and compared to a standard such as the RDA.

Clinical evaluations of individuals include such things as a medical history and physical examination; height, weight, head circumference, and skinfold thickness measurements; dental examination; and X-rays.

Biochemical analyses are used to measure the levels of nutrients and other substances in body tissues and fluids (blood, urine) that reflect current or recent nutritional status. The depletion of body stores of nutrients is the first downward step in the development of nutritional-deficiency disease. Thus, biochemical measurements help to identify risk populations as well as people with actual malnutrition.

Quite obviously, a survey of the nutritional status of a large group of people using these methods would be time-consuming, difficult to conduct, and costly. For these reasons only a limited number of such studies have been done and only on a relatively small scale. So we don't really know what the nutritional status of the people of the United States is.

The most well known of the surveys is the Ten State Nutrition Survey, which was carried out in 1968–70 under the direction of the U.S. Department of Health, Education, and Welfare (HEW). Initially this survey was planned to be a nationwide study, but it was discontinued, for budgetary reasons, after the data from the first ten states were gathered. The results were not considered to be representative of the nutritional status of the total population of the United States because researchers concentrated on studying people living in census tracts having the largest concentration of lower income groups.[2]

Two other large scale studies of nutritional status in the U.S. are the Preschool Nutrition Survey, conducted in 1968–70, and the Health and Nutrition Examination Survey (HANES) conducted in 1971–72 by HEW. Some of the results of the nutrition status studies are included in Chapter 15.

HOW GOOD IS YOUR DIET?

If you wanted to evaluate the nutritional quality of your diet, how might you do it?

To begin with, you would need to keep a careful record of the food you eat, estimating as accurately as possible the amounts eaten, for a period of two or three days. Then you might simply compare your diet with a food guide such as the Four Food Groups to see if you are eating the recommended foods in the recommended amounts. A sample form for making such a comparison is shown in Exhibit 1.7.

For a rough idea of the amounts of the various nutrients that you consumed, look up each food eaten in a food value chart (such as that found in Appendix B), record all the nutrients listed for each food, add them up, and compare your totals for the day with a standard such as the RDA. Remember, however, that there are pitfalls when using the RDA for analyzing individual diets.

If you undertake such a project, you will soon realize that it is tedious and time-consuming, as well as frustrating, because you will not be able to find exactly the foods you ate listed in the chart. But if you are lucky, you may find a college or university or other institution in your

[2]"Highlights from the Ten-State Nutrition Survey." *Nutrition Today*, Vol. 7, No. 4, July-August, 1972, pp. 4-11.

Exhibit 1.7   Score Your Diet: Record the Portion of Serving

FOODS EATEN	AMOUNT	MILK GROUP	MEAT GROUP	FRUIT/ VEGETABLE GROUP	BREAD/ CEREAL GROUP
Morning					
Orange Juice	½ cup			1	
Egg	1		½		
Toast	2 slices				2
Milk	½ cup	½			
Midday					
Peanut Butter Sandwich			½		2
Carrots Sticks				½	
Apple				1	
Milk	1 cup	1			
Late-day					
Meatloaf	4 oz		1½		
Baked Potato	1			1	
Peas	½ cup			1	
Fruit Salad	½ cup			1	
Milk	½ cup	½			
Ice Cream	½ cup	½			
TOTAL NUMBER OF SERVINGS		2½	2½	5½	4
Recommended Number of Servings for Adults		2	2	4	4

area that has available a computer program for analyzing the nutrient value of diets. Using a computer for diet analysis can greatly simplify the task as well as improve the accuracy.

Nutrition scientists have observed that it is not necessary to analyze a diet for every nutrient to evaluate its overall nutritional value. Instead, a diet can be evaluated for the presence of certain *key nutrients* (Exhibit 1.8), which are reliable indicators of the presence of the other nutrients. The key nutrients usually used are protein, vitamin C, niacin, thiamin, riboflavin, vitamin A, calcium, and iron. Exhibit 1.9 shows how these key nutrients are provided by the Four Food Groups.

However, one researcher, J. A. Pennington, has found that there are seven nutrients that more consistently indicate the presence of other nutrients.[3] The *Pennington Index Nutrients*, as they are called, are folacin, vitamin B_6, pantothenic acid, magnesium, vitamin A, calcium, and iron.

[3]S. Lane and J. Vermeersch, "Evaluation of the Thrifty Food Plan." *Journal of Nutrition Education*, Vol. 11, No. 2, April–June, 1979, p. 96.

Pennington found that if the RDA for these nutrients are met in a diet, the other nutrients are likely to be present in adequate amounts as well. A drawback in using the Pennington Index is that several of the nutrients (magnesium, folacin, B₆ and pantothenic acid) are not found on the usual food value charts.

Whatever method you might use for evaluating your diet, remember that this is just a first step in achieving good nutrition. If evaluation shows that your diet is a good one, you will want to try to maintain this standard. And if analysis shows up some deficiencies or excesses, especially calories, you may want to take some action to change your eating patterns to improve your diet.

However, this is often easier said than done. As we will learn in the next chapter, our eating behavior is influenced by many factors not related to the nutritional quality of foods and we may be very resistant to changing our ways.

Summary

The science of nutrition has many dimensions. Although fundamentally concerned with the process of obtaining and utilizing nutrients, it embraces many other elements such as sensory factors, psychological-social influences, and even food purchase considerations. The 40 to 45 essential nutrients discovered to date can be divided into those needed in larger amounts, termed macronutrients (carbohydrates, fats, proteins, and water), and those needed in small amounts, or micronutrients (mineral elements and vitamins).

Scientists are using data from laboratory and the more costly and difficult human nutrition studies in an attempt to determine nutrient needs of people at various stages of life. Those nutrients about which sufficient information has been obtained have been compiled into a table estimating daily nutritional needs. These guidelines for a wide range of age–weight–sex groups are termed *Recommended Dietary Allowances* (RDA). To allow for individual differences, the RDA have a generous margin of safety for most healthy people. An adaptation of the RDA is used as the standard for nutritional labeling of certain foods. Referred to as the U.S. RDA, it consists of a single value for each nutrient, usually the highest for any age group.

Food guides classify foods into basic groups according to similarity of nutrient content and are intended to simplify food selection. A number of food guides have been developed, with advantages as well as criticisms attached to each. *The Basic Four* or Four Food Group guide is in wide use today for planning and evaluating diets. Since all foods in each group are *not* equally nutritious, choose a variety and include as many unprocessed or lightly processed foods as practical.

KEY NUTRIENTS

This chart summarizes the key nutrients, why each is needed, and foods that are good sources of each nutrient. It will help you understand why you should eat a wide variety of food to be well-nourished and healthy.

Nutrient	Why Needed	Some Important Sources
PROTEIN	1. Builds and maintains all tissues. 2. Forms an important part of enzymes, hormones, and body fluids. 3. Supplies energy.	Proteins of top quality for tissue building and repair are found in lean meat, poultry, fish, seafoods, eggs, milk, and cheese. Next best for proteins are dry beans, peas, and nuts. Cereals, bread, vegetables, and fruits also provide some protein but of lower quality.
CALCIUM	1. Builds bones and teeth. 2. Helps blood to clot. 3. Helps nerves, muscles, and heart to function properly.	Milk—whole, skim, buttermilk—fresh, dried, canned; cheese; ice cream; leafy vegetables such as collards, dandelion, kale, mustard and turnip greens.
IRON	1. Combines with protein to make hemoglobin, the red substance of blood which carries oxygen from the lungs to muscles, brain, and other parts of the body. 2. Helps cells use oxygen.	Liver, kidney, heart, oysters, lean meat, egg yolk, dry beans, dark-green leafy vegetables, dried fruit, whole grain and enriched bread and cereals, and molasses.
IODINE	1. Helps the thyroid gland to work properly.	Iodized salt. Saltwater fish and other sea food.
VITAMIN A	1. Helps eyes adjust to dim light. 2. Helps keep skin smooth. 3. Helps keep lining of mouth, nose, throat, and digestive tract healthy and resistant to infection. 4. Promotes growth.	Liver; dark-green and deep-yellow vegetables such as broccoli, turnip and other leafy greens, carrots, pumpkin, sweet potatoes, winter squash; apricots, cantaloupe; butter, fortified margarine.
THIAMINE	1. Helps body cells obtain energy from food. 2. Helps keep nerves in healthy condition. 3. Promotes good appetite and digestion.	Lean pork, heart, kidney, liver, dry beans and peas, whole grain and enriched cereals and breads, and some nuts.

Exhibit 1.8.

20

Nutrient	Why Needed	Some Important Sources
ASCORBIC ACID (Vitamin C)	1. Helps hold body cells together and strengthens walls of blood vessels. 2. Helps in healing wounds. 3. Helps tooth and bone formation.	Cantaloupe, grapefruit, oranges, strawberries, broccoli, Brussels sprouts, raw cabbage, collards, green and sweet red peppers, mustard and turnip greens, potatoes cooked in jacket, and tomatoes.
RIBOFLAVIN	1. Helps cells use oxygen to release energy from food. 2. Helps keep eyes healthy. 3. Helps keep skin around mouth and nose smooth.	Milk, liver, kidney, heart, lean meat, eggs, and dark leafy greens.
NIACIN	1. Helps the cells of the body use oxygen to produce energy. 2. Helps to maintain health of skin, tongue, digestive tract, and nervous system.	Liver, yeast, lean meat, poultry, fish, leafy greens, peanuts and peanut butter, beans and peas, and whole grain and enriched breads and cereals.
VITAMIN D	1. Helps body use calcium and phosphorus to build strong bones and teeth, important in growing children and during pregnancy and lactation.	Fish liver oils; foods fortified with vitamin D, such as milk. Direct sunlight produces vitamin D from cholesterol in the skin.
CARBOHYDRATES	1. Supply food energy. 2. Help body use fat efficiently. 3. Spare protein for purposes of body building and repair.	Starches: Breads, cereals, corn, grits, potatoes, rice, spaghetti, macaroni and noodles. Sugars: Honey, molasses, sirups, sugar, and other sweets.
FATS	1. Supply food energy in compact form (weight for weight supplies twice as much energy as carbohydrates). 2. Some supply essential fatty acids. 3. Help body use certain other nutrients.	Cooking fats and oils, butter, margarine, salad dressings, and oils.
WATER	1. Important part of all cells and fluids in body. 2. Carrier of nutrients to and waste from cells in the body. 3. Aids in digestion and absorption of food. 4. Helps to regulate body temperature.	Water, beverages, soup, fruits, and vegetables. Most foods contain some water.

Exhibit 1.8. (Continued)

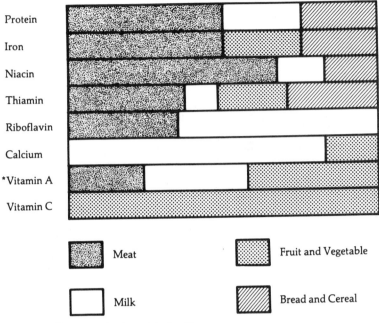

Key Nutrients in the Four Food Groups

Exhibit 1.9. Key Nutrients in the Four Food Groups

Scientists have employed USDA food consumption statistics, surveys of random samples of people, diet diaries, clinical evaluations, and biochemical analyses to study the nutritional status of population groups. Due to cost and other problems, we do not as yet know definitively the nutritional status of the American population. By keeping a careful record of your food intake and comparing it with one of several standards such as the Basic Four or (after determining the key nutrient content) the RDA, you can evaluate your own diet. The next step is to make the changes needed for better nutrition.

WHY WE EAT WHAT WE EAT 2

Highlights

Origins of diverse eating patterns
Influences of family and contemporary society on diet
Emotional values of food
Psychological and physiological responses to food
Motivation to act upon sound nutrition advice

Human beings all need the same basic nutrients, as we learned in Chapter 1. We can eat many different foods and combinations of foods in order to get these nutrients. There is also much diversity between cultures, families, and individuals in what they eat. Our individual food choices and eating patterns are influenced by a complexity of social, cultural, economic, physiological, and psychological factors (see Exhibit 2.1). Each of us processes these external and internal influences into our own unique eating pattern.

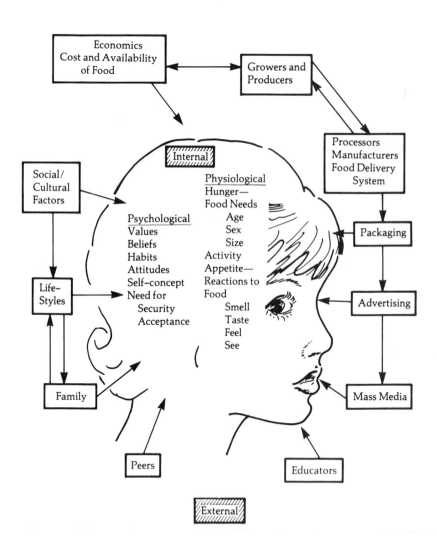

Exhibit 2.1. Influences on Our Food Habits—External and Internal

Social and Cultural Factors

We are all culturally brainwashed from infancy. Our most basic social unit, the family, provides our first enculturation in food experiences. As children we eat what our family eats and we learn to like these foods. We also absorb our family's attitudes towards food: how important food is in providing comfort, satisfaction, relief from boredom or anxiety; whether food is something to be enjoyed or fought over; and how it is used as a status symbol.

The family's food patterns, in turn, reflect those of the larger society of which the family is a part. Economics is also involved at both the family and societal level, that is, what resources are available to the family for either food production or food purchase and what foods are available at a price the family can afford within the agrieconomic system of the society.

Thus, a boy growing up in rural Japan learns to enjoy the fish and rice that his family eats at every meal. These foods are readily available in Japan at relatively low prices. On the other hand, a boy growing up in America, whose Japanese parents are second generation Americans, may learn to enjoy American foods such as meat and bread, perhaps combined as hamburgers, because his family has adopted the food patterns typical of the American culture. And in America these foods are readily available at relatively low prices. If he and his family pay a visit to Japan, they might find it difficult to adjust to their relatives' three meals a day of fish and rice. They may also find that the meat and bread they enjoy are priced very high compared to their cost in America.

Cultural food patterns are determined by the availability of food as well as by family traditions. They are constantly changing as families move, as different foods become available. Yet we have strong feelings that our way of eating is the way, and we may undergo a serious cultural shock if we move from one country or society to another where there are drastic differences in foods.

This was observed among the Vietnamese people who came to the United States at the end of the Vietnam war. American foods were unpalatable to them, and the foods they were accustomed to eating were scarce or not available. Thus, the adjustment to American life was doubly difficult because these people were deprived of the comfort of their accustomed foods.

Because food is so basic to life itself, the study of how a society uses food, its beliefs, values, customs, and food rituals, is a major interest of cultural anthropologists. Anthropologists, in studying a culture, are interested in the kinds of foods eaten, the ways foods are grown or gathered, how foods are prepared and in what sorts of utensils, how foods are served and eaten, how diets are influenced by religious beliefs, and how food is used as a status symbol by different social and economic groups.

In all societies, anthropologists find that food is an important part of the social life, and in each culture, they discern that there are many rituals that involve food. Social customs, religious beliefs, taboos, and superstitions about food may keep some members of the society from eating an adequate diet.

For example, in some cultures, fathers always get to eat first and to have the choicest food. Mothers and children, who may have a greater need for a nutritious diet, get to eat what's left. A taboo on meat eating by pregnant and lactating women, which is found in some societies, can result in protein deprivation for the mother and baby.

A prescribed ritual in many religious traditions is voluntary abstinence from all foods (fasting) or from certain foods. Fasting may be used as a way to liberate oneself from selfish or materialistic concerns or to purify one's body and/or soul. Fasting has also been used as a way to call attention to a grievance or to impress others, for example, the hunger strikes of prisoners and the fasts by United Farm Worker leader, Cesar Chavez.

Social Life. In our own society, food is very much a part of our social life and family rituals. Food is almost always included in major family celebrations: weddings, funerals, christenings, Christmas, Easter, Passover, and so forth. Certain foods such as wedding cake or Thanksgiving turkey become a traditional part of the ritual. And in some events, such as Thanksgiving, the meal becomes the main feature of the celebration, with the original purpose forgotten or downplayed (see Exhibit 2.2).

Daily social events often involve food too: we get together with friends for lunch or dinner; we serve snacks or desserts at meetings and parties; and our work breaks include coffee, doughnuts, and other snacks. The food makes the event more friendly; it helps break the ice. It may provide a reason for getting together, and sometimes the occasion provides an excuse for overeating!

With all this food so readily available in our lives, is it any wonder that the preson who wants to eat less and lose weight has problems avoiding food?

Life-Styles and Social Change

The food patterns in the United States are a blend of the many ethnic food ways brought to this country by the groups who immigrated here from various parts of the world. Regional differences in food patterns often developed because of the differences in ethnic backgrounds of the people living in the various regions.

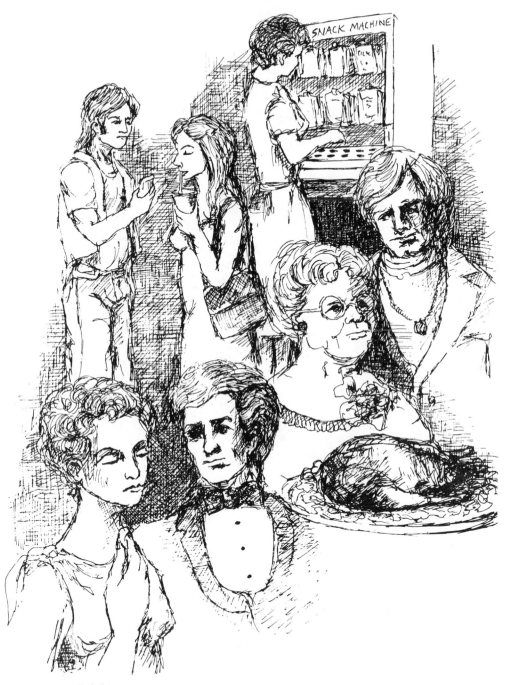

Exhibit 2.2. Food is an important part of our social life.

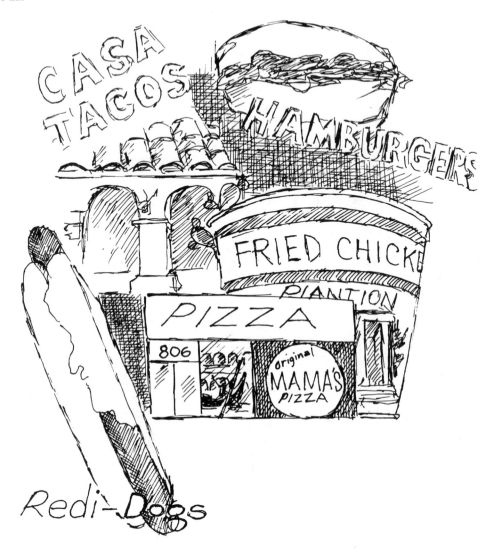

Exhibit 2.3. A variety of ethnic foods are readily available to us.

Today, however, the regional and ethnic differences are disappearing, and the typical American diet may include Oriental, Italian, Mexican, German, and many other ethnic foods within the course of a week (see Exhibit 2.3).

Improved transportation methods, making the wide distribution of food products feasible, have helped bring this about, as has the national promotion of ethnic and regional foods. The upsurge in ethnic-food restaurants and fast-food outlets has contributed to the melding process. Another blending factor has been the growing mobility of American families. Americans vacation across the country, sampling foods from everywhere. They also move often. Current statistics indicate that one-fifth of American families move every year. When families move, they take their food habits with them, but they also learn to eat new foods that are popular in their new location.

Children also sometimes help bring about this change. For example, when a group of Laotian families settled in California after the Vietnam war, the mothers tried to maintain their families' traditional way of eating, even though their accustomed foods were not readily available. But their children attended public school where they participated in the School Lunch Program. Before long the children were rejecting their traditional Laotian foods at home and pressuring their mothers to learn to "cook American." The mothers found this disturbing, for, as many studies have shown, it is easier for young people to change their eating habits than it is for older people to do so.

Fast-Paced Life-Style. "Fast living " has become the "American way of life" and it may be having a negative impact on our nutrition. Time is short, and we are often too busy to eat regular meals. We hurry off in the morning without breakfast, then eat a coffee and doughnut snack. We skip lunch, or we grab a hamburger at a fast-food restaurant. In the evening, worn out from all the rushing we do all day, we may relax before dinner with a cocktail or soft drink and some snack foods. Dinner may not be much because we have not had the time to plan and shop carefully and prepare a balanced meal. So we may need some more snacks in the evening while we sit and watch TV.

And we may not even be aware of what we are doing. The typical American mother, market researchers have found, when asked to describe her family's eating pattern, will reply that it is the traditional "three squares" a day, with after school snacks for the children. But diaries of actual food consumption, recorded by housewives, show a different story that is often surprising to the housewives themselves. The results show that three out of four families do not eat breakfast together, and many have no breakfast at all. And the evening meal together may take place as seldom as three days a week or less and may often be as brief as 20 minutes.[1]

---

[1] J. Hess, "The Unbalanced American's Diet: 20 Partials, Not 'Three Squares.'" The *New York Times*, January 3, 1974, Sec. C, p. 40.

Snacking. The diet records show that snacking is the American pattern from early morning to bedtime. And it may not end at bedtime for people who have problems sleeping and get up at night to raid the refrigerator. One survey showed an average of 20 food contacts a day for individuals instead of three meals a day.

Snacking in itself is not necessarily a poor nutrition practice. Eating more smaller meals throughout the day, instead of two or three larger meals, may be better for some people—the elderly, for example, and young children who may have a small capacity for food. The crucial question is, What do the snacks consist of?

When snacks become an integral part of our daily food pattern, we need to choose them wisely so they too contribute to our total daily food needs. This is especially important when our calorie budget is limited. (More about snacks is included in Chapter 27.)

The Single Life-Style and Single-Parent Families. Because snack foods are quick and easy to serve, they are often the choice of people who live alone, are not motivated, or don't have the skills to cook for themselves. Single adults, as a group, are less likely to eat well than people who live with others. And Census Bureau statistics show that the single life-style is on the increase in the United States due to divorce, postponement of marriage by young adults, and a longer life span of the elderly.[2] Today one out of five American households has just one person. Many singles are elderly or young adults.

The single-parent family is another group that is growing as a result of the increasing number of divorces and family separations. In the mid-1970s about 20 percent of American children under 18 lived in single-parent families, compared to 14 percent in 1970. One percent lived with fathers, 16 percent with mothers, and 1 percent with other adults.[3] This group may be at risk nutritionally because often the single parent is employed and has limited time for shopping or cooking. As a result, the family may rely heavily on fast foods, TV dinners, and other forms of quick and easy foods. Another large group of single parents are unemployed, dependent on welfare aid and food stamps, and have limited food budgets.

Sedentary Life-Style. While the pace of life has speeded up, the amount of exercise we do has slowed down. More and more people work at jobs where they sit most of the day rather than exert themselves. They ride from one place to another rather than walk and take an ele-

[2]P. Glick, "Some Recent Changes in American Families." Current Population Reports: Special Studies, Series P-23, No. 52.U.S. Department of Commerce, Bureau of the Census, Washington, D.C. 1976.

[3]P. Glick, "Some Recent Changes in American Families." Current Population Reports: Special Studies, Series P-23, No. 52. U.S. Department of Commerce, Bureau of the Census, Washington, D.C. 1976.

vator rather than climb stairs. Then they go home and spend the evening sitting in front of television or reading.

The result is that calorie requirements for Americans as a group are decreasing, and the problems of overweight and obesity are increasing because so many of us are taking in more calories in our foods than we're using up in our activities. The solution to this problem appears to be adding more exercise to our lives as well as adjusting our calorie intake downward. Further discussion about calories and weight control is included in Chapter 5.

Alcohol and Drug Use. Alcohol consumption also contributes to the problem of overconsumption of calories. It is estimated that for some people, alcohol accounts for 5 to 10 percent of the total daily calorie intake. Since alcoholic beverages, while high in calories, are low in other nutrients, the regular drinker may be at nutritional risk, getting too many calories and too few of the other essential nutrients. (See Chapter 20.)

Statistics show a growth in both alcoholism and drug abuse among Americans. Both of these addictions, in their more severe forms, have an adverse effect on the nutritional status of the individual. An addict who has a diminished appetite and no interest in food may suffer from general malnutrition, which may lead to serious deficiency diseases. Nutrition counseling and diet therapy are a necessary part of an alcoholic's or drug addict's rehabilitation program.

Economic Factors

The most serious deterrent to good nutrition is poverty. Poverty limits food choices and the availability of food. It exists throughout the world, but is more severe in the developing countries of Asia, Africa, and Central and South America.

According to estimates of the Food and Agriculture Organization (FAO) of the United Nations, 300 to 500 million people in the world do not get enough food, and 800 million are poorly nourished. In developing countries, critical malnutrition (lack of one or more specific nutrients) or undernutrition (not enough food) is found in a high proportion of the poor people. Because of lack of good sanitation, bouts of diarrheal illness and various intestinal parasites add to the seriousness of the situation.

Malnutrition is the largest single contributor to the high death rate of children in developing countries: one out of five children dies before age five and half of these deaths are nutrition related. The Food and Agriculture Organization estimates that 60 percent of preschool children in developing countries suffer from protein-calorie malnutrition. Severe malnutrition in prenatal and infant life may lead to permanently impaired mental and physical development.

The lack of calories is a major problem, because when the calorie intake is below what is needed for the body's energy demands, protein is used to supply energy rather than for its specialized function of building tissue. The result in children is severe retardation of physical growth and delayed sexual development.

Due to inflated food prices, many people in developing countries now spend 70 to 80 percent of their income on food (compared to an average of 16 percent in the United States).[4]

The inability of the agricultural system of a country to produce food at reasonable prices is most often due to overpopulation of an area in relation to its food production capacity. Besides having problems of limited land, antiquated agricultural practices, and lack of transportation and storage facilities, a less developed country is also likely to have a backward economic system with a limited capacity to produce raw materials or products that could be traded for food with other nations. In addition, social, cultural, institutional, and political factors may inhibit food production. In some places, superstitions, customs, and illiteracy act as additional barriers to adequate nutrition.

Worldwide, food production has grown steadily in the last two decades. In developed countries food production has increased much faster than the population; in less developed countries population gains have absorbed nearly all of the production increases.

The FAO reported that for the years 1964–66, developed countries had an average total daily intake of 3,043 calories per person, compared to only 2,097 calories per person in the less developed countries (see Exhibit 2.4).

Another notable difference in food consumption patterns between developed and less developed countries, which you can see in Exhibit 2.4, is in the way the calories were distributed among the food groups.

Note how much more animal food is consumed in the developed countries, particularly North America, and also the large proportion of calories obtained from fats and oils in developed countries. In less developed countries, cereals, corn, rice, wheat, and starchy staples like potatoes, cassava, (tapioca), and yams account for a high proportion of the energy. These foods also provide much of the raw material for livestock production. In the United States, the per capita production of grain is slightly more than one metric ton (2,204 pounds) per person. This is about five times the average amount produced annually per capita in such countries as India, Indonesia, and Bangladesh. The United States now converts two-thirds of the grain produced each year into livestock products and exports half of the remainder.

---

[4]"Consumer Expenditures and Retail Prices for Food: Comparison of the United States with Other Countries." U.S. Department of Agriculture, Office of Communications, Washington, D.C., April, 1974.

Exhibit 2.4   Food Consumption Patterns of Developed and Less Developed
Countries, 1964–66

Developed Countries	Calories Per Day	Cereals CHO	Percent of Calories from: Fruits and Vegetables	Livestock	Fats and Oils
Total Group	3,043	55%	7%	24%	14%
North America	3,155	40%	9%	34%	17%
Western Europe	3,111	46%	8%	28%	18%
U.S.S.R.	3,182	70%	4%	17%	9%
Less Developed Countries					
Total Group	2,097	77%	10%	8%	5%
South America	2,276	68%	7%	17%	8%
China	2,045	80%	9%	8%	3%
Southeast Asia	2,121	82%	8%	7%	3%
Africa South of Sahara	1,730	80%	10%	5%	5%
WORLD	2,386	69%	9%	14%	8%

Source: FAO Food Balances 1964–66, in "Your Food—A Food Policy Basebook." National
Public Policy Education Committee, Publication No. 5, Cooperative Extension Service,
The Ohio State University, Columbus, Ohio, 1975, p. 10.

Poverty and Hunger in the Years to Come. It is forecast that through
1985 the probability is good that world food production in total will keep
a half step ahead of the population growth. However, there will be times
and places of critical shortage. Less developed countries will experience
a chronic tendency of demand growth to outpace supply growth, while
the opposite is expected to happen in the developed world.

However, at current growth rates, the world population will double by about 2000 A.D., and food supplies will also need to double to
keep up. By 1985, 91 of every 100 babies born will begin life in less
developed lands, and by 2000 A.D. this will increase to 93 of 100. This
frightens many experts, who believe that food production and economic
activity in these countries will not expand rapidly enough to fight growing poverty, widespread hunger, and famine. Contributing to the problems of finding enough productive land, with sufficient supplies of good
quality water, will be the growing shortages of fertilizer, petroleum, and
other energy sources.[5]

[5]"Your Food—A Food Policy Basebook." National Public Policy Education Committee,
Publication No. 5. Cooperative Extension Service, The Ohio State University, Columbus,
Ohio, 1975, p. 13.

At a 1974 United Nations World Food Conference in Rome, sponsored by the U.N. Food and Agriculture Organization and attended by world-recognized agricultural and economic experts, the problem of how to solve this dilemma was discussed, but not resolved.[6]

Population control efforts are thought to be the most necessary method for reducing the long-term pressure on the earth's agriculture and other resources. But to date such efforts have not surmounted the social, religious, nationalistic, and moral issues involved in population control. However, recent statistics offer encouragement that there may be a small slowing of the world's rate of population growth. The change is attributable primarily to slackening birth rates, especially among poorer nations. The world population growth rate peaked at 1.9 percent per year in 1970, and by 1977 had fallen to 1.7 percent.[7] At this rate, it will take 41 years for the world population to double, instead of the 36 years it would have taken in 1970.

Poverty in the United States. American agriculture is said to be the most efficient producer of food in the world, providing us with the lowest cost food produced by the smallest number of people. Consumers in the United States presently face no threat of food shortages. We have the ability to produce even more food than we currently produce, and, in addition, we could reallocate our enormous supplies of grain to direct feeding of people rather than to feeding livestock, should this be necessary.

Our living standard is one of the highest in the world. Our people spend a smaller proportion of their income on food than the people of all but a few other countries. Yet there are families in the United States with incomes so low that they must spend as much as 50 percent of their incomes on food. (See Exhibits 2.5 and 2.6.) There are children who are poorly nourished because of their family's limited ability to buy food.

The federal government has accepted some public responsibility to provide food for economically disadvantaged people. In addition to making grants of money ("welfare") to certain needy people, the federal government also operates food assistance programs. The two largest are the Food Stamp Program and the School Lunch Program. Two others of growing importance are the WIC (Women, Infants, and Children) program and the nutrition programs for the elderly (food-serving centers and "Meals on Wheels").

Since the 1960s, expenditures for domestic food-subsidy programs have been one of the fastest growing items in the federal budget. In the

[6]Food and Agriculture Organization of the United Nations. "Assessment of the World Food Situation—Present and Future." United Nations World Food Conference, Documents, Rome, November, 1974.

[7]R. Gillette, "Surprise Slowing of World Population Rise Noted." *Los Angeles Times*, February 15, 1978, Sec. 1, p. 1.

SHARE OF AFTER-TAX INCOME SPENT ON FOOD

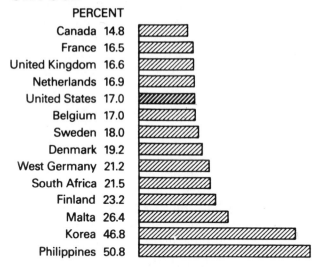

PERCENT

Canada 14.8	
France 16.5	
United Kingdom 16.6	
Netherlands 16.9	
United States 17.0	
Belgium 17.0	
Sweden 18.0	
Denmark 19.2	
West Germany 21.2	
South Africa 21.5	
Finland 23.2	
Malta 26.4	
Korea 46.8	
Philippines 50.8	

1975 data. Canada and United States include nonalcoholic beverages. West
Germany includes alcoholic and nonalcoholic beverages.
Source: U.N. National Accounts of Statistics and National Sources.

Exhibit 2.5. Food Expenditures and Income Relationship

Exhibit 2.6   Percentage of Income Spent for Food

	1972	1973
	Percent	
Under $3,000	40	50
3,000–3,999	30	30
4,000–4,999	25	26
5,000–5,999	23	24
6,000–6,999	20	20
7,000–7,999	19	20
8,000–9,999	17	18.
10,000–11,999	16	17
12,000–14,999	15	15
15,000–19,999	13	14
20,000–24,999	12	13
25,000 and over	8	9 :
All families*	15	16

Source: Handbook of Agricultural Charts. U.S. Department of Agriculture, 1976.

Income is money income before taxes, for families and single persons; food expenditures include both those for food at home and away; includes meals as pay and food on vacation.

*Includes those not reporting complete income.

mid-seventies, about 10 percent of the U. S. population (20 million people) participated in the Food Stamp Program at a cost to the government of some $5 billion annually. The School Lunch Programs cost about $2 billion annually, while the food assistance programs for the elderly cost about one half billion dollars a year. The dollar cost of these programs appears to be high, but the total cost of all U.S. food subsidies adds only about 3 percent to the total farm-level demand for food.

Poverty and Good and Poor Nutrition. While poverty is probably the most likely cause of malnutrition worldwide, it does not mean that the diets of poor people are always poor in nutritional quality.

In many cultures, people have instinctively, or through the natural selection process, developed diets that provide a balance of essential nutrients. For example, in Mexico poor people have thrived on a native diet consisting mainly of corn, legumes, chiles, cactus, squash, and other fruits and vegetables. By soaking corn in lime to soften it, they added calcium. By pounding the corn with limestone, they made chemically formed niacin nutritionally available. By combining corn with beans, they obtained a full complement of essential amino acids. By using large quantities of chiles and cactus they obtained vitamin C and other minerals and vitamins. From squash and other fruits and vegetables they received vitamin A. Diets of low-income people in other countries, such as China, may have a similar good balance of nutrients.

Throughout history food has been used as a status symbol and to show class differences between the rich and the poor. The rich of earlier years could affort the refined white flour, white bread, and white rice, while the poor had to be content with unrefined dark flour, dark bread, and brown rice. Ironically, the unrefined food of the poor was more nutritious than the food of the rich, but it was the food of the rich that everyone desired. Demand and increased supplies eventually brought about the availability of refined cereals and breads to nearly everyone in affluent societies. Today the unrefined grains may cost more, and they are sometimes used by some groups as a status symbol.

In the United States, a national food consumption survey conducted by the U.S. Department of Agriculture in 1965–66 showed a direct relationship between income level and quality of diets.[8] As Exhibit 2.7 shows, as income levels rose, so did the amount of money spent on food and the proportion of people who had diets that were rated as "good" (sufficient in all nutrients) or "fair" (lacking in two or more nutrients).

Note, however, that among even the highest income families surveyed, 9 percent had diets rated as "poor" (severely lacking in two or

[8]"Dietary Levels of Households in the United States, Spring, 1965." Household Food Consumption Survey 1965–66, Report No. 6. U.S. Dept. of Agriculture, Agricultural Research Service, Washington, D.C., p. 5.

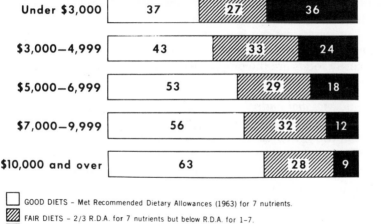

GOOD DIETS – Met Recommended Dietary Allowances (1963) for 7 nutrients.

FAIR DIETS – 2/3 R.D.A. for 7 nutrients but below R.D.A. for 1–7.

POOR DIETS – 2/3 R.D.A. for 1–7 nutrients; is not synonymous with serious hunger and malnutrition.

U.S. HOUSEHOLDS, 1 WEEK IN SPRING, 1965

Exhibit 2.7. Diets at Three Levels of Quality by Income (*Source:* "Dietary Levels of Households in the United States, Spring 1965," Household Food Consumption Survey 1965-66, Report No. 6. U.S. Dept. of Agriculture, Agricultural Research Service, p. 5)

more nutrients), while among the lowest income groups, 37 percent had diets rated as "good."

As a part of this same survey, diets of higher and lower income families living in the Northeastern states were compared to determine the amount of key nutrients obtained per dollar spent on food. The results, shown in Exhibit 2.8, are surprising. In the case of every nutrient, the lower income families got more nutrients for their money. The reason? They spent less for frivolous extras such as soft drinks, snack foods, "gourmet" convenience foods, etc., and more for low-cost but

Exhibit 2.8

NUTRIENTS PER $1 WORTH OF FOOD	UNDER $3,000		OVER $10,000	
Calories	2,430		1,840	
Protein	83	g	65	g
Calcium	870	mg	650	mg
Iron	16	mg	11	mg
Vitamin A	7,330	IU	4,760	IU
Vitamin C	91	mg	78	mg
Thiamin	1.2	mg	.9	mg
Riboflavin	1.9	mg	1.4	mg

Source: "Dietary Levels of Households in the Northeast, Spring 1965." Household Food Consumption Survey 1965–66, Report No. 7. U.S. Department of Agriculture, Washington, D.C. p. 5.

nutritious foods such as liver and organ meats, potatoes, dry beans, poultry and eggs, and enriched cereals and flour.

The lesson we can learn from this study is that spending a lot of money for food does not necessarily guarantee a good diet. Some of the least costly foods are the most nutritious. So the key is careful selection, not how much we spend.

Affluence and Nutrition. This situation is a real paradox: while the poor half of the world goes hungry, the affluent half suffers from malnutrition caused by eating too much. In the United States obesity and overweight are our most common nutritional problems. An even more remarkable paradox is that in affluent countries, obesity often is found among the people with the lowest incomes.

Affluence can be a deterrent to good nutrition, as we can see in the United States where affluence has made it possible for us to:

1. Increase our consumption of meat and other animal foods, with their accompanying saturated fats, well beyond our need for protein. (See Exhibit 4.2, which shows how meat consumption has been increasing.) When our body's need for protein is satisfied, we use the excess for calories or convert it to stored fat.

2. Increase our consumption of high-calorie, low-nutrient-density fats, sugar, and alcoholic beverages. (See Exhibit 4.2.)

3. Increase the amount of eating out we do in restaurants, fast-food outlets, cafeterias, and the like where poor food choices are more likely. (In the United States as much as one-third of the money spent on food is used for food prepared away from home.)

4. Increase our use of high-cost, high-calorie, high-sodium, low-nutrient-density snack foods including soft drinks, potato and corn chips, candy, doughnuts, pastries, and so forth.

5. Increase our use of "gourmet" type convenience foods, like vegetables frozen with sauces, which tend to be higher in fat and calories as well as higher in cost.

6. Increase our pursuit of fad diets and so-called health foods, which may be costly yet no more nutritious than ordinary foods.

Even though the majority of Americans have enough money to buy a nutritious diet, they do not always do so, and in fact, our affluence can sometimes have a detrimental effect on our eating habits and nutritional health.

Technological Changes

In the past 30 years our food consumption patterns have changed profoundly because of vast improvements in food storage, food preservation, and food production methods plus the development of an efficient transportation system for moving fresh, refrigerated, and frozen foods as well as other types of preserved foods rapidly, not only across the country but across the world. Today fresh fruits and vegetables of all kinds are available year-round, to those who are willing to pay the price.

Food Production Changes. The science of food technology was born in the 1930s when scientists began to develop new methods of producing and preserving food. After World War II, research and development in food technology exploded with new processes and products that have brought us an infinite variety of food choices. We now have, in addition to foods preserved by drying, freeze-drying, canning, and freezing, synthesized foods, fabricated foods, and food "analogs" that have literally been put together in the laboratory.

Food industry research and development efforts are motivated by management's desire to improve profits and to gain a larger share of the market. The American public, it seems, has an insatiable desire for new, different, easy foods that provide instant gratification. Enjoyment here and now seems to be what we demand, and the American food industry is geared up to satisfy that desire.

The question we might ask is, Is the food industry, as its representatives claim, responding with new products to consumer demand, or does the industry, through product development and promotion, create the demand? And is this created demand in the best interests of the American consumer?

With the need for profits in the forefront, the concern for nutrition appears to be low on the food industry's priority list. The food quality attributes, as prioritized by food industry research and development experts, are:

1. Safety and purity. Essential to protect consumers, maintain sales, and conform to government standards

2. Organoleptic appeal. How the food looks, smells, tastes, feels when eaten

3. Convenience. Considered of high interest to consumers

4. Shelf life. The food must still be good quality when the consumer uses it

5. Functional performance. The food must behave like it should; a cake mix, for example, must produce a cake when directions are followed

6. Nutritive value

When nutrition scientists express concern to manufacturers that the new foods being produced are high in fat, or sugar, or salt, or are low in essential nutrients compared to the more natural, less processed foods, they are told that the justification for placing nutritive value last on the priority list is that all the other attributes must be there first or people won't eat the food.

To produce the food that people want, food industry researchers first conduct market research to find out consumer preferences. They then proceed to develop a product designed to meet these specifications and also be marketable for a profit. Once developed, new products are test-marketed in selected parts of the country before finally being launched, often with expensive advertising campaigns. In spite of this care, a large proportion of the 6,000 or more new products marketed each year do not bring in sufficient profits and are quietly withdrawn to make way for other new products. Consumers generally are unaware of the enormous costs involved in the process of developing and promoting new food products—costs that are inevitably paid by the consumers themselves. Affluence makes it possible for us to buy these foods; advertising convinces us that we should. However, our nutritional health often is not improved as a result.

Advertising. Food advertising is everywhere: on television, radio, billboards, in newspapers, magazines, window displays, even on food packages. How effective is it in influencing our food habits?

Considering the many ways our eating habits have changed in the past 20 to 30 years and the popularity of the foods that are heavily advertised leads to the conclusion that advertising has played an important role in the change process. In fact, food advertisers appear to be more successful in changing eating habits than educators. Studies show that food practices do not change just because people have accurate, meaningful facts (as provided by nutrition educators) and that, instead, there is widespread lack of correlation between the nutrition facts people know and the application of this information to their own lives.[9]

Food has an emotional rather than an intellectual value to most people. This fact is well known to manufacturers, who use emotional appeals rather than intellectual aspects to sell their products. Thus, advertisements are more likely to emphasize flavor, enjoyment, fun ("Things go better with Coke")—psychological satisfactions—instead of health or nutritional reasons ("it's good for you") for buying the food. Even health or nutritional reasons may be presented with an emotional appeal. For example, a breakfast cereal is promoted by a prominent athlete with the implication that his success as an athlete is related to eating the cereal, a success that can be transferred to other would-be athletes if they too eat the cereal.

Food manufacturers and advertising agencies have for many years employed the services of motivational researchers and psychologists, who have investigated the hidden psyches of consumers to find out what makes them buy. One psychologist, for example, advised advertisers that they need to help consumers overcome guilt feelings about self-indulgence in high-calorie foods like candy, soft drinks, or beer, by

---

[9]J. Pearson, "What Homemakers Know and Do about Feeding Their Families." *Family Economics Review*, Fall, 1973, Washington, D.C., pp. 24–26.

using the "reward yourself, you deserve it" theme, as in the often heard "You owe it to yourself" admonition. Thus, an advertisement portrays a group of working men finishing their work and drinking beer—a hard-earned reward.

Creativity and ego satisfaction are other emotions appealed to by advertisers. Thus, a cake made from a mix is shown receiving the mother's special creative touch, and she then is rewarded by the pleasure and appreciation of her family.

Motivational researchers found that gum chewing provides people with oral comfort, release from tension, and a means of assuaging anxiety. Using this information, advertisers developed ads showing adults using gum chewing as a help in conquering aggravating workaday problems.

As you look at advertisements in magazines or watch them on TV, try to analyze what emotions the advertiser is appealing to, and consider the effectiveness of the approach. Does the ad persuade you to try the product? If so, why? Pay particular attention to advertisements directed to children. What sort of nutrition message do the children receive? Are they learning anything at all about good nutrition from the advertisements?

Advertising on children's television programs has been the target of criticism by numerous nutritionists and concerned parent groups. The average child between the ages of 2 and 11 is thought to see some 20,000 commercials a year while watching 1,300 hours of television.[10] The critics believe that children do not have the maturity to evaluate the information presented and are likely to be persuaded to desire or demand foods having limited nutritional value.[11]

In several studies, TV programming was monitored to count the number of food advertisements and the kinds of foods advertised and to evaluate the sort of nutrition education children received from the ads. One study showed that of 388 network commercials run during 29 hours of children's programs on the three major networks (NBC, CBS, and ABC), 319 or 82 percent were for ingestible items—food, drink, candy, gum, or vitamin pills. Nearly 40 percent of the food ads were for breakfast cereals, almost exclusively the sweetened types. About 17 percent of the food ads were for snack items such as cookies, candy, gum, and popcorn; and another 8 percent were for beverages and beverage mixes. Vitamin pills accounted for 15 percent of the ads, but since that time advertising them on children's television programs has been banned.[12]

---

[10]M. Cimons, "Debate Opens on TV Ads Aimed at Kids." *Los Angeles Times*, March 12, 1978, Part IV, p. 1.

[11]M. Cimons, "Ban Sought for Sugary Ads on Children's TV." *Los Angles Times*, April 17, 1977, Part IV, p. 1.

[12]J. Gussow, "Counternutritional Messages of TV Ads Aimed at Children." Testimony presented to the Subcommittee on the Consumer of the Senate Commerce Committee, March 12, 1972, in *Journal of Nutrition Education*, Vol. 4, No. 2, Spring, 1972, pp. 48-52.

In another similar study conducted in 1976, 580 commercials were monitored during 27 hours of national TV broadcasts: 154 during the Saturday morning "children's time"; 223 during daytime TV, "women's time"; and 203 during the evening hours of 9 to 12 when viewers were both men and women.[13]

During the children's programs, 69 percent of the ads were for food, while 40 percent were for food during the women's programs, and 28 percent were for food during the evening programs. All together, 44 percent of the TV ads monitored were for food. Again, breakfast cereals were at the top of the list of children's advertising—41 percent of the total. Sugar content of the cereals advertised was analyzed and the researchers found that cereals containing 20 percent or more calories as sugar were advertised five times more frequently than were the cereals having less sugar. The cereals were described in the ads in words like "sweet," "fun," "great," or "powerful." Snack items, cookies, candy, popcorn, and gum were a close second with 37 percent of the children's ads. Beverages again averaged 7 percent.[14]

In both of these studies, the researchers concluded that food ads directed to children did not give a balanced nutrition message at all. The Four Food Groups were rarely mentioned, and many nutritious foods were not advertised at all, while the sugary, sweet, "fun" foods were emphasized heavily. All together, the nutritionally oriented TV messages were believed to encourage poor eating habits, rather than good ones.

After examining the results of these kinds of studies, the Federal Trade Commission, in a report published in 1978, proposed that: (1) TV commercials aimed at children be changed to play down the desirability of sugared products and (2) the amount of advertising of sugared products be restricted and accompanied by health messages, for example, on proper dental care.[15] Advertisers and manufacturers objected strongly to this proposal, and a lengthy debate is anticipated before action, if any, is taken.

The key question is, how do children respond to these ads? Do they eat the food that is seen advertised? Logic says they must respond and influence their mothers to buy the advertised foods, or the manufacturers would not continue to spend the enormous amount of money it costs to promote their products on TV.

Studies of children and their response to TV advertising tend to indicate that younger children are much more likely to believe that ads tell the truth. In one limited study of a small sample of children, it was found that children who consume snack foods more frequently also

---

[13]J. Brown, "Graduate Students Examine TV Ads for Food." *Journal of Nutrition Education*, Vol. 9, No. 3, July-September, 1977, pp. 120–2.

[14]*Ibid.*

[15]U.S. Federal Trade Commission, "Children's Advertising Proposed Trade Regulation, Rule Making, and Public Hearing." *Federal Register*, 43: 17967, 1978.

tended to indicate a strong preference for consuming advertised foods.[16] Children whose mothers had better knowledge about the validity of the claims in the ads tended to have lower preference scores for the foods advertised on TV.[17] In other words, informed parents can play a role in counteracting the non-nutritious messages children receive from TV advertising.

However, children can be very persistent naggers and have considerable influence on their mothers' food choices in the supermarket. One study on the effects of television advertising on children showed that most mothers are not able to resist advertising messages beamed at their children. Researchers found that the youngest children paid the most attention to TV commercials, and they were most concerned with products that related to immediate, impulsive needs.

Mothers were found "usually yielding to the child's purchase influence attempts" (see Exhibit 2.9). For five-to-seven-year-olds, mothers yielded 88 percent of the time in buying breakfast cereals, 55 percent of the time for snack foods, 40 percent for candy, and 38 percent of the time for soft drinks.[18]

Even mothers with little money to spend on food are observed buying the foods their children see advertised on TV and giving their children money on a regular basis to buy candy, soft drinks, and other snack foods. Why do mothers do this, rather than use the money for more nutritious foods? For several reasons—the mothers don't have the information they need to determine that this is a poor decision: they believe the TV advertising too. They perceive that these foods have emotional or psychic value: they don't want their children to feel deprived or "different" from their more affluent peers. In essence, they see food as a status symbol, and use it to let others know that their children's status is equal to or better than that of others in the community.

In addition to direct food advertising, many food companies produce educational materials on nutrition that are used mainly by home economics teachers in secondary schools and adult education programs. In 1977–78 a U.S. House of Representatives subcommittee on Domestic Marketing, Consumer Relations, and Nutrition published a report critical of the kind and amount of nutrition education done by food manufacturers.[19]

---

[16]K. Clancy-Hepburn, A. Hickey, G. Nevill, "Children's Behavior Responses to TV Food Advertisements." *Journal of Nutrition Education*, Vol. 6, No. 3, July-September, 1974.

[17]L. Emmons, M. Hayes, "Nutrition Knowledge of Mothers and Children." *Journal of Nutrition Education*, Vol. 5, No. 2, April-June, 1973, pp. 134–39.

[18]S. Ward and O. Wackman, "Television Advertising and Intrafamily Influence: Children's Purchase Influence Attempts and Parental Yielding." *Television and Social Behavior*, Vol. 4, U.S. Department of Health, Education, and Welfare, Washington, D.C., 1972.

[19]Nutrition Education; Hearings before Committee on Agriculture, Subcommittee on Domestic Marketing, Consumer Relations, and Nutrition, House, 95th Congress, 1st Session, Part 1, September 27-28 and October 6, 1977, Washington, D.C.

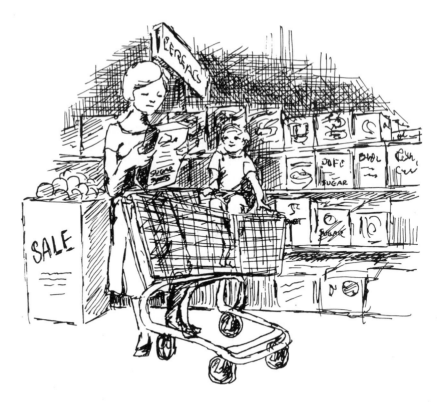

Exhibit 2.9. Mothers usually yield to a child's attempts to influence food purchases.

The report noted that: major U.S. food companies spend very little on nutrition education; what they call nutrition education is no different from product promotion; and this promotion encourages overconsumption. For example, the largest single food company in the United States spent $275 million on advertising in 1976 and allotted a mere $863,000 (less than one percent) for nutrition education.

Nutrition Education and Food Choices

Nutrition education begins at home. A child's first teachers are his parents, and he is more likely to learn from what they do—what foods they serve and eat—than from what they say. How well equipped are parents, mothers in particular, to convey sound nutrition knowledge to their children through the foods they buy and serve? Not much information is available to answer this question, and what little there is, gathered from surveys, is not encouraging.

Since nutrition information of mothers is valuable only to the extent that it is put into practice, the relationship of knowledge to practices is of key importance. A national survey of 2,545 households conducted in 1971 by the U.S. Department of Agriculture showed that homemakers know more facts about food and nutrition than they apply. And even when the homemaker is not satisfied that all family members are eating a desirable diet, she does little or nothing about it.[20] It appears that mothers frequently do not apply their nutrition knowledge fully to feeding the family mainly because of family members' food likes and dislikes, attitudes and customs, and financial and time restraints.

A major problem in providing nutrition education appears to be timing. The most likely time for young people to be exposed to formal nutrition education is when they're in junior or senior high school. But at this time in their lives they usually are not motivated to learn about nutrition, except as it might apply to them; for example, if they are overweight or involved in athletics and believe a better diet might improve their performance. The time of highest motivation for learning about feeding a family or themselves is not when people are young and living at home, but rather when they are faced with the actual problem of providing food for themselves or their own family. When this time comes, they must make an effort to seek out the nutrition information they need, either through reading books or magazines or attending classes. The average person doesn't make this effort and instead may be content to believe what he or she hears from a nonexpert friend, salesperson, or TV advertisement.

Health professionals are often in the position of being available to provide nutrition information to people at times in their lives when they need it, for example, to pregnant women, mothers of babies and preschool children, and people suffering from high blood pressure or obesity. For this reason it's essential that health professionals be well informed about nutrition.

However, the greatest challenge faced by all nutrition educators is motivating people to use the information provided. We do not change our eating habits simply because someone tells us to do so. Only too often people who do change their way of eating, for example, follow a weight reduction diet, do so only temporarily and soon slip back to their old patterns.

Perhaps nutrition educators will not be successful in helping people improve their diets until they take on the methods of the food advertisers and learn to appeal effectively to the emotions rather than the intellect. This is exactly the reason why promoters of food fads have been so successful.

---

[20]J. Pearson, "What Homemakers Know and Do about Feeding Their Families." *Family Economics Review*, Fall, 1973, Washington, D.C., pp. 24–26.

Individuals in our society are bombarded with nutrition messages—from family, peers, educators, and advertisers—on radio, TV, in newspapers, magazines, books, pamphlets, and package labels. All of these messages impact on our inner physiological and psychological responses to food. The physiological and psychological factors in individual food choices are so closely intertwined that it is often impossible to separate them.

Physiological Factors

For almost everyone, eating is fun. The aroma, the flavor, the feeling of food in our mouth, appeals to our hedonistic (pleasure-seeking) instincts. Many physiological functions are involved in our appetite for and our enjoyment of food: sight, smell, taste, touch, and, of course, the feeling of satiety and well-being that follows a good meal (see Exhibit 2.10).

Taste. Our taste buds, which are located on the surface of the tongue, can identify four basic flavors: sweet, sour, salty, and bitter. The number of taste buds, and therefore sensitivity to these flavors, varies from person to person and age to age. The average child is thought to have some 9,000 taste buds. As we grow older, the number of taste buds diminishes. This may explain why children, with many more taste buds than adults, often are more sensitive to and more likely to object to flavors that adults find acceptable.

We taste things only when they are dissolved in water. Saliva often serves the purpose of providing the water for dissolving flavor substances.

Taste blindness for certain flavors, similar to color blindness, has been observed in many people. Apparently, like color blindness, it's an hereditary deficiency.

Smell. Odor is an even more important component of flavor than taste. We are acutely sensitive to odor, much more so than to taste. In some cases we need 3,000 times as much of a substance in order to taste it as we would need in order to detect an odor. However, our sensitivity to odor-flavor becomes "fatigued" with continued exposure. This probably explains why the first few mouthfuls of a food taste so much better than the last few. (In economics this is known as the law of diminishing returns.)

In order to be "smellable," a substance needs to be volatile at ordinary temperatures and be soluble in fat solvents. Most inorganic substances have little odor, while organic substances, which form the basis of foods, are more likely to be odoriferous. No two substances

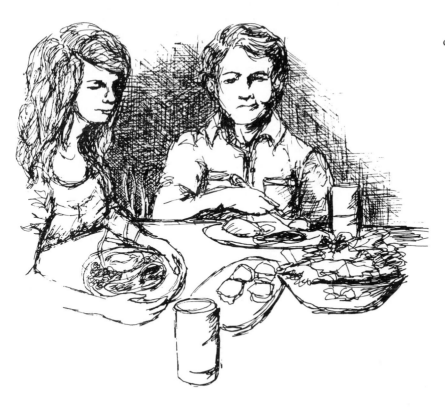

Exhibit 2.10. Many physiological and psychological functions influence our appetite for and enjoyment of food.

smell exactly alike, and scientists have a difficult time categorizing odor-producing food substances. In one simplified system, odors are grouped in four classes: (1) fragrant or sweet, (2) acid or sour, (3) burnt or empyreumatic, and (4) caprylic or goaty.

The importance of odor as a flavor component of food is brought home to us when we can't smell, for example, when we have a head cold, and food consequently has little flavor. "Everything tastes like straw," we're likely to complain.

Because odor and flavor are so essential to our enjoyment of food, they play a vital role in nutrition. People who have lost their sense of smell and taste frequently have poor appetites and tend to be underweight as a result of the lack of pleasure they have in eating.

A good smelling food, bread as it is baking, for example, can set up favorable conditions for digestion by stimulating the secretion of saliva and stomach juices. Even before we start eating that freshly baked bread, we are ready to start digesting it!

Food manufacturers are well aware of the importance of odor and flavor, *organoleptic* qualities, in making their foods saleable. No doubt a great deal more money is spent by manufacturers on the research and development of flavors in new food products than on the nutritional value of these foods. Their rationale is "If the food doesn't taste good, no one will eat it, and you can't have good nutrition unless the food is eaten."

Smell and taste reactions are socially and psychologically influenced. We learn to associate certain smells with enjoyment through a stimulus-response conditioning process. Without this conditioning food odor or flavor may be repulsive instead of enticing. For example, the strong, putrid odor and flavor of fermented fish liquor that is so highly prized by the Vietnamese as a flavoring ingredient in many foods is likely to be abhorrent to a person unaccustomed to it.

Color. The color of food also affects our expectations of enjoyment. We're conditioned through our early experiences to relate certain colors with certain flavors and with desirable foods. Should the food appear in an unfamiliar color, purple potatoes, for example, we would be likely to reject it on the basis of color alone.

Experiments on food colors and flavors have shown that we often judge a food's flavor by its color, rather than by its taste. For example, in one instance, taste testers were given sherbet of three colors, orange, yellow, and green, and were asked to identify the flavor of each. All of the sherbet, regardless of color, was the same flavor, orange. But the taste testers were fooled by the color and identified the flavor of each sherbet based on its color: the orange colored sherbet had an "orange" flavor, they said; the yellow tasted like "lemon"; and the green had a "lime" flavor.[21]

In an informal taste test, adult women were asked to compare two milks for flavor and acceptability. The two samples were identical, reconstituted nonfat dry milk, but one sample had a small bit of blue food coloring added and looked a little "bluish" and the other had a little yellow food coloring and had a slightly "yellowish" cast. Of 30 tasters, only two guessed that the samples were alike, and in fact identified them as reconstituted nonfat dry milk. Eleven women said they preferred the bluish milk because they were used to drinking nonfat milk, liked it better than whole milk, and therefore the blue milk was what they preferred. The remainder of the group, 17, said they preferred the "yellowish" milk because it was "richer, creamier, better tasting." Obviously they were judging flavor on the basis of color.

(There's a lesson to be learned here. If you want to help someone learn to like nonfat milk, add a tiny bit of yellow food coloring, or serve it in a yellow glass, and let that person think he is drinking whole milk!)

[21]R. M. Pangborn, "Speaking of Color." From Your Home Advisor, University of California, Cooperative Extension, Anaheim, CA, November, 1964.

Another study demonstrated the importance of appearance in identification of food. School children were blindfolded and then asked to identify some common vegetables such as cooked carrots and mashed potatoes on the basis of their taste and texture. Very few children could do this accurately when they could not see the food.

Since color has such an important influence on our anticipated enjoyment of food, it is a good tool to use in making foods more appealing. Meals look more appetizing when they contain foods with contrasts in color. Compare, for example, the appeal of a dinner (served on a white plate) consisting of white fish, mashed potatoes, and cauliflower, with another dinner having broiled fish with a sprinkle of paprika, baked potato, and broccoli.

Food manufacturers are well aware of the importance of color and use a great variety of food coloring materials to add eye and sales appeal to their foods. The question of the safety of some of the food colors is discussed in Chapter 24.

Texture. The feel of food in our mouth, texture, is yet another sensory factor that affects our enjoyment of food. Foods that are smooth and creamy or crisp and crunchy tend to have more appeal than foods that are grainy, lumpy, slippery, or stringy. Meals with texture contrasts, some soft, some chewy, and some crunchy foods, have more eating appeal than meals having a monotone of textures.

Crispness as a characteristic of food texture was studied by one researcher who discovered it was not a single texture—many unlike foods are crisp. There are the watery crispness of raw vegetables like celery, carrots, and green peppers; the dry crispness of crackers, dry melba toast, and toasted cereals; the more solid or soggy crispness of nuts; and the fat-fried crispness of french fried onion rings, potato chips, and batter-coated fried chicken or fish.

The researcher finally concluded that the unifying characteristic of these "crisp" foods is they all make a noisy, crunchy sound when chewed. Many crunchy foods are eaten as snacks and many are heavily advertised on TV. Their noisy crunch is part of the sales pitch ("aural thrills") used to sell them, the researcher concluded.[22]

Temperature. The temperature of food sometimes affects its desirability too. Some foods taste better hot; others are best when they are cold; while room temperature is preferred for many foods. Usually, variety of temperature of foods in a meal is more appealing than having everything cold or everything hot. However, the old idea that every meal should have at least one hot food is not related at all to a meal's nutritional value, but rather to its eating appeal.

Summing up, an easy guide to good nutrition is to eat meals with

[22]C. Leroux, "Putting Crispness into Words Is not Easy." Chicago Tribune Service, *Independent Press Telegram*, Long Beach, CA, February 22, 1978, Section F, p. 6.

a contrasting variety of colors, flavors, and textures. Not only will such meals be more enjoyable to eat; they are also likely to provide a good variety of essential nutrients.

Individual Differences. Individuals react differently to all of the sensory aspects of food—color, flavor, texture, temperature. These individual differences show up very early, usually in babyhood, and may continue throughout life. Thus, one baby eats every food offered with gusto and with little regard for texture or flavor; another is selective, rejecting some foods vigorously, accepting others. One child may dislike some foods because of the way they feel in his mouth; another may react adversely to certain flavors; and another child may resist certain foods because he doesn't feel good when he eats them. They may form gas and give him a stomachache because he's allergic to them, for example.

In other words, physical differences between individuals affect their choice of foods. Whether these differences are inborn, the result of conditioning, or a combination of the two, is not always clear. Nevertheless, no two people are alike in their food likes, and trying to impose our likes or dislikes on another person is often futile.

Individuals also differ in the amount and kind of food they need. Age, sex, body size, and how active a person is all affect the body's need for food. There are individual differences in the need for specific nutrients as well.

Hunger and Satiety. Another individual difference is the response to hunger sensations. Hunger as a physiological function that triggers an eating response has been studied in depth, yet still is not thoroughly understood.

Hunger differs from appetite in that it tends to be an unpleasant sensation resulting from lack of food whereas *appetite* is the more pleasant sensation of being aware of a desire for food or an anticipation of enjoyment of food because of its odor, appearance, or taste.

Satiety is the opposite of hunger. It consists of a complex of sensations that tell us to stop eating because hunger and appetite have been satisfied. *Anorexia* is a pathological condition in which appetite and hunger sensations are absent in situations where they are both appropriate.

The word hunger has several other shades of meaning to us besides the simple definition of being desirous for food. It may refer to: (1) the mild discomfort we feel when we have been without food for a short time; (2) a state of nutritional depletion, even starvation, resulting from severe food deprivation; and (3) a psychological experience in which we have complex and unpleasant sensations when we have been deprived of food. Hunger is also used frequently in its broadest sense to refer to groups of people who are starving, as in "world hunger," or to groups of people who may be malnourished, as in "Hunger in America" (a television documentary).

An early theory about hunger, as it occurs in an individual, was that it is a response of the nerve endings in the stomach to emptiness or the absence of food. This theory eventually was disproved. Another theory held that the hunger sensation originated in the brain and was secondarily affected by the sensations of emptiness in the stomach.[23]

The current theory, which is widely accepted as valid, is that physiological changes throughout the body send messages to the visceral centers in the hypothalamus, which processes the information and relays it to the thinking centers of the brain for action.[24] Researchers have determined that two areas of the hypothalamus are involved: the *hunger* or *feeding center* on the left side and the *satiety center* on the right side. Sometimes these centers are referred to as the *appestat*.

A mystery yet to be solved is what triggers the hunger-satiety messages. One theory holds that blood sugar level, or glucose utilization, is a major influence. When blood sugar level or glucose utilization drops, hunger sensations are generated; when it rises, hunger ceases, and satiety sensations are felt.[25]

Another theory focuses on the stomach. Recent studies with rats showed that the stomach is responsible for giving the satiety signal. In a way not yet understood, the stomach appears to sense the amount of nutrients consumed and to tell the brain to end the meal. This finding disputes an earlier theory that it was the release of the hormone *cholecystokinin* in the intestines that turned off the impulse to eat. The signal is not generated by the bulk of food consumed but by the amount of nutrients. (This explains why weight control diets using bulky low- or non-caloric foods to "fill the stomach" are ineffective in curbing appetite.) Researchers are trying to determine exactly what it is that the stomach does measure and how it signals the brain.

Other recent studies with mice show a correlation between obesity and a short supply of cholecystokinin in the brain. Formerly it was thought that cholecystokinin was present only in the intestinal tract, but the new studies show that there is as much cholecystokinin in the brain as there is in the intestines and that it appears to be needed to suppress the appetite. Genetically obese mice were found to have only a third as much cholecystokinin in their brains as their normal weight litter-mates. The cholecystokinin was found in the cortex, the thinking part of the brain, not the hypothalamus. Researchers theorize that lack of cholecystokinin results in the appetite center in the hypothalamus not receiving a strong message to be satiated.[26]

[23] J. Mayer, *"Overweight: Causes, Cost, and Control,* 3rd edition. Prentice-Hall, Inc., Englewood Cliffs," N.J. 1971, p. 15.

[24]"Hypothalamus and Food Intake." *Science News*, Vol. 109, May 29, 1976, p. 266.

[25]J. Mayer, p. 17.

[26]"A Biological Defect Underlying Obesity." *Science News*, Vol. 115, January 27, 1979, p. 57.

But these are just preliminary findings, based on animal studies, which have not been verified as being applicable to humans. Studies of people with severe eating disorders, those who are very obese and who eat too much and those who suffer from anorexia and eat too little, show that such people often have a basic disturbance in the way they experience hunger. They appear to misperceive their bodily sensations and do not recognize when they are hungry or satiated. The unanswered question is whether this is due to psychological causes, physiological causes, or both.

From studying these people, some researchers have concluded that the experience of hunger is not simply innate, inborn, automatic, or chemically induced, but that it has important elements of learning. Somehow, in people with severe eating disorders, the inner awareness of the need or lack of need for food has not been programmed correctly, the researchers theorize. In addition, they may be unable to distinguish between hunger and other states of bodily or emotional need. As a result, they misuse eating to help solve, mitigate, or camouflage complex emotional or interpersonal problems. (More on this in Chapter 5.)

Psychological Factors

In satisfying physiological needs, food also fulfills important psychological needs. To most people, food has emotional rather than intellectual value.

To an infant, food means comfort, love, and the security of being taken care of. All our lives, having food available when we need it satisfies a basic need for security, while being without food, even temporarily, can cause high levels of anxiety.

Even for self-sufficient adults, eating is comforting. The pleasure of eating helps soothe inner tensions and anxieties. And for some people, eating becomes an emotional outlet, a substitute for love, or a psychological crutch for handling tensions, frustrations, depression, loneliness, or boredom. Such people may become dependent on or addicted to food the way others might become addicted to cigarettes, alcohol, or drugs and might have just as much trouble "kicking the habit."

Other people, while not addicted to food, nevertheless eat, not because they are hungry, but because they want something to do while watching TV, movies, or spectator sports. Some simply have an unconscious routine that calls for food at certain times and during certain activities and that is triggered by certain signals such as the time of day or a food advertisement on TV. How do these habits develop?

Parents and Family. Early conditioning in the family appears to be an important factor in the development of food habits. In their families, and most especially from their parents, children may learn:

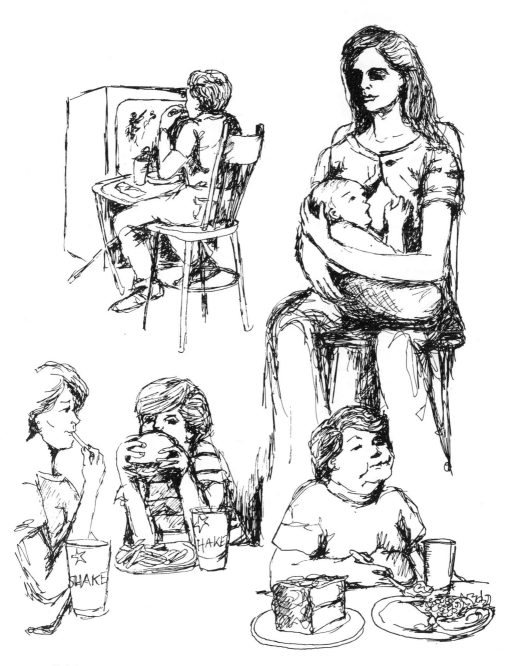

Exhibit 2.11. Eating is doing something; eating is comforting; eating is fun.

To have an excessive fondness for sweets or desserts because these foods are offered as a reward, for example, for good behavior or for eating "good-for-you" foods such as vegetables.

To use food as a substitute for attention or affection when a busy parent gives the complaining child something to eat to keep him quiet, rather than taking the time to love and comfort him.

To hate certain foods such as vegetables because of overanxious coaxing and nagging by worried parents.

To feel they have to live up to certain kinds of fussy eating behavior when parents make constant references to them as "fussy eaters."

To dislike certain foods when one or both parents show a dislike for these foods.

To snack or eat constantly when they are allowed to eat at any time during the day instead of at regularly scheduled intervals.

To depend on their parents' decisions about what and how much they should eat, and to lose or fail to develop their own built-in mechanism that tells them to stop eating.

To always eat everything put in front of them because they are taught to clean their plates.

Peers. There are other influences in a child's life besides his parents. Children are imitative, and they want to be like their friends. So, as they grow older, associate with other children, go to school, they learn food habits from their peers. The pressure to conform to certain behavior norms becomes greater as children grow older. Teenagers especially are known for their need not to "be different" and to conform to peer pressure.

Thus, while a mother might think it a good idea to send her youngster to school with a Thermos of hot soup or cottage cheese with fruit for lunch, the child is likely to refuse to take it if he thinks he's in danger of being ridiculed by his friends or peers because of being "different."

Nutrition educators have long held that children of preschool and elementary age should learn good eating habits that they can follow throughout their lives. However, recent studies have shown that adolescence is an even more important period in acquiring adult dietary patterns. These studies showed that adolescent food intakes are more highly predictive of adult intake than are food patterns in early childhood.[27]

The researchers found that major changes may occur during adolescence and persist into adulthood. Thus, during this period, when the peer group is the adolescent's model, and when teachers, parents, and other adults have much less influence, adult dietary patterns with lifelong implications may be formed.

During the teen years, basic doubts about self-esteem are common.

[27]G. Stewart, "Psychological Aspects of Dietary Change." *Illinois Teacher*, Vol. 19, No. 4, 1976, pp. 191– 97.

A teenager who is unsuccessful in establishing relationships with peers or in achieving scholastically or athletically may use food as a means of bolstering self-esteem. Or eating may become a substitute for other activities and subsequent obesity an excuse for lack of social success. (See Nutrition During Adolescence in Chapter 16.)

Food sometimes has symbolic meanings that affect food choices. Thus the long-held notion that meat symbolizes masculinity and strength may lead young athletes, perhaps encouraged by their coaches, to believe that they need to consume large amounts of meat or protein to develop strength, endurance, aggressiveness, and athletic prowess (see Nutrition for Young Athletes, Chapter 16).

Food habits are also used sometimes as a form of self-expression or even as social protest. Thus, many of the "antiestablishment" young adults of the 1960s and 1970s selected a so-called natural food diet to establish or maintain and present their identity to others. Many of the protestors also became vegetarians as a way of rejecting the affluent, meat-eating American life-style of their parents' generation. Vegetarianism also was an outgrowth of this generation's new religious beliefs. Peer pressure to conform to the diets of the new establishment group was also present among these young people.

Summary

Although all human beings need the same basic nutrients, they obtain them through diverse eating patterns. A complex variety of both internal and external factors interact to shape each individual's eating habits. This molding process begins with exposure to family food patterns and the family's attitudes toward food. The larger society also impacts on families and individuals through social customs, religious beliefs, and food availability.

In American society, the mobility of people and the wide distribution of foods has had a cultural blending effect. Our society is also characterized by fast-paced life-styles and a higher proportion of people living singly at many age levels. This has resulted in more frequent meal skipping, more snacking, and more widespread use of alcohol and drugs. People often do not take time to plan, prepare, and enjoy meals, while they may also be faced with a sedentary life-style requiring fewer calories.

World-wide, the most serious deterrent to good nutrition is poverty, although malnutrition can be observed at all income levels and the diets of poor people are not universally poor in nutritional quality. The key is careful selection.

Food has an emotional, rather than an intellectual, value to most people; this concept is frequently utilized by the food industry in its advertising and food promotion practices. Television advertisements directed toward children are currently under close scrutiny, since critics feel that children lack the maturity to evaluate the information presented and may be strongly influenced to their detriment.

Physiological factors such as taste, smell, and other organoleptic qualities interact with external factors to produce individually unique eating patterns. In addition, people often use food to satisfy a variety of psychological needs. The greatest challenge faced by nutrition educators is motivating people to act upon sound nutrition advice.

THE CONFUSED CONSUMER 3

Highlights

Food advertising and marketing techniques
Pitfalls of impulse buying and its effect on nutrition
Food and nutrition labeling
Use of labels in meal planning and food comparisons
Nutrient density
Calorie labeling
Nutritional Quality Guidelines

To the individual, the nutriton challenge is an *eating* challenge. Good nutrition cannot happen until and unless food is available for our bodies to process. In Chapter 1 we learned that good nutrition means eating the *right foods* in the *right amounts* with both the kind of food and the amount eaten being equally important.

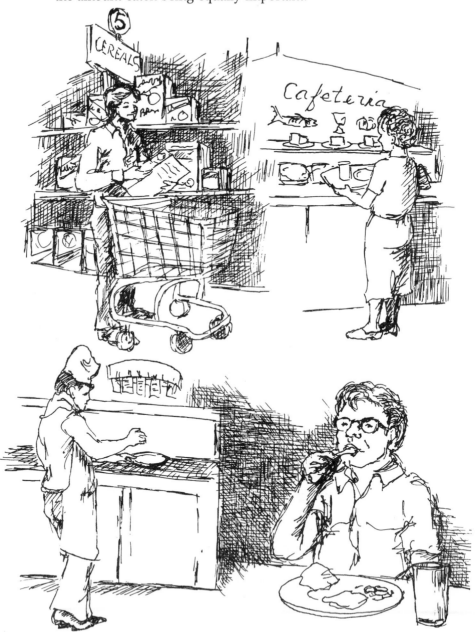

Exhibit 3.1. Your personal nutrition depends on the decisions you make when you choose food to buy or to eat.

What you eat depends, to a great extent, on the decisions you, or the person who prepares food for you, make when you shop for food, store it, prepare it, and serve it, or on the choices you make when you select food from a menu when you eat out.

How much you eat depends mostly on you (although overeaters sometimes try to blame others, such as the cook, for their overindulgence).

In other words, your nutrition depends on decisions relating to food purchase, storage, and preparation, as well as on the ultimate decision of what food you put in your mouth (see Exhibit 3.1). An additional nutrition challenge, especially during times when inflation results in steadily rising food prices, is to choose from among the many alternatives the foods which are "best buys," that is, give the most nutrients for the least cost.

THE FOOD SELECTION CHALLENGE

In America today food shopping has become a complicated decision-making process, and the word that often best describes the food shopper is "confused." (Exhibit 3.2 lists factors that cause confusion and lead to poor nutrition choices.)

Consumers can be confused simply by the sheer numbers of choices available to them: some 10,000 items are sold in an average supermarket (see Exhibit 3.3). Every year hundreds of new products, with new nutritional values, are added, while products that don't sell well or bring in sufficient profit quietly disappear. Many of the foods are packaged to look alike but are different nutritionally; others look different but are basically alike. How are consumers going to tell the difference?

All of the packages on display in supermarkets, with their various pictures, colors, and slogans, can have a mesmerizing effect on shoppers. In one study, in which supermarket shoppers were filmed as they shopped and their eye-blink rate measured, the researcher concluded that many shoppers drifted through the store in a mild hypnotic trance induced by the confusing mass of products.[1] Under these circumstan-

Exhibit 3.2   Reasons Supermarket Shoppers Make Poor Nutrition Choices

Confused by array of products
Don't understand nutrition terms on labels
Don't have time to read labels
Buy on impulse
Misled by advertising
Hear conflicting messages about nutrition and food safety

[1]V. Packard, *The Hidden Persuaders*. Pocket-Cardinal Edition, Simon and Schuster, Inc., New York, 1957, pp. 90–97.

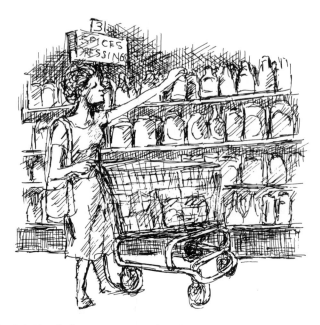

Exhibit 3.3. Food shoppers are confused by the large number of food choices available to them.

ces, decisions are likely to be emotional and impulsive rather than rational.

All too often purchases are not planned ahead of time, and shoppers are highly susceptible to suggestions made through point-of-sales influences in supermarkets. On-the-spot decisions frequently result in the purchase of the high-profit, less nutritious, eye appealing, "self-gratifying" items.

Thus, the confused consumer is prone to buying on impulse, and impulse buying can be a prime enemy of good nutrition. Since impulse buying helps profits, food sellers do what they can to encourage it, by placing high-profit impulse items at eye level, for example, or by putting foods having special appeal to children, such as sugared breakfast cereals, at child-in-the-cart eye level. More nutritious foods and better values are often found on the lower shelves. Bins at the end of the rows of shelves and next to checkout counters are other favored locations for splurge and spur-of-the-moment purchases.

Consumers may also be confused because many of them do not have the knowledge to understand the nutrition terms used on labels and many more do not read well enough to even bother looking at them. A survey testing the basic verbal and mathematical literacy of American adults which was conducted by the U.S. Office of Education in the mid-1970s showed that less than half are really proficient enough to handle their daily affairs. One-third have just the minimum competency, and

20 percent simply cannot function effectively.[2] Only 37 percent were rated proficient at picking the best buy from a grocery shelf, while 30 percent were rated incompetent. The current sophisticated nutrient information used on lables has no meaning for this large group of American consumers who lack basic reading and mathematical skills.

Even proficient consumers can be confused by misleading information presented in food advertisements. Many consumers are easily fooled by subtle techniques such as the omission of a key fact or the use of unrealistic or unfair comparisons. For example, an advertisement for a nondairy liquid coffee creamer declared in boldface type that the product contained "only seven calories per teaspoon." This was factual, but it was designed to mislead because it implied, but did not say, that the substitute was lower in calories than other products. Consumers were not expected to consider what a small amount a teaspoon contains nor to know that half and half, or coffee cream, also has just seven calories per teaspoon.

As this example illustrates, many consumers also are confused about serving sizes, and especially so when they are expressed in ounces or grams. Many have no idea what a three-ounce serving of meat looks like, for example, and many do not know that a one-ounce serving of breakfast cereal can vary in volume from as little as a quarter of a cup (some types of granola) to as much as two and one-half cups (puffed wheat or rice), depending on the density of the product. Thus serving sizes on labels need to be stated in terms that are meaningful to the average person (for example, "ten medium-sized potato chips" instead of "one ounce"), but often they are not.

Because they lack sufficient knowledge of nutrition facts, consumers also may be confused by the conflicting messages they receive about nutrition and food safety. A survey of 1,500 people with primary responsibility for family food purchases conducted in the mid-1970s by the Food and Drug Administration revealed that consumers have many misconceptions about the nutritive value of foods and that a few widespread myths stand in the way of making wise choices. For example, 40 percent said they believed that if a person knows little about nutrition, but simply eats a variety of foods, he will be likely to be well nourished, and 40 percent also believed that between-meal snacks are never as valuable as food eaten at meals.[3]

One of the government's major efforts to improve the nutrition knowledge of consumers is regulation of food labeling, especially the implementation of nutrition labeling. But labels alone cannot possibly give consumers the nutrition education they need to understand how to manage their nutritional well-being.

[2]"Why 1.4 Million Americans Can't Read or Write." *U.S. News*, Vol. 77, August 19, 1974, pp. 37–38.

[3]FDA Consumer Nutrition Knowledge Survey Report, II, 1975, U.S. Department of Health, Education, and Welfare, Public Health Service, Food and Drug Administration, DHEW Publication No. (FDA) 72-2059, Washington, D.C., 1976.

Food labeling comes under the jurisdiction of several different federal agencies: the U.S. Department of Agriculture (USDA) regulates the labeling of fresh and processed meat and poultry products and dairy products; the Food and Drug Administration (FDA) regulates the labeling of all processed foods shipped across state lines (interstate commerce) except those containing meat or poultry; and the Federal Trade Commission (FTC) regulates false or misleading labels, packaging, and the advertising of food (and other products). Foods grown and shipped *intrastate*, within a single state, are regulated by state laws rather than the federal government, except for meat and poultry products. State regulations vary greatly, from excellent to inadequate.

Both the USDA and FDA require certain basic information to be present on all labels:

Name of product, its form or style, and packing medium, for example, sliced peaches in heavy syrup.

Net weight in pounds and ounces and in total ounces, for example, 1 lb 6 oz (22 oz). Net weight includes everything edible in the container—liquid, oil, sugar, etc. It is *not* a drained weight.

Ingredient list, with ingredients listed in descending order of predominance by weight. The first ingredient is present in greatest amount, and so on down the list. An exception is *standardized foods,* made by standard recipes approved by the FDA, on which no ingredient list is required. Standardized foods are being phased out, and some states now require that all processed foods be labeled with ingredient lists.

Any special treatment the food has undergone, for example, concentrated or evaporated means water removed; enriched or fortified means nutrients added, and so on.

Name and address of packer.

"USDA Inspected and Passed." This symbol is mandatory on all processed meat and poultry products, but is voluntary on other types of food. It indicates that the product has been inspected for wholesomeness by USDA inspectors. USDA *quality grading*—for example, "USDA Choice" on beef, "USDA Grade A" on fruits—is voluntary for all food, and may be used if the packer pays to have the grading service of USDA. USDA quality grading may not be used on products unless the USDA inspection is also provided. USDA inspection and quality grading do not denote nutritional value. They relate only to wholesomeness and eating quality of the food, that is, flavor, color, texture, tenderness. A lower grade food could be just as nutritious as a higher grade one, although for fruits and vegetables, top quality and top nutritional value usually go together. In the case of beef, a lower grade meat might have

less fat and be preferable from the calorie and saturated fat standpoint than a higher grade meat.

Nutrition Labeling

In January 1975, a new FDA regulation for nutrition labeling of processed foods went into effect. It required that nutrition information be displayed on the labels of all foods that are fortified or enriched, or for which any sort of nutrition claim is made ("low calorie," "high protein," "vitamin D added," etc.) on either label or in advertising. For other ordinary foods this nutrition labeling is voluntary. It is also voluntary if nutrients are added during the manufacturing process for some purpose other than enrichment or fortification, for example, when vitamin C is added to fruit to prevent browning.

The nutrition information must appear in a standard format, on the part of the label immediately to the right of the main panel. It must be given per serving with the serving size and number of servings per container clearly stated. Information must be given on:

The number of calories.

The grams of protein, carbohydrate, and fat.

The percentage of the U.S. Recommended Daily Allowances (U.S. RDA) for protein, vitamin A, vitamin C, thiamin, riboflavin, niacin, calcium, and iron. If the product has less than 2 percent of the U.S. RDA for any of these nutrients, opposite the nutrients zeroes or asterisks can be used that relate to a footnote stating "contains less than 2 percent of these nutrients." A sample label is illustrated in Exhibit 3.4.

The listing of 12 additional minerals and vitamins such as iodine, folic acid, vitamin E, etc., as a percentage of the U.S. RDA is optional.

The percentage of calories that comes from fat and the grams of cholesterol, polyunsaturated and saturated fat may be listed, but if they are listed, the label must include the statement, "Information on fat and cholesterol content is provided for individuals who, on the advice of a physician, are modifying their total dietary intake of fat and cholesterol." The sum of saturated and polyunsaturated fat may not always equal the total grams of fat because the monounsaturated fats are not included. However, the actual amount of polyunsaturated fat and the ratio of polyunsaturated to saturated fats would be listed.

The amount of sodium may be listed on an ingredient list without triggering a full nutrition statement, but if an amount of sodium is given, the label must include the statement, "The information is intended for persons who are limiting the amount of salt in their diets on the advice of a physician."

Nutrition labels show amounts of nutrients in grams and milligrams rather than the familiar ounces because they are a smaller unit of

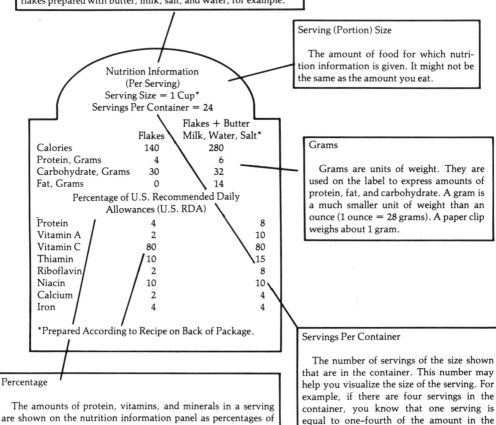

Nutrition Information

Information must be given for a specified serving of the product as found in the container. This label shows information for a serving of potato flakes. Additional information may be listed for the product in combination with other ingredients— flakes prepared with butter, milk, salt, and water, for example.

Serving (Portion) Size

The amount of food for which nutrition information is given. It might not be the same as the amount you eat.

Nutrition Information
(Per Serving)
Serving Size = 1 Cup*
Servings Per Container = 24

	Flakes	Flakes + Butter Milk, Water, Salt*
Calories	140	280
Protein, Grams	4	6
Carbohydrate, Grams	30	32
Fat, Grams	0	14

Percentage of U.S. Recommended Daily Allowances (U.S. RDA)

Protein	4	8
Vitamin A	2	10
Vitamin C	80	80
Thiamin	10	15
Riboflavin	2	8
Niacin	10	10
Calcium	2	4
Iron	4	4

*Prepared According to Recipe on Back of Package.

Grams

Grams are units of weight. They are used on the label to express amounts of protein, fat, and carbohydrate. A gram is a much smaller unit of weight than an ounce (1 ounce = 28 grams). A paper clip weighs about 1 gram.

Servings Per Container

The number of servings of the size shown that are in the container. This number may help you visualize the size of the serving. For example, if there are four servings in the container, you know that one serving is equal to one-fourth of the amount in the container.

To find the cost of a serving, divide the price for the container by the number of servings per container.

Percentage

The amounts of protein, vitamins, and minerals in a serving are shown on the nutrition information panel as percentages of the U.S. Recommended Dietary Allowances (U.S. RDAs).

Percentages of the U.S. RDA are given in increments of 2 percent (2, 4, 6, etc.) up to 10 percent; of 5 percent (10, 15, 20, etc.) up to 50 percent; and of 10 percent (50, 60, 70, etc.) above 50 percent.

Exhibit 3.4. (*Source:* B. Peterkin, J. Nicholas, and C. Cromwell, "Nutrition Labeling: Tools for Its Use." Agricultural Information Bulletin No. 382, U.S. Department of Agriculture. Washington, D.C.: U.S. Government Printing Office, April 1975, p. 3.)

measurement and therefore provide more precise information. (One ounce equals 28.35 grams; a milligram is 1/1000 of a gram.)

Nutrition information also may be given for a serving of the food as cooked or prepared in combination with other foods, according to directions given on the label (for example, soup made with milk), or according to the way the food is usually eaten (for example, cereal with milk).

To have accurate information about nutrient content of their foods, manufacturers must have a laboratory analysis made of each food to be labeled. The FDA regulations include the details of testing compliance, including statistical guidelines.

The compliance section provides ample range of nutrient content naturally found in foods to allow for natural variations. To be in compliance a naturally occurring nutrient must be present at 80 percent of the declared value. Tolerances for added nutrients are considerably more strict, but still provide room for reasonable variation consistent with good manufacturing practices. To be in compliance, a manufacturer is likely to somewhat understate nutrient values of products.

This means that nutrition labels tell you approximately, but not exactly, what nutrients are present in the food when you buy it.

Nutrition labeling also takes into account the quality of the protein in food as well as the quantity. (See Chapter 9 for an explanation of protein quality and the PER value.) Two adult U.S. RDA values for protein have been set. The U.S. RDA values for adults are listed as 65 grams if the PER of the protein is less than that of casein and 45 grams if the PER is equal to or better than that of casein. This is because when we eat a "better than casein" protein, we need less protein to get the U.S. RDA value than when we eat a protein with a PER value below casein.

The "better than casein" group would be the traditional high quality proteins from meat, fish, eggs, and dairy products. Other protein products such as vegetable proteins and mixtures of cereal and animal proteins would be expected to fit the higher (65 gram) U.S. RDA value.

The regulation also is written so that protein that has a value less than 20 percent of the PER of casein cannot be counted as a contributing protein at all. This would refer to a protein like gelatin that is of little value as a protein contributor.

Meat and poultry products, for which the labeling is regulated by the USDA rather than the FDA, also are covered by a voluntary nutrition-labeling regulation. Manufacturers who elect to nutritionally label their products must follow the labeling requirements providing for a uniform format. All meat and poultry products that are nutritionally labeled must provide nutrition information on an "as purchased" basis. Nutritionally-labeled products requiring cooking before they are eaten must also include nutrition information on an "as prepared" basis, with a specific method of cooking shown in a statement adjacent to the nutrition statement.

This additional information is required because in many instances cooking results in significant nutritional changes, especially in fat and calorie values, and these are considered to be of widespread consumer interest and concern.

A few kinds of foods with added nutrients are exempted from nutrition labeling. These include infant formulas, which are regulated under foods for "special dietary use." Other baby and junior-type foods marketed for infants or very young children are included in the voluntary FDA nutritional-labeling program. For such foods, the "serving" means a reasonable quantity for an infant or young child and the nutrient content information is based on one of two special sets of the U.S. RDA for infants and children under age four instead of the adult allowances.

Other exemptions are foods that are represented for use as the sole item of a diet (not a meal) and food products that are represented for use under medical supervision for the dietary management of specific diseases.

The use of iodized salt does not require nutrition labeling as long as neither iodine nor iodized salt is otherwise referred to on the label.

Using Nutrition and Ingredient Labeling

On nutrition labels, the levels of protein, minerals, and vitamins are expressed as a percentage of the U.S. RDA for adults (see Exhibit 3.5).

Most people do not need to get 100 percent of the U.S. RDA for every nutrient since the U.S. RDA for adults are based on those of the group (usually teenage boys) with the highest need for each nutrient. Use of 100 percent of the U.S. RDA as a nutritional goal is in no way dangerous, but it may lead to unnecessary changes in diet and food spending, as well as causing unwarranted concern about shortages of nutrients. In some cases, there can be differences of as much as 50 percent between an individual's need for a nutrient and the U.S. RDA.

Exhibit 3.5   U.S. Recommended Daily Allowances of Protein, Minerals, and Vitamins for Adults

NUTRIENT	AMOUNT
Protein	65 grams (PER less than casein)
	45 grams (PER equal to or better than casein)
Vitamin A	5,000 International Units
Vitamin C	60 milligrams
Thiamin	1.5 milligrams
Riboflavin	1.7 milligrams
Niacin	20 milligrams
Calcium	1.0 grams (1,000 milligrams)
Iron	18 milligrams

Therefore if you want to use the U.S. RDA in planning meals tailored to nutrient needs, use the appropriate goals for your age and sex listed in Exhibit 3.6. For example, a 60-year-old woman's need for iron is 60 percent of the U.S. RDA. Therefore, her goal for meal planning could be to include food for a day that provides 60 percent or more of the U.S. RDA for iron.

If all foods had nutrition labels, a person could, if he had the time and patience, add up the percentages of the U.S. RDA supplied by each food to see if his total for the day was equal to his requirement. However, this use of the nutrition-labeling information is not practical since only some foods carry the nutrition labels and few, if any, consumers would be willing to take the time to make the necessary calculations.

Exhibit 3.6   Allowances for Food Energy and Percentages of the U.S. RDA Needed to Meet the RDA for Children, Men, and Women of Different Ages

AGE	FOOD ENERGY[1]	PROTEIN[2]	VITAMIN A	VITAMIN C	THIAMIN	RIBO-FLAVIN	NIACIN[3]	CALCIUM	IRON
Years	Calories	-------- Percent of U.S. Recommended Daily Allowance --------							
Child:									
1–3	1,300	35	40	70	50	50	30	80	85
4–6	1,800	50	50	70	60	65	35	80	60
7–10	2,400	55	70	70	80	75	50	80	60
Male:									
11–14	2,800	70	100	75	95	90	55	120	100
15–18	3,000	85	100	75	100	110	55	120	100
19–22	3,000	85	100	75	100	110	60	80	60
23–50	2,700	90	100	75	95	95	45	80	60
51+	2,400	90	100	75	80	90	35	80	60
Female:									
11–14	2,400	70	80	75	80	80	45	120	100
15–18	2,100	75	80	75	75	85	30	120	100
19–22	2,100	75	80	75	75	85	35	80	100
23–50	2,000	75	80	75	70	75	30	80	100
51+	1,800	75	80	75	70	65	25	80	60
Pregnant	+300[4]	+50[4]	100	100	+20[4]	+20[4]	35	120	100+
Nursing	+500[4]	+35[4]	120	135	+20[4]	+30[4]	35	120	100

Source: B. Peterkin, J. Nicholas, and C. Cromwell, "Nutrition Labeling: Tools for Its Use." Agricultural Information Bulletin No. 382, U.S. Department of Agriculture. Washington, D.C.: U.S. Government Printing Office, April, 1975, p. 47.

[1] Calorie needs differ depending on body composition and size, age, and activity of the person.

[2] U.S. RDA of 65 grams is used for this table. In labeling, a U.S. RDA of 45 grams is used for foods providing high-quality protein, such as milk, meat, and eggs.

[3] The percentage of the U.S. RDA shown for niacin will provide the RDA for niacin if the RDA for protein is met. Some niacin is derived in the body from tryptophan, an amino acid present in protein.

[4] To be added to the percentage for the girl or woman of the appropriate age.

However, food labels *can* serve some useful purposes in helping consumers make wise food choices. By using ingredient lists in conjunction with nutrient labels, consumers can find out some important facts about foods.

Say, for example, you are comparing two types of prepared breakfast cereal. The *ingredient list* of one has sugar and fat listed as the first two ingredients, meaning they are present in the largest amount by weight, and oats as the third ingredient. The nutrient label tells you the product has 140 calories in a one-ounce (¼ cup) serving. From this information, you can conclude that the bulk of the calories in this product come from the sugar and fat and also that it is a very concentrated food since just ¼ cup weighs an ounce.

The ingredient list on the second cereal lists oats first, then wheat, then sugar, while the nutrient label tells you the product has 100 calories in a one-ounce (1½ cup) serving. With this cereal you can conclude that the bulk of the calories comes from starch in the oats and wheat and that you will have to eat a rather large bowlful to get a one-ounce serving.

While comparing these cereal labels, you might also be checking the percentage of the U.S. RDA for iron and B vitamins in each cereal and perhaps discovering that one product is fortified with these nutrients to as much as 25 or 50 percent of the U.S. RDA, while the other product is not fortified at all (perhaps because it's supposed to be "natural") and has relatively little iron and B vitamins.

This example shows how the ingredient list and the nutrient label are useful in helping evaluate foods on the basis of *nutrient density*. Nutrient density refers to a food's nutrient content in relation to its energy value or calorie content. To determine nutrient density you look at (1) the number of calories in a serving and (2) the amount of other nutrients, especially minerals and vitamins, that are present.

A food with a low nutrient density would have many calories and few, or small amounts of, other nutrients; so if you wanted to get many other nutrients, you would have to eat it in large quantities at a high-calorie cost. In contrast, a food with a high nutrient density is one that supplies significant amounts of one or more nutrients along with relatively few calories.

High-sugar and high-fat foods tend to fall in the low-nutrient-density category, while watery, fibrous foods such as vegetables, which are low in sugar and fat, fall in the high-nutrient-density category. Exhibit 3.7 shows some examples of the differences between high- and low-nutrient-density foods.

Nutrition labeling can be especially helpful when comparing the nutrient value of plain foods versus fancy prepared foods. For example, look at the nutrition labels for two types of frozen broccoli (Exhibit 3.8). The plain frozen broccoli, which has no added ingredients, has half the calories of the frozen broccoli with hollandaise sauce and more vitamins A and C—and it costs just half as much. As a general rule, the plain

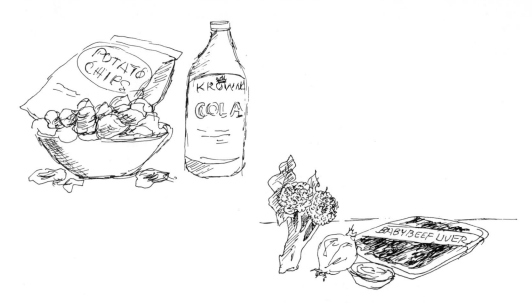

Exhibit 3.7. Low-nutrient-density foods have many calories in proportion to other nutrients. High-nutrient-density foods have significant amounts of one or more nutrients and relatively few calories.

Exhibit 3.8   Two Nutrition Labels

	CHOPPED BROCCOLI	BROCCOLI WITH HOLLANDAISE SAUCE
Serving size	3.3 oz (100 g)	3.3 oz (100 g)
Calories	25	100
Protein	3 g	3 g
Carbohydrate	4 g	3 g
Fat	0	9 g
Sodium	15 mg	115 mg
Potassium	205 mg	180 mg

PERCENTAGES OF U.S. RECOMMENDED DAILY ALLOWANCES (U.S. RDA)

Protein	4%	4%
Vitamin A	45	20
Vitamin C	90	70
Thiamin	4	2
Riboflavin	4	4
Niacin	*	*
Calcium	4	2
Iron	2	4
Vitamin B_6	6	6

* Contains less than 2% of U.S. RDA

foods are not only cheaper but are also lower in calories and have a higher level of nutrients. But, in spite of this, you may choose the more expensive product because you or your family prefers the taste!

Nutrient and ingredient labeling can be especially helpful to people who must eat modified diets such as: (1) low calorie; (2) controlled fat; (3) low sodium; (4) high iron; and so on. However, remember that the type of fat and the amount of cholesterol and sodium are not required on nutrition labels; this information is voluntary.

With the advent of nutrition labeling, manufacturers have had to be more precise about the words they use on labels and in advertising. For example, if they claim a food is "low calorie" this triggers a nutrition statement in which they must tell you how many calories are in what size serving and how many servings are in the container.

Information on labels can be used to compare the protein, vitamin, and mineral content of foods you might substitute for each other in meals or snacks. However, it's important to remember that the foods with the highest percentages of U.S. RDA on their labels are not always the best selections, and a food with a high percentage improves your diet only if your diet is short in that nutrient. A food with a 100-percent U.S. RDA of one nutrient may be totally lacking in other important nutrients. And if you looked for just large percentages on labels, you might end up with excess amounts of some nutrients and a total lack of other nutrients. You might also end up with expensive foods or foods that are less acceptable to you or your family.

With the exception of some highly fortified foods, no one food provides recommended amounts of all the nutrients, or even large percentages of single nutrients. A variety of foods of different types is needed to obtain a daily supply of recommended nutrients. Thus, nutrition labeling, while an important aid in evaluation of foods, does not offer the shopper a simple approach to selecting nutritious diets.

Calorie Labeling

In 1978, the FDA finalized a regulation setting new rules on how "low calorie," "reduced calorie," and "diabetic" foods must be labeled. The purpose of the regulation was to ensure that foods called "low calorie" or "reduced calorie" really are lower in calories than their nonreduced-calorie counterparts (see Exhibit 3.9).

Under this regulation:

1. A food labeled as "low calorie" may contain no more than 40 calories per serving. This means the term cannot be used for foods that may have few calories per piece (for example, a potato chip) but are normally eaten in large amounts.

2. A food may be called "reduced calorie" only if its caloric content is at least one-third lower than a similar food for which it can substitute.

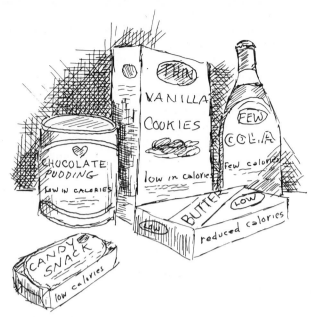

Exhibit 3.9. A Food and Drug Administration regulation ensures that foods whose labels state that they are low or reduced in calories really are lower in calories.

3. Labels on all foods that claim to be reduced in calories must describe the comparison on which the claim is based. For example, "artificially sweetened peaches packed in water, 38 calories per ½-cup serving, 62 percent less than Brand X peaches in heavy syrup."

4. Foods that are normally low in calories, such as celery, cannot have the term "low calorie" immediately before the name because this would suggest that one particular celery has fewer calories than another. However, the label may state "celery, a low-calorie food."

5. A food cannot be labeled as "diabetic" unless it is useful in the diets of diabetics.

6. For a food to be labeled as "sugar free," "sugarless," or "no sugar," it must also be labeled as "low calorie" or "reduced calorie" and meet the labeling requirements of those categories, or be accompanied by such statements as "not a reduced calorie food" or "not for weight control."

Nutritional Quality Guidelines

Besides the nutrition-labeling rules, the FDA has also issued Nutritional Quality Guidelines for several food products. The purpose of the guidelines is to prescribe basic levels of nutrient composition for food classes. A food that complies with these guidelines may carry the statement, "This product provides nutrients in amounts appropriate for this class of food as determined by the U.S. Government." A food so labeled must include nutrition labeling and make no special claim for nutrients that were added to make it meet the guideline. However, the nutrients added would be included in the ingredient list.

The first nutritional guideline was for frozen "heat and serve" dinners. To qualify as a dinner the product must consist of three parts, which include: (1) one or more protein sources from meat, poultry, fish, cheese or eggs; (2) one or more vegetables or vegetable mixtures other than potatoes; and (3) potatoes, rice, or cereal products or another vegetable or vegetable mixture. Other items may be added but are not counted as fulfilling the basic nutrient content. The use of iodized salt is also prescribed where feasible.

Do Consumers Use Food Labels?

Through nutrition labeling, manufacturers and the government acknowledge that consumers have a right to know about the nutritional qualities of foods. Consumers receive some benefits even if they totally ignore nutrition information on labels. Because of labeling, food companies are becoming more concerned about the nutritive value of the foods they produce. In addition, the analysis of foods now being performed by the companies to determine nutritive value for labeling is providing scientists with a great deal of information that formerly was not available.

Numerous surveys show that consumers' interest in having this nutrition information available to them on labels is high, but that the actual use of it is low (see Exhibit 3.10). Consumers report that they don't have time to read labels when they are shopping and that they find the information confusing. They don't understand words such as carbohydrate, sodium, cholesterol; they don't know the meaning of "U.S. RDA"; nor do they have any concept of quantities of nutrients when given in terms of grams or milligrams.[4]

A survey conducted in the mid-1970s by the Food and Drug Administration among 1,600 food shoppers showed that about 33 percent of those surveyed said they used nutritional labeling in choosing some foods and beverages and about 50 percent said they checked the ingredient list of foods the last time they shopped. Persons found to be most likely to read and use labels are generally the younger, better educated, higher income group. In another study where consumers were interviewed in stores while shopping, only 9.2 percent said they used labels to make purchase decisions.[5]

[4]"1978 Consumer Food Labeling Survey—Summary Report." Consumer Research Staff, Division of Consumer Studies, Bureau of Foods, Food and Drug Administration, Washington, D.C., May, 1979.

[5]E. Kaitz, *National Food Situation.* U.S. Department of Agriculture, Washington, D.C., June, 1977, pages 17–18.

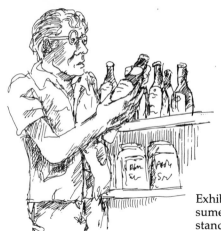

Exhibit 3.10. Food labels do not help consumers unless consumers read, understand, and use them.

Thus, while food labels do provide useful information for decision making, the labels do not help consumers unless they read them, understand them, and use them. It appears that nutrition education has a long way to go before a major portion of consumers benefit notably from the information provided on nutrition labels.

Summary

Today's food shopper is confronted with a confusing array of products making competing claims. This often leads to impulsive decision making. Emotional impulse buying can be a prime enemy of good nutrition.

The U.S. Department of Agriculture (USDA) and the Food and Drug Administration (FDA) require that certain basic information be present on all labels. This includes the ingredient list, which ranks ingredients in descending order of predominance by weight. Since 1975, the FDA has required nutrition labeling on food to which nutrients have been added or to which a nutritional claim is attached. Although nutrition labeling is not required for all food products, many companies have voluntarily implemented it. Information appears in a standard format to simplify comparisons. Both ingredient lists and nutrition labeling are useful in evaluating the nutrient density of foods for people whose diets must be modified.

A relatively new labeling guideline defines use of the terms "low calorie," "reduced calorie," and "diabetic foods"; FDA regulations must be met by manufacturers to ensure that these foods really are lower in calories than the standard food. The FDA has also issued Nutritional Quality Guidelines for certain classes of food. To benefit from food labels, consumers must read, understand, and use them.

Part II

ENERGY
AND
BODY
WEIGHT

OUR NEED FOR ENERGY 4

Highlights

Balance of energy intake with energy needs of the body
Energy sources, fat storage, and adjustment of energy balance
Adipose tissue, calories, and basal metabolic rate

All the functions of food in the body—growing and repairing body tissue, regulating body processes, and supplying energy—are essential. However, our first nutritional priority is for energy. Without fuel bodies cannot function, just as without gas automobiles cannot run.

ENERGY AND OUR BODIES

The sun is the original source of our energy, but our bodies are not capable of converting sun energy into usable fuel. This task is done by green plants through the process known as *photosynthesis*. Using chlorophyll and sunlight, plants synthesize carbohydrate (*glucose*) from carbon dioxide and water. From this simple sugar, plants manufacture complex carbohydrates, fats, and proteins. These nutrients serve as a source of fuel to animals. And we, in turn, obtain fuel by eating either plants or animals (see Exhibit 4.1).

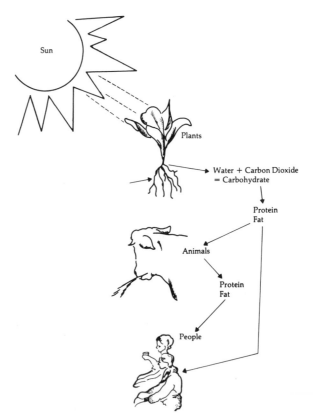

Exhibit 4.1. The Energy Cycle: From sun to plants to animals and people.

Foods for Energy

Our fuel foods are fats, proteins, and carbohydrates, and they are basically interchangeable in meeting energy needs. However, our bodies prefer to use carbohydrates and fats for energy and protein for building, repairing, and maintaining body tissue. Protein is used for energy (1) when there is insufficient intake of calories in our diets from carbohydrates and fat, or (2) when there is more protein available than needed for building, repairing, and maintaining body tissues. Since protein foods are more costly than other foods, eating excess protein is an expensive way to obtain energy.

In the American diet, protein supplies 11 to 12 percent of our energy, and carbohydrates and fats make an almost equal contribution of 46 percent and 42 percent, respectively (see Exhibit 4.2). For some people, alcohol supplies 5 to 10 percent of energy.

Our body's use of energy conforms to the *law of conservation* of energy: energy can neither be created nor destroyed; it can only change form. When one form of energy is produced, another form is reduced by exactly the same amount.

Plants convert sun energy to chemical energy in the form of carbohydrates, fats, and proteins. Our bodies use oxygen to "burn" these fuel foods and produce other forms of energy plus carbon dioxide and water. The other forms of energy produced in the body include: mechanical, for muscle contraction; osmotic, for transporting fluids and nutrients; electrical, for transmitting nerve impulses; chemical, for synthesizing new compounds; and thermal, for heat regulation (see Exhibit 4.3).

Storage of Energy

Energy not immediately needed is stored in the body for future use, primarily as fat. Plants store much of their energy as carbohydrate, but humans store very little in this form. We store only a small amount of carbohydrate in the form of *glycogen* in the liver and muscles to supply "instant energy." Our main reserve supply of energy is in the form of fat cells known collectively as *adipose* tissue. We have very little ability to store protein, but muscles and organs are rich in protein and can serve as an emergency source of energy. However, this use can result in the depletion of body tissue.

Of the three nutrients, fat stores energy most efficiently. A gram of fat will supply 9 calories—two and one-fourth times as many as an equal weight of either carbohydrate or protein, which both yield 4 calories per gram (see Exhibit 4.4). In nonmetric terms, an ounce of fat has about 250 calories; an ounce of protein or carbohydrate has about 110 calories.

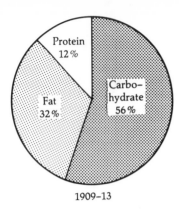
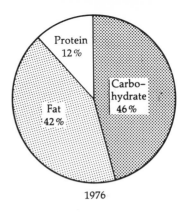

1909–13   1976

Per Capita Civilian Consumption.

Food Energy (Calories) From Food Groups

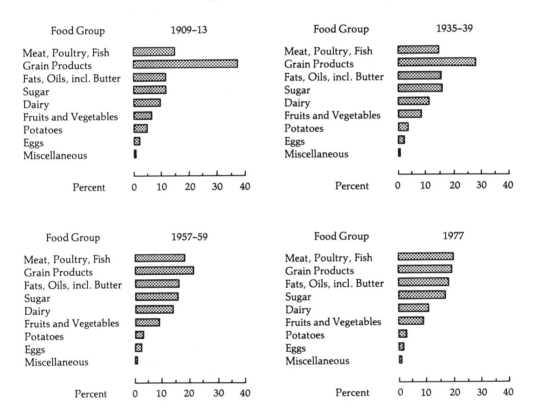

Food Group	1909–13
Food Group	1935–39
Food Group	1957–59
Food Group	1977

Meat, Poultry, Fish
Grain Products
Fats, Oils, incl. Butter
Sugar
Dairy
Fruits and Vegetables
Potatoes
Eggs
Miscellaneous

Percent   0   10   20   30   40

Source: 1978 Handbook of Agricultural Charts. U.S. Department of Agriculture, Agricultural Handbook No. 551

Exhibit 4.2. Where Calories Come From

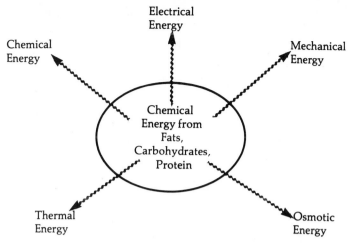

Exhibit 4.3. Our bodies convert chemical energy in foods into other forms of energy.

Calories Measure Energy

The energy value of food and the energy our bodies expend are measured in calories. A *small calorie*, used in most fields of science, is the amount of heat needed to raise the temperature of one cubic centimeter (cc) of water one degree celsius (centigrade). In nutrition, we use the *large calorie* (C), which is 1,000 times larger than the small calorie (c). The large calorie is the amount of heat needed to raise the temperature of one kilogram of water one degree celsius. The official designation for the large calorie is *kilocalorie* or *Kcal*, but for the sake of simplicity the term calorie will be used in this book to designate the large calorie. Conversion to the metric term *joule* in place of calorie is underway in the scientific world. One joule is equivalent to 4.184 calories; one *kilojoule* (kJ) equals 4.184 Kcal.

Exhibit 4.4   Nutrient Energy Storage

NUTRIENT	ENERGY IN CALORIES	
	PER GRAM	PER OUNCE
Protein	4	110
Carbohydrate	4	110
Fat	9	250

A gram of fat supplies two and one-fourth times the amount of calories as a gram of protein or carbohydrate.

A calorie, as a unit of measure, is not in itself a nutrient or something we eat. Thus, it is technically incorrect to say that a food "contains calories." It contains nutrients, whose energy value is measured in calories. But this language is commonly used and accepted because it is simpler. The same is true of "you need calories" and similar phrases.

ENERGY USE IN THE BODY

We use energy *involuntarily* to maintain our life processes and *voluntarily* to conduct our activities. Our total energy requirement is a combination of energy needed for involuntary functions and voluntary activities.

Energy for Body Processes

The amount of energy used to carry out the involuntary, internal work of the body, the functioning of the heart, liver, lungs, kidney, etc., is known as our *basal metabolic rate* (BMR). Basal metabolic rate also is defined as the amount of energy the body uses at rest. It accounts for over half of our calorie needs.

The prime regulators of BMR are the secretions of the endocrine glands, the thyroid, adrenal, and pituitary. Size, shape, weight, sex, age, rate of growth, body temperature, amount of sleep, and state of nutrition are all variables that affect BMR.

Sex differences in BMR are caused by the activity of male and female sex hormones, particularly their effect on fat deposition. Thus, a man requires 10 to 20 percent more energy per kilogram of body weight to maintain his body at rest than a woman requires. The average man requires one calorie per kilogram of body weight, 1,600–1,800 calories, to maintain his body at rest. The average woman needs 0.9 calorie per kilogram of body weight to maintain her body at rest. To determine total calorie requirements, the calorie needs for activities are added to the BMR. Because men often are more active than women, their calorie needs for activities may be greater.

Children need additional calories for growing and increasing body weight. Thus, BMR is higher in younger people than in older people and is highest during periods of rapid growth. Active males ages 15 to 22 and females ages 11 to 14 have the highest calorie requirements of all age groups. During pregnancy there is an increase in BMR as well as a need for additional energy to build new tissue for both mother and fetus (see Chapter 13). In lactation, additional energy requirements are proportional to the amount of milk produced (see Chapter 13).

AGE GROUPS	PERCENTAGE REDUCTION IN BMR CALORIE REQUIREMENTS
22–35	5
35–45	3
45–55	3
55–65	5
65–75	5
Each decade past 75	7

As we age, our BMR gradually declines, as illustrated in Exhibit 4.5, and we need less energy.

Energy for Activities

Although many variables affect involuntary energy needs, even more individual differences influence the energy expended in activities. For example, a small, relatively inactive woman might expend 1,200 BMR calories and 600 activity calories—a total of 1800 calories. A young, male athlete, on the other hand, might require 1,800 BMR calories and 2,700 activity calories—a total of 4,500 calories.

Variables affecting activity energy use include: weight (it takes more energy to move a heavy body than a light one), occupation, recreational pursuits, age (older people tend to be less active than younger people), the amount of time spent sleeping, and even personality (calm, placid people tend to use fewer calories than nervous, hyperactive types).

The brain is always active and uses about one-fifth of a person's BMR calories. So complex mental work does not affect energy use, except if we are physically active while doing it (for example, if we are tense, jittery, and wiggle a lot while we think).

The strenuousness of activities and the amount of time devoted to them are the two most important factors in determining how much energy we use. Exhibit 4.6 shows differences in the energy expended by people in various occupations and activities.

How Many Calories Do We Need?

A number of methods have been devised to help estimate calorie needs. The simplest method is to use a table showing calorie needs by age, sex, and weight such as Exhibit 4.7, remembering to adjust it to suit level of activity.

Exhibit 4.6   Calories Expended in Various Types of Activities

TYPE OF ACTIVITY	CALORIES PER HOUR
Sedentary activities, such as: Reading; writing; eating; watching television or movies; listening to the radio; sewing; playing cards; and typing, office work, and other activities done while sitting that require little or no arm movement.	80 to 100
Light activities, such as: Preparing and cooking food; doing dishes; dusting; handwashing small articles of clothing; ironing; walking slowly; personal care; office work and other activities done while standing that require some arm movement; and rapid typing and other activities done while sitting that are more strenuous.	110 to 160
Moderate activities, such as: Making beds, mopping and scrubbing; sweeping; light polishing and waxing; laundering by machine; light gardening and carpentry work; walking moderately fast; other activities done while standing that require moderate arm movement; and activities done while sitting that require more vigorous arm movement.	170 to 240
Vigorous activities, such as: Heavy scrubbing and waxing; handwashing large articles of clothing; hanging out clothes; stripping beds; walking fast; bowling; golfing; and gardening.	250 to 350
Strenuous activities, such as: Swimming; playing tennis; running; bicycling; dancing; skiing; and playing football.	350 or more

Source: Food and Your Weight. U.S. Department of Agriculture, Agricultural Research Service, Home and Garden Bulletin No. 74, Washington, D.C., 1977, p. 4.

The Recommended Dietary Allowances for calories, on which Exhibit 4.7 is based, do not allow an excess as a "margin or error," as do RDA for other nutrients. The recommendations are made at the *lowest level* consonant with good health of the average person in each age group at a light level of activity. The recommendations are based on *averages* and there are wide individual variations within each range.

A simple "rule of thumb" method for calculating energy needs, which gives reasonably accurate results for an average adult, is to take the midpoint of desirable weight range (from Exhibit 4.8) and multiply it by 18 for a man or by 16 for a woman. The answer will be the approximate number of calories used daily by a young adult of average activity. Older adults will need to adjust the figure downward.

Some people use the energy expenditure method of determining calorie needs. This involves estimating the number of hours and/or minutes spent at various levels of activity, including sleeping (as listed in

Exhibit 4.7 Daily Calorie Allowance

85
Energy Use
in the Body

WEIGHT	WOMEN	AGE IN YEARS		WEIGHT	MEN	AGE IN YEARS	
(LBS)	22	45	65	(LBS)	22	45	65
88	1,550	1,450	1,300	132	2,500	2,300	2,100
99	1,700	1,550	1,450	143	2,650	2,400	2,200
110	1,800	1,650	1,500	154	2,800	2,600	2,400
121	1,950	1,800	1,650	165	2,950	2,700	2,500
128	2,000	1,850	1,700	176	3,050	2,800	2,600
132	2,050	1,900	1,700	187	3,200	2,950	2,700
143	2,200	2,000	1,850	198	3,350	3,100	2,800
154	2,300	2,100	1,950	209	3,500	3,200	2,900
				220	3,700	3,400	3,100

Source: National Academy of Sciences, National Research Council, Food and Nutrition Board, *Recommended Dietary Allowances,* Eighth Edition. Washington, D.C., 1974, p. 29.

Exhibit 4.6), multiplying by the estimated calorie expenditure for each level, and adding up the total. Because of the difficulty of making an accurate estimate of activity level and calorie use, this method is least likely to give reasonable results. But it may help a person evaluate his energy patterns and show him how they relate to his weight.

The Energy Balance

Why should we be concerned about our calorie requirements? Simply because to maintain our weight, we need to keep energy needs in balance with energy intake. When we take in more energy than we use, our bodies squirrel away the excess in the form of fat, and we gain

Exhibit 4.8 Desirable Weights for Heights

WOMEN		MEN	
HEIGHT (IN)	WEIGHT (LB)	HEIGHT (IN)	WEIGHT (LB)
60	109± 9	64	133±11
62	115± 9	66	142±12
64	122±10	68	151±14
66	129±10	70	159±14
68	136±10	72	167±15
70	144±11	74	175±15
72	152±12	76	182±16

Source: National Academy of Sciences, National Research Council, Food and Nutrition Board, *Recommended Dietary Allowances,* Eighth Edition. Washington, D.C., 1974, p. 29.

* Weights indicated are without shoes or outer clothing.

weight. If we take in less energy than we use, we withdraw some from our stored fat, and we lose weight.

For the average person, it takes approximately 3,500 extra calories to produce a pound of stored fat; and, conversely, a 3,500 calorie deficit to use a pound of stored fat. So for each pound of weight that we want to gain or lose, we need 3,500 calories more or 3,500 calories less than we are using. As with other averages there are wide individual variations from this 3,500 calorie-per-pound rule.

Weight as a Guide. If we are adults, our weight is a fairly reliable gauge that tells us how we are balancing our energy intake and output (see Exhibit 4.9). When weight remains fairly constant, it means calorie

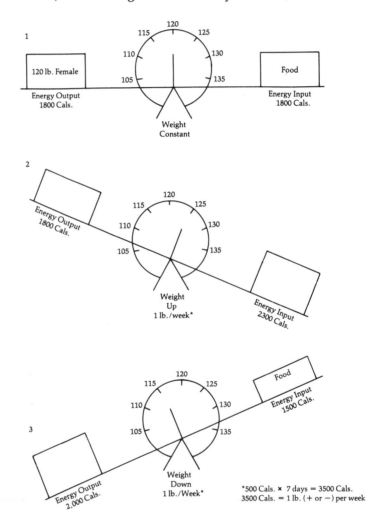

Exhibit 4.9. Your weight is a guide to how you should balance energy intake and energy output.

intake and output are in balance; when weight goes up, calories consumed are in excess of need; when weight goes down, calorie intake is less than need.

Weight is not an exact measure of energy balance, especially on a short-term basis, because of day-to-day variations in water balance—the amount of water retained in body tissues. Moreover, we may be gaining *weight,* but not *fat,* if we are exercising a lot and developing our muscles. Nor does our weight go up and down with mathematical precision as the formula might lead us to believe. Weight changes tend to be erratic, with ups, downs, and plateaus. However, the trend of our weight over time—constant, up, or down—does clearly show how we are balancing energy input and output.

Exhibit 4.9 illustrates that there are two ways to adjust our lives to change our energy balance: eating and exercising. We can eat more or exercise less to gain weight; eat less or exercise more to lose weight; or combine the two. If we need to lose weight, we will be more successful if we both eat less and exercise more.

The Food and Nutrition Board of National Research Council in the 1974 Recommended Dietary Allowances recommends that adults or children who gain excessive amounts of fat while habitually consuming the calories recommended for their age group (see Exhibit 5.6) should *increase their physical activity* rather than use fewer calories to attain a balance because:

1. We need sufficient energy for efficient utilization of protein.

2. We will not obtain enough of the essential nutrients on diets too low in energy, unless we restrict fats, sugar, and alcohol consumption more rigidly than is customary in the American diet.

3. We may be more prone to arterial disease and diabetes if we maintain a sedentary life-style.[1]

Summary

Our body's highest nutritional priority is for energy. The original source of the energy we use is the sun, and through the process of *photosynthesis,* plants ultimately build the energy-supplying nutrients: carbohydrates (sugars and starches), proteins, and fats. Our body, in turn, breaks these nutrients apart, obtaining energy to power itself. Energy not immediately used is primarily stored as fat in fat cells, termed *adipose tissue.*

The energy value of food as well as the energy expenditure of the body is measured in *calories.* In nutrition, the kilocalorie or "large calorie" is most commonly used. Proteins and carbohydrates give us 4 calories per gram (110 calories per ounce); fat, a more concentrated source

---

[1]National Academy of Sciences, National Research Council, Food and Nutrition Board, *Recommended Dietary Allowances,* Eighth Edition. Washington, D.C., 1974, p. 26.

of energy, supplies 9 calories per gram (250 calories per ounce). It takes approximately 3,500 calories to gain or lose one pound of fat.

Energy is needed both for the *involunatry* activities of maintaining basic life processes and for the *voluntary* activities of movement and exercise. The *basal metabolic rate* (BMR) refers to the amount of energy needed to maintain the involuntary activities, i.e., the energy needed by your body at rest. Basal metabolic rate is affected by a number of factors and generally declines with age. In order to maintain weight, energy intake must be kept in balance with energy needs. Eating and exercise are two ways we can change our energy balance.

THE CHALLENGE OF MAINTAINING IDEAL WEIGHT 5

Highlights

Risks, diagnosis, and causes of obesity
Factors associated with effective weight loss diets
Behavior modification approaches to dieting
Questionable weight control techniques

Probably the single most important nutritional challenge facing us in the United States today is to maintain our ideal weight throughout life. The evidence is clear that being of normal or below-average weight greatly reduces the risks of illness and death from coronary heart disease, arterial disease, high blood pressure, stroke, kidney disease, diabetes, gallbladder disease, and cirrhosis of the liver.

Overweight people often have elevated blood triglycerides and cholesterol levels and a reduced tolerance for carbohydrates. The effects of degenerative arthritis and gout are more serious when one is overweight. Respiratory problems—decreased lung volume and pulmonary hypertension—increase with excess weight. The hazards of surgery, pregnancy, and childbirth are multiplied in the obese, and heavy people, being less agile, are even more prone to accidents than people whose weight is normal.

The obese also suffer from other physical handicaps, such as increased discomfort in hot weather and fatigue, backache, and foot problems. Most people don't enjoy being fat. The picture of the happy fat person is a myth.

While most overweight people are psychologically normal, obesity can cause anxiety, social alienation, low self-esteem, mistrust, behavioral immaturity, and hypochondria. Being fat can breed more fat in a vicious cycle sometimes referred to as the *obesity syndrome.* Overeating can disrupt normal metabolism and the increased mass of fatty tissue can lead to endocrine and metabolic changes. More fat, for example, triggers greater insulin production, which increases a person's hunger and eating capacity.

Obesity also contributes to physical inactivity, which in turn leads to more fatness. And being fat leads to unhappiness and emotional problems, which in turn may lead to more fatness in the case of people who eat when they are upset or distressed.

In sum, there are many valid reasons for maintaining ideal weight: we look better, feel better about ourselves, are healthier, and are more likely to live longer. We will also save money by eating less, being healthier, and not squandering resources on costly weight control products.

Getting rid of excess weight, once we have it, is exceedingly more difficult than keeping it off in the first place. The success rate of obese people who diet and keep weight off permanently is estimated at a mere two percent or less. This is the most important reason of all for making *prevention* of overweight our goal.

OVERWEIGHT AND OBESITY

The difference between obesity and overweight is one of degree. Obesity usually means a weight 20 percent or more above ideal body weight; overweight indicates a weight 10 to 20 percent above the ideal.

Some 15 million Americans are estimated to be obese, and 30 million are estimated to be overweight. And we are getting fatter.

A mid-1970s survey of 10,000 people by the National Center for Health Statistics showed that women younger than 45 and all adult men were approximately 4 pounds heavier than their counterparts surveyed in 1960–62. Across ages, income levels, and races, a greater percentage of women than men are obese. The average U.S. male was found to be 20 to 30 pounds overweight, the average American female from 15 to 30 pounds overweight. (See Exhibit 5.1.)

Exhibit 5.1 Average Weights for Heights and Age of 10,000 Persons Surveyed in the National Health and Nutrition Examination Survey*

	AGE GROUP IN YEARS					
SEX AND HEIGHT	18–24	25–34	35–44	45–54	55–64	65–74
Men	Weight in pounds					
62 inches	130	141	143	147	143	143
63 inches	135	145	148	152	147	147
64 inches	140	150	153	156	153	151
65 inches	145	156	158	160	158	156
66 inches	150	160	163	164	163	160
67 inches	154	165	169	169	168	164
68 inches	159	170	174	173	173	169
69 inches	164	174	179	177	178	173
70 inches	168	179	184	182	183	177
71 inches	173	184	190	187	189	182
72 inches	178	189	194	191	193	186
73 inches	183	194	200	196	197	190
74 inches	188	199	205	200	203	194
Women						
57 inches	114	118	125	129	132	130
58 inches	117	121	129	133	136	134
59 inches	120	125	133	136	140	137
60 inches	123	128	137	140	143	140
61 inches	126	132	141	143	147	144
62 inches	129	136	144	147	150	147
63 inches	132	139	148	150	153	151
64 inches	135	142	152	154	157	154
65 inches	138	146	156	158	160	158
66 inches	141	150	159	161	164	161
67 inches	144	153	163	165	167	165
68 inches	147	157	167	168	171	169

Source: S. Abraham, F. W. Lowenstein, D. E. O'Connell, "Preliminary Findings of First Health and Nutrition Examination Survey, U.S. 1971–72, Antrhopometric and Clinical Findings." National Center for Health Statistics, U.S. Department of Health, Education and Welfare Publication No. (HRH) 75–1229, Rockville, MD, August, 1975.

* The averages: ". . . not presumed to indicate 'ideal' or 'desirable' weight."

Diagnosing Obesity

Obesity is not a disease—it is a symptom of an improper energy balance, typified by an excess of adipose tissue. Adipose is fat stored in the loose connective tissue distributed throughout the body.

One relatively simple and inexpensive way to diagnose obesity is to measure the thickness of a pinch of skin with a special caliper (see Exhibit 5.2). Skinfold thickness may be measured in several locations on the body, such as the upper back, abdomen, chest, arms, and legs. Often just a single measure is taken using the skin at the triceps on the upper arm. Mathematical formulas can be used to estimate body fat from skinfold measurements. But in general, when a skinfold measures above an inch in thickness, the person is considered to be overweight. In the National Center for Health Sciences survey referred to above, people were considered obese if this thickness was greater than that found in 85 percent of men or women 20 to 29 years old. This standard was based on the concept that a healthy adult should not become fatter with age.

However, as illustrated in Exhibit 5.1, adults *do* become fatter with age. Average weights of men were found to increase most rapidly until 25 to 34 years of age and eventually peak between 35 and 44 years of age for tall men and between 45 and 54 years of age for men shorter than 5'8". Average weights of women were found to increase rapidly until 35 to 44 years of age, but did not peak until 55 to 64 years of age.

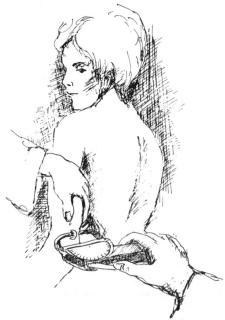

Exhibit 5.2. Measuring the thickness of a pinch of skin with a special caliper is a relatively simple way to diagnose obesity.

Causes of Obesity

To say that obesity is caused by overeating and inactivity is an oversimplification of a much more complex problem. There is no single kind of obesity and no single cause or cure.

After years of research, scientists still do not know exactly why people become obese. The causes are complex and vary with individuals. They include heredity, eating behavior, dietary patterns, lack of exercise, life-style, personality, and physiological malfunctioning that may be psychological in origin.

Scientists are able to count fat cells and measure their size. They have found that both the *number* of fat cells and the *size* of fat cells are involved in obesity. Some people are obese because their number of fat cells is much greater than average; some because they have an average number of fat cells, but the cells are excessively large, that is, overfilled with fat; and some because they have both many fat cells and extra large ones (see Exhibit 5.3).

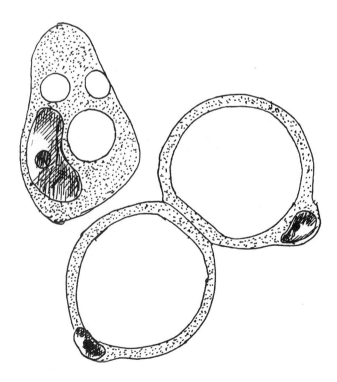

Exhibit 5.3. Both the number of fat cells and the size of fat cells are involved in obesity.

Once a fat cell is formed, it does not disappear. If weight is lost, the cells get smaller, but they are on "standby"—ready and waiting to gather up any extra fat that is available in the bloodstream.

After a person loses weight because of illness, dieting, or deprivation, his subsequent normal reaction is to eat large amounts of food. His appetite will not fall off until he has eaten enough to bring his weight back to where it was before or even sometimes a little higher. For the dieter, this means it will take a great deal of willpower, after successfully losing weight, to overcome this increased appetite and keep from regaining the lost weight. This helps to explain why people who diet and lose weight are so seldom successful in keeping their weight down.

Effect of Heredity. Studies of genetically obese rats clearly show abnormal fat cell development. These fat rats have more fat cells and also much bigger fat cells. When normally lean rats were made obese by making them overeat, the fat cell numbers were stable. The only increase was in cell size.

When genetically obese rats were overfed after being underfed and kept lean during early life, later overfeeding caused an increase in fat cell numbers. In other words, unlike normally lean rats, the underfed-overfed genetically fat rats made more fat cells after weaning. Further study showed that lean rats stopped making fat cells at 4 to 6 weeks; genetically fat rats were still making them at 18 weeks. The researchers theorized that failure to stop making fat cells may be the problem in animals that are genetically fat.[1] Some scientists theorize that a defect in genetically obese people also may be due to failure to shut down fat-cell proliferation.[2]

With people, research and statistics show that there is evidence of a genetic basis for obesity although it is difficult to know if a child *inherits* his obesity or *develops* it because of the eating habits he learns from obese parents. Statistics show that when both parents are obese, a child has an 80 percent chance of becoming obese; if one parent is obese, a 40 percent chance; and if both parents are lean, a 9 percent chance. Obese children generally go on to become obese adults.[3]

Effect of Exercise. Rats that are genetically fat get very inactive after weaning. Yet if their food is restricted, they become normally active. One study showed that genetically fat rats, given access to activity wheels early in life, didn't become inactive and didn't become obese.[4]

[1]J. Hirsch, "Cell Number and Size as a Determinant of Subsequent Obesity," in *Symposium on Childhood Obesity*, M. Winick (ed.). Interscience Publishers, Inc., New York, 1975, pp. 15–21.

[2]J. Knittle, "Basic Concepts in Control of Childhood Obesity," in *Childhood Obesity*, M. Winick (ed.). John Wiley & Sons, New York, 1975.

[3]"Will a Fat Baby Become a Fat Child?" *Nutrition Reviews*, Vol. 35, No. 6, June, 1977, pp. 138–40.

[4]J. Stern and P. Johnson, "Spontaneous Activity in the Zucker Obese Rat." *Federal Processor*, Vol. 33, 1974, p. 677.

Human studies also show definite relationships between the lack of exercise and obesity. Studies of obese teenagers have shown that they are much less active than their lean friends. Even obese infants have been found to be less active than lean babies. One study involving 4- to 5-year-old normal-weight children showed that those having obese parents expended only about half as much energy on physical activity as did the children of normal-weight parents.[5] Researchers did not know whether this was due to genetic or environmental factors, however.

For an adult who has been lean and becomes fat, an important factor appears to be activity level. In one study, the amount of walking people did during a normal day was measured. The results showed that obese women walked an average of 2 miles a day, while lean women walked 3.9 miles; obese men walked an average of 4 miles a day, while lean men walked 6 miles.[6]

Prevention of Obesity

The results of nearly every study support the conclusion that the emphasis should be placed on the prevention of obesity in childhood. Children at risk—for example, those having obese parents, those with stocky builds (*endomorphs*, who are more prone to being obese than the tall, slender *ectomorphs*), and those who show early onset of weight gains above those expected for their height—should be identified at an early age.

The calorie intake of children at risk should be reduced, particularly during times when obesity is most likely to develop—during the first year of life and during the teenage growth spurt—but not so much that normal growth is affected. These children also should be encouraged to make exercise and vigorous activity a regular part of their life-style.

Since the treatment of obesity is so rarely effective, prevention of overweight at all ages should be our goal. The formula is simple: we must balance the intake of energy foods with our body's output of energy. Putting it into effect is a challenge of major proportions for many people.

The two success factors are: (1) establishing eating patterns in which high-nutrient-density foods are emphasized and high-calorie, low-nutrient-density foods (fats, sugars, alcohol) are limited and in which all foods are eaten in moderation and (2) maintaining a life-style that regularly includes some moderate to strenuous exercise.

[5]"Obesity in the Family." *Science News*, Vol. 109, May 8, 1976, p. 297.

[6]A. Chirico and A. Stunkard, "Physical Activity and Human Obesity." *New England Journal of Medicine*, Vol. 263, 1960, pp. 935–40.

Americans are obsessed with trying to cure their real or imagined overweight problems with "quick," "easy," "no will-power" methods. We spend some $10 billion a year on fad diets, diet foods, devices, drugs, books, reducing salons and health spas, and other gimmicks (see Exhibit 5.4). Yet our fatness continues and even worsens. Why? Because none of these "wishful thinking" methods can melt away fat.

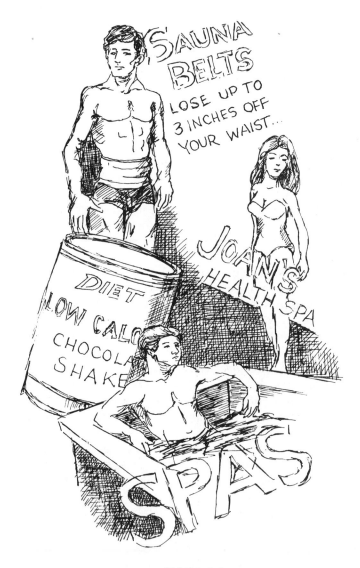

Exhibit 5.4.

To lose weight, we must apply the energy formula: eat less, exercise more. We must change eating behavior, not just temporarily, but forever, if we are going to lose weight and keep it off permanently, for obesity is controllable but not curable. Let's face it, there is no easy way to lose weight. It is difficult, often discouraging, and requires a great deal of inner strength to stay on a good weight loss program. Forever.

Weight Loss Diets

A person can lose weight on just about any diet if calories consumed are less than calories expended. But many fad-type diets are not nutritionally well balanced, may be unhealthful, and offer but a temporary solution to a permanent problem. An effective diet plan is one that will maintain a healthful level of nutrients and will teach new eating habits that can continue to be followed, with modification, after weight is lost.

A weight control diet that includes a wide variety of foods will not become monotonous and is more likely to be followed than one that severely restricts the kinds of foods that can be eaten. The diet needs to be low enough in calories so weight can be lost on it, but not so low that a person will be undernourished or hungry all the time.

An important criterion for choosing foods for a weight control diet is their calorie content. The energy value of foods depends on their composition; that is, the relative amount of fat, protein, and carbohydrate they have in proportion to the noncaloric components of water and fiber. Watery, fibrous foods such as vegetables and fruits have fewer calories per portion than such foods as fatty meats, whole milk, cheese, ice cream, nuts, etc., which have proportionately large amounts of fat, protein, sugar, and starch.

Another factor to consider in choosing foods for a diet, in addition to their energy value, is their satiety value—their ability to keep you feeling satisfied for a period of time. Fats and protein have the greatest satiety value, while carbohydrates, especially sugars, are quickly digested. Watery, fibrous foods lack satiety value. Studies show that the body is not "fooled" into feeling satisfied when the stomach is filled with fibrous, nonnutritive foods. The crisp, fibrous foods provide lots of chewing action for the dieter or nervous eater who needs constant mouth motion, but this may stimulate the appetite rather than satisfy hunger. Thus, the diet that is based on large amounts of low calorie, watery, fibrous foods may soon be discarded by the dieter.

Diets containing a reasonable balance of carbohydrates, proteins, and fats, rather than a drastic reduction of any one of these nutrients, seem to be best for most people. However, often an overweight person's diet is overly high in fat, and cutting down on this nutrient can result in the greatest calorie savings. Keeping a diet diary can help a person identify the sources of calories in his meals to determine what changes should be made.

Often, if a person's normal diet is reasonably well balanced among the food groups, the best way to achieve calorie reduction is simply to eat less of everything, to reduce serving sizes, forego second helpings, and trim away as many as possible of the high-calorie extras such as butter, margarine, gravies and sauces, salad dressing, cream, and the like. Snacks for the dieter should be selected from the Four Food Groups rather than being foods such as chips, nuts, cookies, candies, doughnuts, and soft drinks. (See Chapter 27 for more on snack selection.)

Cutting down, but not out, is a good rule to follow in planning a weight control diet. No food is so innocent that you can eat all you want, but on the other hand, no food is so bad that you cannot have some of it, at least occasionally.

For some people, the "casual diet plan" of simply cutting down on all foods does not work. They need a more structured, calorie-counting type of diet. Usually a diet of 1,200 calories for women and 1,500 to 1,800 calories for men is conducive to a healthful weight loss of 1 to 2 pounds a week. Diets below 1,000 calories are unlikely to provide all of the necessary nutrients and will leave a person constantly hungry. However, in especially difficult cases of obesity, very low-calorie diets may be used, along with vitamin and mineral supplements. Close medical supervision is recommended with such a diet.

The Four Food Groups, eaten in the minimal recommended amounts for adults, with few added extras (fats, sugars, alcohol), provide a good basic plan for the 1,200-calorie diet, as illustrated in Exhibit 5.5. The person who needs a calorically planned diet can easily fit foods into each group, as illustrated on the sample menu for a 1,200-calorie diet (Exhibit 5.6). While some people can happily follow a standard, preplanned diet, such as this one, most dieters need to make their own plan, to fit their food preferences and to learn exactly how much food they can eat for their calorie allotment.

When planning a diet, keep in mind that the first criterion should be that it is well balanced nutritionally. The person with few calories to "spend," just like the person with a limited budget, must spend his

Exhibit 5.5   A Four Food Group 1,200-Calorie Diet Pattern

	Lean Meat, Poultry, Fish, Eggs, Legumes	Nonfat Milk or Cheese	Enriched or Whole-Grain Cereals, Bread	Fruit	Vegetable	Extras
Minimum Recommended Daily	6 ounces	2 cups	3–4 servings	2	2–4	
Calorie Range	320–350	180–230	250–325	200–250		75–100

calories where they count—on the foods that give the highest nutrient return for their calorie cost. A good rule to remember is, "Count your calories by the company they keep," and choose those with many nutrient "friends."

Changing Eating Behavior

In addition to changing the kinds and amounts of foods they eat, most overweight people also need to change their eating behavior: how often they eat, how fast they eat, and what they are doing when eating. They also need to know what cues trigger their eating.

Studies have shown that obese people often are unaware of or have a totally inaccurate idea of how often they eat and how much food they eat. When queried, they proclaim that they eat very little. Yet diet

Exhibit 5.6   Sample Menu for 1,200-Calorie Diet

| | FOOD GROUP CALORIES | | | | |
	MEAT	MILK	BREAD	F & V	EXTRAS
BREAKFAST: 240 CALORIES					
½ cup Tomato juice				25	
¾ cup Cooked oatmeal, with 1 t sugar			100		15
½ cup Nonfat milk for cereal		45			
2 medium Graham crackers			55		
LUNCH: 395 CALORIES					
1 Tuna sandwich: 2 slices bread, 2 oz tuna, 2 t dressing	105		120		40
1 Carrot (sticks)				30	
½ Fresh orange				30	
¾ cup Nonfat milk		70			
DINNER: 440 CALORIES					
4 oz Baked chicken, skinned	210				
½ Baked potato with 1 t Margarine				70	30
½ cup Cooked broccoli with lemon juice				20	
¼ Cantaloupe				40	
¾ cup Nonfat milk		70			
SNACKS: 125 CALORIES					
1 cup Popped Popcorn, no fat			40		
3 Celery stalks				10	
½ Fresh orange				30	
½ cup Nonfat milk		45			
DAY'S TOTAL: 1,200 Calories	315	230	315	100 155	85

Exhibit 5.7   One Menu Can Vary by 2,000 Calories

	MENU	AMOUNTS FOR FAMILY MEMBERS			
		ADULT WEIGHT WATCHER	CHILD 6 TO 9 YEARS	BOY 15 YEARS	ADULT MALE
Breakfast	orange juice	½ cup	½ cup	½ cup	½ cup
	soft-cooked egg	1	1	1	1
	bacon slices	—	—	2	2
	whole-wheat toast	1 slice	1 slice	2 slices	2 slices
	butter or margarine	1 t	1 t	2 t	2 t
	whole milk	—	¾ cup	1 cup	—
	coffee	1 cup	—	—	1 cup
Lunch	tomato soup	—	½ cup	1 cup	1 cup
	sandwich				
	enriched bread	2 slices	2 slices	4 slices	2 slices
	boiled ham	1½ oz	1½ oz	3 oz	2 oz
	mayonnaise	2 t	2 t	3 t	2 t
	lettuce	1 leaf	1 leaf	2 leaves	1 leaf
	celery	1 stalk	1 stalk	1 stalk	1 stalk
	radishes	4	4	4	4
	dill pickle	½	½	½	½
	apple	—	—	1 medium	1 medium
	skim milk	1 cup	—	—	—
	whole milk	—	¾ cup	1 cup	1 cup
Dinner	beef roast	3 oz	2 oz	4 oz	4 oz
	rice	½ cup	½ cup	⅔ cup	⅔ cup
	spinach	¾ cup	⅓ cup	⅔ cup	⅔ cup
	lemon	¼	¼	¼	¼
	salad				
	cottage cheese	⅓ cup	⅓ cup	⅓ cup	⅓ cup
	peaches	1 half	1 half	2 halves	2 halves
	lettuce	1 leaf	1 leaf	1 leaf	1 leaf
	rolls	—	1	1	1
	butter	—	1 t	1 t	1 t
	plain cake iced	—	1″ piece	2″ piece	2″ piece
	skim milk	1 cup	—	—	—
	whole milk	—	¾ cup	1 cup	—
	coffee	—	—	—	1 cup
Snack	apple	1 medium	—	—	—
	soda crackers	—	4	4	—
	peanut butter	—	2 t	2 t	—
	cookies—3″	—	—	—	2
	nonfat milk	—	—	—	1 cup
	whole milk	—	¾ cup	1 cup	—
	coffee	1 cup	—	—	—
TOTAL CALORIES		1,219	2,039	3,229	2,571
CALORIES RECOMMENDED		1,100–1,400	2,100	3,200	2,600

Source: University of California, Cooperative Extension, *Calorie Control*, Berkely, CA, p. 10.

records usually tell a different story. They show that people who are overweight tend to: (1) eat fewer meals (often skipping breakfast, eating little or no lunch, then eating enormous amounts from dinner to bedtime); (2) eat more at each meal; and (3) eat faster.[7]

Studies also show that overweight people respond more readily to the sight, smell, and taste of food and may eat without being conscious of it.[8] Their eating may be triggered not by hunger, but by other cues—clock time, television advertising, the sight of food when walking past a bakery, etc. They may be addicted to food the way others are addicted to drugs or alcohol and abuse it in a similar way, using it as a means of coping with emotions such as depression and anger.

Thinner people have been found to be more sensitive to knowing when they are really hungry; to feel satisfied by food sooner; and to quit eating when they have had enough.

From these studies, a type of weight reduction program was developed by psychologists to help the overweight person make necessary behavior changes. Called behavior modification or behavior self-management, these systems are based on the belief that the overweight person needs to learn to exercise conscious control over his eating behavior by finding out what his eating habits are, unlearning bad habits, and developing new ones. This system, like all other forms of learning, is effective only if an individual really wants to change. The would-be dieter must be motivated and energized into action.

Two aspects of behavior modification are for the person to reprogram himself and to reprogram his environment. The usual first step is for the dieter to learn about his habits by means of a diet diary. The person keeps a detailed record of every food eaten during the day: what is eaten, how much, when, where, with whom, while doing what else, what triggered the eating, and, perhaps, what mood the person was in at the time.

The second step is for the dieter to analyze his food record carefully for the purposes of: (1) identifying the stimuli that lead to eating, (2) identifying the kinds of foods he abuses, (3) determining what habits should be changed, and (4) determining what changes can be made in the environment to reduce the number of things that make the person want to eat.

Some examples of behavior changes are that the dieter:

1. Eats only when hungry; when hungry, postpones eating for a period of time.

---

[7]J. Mayer, *Overweight, Causes, Cost, and Control.* Prentice-Hall, Inc., Englewood Cliffs, N.J., 1968, p. 94.

[8]J. Greenberg, "The Fat American." *Science News*, Vol. 113, No. 12, March 25, 1978, pp. 188–89.

2. Guards against becoming too hungry, too fatigued, too bored.

3. Learns to cope with feelings such as frustration, boredom, anger, or depression using means other than food.

4. Substitutes some other activity for eating. For example, runs in place in front of refrigerator instead of opening it!

5. Eats three regular meals in morning, midday, and evening.

6. Learns to estimate the amounts of allotted servings by weighing or measuring food.

7. Takes only the amount of food allotted and does not eat out of containers of food.

8. Consciously slows down eating by chewing slowly and setting down utensils between each mouthful, consciously savoring the aroma and flavor of each mouthful.

9. Eats in only one place in the house and not anywhere else.

10. Does nothing else while eating.

11. Keeps a food diary, writing down food and calories contained therein before eating to stop unconscious eating.

Some environmental changes which might be made include:

1. Food is kept out of sight. No serving dishes are placed on the table.

2. Tempting high-calorie foods are not bought.

3. Family members refrain from urging the dieter to eat and from providing foods the dieter is trying to avoid.

4. Family members provide support for successes (for not eating) and refrain from nagging or reminding dieter of his backsliding.

In this weight control system, a dieter is encouraged to set *behavior goals* rather than weight loss goals—the rationale being that weight loss will eventually follow after behavior leading to overeating is changed. Keeping the diet diary provides the dieter with feedback for evaluating his progress in making behavior changes. Often, just by keeping a food diary a dieter will reduce intake by an appreciable amount (see Exhibit 5.8). The dieter also is encouraged to develop a system for rewarding himself immediately and often for reaching behavior goals.

The behavior modification system is an adjunct to, not a substitute for, a reduced calorie diet and an increased exercise program. The emphasis is on unlearning habits that lead to overeating and replacing them with new habits that include eating a balanced, low-calorie diet. The system has been employed successfully both with individuals and on a group counseling basis and has been shown to be more effective than other methods of weight reduction. Many of the techniques have been adopted by well-known weight control groups such as Weight Watchers.

Diet Diary

Eating Behavior Diary

Time of Day	Length of Eating Time	Place	Physical Position	Eat Alone	Eat With Whom	Other Activity While Eating	Mood*	Hunger**	Food	Amount	Calories

*Mood: 8–Very Happy; 7–Happy; 6–"So–So"; 5–Bored; 4–Tense; 3–Unhappy; 2–Depressed; 1–Very depressed.
**Hunger: 6–Very Hungry; 5–Hungry; 4–Not Hungry; 3–Partly Full; 2–Full; 1–Stuffed.

Source: University of California. Cooperative Extension, Anaheim, CA.

Exhibit 5.8. Weight Control Diary

Questionable Weight Control Techniques

While the American overweight problem is real, our obsession with curing it may in large part be due to the overeager propaganda about reducing diets and their cure. Time and again someone "discovers" a new weight control method that will miraculously melt away fat. It becomes a fad with many followers. But the end results are always the same: disillusionment and loss of dollars for dieters, not permanent weight loss, and enrichment of the authors, producers, and promoters of the weight control book, product, or service.

All such diets and products are promoted as "easy," "foolproof," and "quick." The need for unpleasant things such as exercise, willpower, and changing diets and eating behavior is ignored or downplayed. The fad program or product may be presented as a "new scientific discovery," and promotions often include testimonials and success stories of people who have lost weight or amazing "before and after" photographs. (A good rule to remember here is that if something seems too good to be true, it probably isn't.)

Fad Diets. These come and go with predictable regularity. While each is promoted as offering something new or unique, many are simply a new form of an old, well-worn idea. Thus, there are the many varieties of the low-carbohydrate diet, which are, in effect, high-protein, high-fat diets, including the "Calories Don't Count Diet," the "Mayo Diet" (no connection with the Mayo Clinic), the "Doctor's Quick Weight Loss Diet," and the "Adkins Diet." These diets create an illusionary quick weight loss because they cause water to be lost from the tissues. But this is not fat tissue loss, and weight is quickly regained when the diet is discontinued. Some of these diets are so seriously lacking in carbohydrates that they upset the metabolism and can lead to serious health problems if followed for any length of time.

Other popular types of diets include the low-protein diets, the high-roughage (fiber) diets, the vegetarian diets (which generally are low in fat and high in carbohydrate and fiber), the special formula diets, the "eat all you want" diets, the one- or two-food emphasis diets (skim milk-bananas and prune-egg diets), and the diets that have a "secret ingredient that burns fat" (such as the grapefruit diet and the lecithin, kelp, vinegar, and vitamin B_6 diet). These diets are based on false premises. For example, there is no ingredient in food that will burn fat or prevent us from using the energy in other foods.

Fad diets often are unhealthful because they are not nutritionally balanced. They may be costly if special products must be purchased. They are tiresome, and fortunately (since the hazards increase with length of use) most people soon give them up. Most importantly, because these diets do not help an overweight person learn new eating habits, any weight lost is gained back quickly when the dieter goes back to his old way of eating. If this is the case, why bother? Why go through

Exhibit 5.9   Questions to Ask Yourself About a Weight Control Diet

105
Losing Weight
the
American
Way

Is it nutritionally balanced?
Is it really low in calories?
Does it provide a variety of well-liked foods?
How much does it cost?
Will it teach me new eating habits?
Can I continue to follow it, with modifications, after I lose
    weight?

the agony of a weight loss regime, only to return swiftly to the point
you started from? Again, to be effective weight loss diets must be *well
balanced,* and the dieter must change *behavior* as well as *food intake* (see
Exhibit 5.9).

Nonprescription Diet Aids. Sold over the counter in many drug-
stores, these include hundreds of brands that can be grouped into a few
basic types: the bulk-producing aids, such as *methylcellulose,* which are
supposed to make the dieter feel full without eating so much; diuretic
pills, which increase water excretion from the body—an illusionary
weight loss; reducing candy (nothing but sweets that may be fortified
with extra nutrients), which is supposed to take your appetite away if
you eat it before a meal; and fad pills, which may be a combination of
some of the above substances. With all these substances, the dieter will
not lose weight unless he actually eats less. They don't melt away fat.

Prescription Drugs or Injections. These include appetite depressants,
such as amphetamines; metabolic stimulators, such as thyroid hormone;
more potent diuretics; and *human chorionic gonadotropin* (HCG). The
drugs can be addictive, have serious side effects, and be ineffective in
reducing appetite or weight, and they can lose effectiveness in time. For
these reasons their use as an aid to losing weight is not considered wise
except in special circumstances.

Wearable Products. All items in this category, such as sauna shorts,
belts, body wraps, and the like, are ineffective, and some are dangerous.

Exercise Machines. These are of two types: those with which the
dieter does something, i.e., rows, bicycles, walks a treadmill, lifts
weights, and those which do something to the dieter, for example, vibrators or rollers that knead fatty tissue. As indicated earlier, exercise—
by the dieter—does have its place in a weight loss program. However,
the value of exercise in losing weight is in using extra calories, not in
spot-reducing, even when certain muscles are emphasized. Studies
show that spot-reducing of fatty deposits does not take place through
any form of exercise. Machines, such as vibrators and the like that involve a passive dieter, are ineffective in causing weight loss and often
are promoted by false and misleading claims. Massage and rollers will

not remove fat deposits under the skin, for example. These disappear only after a person loses weight through active exercise and diet.

Medical-Surgical Weight Control Techniques. Surgery usually is used only as a last resort for treating grossly obese people who have not responded to traditional methods of weight control and whose obesity is considered life-threatening.

Bypass surgery is still considered to be experimental. The most widely performed procedure is the *jejunoileal bypass,* where a portion of the intestine is removed. As a result, an individual's ability to absorb nutrients is reduced drastically. Appetite and food intake also tend to be reduced. This process is considered dangerous, with the potential for death resulting from the surgery itself or from postoperative complications such as liver failure, pulmonary embolism, and cardiac failure. Serious side effects that may develop after recovery include liver disease, intractable diarrhea, and nutritional deficiency.

Gastric bypass surgery is beginning to be recognized as preferable to the jejunoileal bypass because it limits food intake but allows a more normal digestion and absorption and fewer complications are observed.

Surgical removal of adipose tissue and some skin has also been done as a form of cosmetic surgery. Although this has the immediate effect of improving the obese person's appearance, it does not cure the person's eating and weight-gain problems.

Jaw-wiring so that a person cannot chew and must limit food intake to liquids has been tried as a way to bring about weight loss. This, too, is a temporary measure with no assurance that the dieter will eat prudently in order to stay slim when the wires are removed.

Fasting and Semistarvation. Total abstinence from food and semistarvation are two other methods that have been experimented with for treating hard-core obesity. Usually patients are hospitalized and closely monitored for metabolic changes that could be life-threatening.

Short-term fasting generally causes no serious metabolic disturbances, but prolonged fasting can have serious repercussions. Even though the loss of body fat exceeds the loss of structural protein, the loss of muscle and organ tissue is the most serious result of fasting.

During the late 1970s a semistarvation diet, usually known as the *liquid protein diet*, was widely promoted. This diet called for the elimination of food for one or more months. In place of food, dieters were given a 300-calorie formula—the liquid protein (sometimes called *predigested* because it had been broken down into amino acids). The liquid protein, often hydrolyzed collagen, an incomplete protein derived from animal bones and connective tissue, contained added minerals and vitamins.

The purpose of using the formula was to bring about rapid loss of body weight without the severe loss of tissue protein that results from total fasting. For this reason it was labeled the "protein-sparing, modi-fied-fast, diet."

After numerous deaths occurred among women who had been fol-lowing this diet, the liquid protein product and diets were declared un-safe by the Food and Drug Administration and warning labeling was required.[9]

This diet, and other total fasting and semistarvation diets, alter body chemistry and can, for example, cause ketosis, loss of electrolytes such as potassium, and increased blood uric acid levels. Such changes may trigger disorders in susceptible individuals, such as gout or kidney, liver, cardiac, vascular, or metabolic disease, or may even lead to death. Unpleasant side effects include weakness and fainting, increased sus-ceptibility to infectious and noninfectious diseases, nausea, dehydra-tion, hair loss, dry skin, bad breath, constipation, and fatigue. Patients who survive the diets and lose weight face the problem of keeping off the lost weight, which means they will need a new set of eating habits. And as with so many other methods of weight control, these eating habits are not learned during fasting.

There's No Easy Way to Lose Weight

After reviewing all of the methods that have been promoted and tried, we have to conclude that there are no shortcuts to weight reduc-tion and weight control that are safe and permanent. People who are overweight must get over the idea that someone can do something for them (the "doctor put me on a diet" syndrome) and realize that losing weight is a do-it-yourself effort. The only way a person can achieve last-ing weight reduction is by cutting down on the total number of calories consumed and increasing the amount used. Maintaining thinness takes a lifetime commitment and constant monitoring to keep energy con-sumption in balance with energy output. This is most Americans' num-ber one nutrition challenge!

Summary

A large percentage of Americans are overweight, and the many physical and psychological consequences of obesity make this a major nutritional problem. Causes of obesity are complex and vary with indi-viduals. Research on fat cell development indicates that the relative number as well as the size of fat cells may vary from one individual to another. Obese children often become obese adults, and it is difficult to separate an inherited from a learned tendency toward being overweight. Two success factors in prevention of obesity are establishing good eating patterns and maintaining a life-style that includes at least moderate ex-ercise.

[9]"Liquid Protein: A Deadly Diet." *Science News,* Vol. 114, No. 5, July 29, 1978, p. 70.

An effective diet plan must contain a healthful level of nutrients, teach good eating habits, include a wide variety of foods, provide satiety value, and be at a reasonable reduced-calorie level. Behavior modification or behavior self-management systems can help individuals reprogram their eating responses and their environment in order to control overeating. An increased exercise program should also be a part of weight management.

A wide variety of questionable weight loss techniques are available, most causing a greater loss of money than weight. Many cause an illusionary quick weight loss of water, some are dangerous, and most do not result in a long-term weight loss.

UNDERWEIGHT 6

Highlights

Benefits and hazards of being underweight
Causes and treatment of underweight
Anorexia and anorexia nervosa

Underweight is the opposite of overweight. It results when energy intake does not fully meet energy requirements. While an overweight person is always considered to be malnourished (*mal* meaning poorly or badly), this is not necessarily true for those who are underweight.

BENEFITS AND HAZARDS OF BEING UNDERWEIGHT

Being slightly underweight can be an advantage to the health of mature adults and provide the benefit of increased life expentancy. But frequently an underweight person is malnourished because the food intake is insufficient to provide all needed nutrients. The underweight person may have a physical ailment, for example, an intestinal malfunction that interferes with digestion and absorption and that causes a deficiency of all nutrients including calories. On the other hand, people who are very active, tense, and nervous may not be malnourished because their diet is sufficient except for calories. Irregular eating habits and insufficient rest may contribute to an underweight problem.

Children and young adults who are seriously underweight (more than 7 to 10 percent below their recommended weight) are more likely than adults to incur health problems from being underweight. Their self-image may suffer, too, if they are teased about being "skinny."

Fat deposits serve as padding for organs and nerve plexes and provide a reserve supply of energy to draw on in times of stress. Very thin children chill easily. They may suffer from physical fatigue more readily and be more susceptible to the effects of infections than normal-weight children.

In cases of severe underweight, for example, from starvation, there is depression, anemia, loss of muscle tissue, edema due to lack of plasma, and reduced ability to resist infectious diseases such as tuberculosis.

An excessive concern with slimness and weight loss, exhibited by some Americans, particularly teenage girls and young women, and the resulting use of fad diets and semistarvation can lead to nutritional inadequacy and detrimental effects on health. Especially serious are the effects of dieting prior to or during pregnancy. A girl or woman who is underweight at the beginning of pregnancy and fails to gain weight at a sufficient rate has an increased likelihood of delivering a premature baby. (See Chapter 13 for more information on diet during pregnancy.)

"Thin-fat" people, who constantly starve themselves in order to be abnormally thin, make both a physical and emotional sacrifice to maintain this unnatural condition. They are likely to be chronically fatigued, listless, irritable, depressed, dissatisfied, and suffering from chronic malnutrition because of their abnormal preoccupation with weight.

Psychological and physiological factors can affect appetite and result in severe undernutrition. *Anorexia* refers to the loss of a desire to eat and is seen as a prominent symptom of many illnesses and other physical and emotional disorders. Diseases of the gastrointestinal tract, liver, heart and circulatory systems, kidney, lungs, adrenal glands, and thyroid all may cause this disorder. In infants and children, almost any acute illness causes anorexia, and such chronic diseases as leukemia and arthritis often are associated with this problem.

Serious psychological problems can lead to a condition known as *anorexia nervosa.* This is a self-imposed state of starvation, which may become life-threatening. Seen primarily in girls and young women, often from higher income groups, the condition seems to have become more common in recent years.

In anorexia nervosa, psychological disturbances result in an abnormal desire to lose weight. Excessive concern about personal appearance may lead to pathological fear of overeating or becoming fat. The result is a profound loss of weight in the absence of other signs of illness. Denial of fatigue, overzealous exercising, and hyperalert, hyperactive behavior accompany many bizarre eating habits such as alternating starvation and an uncontrollable urge to eat. Enormous eating binges may be followed by self-induced vomiting and fasting. Enemas, laxatives, and diuretics also may be used excessively. People having anorexia nervosa may appear to be indifferent to changes in temperature, for example, to be blue with cold and deny feeling cold.

Anorexia nervosa patients may gradually develop severe signs of malnutrition, multiple vitamin deficiencies, and changes in body metabolism to the extent that death may be the outcome. Psychiatric as well as medical treatment and hospitalization generally are required, and results often are far from satisfactory.

TREATING UNDERWEIGHT

In general, the way to overcome an underweight problem is to do the opposite of what you would do to overcome an overweight problem: increase the intake of energy foods and/or decrease the output of energy through activities. To gain a pound a week, a person needs to take in about 500 more calories than he uses every day. (Remember the formula: it takes about 3,500 extra calories to form a pound of fat.)

The goal is not a rapid weight gain, but rather a gradual building of fat deposits. If the objective is to build muscles, then these muscles need to be exercised.

To provide more calories, a diet needs to include more food and more liberal amounts of fat, protein, and carbohydrate, preferably in combination with other nutrients. Using large amounts of low-nutrient density foods just as a way of adding calories is not recommended. The added calories should have nutrient "friends."

Some high-nutrient, high-calorie choices might be: nuts; peanut butter; sunflower seeds; dried beans and peas; dried fruit; whole milk; milk fortified with additional nonfat milk solids; milk shakes and malts; ice cream; whole milk cheese; crackers with cheese, peanut butter, or butter/margarine; meats containing fat; bologna, hot dogs, and other sausage; and vegetables with sauces, salad dressing, or dips (see Exhibit 6.1).

An underweight person probably will have to force himself to eat in excess of his appetite. Usually frequent, small meals are tolerated better than large meals, and the individual may need to eat by the clock instead of when his appetite tells him to eat.

The calories need to be increased gradually since a sudden excess of food eaten by a person who has been eating very little may lead to vomiting, intestinal disturbances, and even shock.

The person who is anorexic to the point of refusing food may need to be force-fed intravenously or by means of a nasal tube to be kept

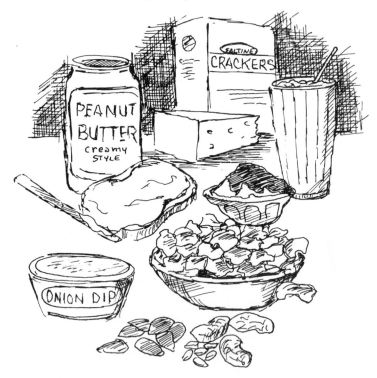

Exhibit 6.1. To gain weight, eat snack foods that are high in both nutrients and calories.

alive. Such drastic measures are generally stopgap and temporary, unless the patient is unconscious for a long period of time, and are discontinued when the cause of the patient's inability to eat is overcome.

Although underweight problems are rare in comparison to problems of overweight and obesity, they can be serious and need to be ameliorated as soon as possible.

Summary

Slightly underweight adults may be at an advantage healthwise, with lower stress on body organs contributing to a longer life expectancy. However, severe underweight, especially in children and young adults, can be hazardous. The underweight person may have a physical ailment, psychological problems, or simply a life-style that does not lend itself to obtaining sufficient calories.

Loss of the desire to eat is termed *anorexia* and is associated with acute illness. Serious psychological disturbances may lead to *anorexia nervosa*, a self-imposed starvation state.

The goal in treatment of underweight is a gradual weight gain by increasing energy-containing foods and/or decreasing activity. High-calorie food choices should also have a high nutrient density and should be introduced gradually.

Part III

THE NUTRIENTS AND THE FOODS THAT SUPPLY THEM

CARBOHYDRATES AND FIBER 7

Highlights

Trends and theories of carbohydrate consumption

Forms of carbohydrate

Food sources and bodily functions

Digestion, absorption, and metabolism

Role of enzymes and processes of anabolism and catabolism

Insulin's role in diabetes and hypoglycemia

Types, effects, and sources of fiber

Supermarket Nutrition: Choosing foods in the bread and cereal group and choosing sugars and sweeteners

Carbohydrates, the major constituents of grains, legumes, and potatoes, are the world's least expensive source of calories. In some cultures carbohydrates may supply 80 percent or more of calories consumed, compared to the United States where they supply an average of 40 to 50 percent of calories.

Which is better for us, the higher carbohydrate diet or the lower one? Scientists today cannot answer that question: they do not know exactly what level is most conducive to health, for it appears that people can exist healthfully on a wide range of carbohydrate intake.

Popular, fad weight-control diets based on low-carbohydrate intake (Chapter 5) and the recommendation to count carbohydrates rather than calories have given many people the false impression that carbohydrates are basically bad for us and should be avoided. More recently, this anticarbohydrate philosophy has been counteracted by the antifat proponents, who recommend reducing fat and protein intake and increasing carbohydrate intake as a way to reduce the risk of coronary heart disease and cancer.

Is it any wonder that consumers are confused when they hear two such diametrically opposed dietary recommendations? The wise will reject extremes and adhere to the path of moderation, realizing that carbohydrate is an essential nutrient that is low in cost and readily available.

What Are Carbohydrates?

Carbohydrates derive their name from the fact that they are made up of carbon, hydrogen, and oxygen with the proportion of hydrogen to oxygen being the same as that found in water, that is, two parts hydrogen to one part oxygen. In essence, carbohydrates are hydrated carbons.

While all carbohydrates are made up of these three elements, they vary greatly in complexity and in the way the elements are linked together. All carbohydrates can be broken down into simple sugars, which is the form in which they are used in the body. Simple sugars are *monosaccharides* (one sugar), *glucose, fructose,* and *galactose.* All have the same chemical formula, that is, 6 atoms of carbon, 12 atoms of hydrogen, and 6 atoms of oxygen ($C_6H_{12}O_6$), but each is structured differently. When two simple sugars are hooked together they form a *disaccharide:* glucose and fructose form *sucrose,* ordinary table sugar; glucose and galactose form *lactose,* milk sugar; and glucose and glucose form *maltose* when starch ferments or is digested.

When many sugars are linked together, in either straight or branched chains, the substance is called a *polysaccharide,* and it can be very complex. Starch, a carbohydrate formed by plants, is a polysaccharide that has over 300 simple sugars hooked together. It is composed of the straight-chain carbohydrate, *amylose* (20 percent) and the branched

118

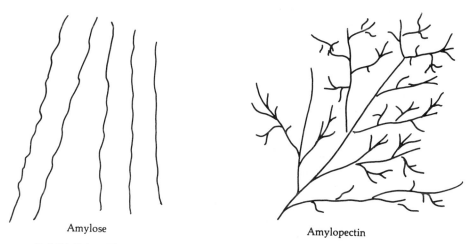

Amylose   Amylopectin

Exhibit 7.1.   The two most common constituents of starches are the straight-chain *amylose* and the branched-chain *amylopectin*.

chain, *amylopectin* (80 percent)—(see Exhibit 7.1). When starch is broken down, it forms an intermediary polysaccharide called *dextrin*. Dextrin in turn breaks down into maltose, and finally to glucose.

Glycogen is a very complex polysaccharide formed by animals and is broken down into glucose. Fibers are another type of polysaccharide but differ from starch and glycogen in that humans cannot digest them.

You can see from Exhibit 7.2 that the differences between the digestible carbohydrates are that the monosaccharides and disaccharides are sweet tasting and soluble in water, while the polysaccharides do not taste sweet and are not soluble in water. When starch is cooked in water, the starch granules *take up* water and swell. In this form, starch is more readily digested.

Exhibit 7.2   Forms of Carbohydrate in Human Diet

CLASS	TYPE	DIGESTED BY HUMANS?	SWEET TASTE?	WATER SOLUBLE?
Monosaccharides	Glucose, fructose, galactose	yes	yes	yes
Disaccharides	Sucrose, lactose, maltose	yes	yes	yes
Polysaccharides				
Plant Sources	Dextrins, starch	yes	no	no
Cell contents	Gums, mucilages	no	no	yes
	Algal polysaccharides	no	no	no
Cell walls	Pectins	no	no	yes
	Hemicellulose	no	no	no
	Cellulose	no	no	no
	Lignin (not a carbohydrate)	no	no	no
Animal Sources	Glycogen	yes	no	no

Sources of Carbohydrates

Plants are the world's original source of carbohydrates. They form glucose in the process of photosynthesis and from glucose manufacture other carbohydrates, such as fructose, sucrose, maltose, starch, dextrins, and fibers (see Exhibit 7.3). Animals, using plant carbohydrates as food, produce glycogen and lactose or convert complex carbohydrates to such simple sugars as glucose and galactose.

Starch is stored by plants as an energy source and is found in seeds such as wheat, rice, oats, corn, peas, and beans; in tubers (underground stems) such as potatoes; and in roots such as yams, sweet potatoes, and cassava.

Sucrose is found principally in sugar cane, sugar beets, and maple syrup; lactose is found in milk; fructose in fruits. In some instances starch changes to sugar, as when fruit ripens. In other instances sugar may change to starch, for example, in sweet corn after it is picked or in potatoes stored at too cold a temperature.

Functions of Carbohydrates

As indicated earlier, the chief function of carbohydrate in the body is to supply energy (see Exhibit 7.4). There has been no specific Recommended Dietary Allowance (RDA) for carbohydrate because it can be

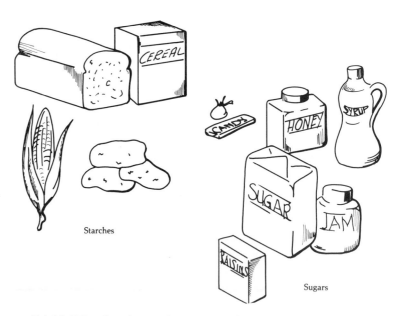

Starches

Sugars

Exhibit 7.3. Starches and sugars are the two main forms of carbohydrates.

Exhibit 7.4   Functions of Carbohydrates

121
Carbohydrates
in our Diets

Supply Energy—
  Essential for Brain
  Spare Protein
Help Make Nonessential Amino Acids
Prevent Dehydration

made in the body from some amino acids and from the glycerol of fats. However, if we receive an insufficient amount of preformed carbohydrate, we are unable to metabolize fats completely, and ketosis can result (see Metabolism of Fats in Chapter 8). It has been found that a minimum of 50 to 200 grams or 15 percent of total calories of digestible carbohydrate per day is sufficient to offset the undesirable effects of ketosis.

A diet that is low in carbohydrates, because it causes a loss of water from tissues, can result in an excessive loss of the minerals, especially sodium and potassium, in the urine and can also lead to involuntary dehydration.

Carbohydrates aid in the manufacture of certain nonessential amino acids when they are in short supply. They also are said to have a "protein sparing" effect. This means that when carbohydrates are plentiful in the diet we will use them as a source of energy instead of protein, thereby making the protein available for building and repairing body tissue. It is much more efficient and less costly to use carbohydrates for energy than to use protein. Carbohydrates and proteins combine to form several compounds that have important functions in the body, for example, serving as lubricants for joints and as the component of nails, bone, cartilage, and skin.

Carbohydrates are also an essential source of energy for the central nervous system. Approximately one-fifth of the energy requirement of our basal metabolic rate (Chapter 5) is for brain function, and glucose only, not fat, is required. Recent studies with laboratory animals showed that after a meal rich in carbohydrates there is an increase in the rate at which the brain synthesizes *serotonin*. Serotonin is one of six compounds, called *neurotransmitters*, known to be present in the neurons of mammals that, when released, transmit signals across nerve synapses to other neurons within the brain or muscle cells or secretory cells outside the brain. Researchers theorize that this increased secretion of serotonin after rats eat a high-carbohydrate meal modifies brain function.[1] However, whether the high-serotonin levels will improve the learning ability of a rat is not known, nor is it known if these data are applicable to humans.

[1] J. Fernstrom and R. Wurtman, "Nutrition and the Brain." *Scientific American*, Vol. 230, February, 1974, pp. 84-91.

Diets that are low in carbohydrates are necessarily high in protein and fat and appear to produce high levels of cholesterol and fat in the blood (*hyperlipidemia*), which are believed to be related to coronary heart disease (see Chapter 19). Low-carbohydrate diets also promote the retention of uric acid, which may lead to the development of gout in susceptible individuals. Most population groups with a low incidence of coronary heart disease consume diets having 65 to 85 percent of total energy as carbohydrates from whole grains and potatoes. Current thinking, however, does not attribute the low rate of coronary heart disease in these people to the presence of large amounts of carbohydrates, per se, but rather to the absence of large amounts of fat.

An opposite viewpoint regarding carbohydrate intake has been taken by some researchers who asserted that people should restrict carbohydrates rather than increase them in order to control hyperlipidemia. However, this theory is not considered to be based on good evidence. The strongest evidence available to date shows that low-carbohydrate diets are more likely to cause elevated levels of cholesterol and fatty acids in the blood.[2]

Statistical studies of populations show a good correlation between the amount of sugar consumed and death from coronary heart disease.[3] A cause and effect relationship between sugar itself and heart disease has yet to be proven, however. From the evidence currently available, it is not possible to separate the effects of sugar intake from the effects of increased energy intake and obesity as causes of coronary heart disease.

However, there is general agreement among nutrition scientists that Americans would be healthier if they ate less sugar and more of the complex carbohydrates instead. This was one of the recommendations included in the Dietary Goals for the United States (Chapter 18). The Dietary Goals recommendation was based on:[4]

(1) The theories (discussed above) that a diet high in complex carbohydrates may reduce the risk of heart disease and that a diet high in refined sugar may contribute to heart disease.

(2) The fact that foods having complex carbohydrates are likely to carry more of the other important nutrients, particularly vitamins and minerals, plus fiber, while the refined sugars have little nutritional value other than their energy value.

(3) The recent finding that a complex carbohydrate diet is likely to be helpful to diabetics in reducing the threat of atherosclerosis and hyperlipidemia.

[2]W. Connor and S. Connor, "Sucrose and Carbohydrate," in Nutrition Reviews' *Present Knowledge of Nutrition*, 4th edition. The Nutrition Foundation, Inc., New York and Washington, D.C., 1976, pp. 33-41.

[3]*Ibid.*

[4]"Dietary Goals for the United States." Report of the U.S. Senate Select Committee on Nutrition and Human Needs in *Nutrition Today*, Vol. 12, No. 5, September-October, 1977, p. 22.

(4) The fact that sugars are more likely to cause tooth decay than complex carbohydrates.

The digestion, absorption, and metabolism of the major nutrients, fats, carbohydrates, and protein are all interrelated. In some respects the processes are similar and in other respects they are different. In this chapter we will examine the processes for carbohydrates; fats and proteins will be discussed in Chapters 8 and 9.

DIGESTION, ABSORPTION, AND METABOLISM OF CARBOHYDRATES

Three processes take place in our bodies to convert the food we eat into usable forms and either make it part of our tissues or "burn" it for energy. These processes are digestion, absorption, and metabolism (see Exhibit 7.5).

The first step, digestion, is a mechanical and chemical process whereby food is broken down into component parts that our bodies can absorb. In the second step, absorption and transport, these component parts of food are moved from the digestive tract to the sites in the body where they are to be used. In the third step, metabolism, which takes place inside of the cells, the food elements are converted into substances the body needs or are broken down to supply energy.

Digestion and Absorption of Carbohydrates

About 97 to 98 percent of the carbohydrate in the American diet is digested and absorbed. The undigested portion consists of the various types of fiber.

During digestion, long chains of complex carbohydrates must be broken down in a series of steps to smaller and smaller units and finally into simple monosaccharides that can be absorbed in the intestine. The breakdown process is called *hydrolysis* since it is literally a splitting of the bond by the addition of water. Monosaccharides in our foods do not need to be broken down to be absorbed.

The digestion of carbohydrate begins in the mouth when food is chewed and mixed with saliva (see Exhibit 7.6). The saliva contains the first starch-digesting enzyme, *salivary amylase* (also called *ptyalin*), which converts some of the cooked starches into dextrins and other shorter chain sugars (oligosaccharides). This action is not extensive, since the food does not remain in the mouth very long. However, salivary amylase continues to work on digesting starch while the food moves into the stomach until the acidity level of the stomach contents inactivates it.

Digestion: Food is broken down into parts.

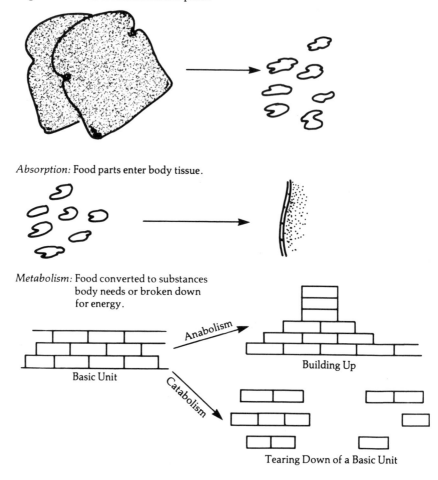

Absorption: Food parts enter body tissue.

Metabolism: Food converted to substances body needs or broken down for energy.

Anabolism

Building Up

Basic Unit

Catabolism

Tearing Down of a Basic Unit

Exhibit 7.5.

Most of the digestive action on starch takes place in the intestinal tract. Here the pancreatic enzyme, amylase, works effectively in a slightly alkaline environment to convert starch to dextrins, then to other complex sugars, and finally to the disaccharide maltose. Three more enzymes are present in the walls of the intestines: *sucrase,* which breaks down sucrose to glucose and fructose; *maltase,* which splits maltose into two molecules of glucose; and *lactase,* which splits lactose into glucose and galactose (see Exhibit 7.7).

These three monosaccharides, glucose, fructose, and galactose, are almost completely absorbed in the small intestine. Small amounts of these single sugars also may be absorbed in the stomach. The sugars enter the bloodstream and are carried to the liver by the portal vein. In

Exhibit 7.6 Digestion of Carbohydrates

125

Digestion,
Absorption,
and
Metabolism
of
Carbohydrates

ORGAN	SOURCE OF SECRETION	ENZYME OR DIGESTING AGENT	SUBSTRATE	PRODUCT
Mouth	Salivary glands	Salivary amylase	Starch (cooked) Dextrin Glycogen	Oligosaccharides Dextrins and some maltose
Stomach	Gastric glands	Hydrochloric acid	Sucrose Starch	Glucose Fructose Oligosaccharides
Intestinal Tract	Pancreas	Pancreatic amylase	Starch Oligosaccharides Dextrins	Maltose Glucose
	Mucosal cells of villi (cells lining the intestine)	Sucrase Maltase Lactase	Sucrose Maltose Lactose	Glucose, fructose Glucose Glucose, Galactose

the liver, most of the galactose and fructose are converted to glucose. The liver then converts some glucose to glycogen or fatty acids and dispatches some glucose to other tissues as needed.

Glycogen is the storage form of carbohydrate in our bodies, while glucose is the active form. Glycogen is stored in relatively small amounts in the muscles and the liver and can be used for energy during exercise. Glucose is the normal sugar circulating in the blood, available for instant

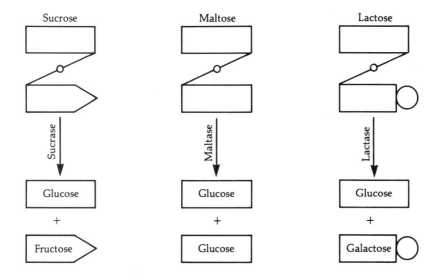

Exhibit 7.7 Digestion of disaccharides to monosaccharides.

conversion to energy in the cells. The total amount of glucose in the blood is relatively small: only about 6 grams, or less than one-fourth of an ounce. In fasting, the amount varies between 70 and 100 milligrams per 100 milliliters of blood. After we eat a high-carbohydrate meal, our blood glucose rises to approximately 120 to 130 milligrams per 100 milliliters but will return to the normal fasting level, under normal conditions, in one to one and one-half hours.

The maintenance of normal blood glucose levels, regulated by the liver, is very important and is controlled by hormones secreted by the pancreas, thyroid, adrenal, and pituitary glands. The most important blood-glucose-controlling hormone is *insulin,* which is produced by the pancreas. It is the only hormone known to lower blood glucose levels. Insulin triggers the action of the liver to produce glucose from stored glycogen, if the blood sugar level falls, and to remove glucose from the blood if the level goes too high. If insulin is lacking, the process does not function well and *hyperglycemia,* high-blood sugar, may result. This is what happens in people who have diabetes. The opposite condition, low blood sugar, is known as *hypoglycemia* and may take place if there's too much insulin or if the liver or pancreas is malfunctioning. This may affect the central nervous system in varying degrees from dizziness to unconsciousness. (See Chapter 19 for more information about diabetes and hypoglycemia.)

Metabolism of Glucose

The metabolism of nutrients may take one of two pathways, as illustrated in Exhibit 7.5: (1) anabolic pathways, or anabolism, in which molecules are built up and energy is consumed; and (2) catabolic pathways, or catabolism, in which molecules are broken down or degraded and energy is released. Both processes are necessary and take place concurrently in the body.

In anabolic pathways, glucose may be converted to glycogen by the liver or muscles for storage as a quick energy reserve, or to fat by the liver or *adipose* (fat) tissue. Glucose also combines with proteins to form essential body compounds and may be used to form certain nonessential amino acids. The steps in these processes are very complex and are controlled by various hormones.

In catabolic pathways, glucose is oxidized to release energy. This process also is highly complex and takes place, not as one explosive reaction, but rather as a series of stages and steps in which many intermediate compounds are formed.

In the cells, the oxidation of glucose takes place in one of two general ways, depending on how much oxygen is available. Normally the necessary amount of oxygen is present, and glucose is first broken down into a three-carbon substance called *pyruvic acid* and two molecules of a high-energy compound called *ATP, adenosine triphosphate* (see Exhibit

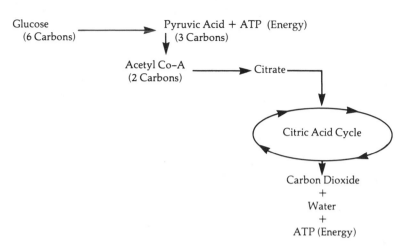

127
Digestion,
Absorption
and
Metabolism
of
Carbohydrates

Exhibit 7.8.   A simplified version of how glucose is metabolized when sufficient energy is present.

7.8). ATP is the most energy-rich of several high-energy phosphate compounds found in the body and is the most important substance formed when glucose is broken down.   By releasing phosphorus, ATP supplies energy in almost every place in the body where energy is needed, for example, in muscles. When ATP releases energy it becomes *ADP, adenosine diphosphate.* This action is reversible so that ADP can become ATP when energy-rich phosphate is available.

After pyruvic acid and ATP are formed from glucose, the pyruvic acid is further broken down: first to a two-carbon substance called *Acetyl Co-A* (Co-A stands for coenzyme A), then to citrate. The citrate goes into a major cycle called the *citric acid cycle,* the *Krebs cycle,* or the *tricarboxylic cycle,* in which many intermediate compounds are formed, and the end result is carbon dioxide and water. The total process, from pyruvic acid to carbon dioxide and water releases 36 ATP molecules, illustrating its high-energy potential.

Enzymes and coenzymes are required throughout the breakdown process. Enzymes bring about—*catalyze*—chemical reactions without themselves being changed; coenzymes are compounds needed for the functioning of enzymes. Vitamins, especially pantothenic acid, thiamin, niacin, and riboflavin, and minerals, such as iron, copper, and magnesium, are an essential part of the coenzymes necessary to catalyze these reactions.

The carbon dioxide produced when glucose is oxidized is removed from the cells by the blood and carried to the lungs where it is expelled when we exhale. Some of the water also is removed by this route as well as through perspiration and kidney action. Some of the hydrogen produced in the oxidation of glucose, plus the coenzymes that catalyze the reaction, enter another cycle called the *electron transport cycle.* In this cycle more energy is released in the form of ATP, and the coenzymes are regenerated so they can be used again in the metabolism of glucose.

Sometimes oxygen is not available in sufficient amounts for the complete oxidation of glucose, for example, during prolonged or strenuous exercise when muscle oxygen supplies are depleted. When this *anaerobic* (no oxygen) situation exists, glucose is broken down to form *lactic acid*, instead of pyruvic acid, along with two molecules of ATP. When lactic acid accumulates in muscles, we feel the well-known cramping symptoms of muscular fatigue. Some of this lactic acid may be further oxidized to carbon dioxide and water, but most of it is resynthesized into glycogen to reestablish muscle glycogen stores.

As mentioned earlier, metabolism of the major nutrients is interrelated. Thus, glucose metabolism cannot be considered separately from fat and protein metabolism. These two substances are potential sources of glucose. Conversely, glucose can be converted to fatty acids, glycerol, and certain amino acids. So at a number of points in the metabolic pathways there are crossroads where the metabolism of fats, proteins, and glucose interact, and in some cases one nutrient may substitute for another. Minerals and vitamins also are involved. Thus we see the interdependence of all the nutrients and the importance of having a balance of them available in the body at all times.

FIBER: THE UNDIGESTABLE CARBOHYDRATES

While we speak of fiber as if it is a single entity, the term actually refers to a number of complex substances derived from plants, most of which are part of the carbohydrate family. Fibers are not classed as nutrients because humans do not digest them to any great extent. However, we know that fibers are a necessary element in our diets, performing important functions, such as their "scrub brush" action in the teeth and intestines.

Scientists have found some evidence that there may be a relationship between the amount of fiber in the diet and several diseases of the digestive system, particularly diverticular disease and cancer of the colon. However, much of this information is still hypothetical, and more research is needed.

Even though the need for fiber, or "roughage," in the diet to help prevent constipation has been known for generations, in the mid-1970s fiber was rediscovered and touted widely as the new miracle food that would cure or prevent just about everything from cancer to heart disease. Unfortunately, the fiber fad is one of many examples of how a little research evidence is blown up all out of proportion to known facts by authors, manufacturers, and sellers who are profit oriented.

Nutrition researchers in general believe that many Americans today may not be getting enough fiber because our diets are so high in fat, sugar, and refined cereals and so low in fruits, vegetables, and whole grains. But because scientists have found some evidence that too much fiber can have harmful effects, they are saying, "Go slow in changing your diet. Don't overdo the fiber." That old adage that applies to so many elements in our diets, "moderation in all things," also applies to fiber.

What is Fiber?

Plant constituents resistant to digestion by secretions of the human gastrointestinal tract make up the compounds known collectively as *fiber*. While they are not broken down by the digestive juices of humans, some fibers may be absorbed to some extent, however, because they are partially digested by intestinal bacteria.

The different types of fiber include:

1. Those found in the cell walls of plants (*cellulose, hemicellulose, pectins, and lignin.*)

2. Non-cell-wall fibers, including *plant gums (gum arabic, agar, and mucilages).*

All of these substances are classed as carbohydrates except lignin. Pectins, gums, and mucilages are water soluble. Cellulose, hemicellulose, and pectin are partially digested by intestinal bacteria. In this process methane gas, carbon dioxide, hydrogen, ammonia, and other substances are produced which contribute to *flatulence*, intestinal "gas." Lignin, on the other hand, impairs bacterial digestion of fibers.

Sources of Fiber

Since the interest in fiber is relatively recent, and analytical methods for obtaining data on fiber content are complicated and expensive, data on the fiber content of foods are limited and inadequate. In food composition tables, fiber in foods is usually listed as *crude fiber*, which is defined as the insoluble material remaining after severe acid and base hydrolysis (boiling the food with solutions of sulfuric acid and sodium hydroxide). *Dietary fiber* is not the same, since the acid-base solvents dissolve some fiber elements, including most or all of the hemicelluloses and pectin, and often part of the lignin and cellulose as well. For this reason the crude fiber of the tables probably represents only one-fourth to one-half of the true dietary fiber present in foods. Exhibit 7.9 shows a comparison of the crude fiber in some common foods.

Whole grains, wheat bran in particular, are high in hemicellulose and cellulose. Other foods high in hemicellulose include carrots, corn-germ meal, beet pulp, and cabbage. Leafy vegetables, cauliflower, celery, peas, beans, peaches, apples, pears, melons, and berries also are good sources of hemicellulose. Whole fruits and vegetables, especially

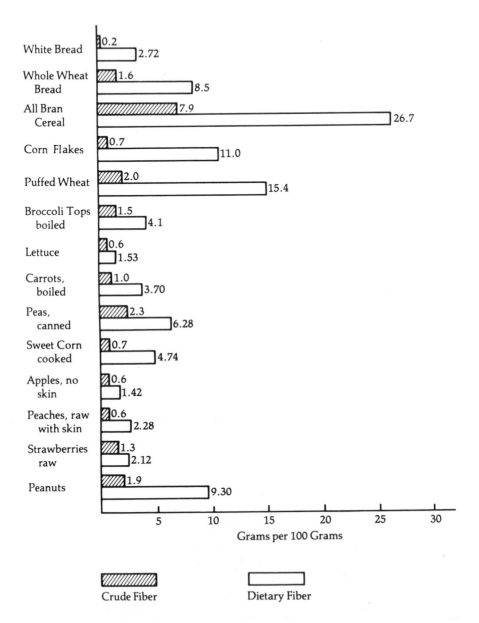

White Bread — 0.2 / 2.72
Whole Wheat Bread — 1.6 / 8.5
All Bran Cereal — 7.9 / 26.7
Corn Flakes — 0.7 / 11.0
Puffed Wheat — 2.0 / 15.4
Broccoli Tops boiled — 1.5 / 4.1
Lettuce — 0.6 / 1.53
Carrots, boiled — 1.0 / 3.70
Peas, canned — 2.3 / 6.28
Sweet Corn cooked — 0.7 / 4.74
Apples, no skin — 0.6 / 1.42
Peaches, raw with skin — 0.6 / 2.28
Strawberries raw — 1.3 / 2.12
Peanuts — 1.9 / 9.30

Grams per 100 Grams

Crude Fiber   Dietary Fiber

Exhibit 7.9.   Comparison of crude fiber and dietary fiber in certain foods. (*Source:* "Dietary Fiber." Scientific Status Summary by Institute of Food Technologists Expert Panel on Food Safety and Nutrition, Jan. 1979).

unpeeled ones, are considerably higher in fiber than juices, since most of the fiber remains behind in the pulp when juices are made. Fruits and their juices, such as citrus, apples, and others, are high in pectin, which is often used because of its thickening ability in making jellies and jams.

Effects of Fiber

Because of the variable characteristics of the different types of fiber, their effect on the body must be considered individually. Such generalizations as all fibers prevent constipation, all fibers reduce cholesterol, and so forth are inaccurate (see Exhibit 7.10).

The water-binding capacity of fibers is one of the main reasons why fibers help prevent constipation. By binding water, fibers increase stool bulk and make it soft so it moves through the intestine quickly and without increased pressure. A low-fiber diet results in small, hard, compact, infrequent stools.

Exhibit 7.10   Functions of Fibers

✓ Bind Water

? Lower Blood Cholesterol
    (certain fibers)

? Bind Toxic Substances
    (certain fibers)

But not all fibers bind water. Hemicellulose is the most able to bind water and is the one most useful in preventing constipation. Cellulose is somewhat effective in binding water. On the other hand, residues high in lignin are constipating.

Hard stools are believed to aggravate the colon by making the colon muscle work harder, thereby thickening the colon wall. This leads to temporary obstructions and small outpouchings, or hernias, known as *diverticula*. Inflammation of these protrusions is called *diverticular disease* or *diverticulitis*.

Formerly it was thought that diverticulitis was caused by small, hard pieces of food lodged in the colon causing inflammation, and the condition was usually treated with a bland, low-residue diet. Now most gastroenterologists believe that the low-residue diet aggravates, rather than helps, this problem. So they are recommending that patients suffering from diverticular disease and irritable colon be treated with a high-fiber diet.

The effect of fiber on blood cholesterol varies with the kind of fiber. Pectin, lignin, caragean, metamucil, and foods such as rolled oats, legumes, and locust bean reduce cholesterol levels. Wheat bran and cellulose have no effect or raise cholesterol slightly. Gum arabic and agar elevate cholesterol. The fact that certain fibers do have a lowering effect on blood cholesterol has led to the theory that a high-fiber diet might help to prevent coronary heart disease. However, sound evidence is lacking at this time to support this idea.[5]

Too much pectin may cause vitamin B$_{12}$ depletion, according to a recent study, and this could lead to pernicious anemia.[6] For people who consume animal foods and get plenty of vitamin B$_{12}$ this is not a problem. But it could be a problem for strict vegetarians who eat no animal foods and who ingest much pectin and no B$_{12}$ in their fruit, vegetable, and cereal diets.

Certain fibers may bind toxic substances chemically in the intestines and prevent or impair their absorption and their potential carcinogenicity. For this and other reasons (discussed in Chapter 19), fiber is thought by some experts to be a preventive factor in cancer of the colon.[7] Proof of this theory is currently lacking, however.

Fiber reduces the absorption efficiency of the small intestine by reducing the time it takes for food to move through the intestine. Thus, only about 92 percent of the calories in high-fiber foods are available, compared to 97 percent in refined foods. Because fiber reduces absorption efficiency, because it requires more chewing and may cause a person to eat less, and because bulky fibrous foods tend to be low in calories, high-fiber diets may be helpful in a weight control diet, even though they have very low satiety value.

Phytic acid is associated with non-cell-wall fibers and binds essential minerals such as zinc, iron, calcium, magnesium, manganese, and copper, thereby reducing their availability. Phytic acid is found in whole grains and bran. Other fiber components also decrease absorption of certain minerals such as calcium, zinc, and iron. Thus, overuse of high-fiber diets could deplete the body of these essential minerals.

Ways to Add Fibrous Foods to the Diet

Because the American diet tends to be low in fiber, many experts believe that moderately increasing the amount of fiber in our diet would be helpful. Here are some suggestions:

1. Eat 100-percent whole wheat bread or wheat or cracked wheat bread.

[5]"Dietary Fiber." A Scientific Status Summary by the Institute of Food Technologists Expert Panel on Food Safety and Nutrition and the Committee on Public Information, January, 1979.

[6]S. Oace, R. Cullen, "Vitamin B$_{12}$ Loss May Result from High Fiber Diet." Report presented at American Institute of Nutrition, Chicago, Ill., April 5, 1977.

[7]"Dietary Fiber." A Scientific Status Summary by the Institute of Food Technologists Expert Panel on Food Safety and Nutrition and the Committee on Public Information, January, 1979.

2. Add bran to quick breads, muffins, pancakes, and homemade granola.

3. Eat bran cereal, for example, 100 percent bran, branflakes (40 percent bran), or raisin bran, or add a spoonful of bran to your favorite cereal.

4. Eat whole-grain cooked cereals such as oatmeal, cracked wheat, wheat berries, rolled wheat flakes.

5. Use brown rice, cracked wheat, or bulgur wheat in place of white rice.

6. Eat sunflower seeds, pumpkin seeds, peanuts, soynuts, and other nuts.

7. Add millet or barley to soups; use these grains for casseroles in place of pasta or white rice.

8. Use dried peas and beans for soup, casseroles, and dips.

9. Eat whole fruits, including peels where practical, instead of drinking juice.

SUPERMARKET NUTRITION: CHOOSING FOODS IN THE BREAD AND CEREAL GROUP

"Starchy foods" is the name often given to foods in the bread and cereal group, and with good reason. Of the solid material in breads and cereals, 70 to 80 percent is starch, while 7.5 to 19 percent is protein. Because of their relatively low cost, the foods in this group, which include not only breads and breakfast cereals, but also rice, cornmeal, hominy, crackers, rolls, tortillas, biscuits, macaroni, spaghetti, noodles, cakes, and cookies (Exhibit 7.11), are an inexpensive source of energy and protein.

Other nutrients provided in important amounts by this food group include iron, niacin, and thiamin and lesser amounts of riboflavin and trace minerals. Whole grains and bran are a good source of fiber. Nutrients not found in this group are vitamins C and A, and calcium is present in only small amounts. The protein is not complete because it is limited in the amino acids lysine and tryptophan. When milk solids, soy solids, or peanut flour are added to products made from cereals, the protein value improves appreciably since these foods supply lysine and tryptophan as well as additional amounts of calcium.

Because of the common notion that "starchy foods" are high in calories, dieters frequently omit or cut way back on foods in this group. This can be unwise as it can result in deficiencies of iron, niacin, and thiamin as well as carbohydrate. The problems encountered with low-carbohydrate diets are discussed in Chapter 5. What dieters need to remember is that basic breads and cereals are not excessively high in calories until we begin adding the extras—butter, margarine, jelly, honey, syrup, cream, etc.— that usually accompany these foods.

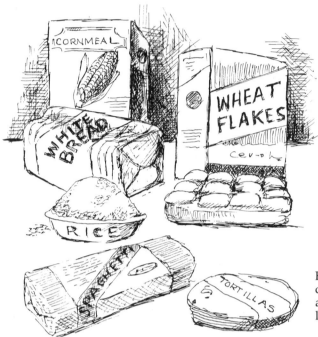

Exhibit 7.11. Foods in the bread and cereal group are high in starch and are an inexpensive source of energy and less complete protein.

Cereal Grains

The most popular cereal grains used for consumption as cereals and as ingredients in breads and pasta are wheat, rice, oats, corn, rye, and barley. All are the seeds of grasses, and each type of seed has a structure similar to that of the wheat grain pictured in Exhibit 7.12.

The outer layer, or *hull*, is coarse and inedible; under it is the fibrous *bran* layer, which is rich in iron and B vitamins. Next is the *aleurone* layer, which contains protein, niacin, and iron. Then comes the white starchy *endosperm*, which also contains some protein, but less of the other nutrients. The innermost part is the *germ*, which is the source of

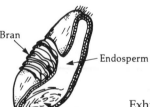

Bran

Endosperm

Germ

Exhibit 7.12. Whole wheat contains the bran, germ, and endosperm, while refined wheat contains only the endosperm.

134

growth for the new plant and which contains protein and fat and is rich in iron, other trace minerals, and B vitamins.

A *whole-grain cereal* is one that contains all of these parts except the outer hull. When a grain is fully milled, or refined, all parts are removed except the least nutritious endosperm portion.

After nutrition researchers discovered the importance of the B vitamins found in whole-grain cereals, widespread efforts were made to educate consumers and to encourage consumption of whole-grain instead of refined cereals. When these efforts were unproductive, the federal government launched the cereal enrichment program to put back into refined cereals the iron, thiamin, niacin, and riboflavin that were removed in the milling process. Legal standards were established for enrichment: for each pound of bread or cereal are added 1.1 to 1.8 mg thiamin, 0.7 to 1.6 mg riboflavin, 10 to 15 mg niacin, and 8.0 to 12.5 mg iron. The additions of calcium and vitamin D are optional. The effect of enrichment is shown in Exhibit 7.13, which compares three types of wheat flour.

Exhibit 7.13   Comparison of Selected Nutrients in Three Different Types of Wheat Flour

NUTRIENT MG PER LB	UNENRICHED	FLOUR ENRICHED	WHOLE GRAIN
Iron	3.6	13.0	15.0
Niacin	4.1	16.0	19.7
Thiamin	0.28	2.00	2.49
Riboflavin	0.21	1.20	0.54
Calcium	73.0	73.0	186.0

Source: B. Watt, A. Merrill, *Composition of Foods, Raw, Processed, Prepared.* Agriculture Handbook No. 8. U.S. Department of Agriculture, Washington, D.C., 1965, p. 66.

While enrichment of refined cereals and breads does provide major nutrients, it does not add trace minerals such as zinc, magnesium, and copper, and other B vitamins such as pyridoxine (B_6), which are found in the bran and germ but not in the endosperm. Whole grains also are higher in protein and fiber than milled cereals.

On the other hand, refined cereals do not contain the phytates, or phytic acid, found in the whole grains, which bind minerals such as iron, calcium, and zinc and make them less available to the body (see Chapter 23). They also stay fresh longer. The germ portion of whole wheat cereals, which contains fat, does not keep well, since the fat tends to turn rancid in storage.

During World War II cereal enrichment was mandated by the federal government. However, this requirement was later changed from a mandatory one to a voluntary one. Now the requirement of enrichment is by state law, and not every state requires it. So it is up to the consumers in states where enrichment is not required to read labels on all packages of bread, cereal, flour, rice, pasta, and the like to determine if the product to be purchased has been enriched. The nutrition-labeling law requires that when a product is enriched, the full nutrition statement must be included on the label.

Bread Products

A form of bread is found in many cultures of the world because man can easily grow and store grains and by simple processes turn them into bread. The raised or leavened bread, in which fermentation of yeast or bacteria produces carbon dioxide gas, is thought to have been discovered by accident, perhaps in ancient Egypt.

Wheat flour is preferable for making leavened bread because it contains the protein *gluten*, which becomes elastic when mixed with water and is developed through stirring and kneading. The elasticity of gluten allows the bread dough to rise. Baking coagulates or sets the gluten so the dough holds its shape. Whole wheat flour tends to yield a more compact, solid bread because the proportion of gluten is lower than in white flour.

Other grains do not contain any or much gluten, which is why they do not make good bread. Recently, however, two gums, *xanthan gum* and *hydroxypropyl methylcellulose*, have been found to serve as effective substitutes for gluten in doughs and batters made from rice flour, starch, soybean protein, and other nongluten flours. These nongluten breads are useful to persons who are allergic to gluten.

The most popular bread in the United States is *white enriched bread*, made from white enriched flour. Nutrient value is improved if nonfat milk solids are added (at the rate of two to six percent per pound).

Whole wheat bread must be made from 100 percent whole wheat flour, but this is less commonly sold than *wheat bread* or *cracked wheat bread*, both of which are made from a mixture of white flour and whole wheat flour. Label reading will tell which flour is present in the greatest amount, since ingredients must be listed in order of predominance by weight. Breads made from half white and half whole wheat flour have a lighter texture than those made with whole wheat because of the higher gluten content.

Many other specialty breads that have other ingredients are available:

Rye bread—which generally has a considerable amount of wheat flour added to provide gluten

Potato bread—which contains at least 3 parts potato flour to 100 parts white flour

Raisin bread—which will have about 50 pounds of raisins per 100 pounds of flour

Sourdough bread—in which fermentation by a special culture of acid-producing bacteria provides a sour flavor

Butter bread—having a small amount of butter

Egg bread—having a small amount of egg

Gluten bread—which is made from gluten flour so it has a somewhat higher proportion of protein and lower proportion of starch, but not enough of an increase in protein to warrant paying a high price for it.

The nutritional value of all of these speciality breads is roughly comparable to breads in which enriched flour has been used throughout. Differences in cost can be great, however, and what you get for your extra money is a flavor change, not more nutrition.

To compare the costs of different breads, determine the cost per ounce by dividing the total cost of a loaf by the number of ounces it contains. Because many of the popular white breads have been puffed up with air through extra rising, they look like a large one-and-one-half pound loaf of bread, but actually weigh only one pound. Known as *balloon loaves*, they may be more costly than ordinary loaves. Each slice will be lower in calories and other nutrients, because it weighs less (see Exhibit 7.14).

Popular with dieters has been the so-called *diet bread*, which usually has added protein and ingredients such as honey, seeds, and vegetable flours. The price is high, and many people think they are getting more nutrition for fewer calories. However, the nutritional difference, compared with enriched white or wheat bread, is small, and the calories

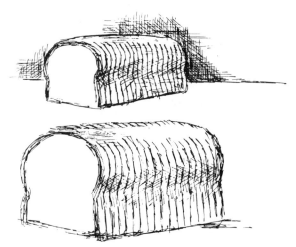

Exhibit 7.14. A balloon loaf, which has more air, gives more slices per pound, but each slice has less food value (and fewer calories).

per pound are the same. The reason for fewer calories per slice is that the bread is sliced much more thinly. Eating half a piece of lower priced bread can save money as well as calories—with less surface area on which to spread butter, jelly, etc.

Recently, a lower calorie, *high-fiber* bread has been promoted, which contains cellulose, usually produced from wood pulp. The cellulose reduces the proportion of other ingredients and thereby does reduce the number of calories per slice by about one-third. The wood pulp is a purified plant fiber that is accepted for use by the Food and Drug Administration. It is listed on the label as "powdered cellulose" (fiber). Some scientists have expressed concern about its safety.

Most white wheat flour has been *bleached* before being made into bread or packaged as flour. Bleaching is a natural oxidation process that takes place as flour is stored and improves its baking qualities. To speed up the bleaching process, oxidizing agents are added. Bleaching does not destroy nutritional value or add residues to the flour. However, many people have the idea that unbleached flour is more nutritious, and, as a result, manufacturers have provided it to meet this demand.

Another unfounded notion people have is that flour that is *stone ground* as opposed to that which is ground by steel grinders is more nutritious. As a result, they are willing to pay a higher price for stone ground flour and bread made with this flour and get less nutrition for their money.

Homemade bread costs about half as much per ounce as purchased bread and can be improved nutritionally by adding such ingredients as nonfat dry milk, whole wheat flour, wheat germ, soy flour, oatmeal, or bran. Because it is usually more compact than purchased bread, each slice is heavier and provides more nutrients and calories. However, you may not save money by making your own bread if it tastes so good that everyone eats twice as much!

Other fancier bakery products—biscuits, rolls, cakes, pies—all have more calories, as illustrated in Exhibits 7.15 and 7.16, and cost more than plain bread. Two ingredients, sugar and fat, add the calories.

Exhibit 7.15   Calories and Costs for Various Bread Products

BREAD	CALORIES	COST
1 slice bread or toast	65	2¢
1 flour tortilla	80	4¢
1 toaster tart	210	10¢
1 doughnut	150	12-15¢
1 sweet roll	275	25¢
1 biscuit or muffin	120	5¢
1 english muffin	140	10¢
1½ t butter or margarine adds—	50	2-3¢
1 T jelly or honey adds—	50-65	3¢

1975 estimated prices

Exhibit 7.16   Calories of Selected Desserts

DESSERTS	CALORIES
1 piece apple pie	345
1 baked apple	105
1 piece chocolate cake, iced	445
1 piece angelfood cake, uniced	110

With these products the ready-made, either fresh or frozen, are notably higher priced than those made from mixes or "from scratch." In many instances the mixes are the cheapest of all. From a calorie standpoint, the best cakes to eat are angel food or sponge cake, because these are made without fat or oil.

Breakfast Cereals

Breakfast cereals provide a quick, easy, and nutritious answer to the daily question, "What should I have for breakfast?" A breakfast consisting of fruit, a bowl of cereal with milk, toast, and some milk to drink will supply one-fourth to one-third of your day's nutritional requirements—if you choose your cereal wisely.

Nutritional values and costs of cereals vary greatly. With the vast array of different types of cereals found on supermarket shelves today, and there are probably more of them than of any other single product, no wonder many consumers are confused about which products are the best nutritional choice (Exhibit 7.17).

You can choose cereals that are:

To be cooked and served hot—long cooking, quick cooking, and instant

Ready to eat and served cold—flaked, puffed, granular, and shredded

Made of corn, wheat, oats, rice, barley—alone or in combination

Made of whole grains or refined grains

Made of just cereal or of cereal plus ingredients such as sugar, oil, dry milk, soy protein, dry fruit, malt, salt, and other flavorings as well as preservatives

Enriched with minerals and vitamins such as the iron and B vitamins lost in milling

Superenriched (fortified) with minerals and vitamins to the point that you are getting what amounts to a vitamin pill with your cereal

Packaged in varied sizes from "large economy" to convenient, small, individual servings.

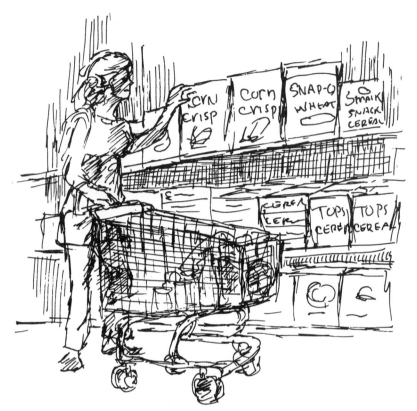

Exhibit 7.17.   Today's shopper faces a confusing variety of break-fast cereals from which to choose.

Guidelines for choosing cereals to obtain the best nutritional value include the ingredient list, the nutrition label, and the price.

Ingredient List. Remembering that ingredients must be listed on labels in order of predominance by weight, look for nutritious ingredients such as whole grains, bran, wheat germ, soy protein, and nonfat milk to see if they are near the top of the list. Then look for sugar in all its varied forms: sucrose, white sugar, brown sugar, corn syrup solids, molasses, honey, etc. The product may contain more sugar than cereal if sugar is listed first, or if several types of sugar are used even though a form of grain is listed first. Some sugared cereals contain 30 to 50 percent sugar. The sugar adds calories and dilutes the quantity of the cereal and the level of cereal nutrients.

Also look for vegetable oil; it adds many calories. Some cereals, particularly the "natural" or "granola" types have as much as 20 percent oil (hardly a natural ingredient of cereal!). Oil is used because it makes the products crunchy. This type of cereal often contains no enrichment nutrients, since it is made from whole grains, particularly oats, but it may have less iron and B vitamins than ordinary enriched cereals.

When ready-to-eat cereals are manufactured, processing includes hot, dry heat to make them crisp. This type of heat destroys nutrients such as protein and B vitamins to a much greater extent than the moist heat in which hot cereals are cooked. So cooked cereals may have a higher quality protein than ready-to-eat cereals if the ready-to-eat ones have no other added protein sources such as soy or dry milk.

Most of the ready-to-eat cereals are enriched, and some are fortified with minerals and vitamins to a much higher level than called for under enrichment regulations. Most whole-grain cooked cereals are not enriched, but those made of refined cereals, such as cream of wheat and cream of rice, and those made for infants are enriched.

Nutrition Information Statement. This provides a basis for comparing the nutrients in one brand of cereal with those in another, as seen in the comparison of two typical cereals in Exhibit 7.18. This label also tells you the size of a one-ounce serving, which may range from ¼ cup to 2½ cups depending on the density of the product, and how many calories you will get in that one-ounce serving. You can compare your serving size to this and determine the caloric content. For example, if you eat one cup of a cereal that weighs one ounce per ¼ cup and has 140 calories per ounce, multiply 140 times 4 to obtain 560, the total calories in your one-cup serving.

Price. By dividing the price of the package by the number of servings it contains (as listed on the nutrition statement), you can determine the price per serving. In general, the cereals that offer the most food value for the least cost are the whole grain cereals that are to be cooked, such as rolled oats (with the instant costing twice as much as the quick cooking), toasted or cracked or rolled wheat, and unrefined corn meal. These are 100 percent cereal and have all of the minerals, vitamins, and fiber of the natural cereal.

Also a good choice are the to-be-cooked, milled, enriched cereals such as farina, cream of rice, and degermed corn meal. Of the ready-to-eat cereals, the best values are those with the least amount of sugar and fat, those made with whole grains, and those having nutritious added ingredients such as soy protein, dry milk, wheat germ, bran, or raisins. Cereals which provide the least nutrition for the money are those sold in small individual serving-size packages (you pay for the extra packaging materials) and the heavily sugared cereals, particularly those advertised on TV.

Rice

Rice is the mainstay of life for about one billion of the world's people. Many varieties are eaten, but the most common in the United States are the short grain, which when cooked is tender, moist, and sticky; the medium grain, which is similar to short grain when cooked;

Product Information from
GENERAL FOODS CONSUMER CENTER

A nutritious Post breakfast consists of juice or fruit cereal with milk, toast with butter or margarine, and milk to drink.

NUTRITION INFORMATION PER SERVING

SERVING SIZE: 1 OZ.
(ABOUT ¼ CUP)
SERVINGS PER PACKAGE: 24

	CEREAL ALONE	WITH 1-2 CUP VITAMIN D FORTIFIED WHOLE MILK
CALORIES	100	180
PROTEIN	3 G.	7 G.
CARBOHYDRATE	23 G.	29 G.
FAT	0	4 G.

PERCENTAGES OF U.S. RECOMMENDED DAILY ALLOWANCES (U.S. RDA)

PROTEIN	4%	10%
VITAMIN A	25%	30%
VITAMIN C	*	*
THIAMINE	25%	30%
RIBOFLAVIN	25%	35%
NIACIN	25%	25%
CALCIUM	*	15%
IRON	4%	4%
VITAMIN D	10%	25%
VITAMIN B₆	25%	30%
FOLIC ACID	25%	25%
VITAMIN B₁₂	25%	30%
PHOSPHORUS	6%	15%

*CONTAINS LESS THAN 2% OF THE U.S. RDA OF THESE NUTRIENTS.

INGREDIENTS: WHEAT, MALTED BARLEY, SALT, YEAST, AND FORTIFIED WITH THE FOLLOWING NUTRIENTS: NIACIN, VITAMIN A PALMITATE, VITAMIN B₆, RIBOFLAVIN (VITAMIN B₂), THIAMINE MONONITRATE (VITAMIN B₁), VITAMIN D₂, FOLIC ACID AND VITAMIN B₁₂.

680 G.

GENERAL FOODS CORPORATION WHITE PLAINS, N.Y. 10625, U.S.A.

GENERAL FOODS

CARBOHYDRATE INFORMATION

	1 OZ CEREAL	WITH ½ CUP WHOLE MILK
STARCH AND RELATED CARBOHYDRATES	20 G.	20 G.
MALTOSE AND OTHER SUGARS*	3 G.	9 G.
TOTAL CARBOHYDRATES	23 G.	29 G.

*All sugar in GRAPE-NUTS is derived naturally from whole wheat and malted barley flour.

This package is sold by weight not by volume. Some settling of content may have occurred during shipping and handling.

CONSUMER: PLEASE INCLUDE THE DATE PORTION OF THIS GRAPE-NUTS® BOX TOP ON ALL CONSUMER CORRESPONDENCE.

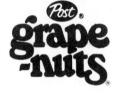

Exhibit 7.18. By using both the ingredient list and the nutrition statement, the consumer can determine the relative nutritional value and sugar content of a prepared cereal.

142

and the long grain, which is firm and dry when cooked and has kernels that do not cling together.

Commonly, rice is milled to remove bran and husk so only the white portion of the kernel remains. The kernels are washed, cleaned, graded, polished, and finally enriched by coating them with thiamin, niacin, and iron, using 1 part of each to each 200 parts of rice. Riboflavin is not added in this process as it causes the rice to turn yellow. This type of white rice *should not be washed before using*. Washing will remove the added nutrients and is unnecessary since the rice has been thoroughly washed before packaging.[8] Cook this white rice in just the amount of water it will absorb. If extra water is used and poured off, nutrients dissolved in the excess water will be lost. Usually package directions tell you just how much water to use.

Another form of rice is "converted rice," which is parboiled in a special steam pressure process before milling. This process forces much of the B vitamin content into the grain so these nutrients are not lost when the bran is removed. Enrichment of converted rice increases the nutrient level above that of regular white enriched rice.

Brown rice is the whole grain with only the outer husk and a small amount of the bran removed. It has a nutlike flavor, is slightly chewy, and requires more water and longer cooking than regular white rice. Normally brown rice is not enriched since it contains the natural nutrients of the whole grain.

All of these types of rice—white, converted, and brown—can be purchased in convenient, precooked forms, dehydrated, canned, and frozen, with and without added flavoring and other ingredients. The quick cooking or instant rice is first cooked, then dehydrated, then enriched. Cooking time is thereby reduced to just 5 to 10 minutes. The precooked, dehydrated rice has an expanded volume but a lighter weight than raw rice. It requires less water and yields a much smaller amount of rice per measure of dry rice. Therefore, package sizes are deceiving, and it is necessary to compare prices between raw and precooked rice on the basis of cost per cooked serving. A nutrition label will list the number of servings of cooked rice per package. Divide this number into the cost of the package to get cost per serving, but be sure to compare equal serving sizes. You will probably find that plain precooked rice costs about twice as much as plain raw rice, and the seasoned varieties may be three or more times more costly than plain raw rice.

Canned and frozen varieties of rice may be even more convenient since they need only to be reheated. However, they cost even more than

---

[8] An exception to the rule about not washing rice is the unenriched rice imported from the Orient, which is coated with talc. Since talc contains asbestos, which can be harmful if ingested, the talc-coated rice should be thoroughly washed before being cooked. Rice sold in bulk form generally is not enriched and should be washed before cooking.

precooked rice because you're paying for water as well as convenience when you buy them. Since all the different types of rice offer comparable amounts of nutrients if all are enriched, you receive less nutrition for your money when you choose the more convenient, time-saving forms.

Macaroni or Pasta

Spaghetti, vermicelli, pastina, egg noodles, macaroni, of all shapes and sizes, are known collectively as macaroni or pasta. All are made from the same basic dough made from semolina, which is composed of duram wheat. To make semolina, duram wheat is cleaned, the bran and germ are removed, and the wheat is ground to a granular consistency. Its natural yellow color imparts a desirable yellow to pasta products.

Some states require enrichment of pasta products with thiamin, niacin, riboflavin, and iron, and if this is done, such products will be labeled "enriched" and have a nutrition statement of the label. Macaroni enriched with fortified protein is now marketed in some areas. In addition to the enrichment with B vitamins and iron, this type of pasta is fortified with protein, usually in the form of soy flour and/or nonfat dry milk solids. The ingredient list will show what has been added. Noodles are often labeled "egg noodles," but the amount of egg added is not enough to make a significant difference in the protein content.

Since all of these products, except for the protein-enriched varieties, are comparable in nutritional value, the best buys are those that sell for the lowest price per pound. Noodles are generally about twice as costly as spaghetti or macaroni. When you buy ready-cooked pasta, for example, canned spaghetti or frozen macaroni and cheese, you pay for the water used in cooking it.

When buying the prepared pasta mixes for main dishes and casseroles, to which you add protein food such as meat or tuna, you pay a high price for the pasta, compared to buying it plain and adding your own seasonings. However, these products are convenient and provide a variety of ways to serve lower cost meats such as ground beef.

To Sum Up. The foods in this group that give more food value for the money, especially in large "family pack" sizes, include: uncooked breakfast cereals and ready-to-eat cereals with little sugar, whole wheat and enriched bread and flour; homemade rolls and biscuits; cakes made from mixes; enriched uncooked rice, macaroni, and spaghetti; and plain crackers such as saltines or graham crackers.

Foods that give you less food value for the money include: stone ground and unenriched white flour; specialty and diet breads; ready-made fresh and frozen cakes, pies, coffee cakes, rolls, and muffins; unenriched and canned or frozen macaroni, spaghetti, and noodles; quick-cooking, canned, or frozen rice and unenriched rice, sugared, puffed, and individual serving-size packs of ready-to-eat cereal; and specialty crackers and wafers.

Starches and sugars comprise the carbohydrate group and together are the number one source of calories in the American diet. Over the years, the proportion of calories Americans obtain from starches and sugars has been changing. In the early 1900s, starch provided about 68 percent of carbohydrates and sugars 32 percent. Since then our total carbohydrate consumption has decreased so that by the mid-1970s, sugars made up 53 percent of our total carbohydrate intake and starch only 47 percent. This means that sugar and syrups supply roughly 24 percent of our total calories. Of these, 18 percent are from sugar added to food, only 3 percent are from fruits and vegetables, and just 3 percent are from milk sugar (lactose). The changing picture of sugar consumption since 1910 is illustrated in Exhibits 7.19 and 7.20. Our total consumption of sugar and syrup was not much different in the mid-1970s than it was in the mid-1920s. However, the sources of sugars changed notably between 1966 and 1976, as is shown in Exhibit 7.24, with dextrose and corn syrup moving from 15 percent to 25 percent of total sweeteners during that time.

Another major shift is in the way we buy sugar. In 1930, 64 percent of sucrose consumed in the United States was purchased directly by consumers for home use and 30 percent by industry for prepared foods. By 1970 these figures were nearly reversed: only 24 percent of sucrose was purchased for home use and 65 percent was bought by industry,

Consumption of Total Sugars, Refined
Sugar, Starch, and Carbohydrate
% of 1909–1913 Avg.

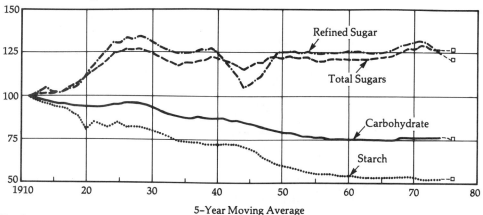

5–Year Moving Average

Per Capita Civilian Consumption.

Exhibit 7.19. (*Source: 1977 Handbook of Agricultural Charts.* U.S. Dept. of Agriculture, Agriculture Handbook No. 524, Washington, D.C., p. 53).

SOURCES OF
CARBOHYDRATE

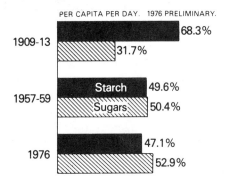

PER CAPITA PER DAY. 1976 PRELIMINARY.

1909-13   68.3%   31.7%

1957-59   Starch 49.6%   Sugars 50.4%

1976   47.1%   52.9%

Exhibit 7.20. (*Source: 1977 Handbook of Agricultural Charts.* U.S. Dept. of Agriculture, Agriculture Handbook No. 524, Washington, D.C., p. 52).

with the remainder purchased by restaurants and the like.[9] Because sugar is already added to foods and therefore not visible, many people are unaware of the large amount of sugar they consume every day. The sugar content of some popular foods tells the story (see Exhibit 7.21).

Unfortunately, nutrition labeling does not help promote awareness of sugar content because it shows only total carbohydrate and not the percentage of sugar and starch in a product. Another problem is that many different types of sugar may be listed by name on an ingredient label, for example, sucrose, glucose, lactose, maltose, words unfamiliar to the average consumer, plus brown sugar, honey, molasses, corn

Exhibit 7.21   Sugar Content of Some Popular Foods

FOOD	PERCENTAGE SUGAR
Canned fruit, heavy syrup	18
Sweet/sour type salad dressing	25-30
Catsup	29
Fruit-flavored yogurt	14
Ice cream	21
Frozen whipped topping	21
Powdered coffee creamer	60
Powdered gelatin dessert mix	82
Sugared cereal	40-55
Granola-type cereal	25
Soft drinks	9
Breakfast bars	22
Powdered instant breakfast	34

[9] "Too Much Sugar?" *Consumer Reports*, March, 1978, Vol. 43, No. 3, pp. 136-42.

syrup, and so forth. The consumer, focusing on the word "sugar," and finding it well down the list of ingredients or not present at all, may think the product does not contain much sugar when, in truth, sugar may be the most prominent ingredient in the food because of all the different forms of it that are used. A simple percentage statement of sugar content could solve this problem.

The words "no sugar added" on a label may be comforting to a person who is trying to reduce sugar consumption. However, this does not mean that no sugar is present, since many foods contain natural sugars. A juice such as apple juice, for example, may have slightly more natural sugar than the sugar added to a soft drink. The difference, of course, is that the fruit juice will have some other nutrients that will not be found in the soft drink.

Sugar in Any Form Equals Calories

Sugars and syrups are notably low in nutrient density, having mostly energy value and only minute amounts of minerals and vitamins (see Exhibit 7.22). Exceptions are dark and blackstrap molasses, which have worthwhile amounts of iron, calcium, and potassium. Corn syrup and brown sugar have slightly more iron than refined white sugar.

Excess sugar can make our diets too high in calories, or if sugar replaces other more nutritious foods in our diets, we may shortchange ourselves on essential nutrients. People on weight control diets particularly cannot afford to spend their limited calorie budget on such "naked calorie" foods (see Chapter 5). Another problem is the contribution of sugary foods to tooth decay (discussed in Chapter 15).

However, sugars do have their place in the diet as a relatively low priced, readily digested, and quickly available energy source. Their low price, in comparison to other ingredients, and flavor appeal are the two principal reasons for their large use in manufactured foods. In many cases, it would be less costly for consumers to buy sugar as sugar and

Exhibit 7.22   Chief Nutrients in Some Popular Sweeteners

SWEETENER (1 TABLESPOON)	WEIGHT (G)	CALORIES	CALCIUM (MG)	POTASSIUM (MG)	IRON (MG)	MAGNESIUM (MG)
White sugar (granulated)	12	46	trace			
Dark brown sugar	14	52	11	32	0.4	
Light molasses	20	50	33	200	0.8	9
Medium molasses	20	46	60	213	1.4	16
Blackstrap molasses	20	43	137	600	3	52
Strained honey	21	64	4	11	0.2	0.6
Corn syrup	20	57	6	trace	0.8	

add it to foods, for example to unsweetened cereals, instead of buying the foods to which manufacturers have added sugar.

An effective way to reduce calories in our diets is to limit our consumption of sugar, syrups, jams, and jellies and other high-sugar foods. However, if we substitute raw or brown sugar, honey, corn syrup, or molasses for white sugar, we are not eating less sugar. We are merely substituting one kind of sugar for another and the calories will be just as high or higher, as Exhibit 7.22 shows. Learning to like foods that are less sweet, to enjoy foods such as fruit "as is" without added sugar, and to choose snacks and desserts that are not loaded with sugar is a more healthful alternative.

Dried fruits—prunes, apricots, raisins, dates—make good sweet foods to eat in place of candy. While their sticky sweetness clinging to the teeth is just as likely to cause tooth decay and needs to be removed immediately by tooth brushing, this sugar is accompanied by other nutrients such as iron, niacin, and vitamin A. While dried fruits are high in calories and seem costly, they have much more nutritional value than candy and are not as expensive as they seem, since most of the water is removed to make them concentrated foods.

The Honey and Raw Sugar Myths

Many consumers not only have the mistaken notion that honey and raw sugar are lower in calories than white sugar (sucrose), but also think that they are less likely to cause tooth decay and are more nutritious. Dental research has shown that bacteria thrive and plaque forms on teeth in the absence of sucrose when other sugars are used (see the discussion of dental disease during childhood in Chapter 15). (Raw sugar contains sucrose; honey contains glucose and fructose.) As the comparison in Exhibit 7.22 shows, honey has few nutrients in proportion to calories and is lower in nutrients than molasses, brown sugar, and corn syrup. A tablespoon of honey has more total sugar and calories than a tablespoon of granular sugar. A rational reason for eating honey is for its good taste and not because it's more nutritious than other sugar products.

Actually, sugar sold as "raw sugar" is not raw sugar at all. True raw sugar cannot be sold in the United States because it contains contaminants such as insect parts, soil, molds, bacteria, lint, and waxes. Raw sugar crystals are separated from these impurities in a centrifuge, then washed with steam. The resulting offwhite product is turbinado sugar, which is sometimes labeled "raw sugar." It is 99 percent sucrose and nutritionally comparable to refined white sugar. The consumer's paying a high price for it makes good sense for the seller, but not for the buyer.

Refined white sugar comes from the same source, sugar cane or sugar beets. Processing causes sugar crystals to form in the syrup. The two are mechanically separated into raw sugar and molasses. The crystals are washed, filtered, and eventually turned into refined white sugar. Brown sugar is made by coating a mass of fine sucrose crystals with highly refined, colored, molasses-flavored syrup. Molasses is separated as a thick liquid from the sugar crystals and has more nutrients because it contains other substances besides sucrose. The darker the molasses, the higher the level of these nutrients.

Corn syrups are produced by partially hydrolyzing corn starch. They contain dextrose, maltose, and other higher saccharides, along with some iron and small amounts of other minerals. Two relatively new products developed for industrial use are high-fructose corn syrup and superhigh-fructose corn syrup. Because fructose is sweeter than both glucose and sucrose, less of it can be used to achieve the sweetness desired (see Exhibit 7.23). The product is then somewhat lower in calories. The high-fructose products are used, in only limited amounts, in a few foods such as cakes, candies, and soft drinks. Too much fructose causes excessive browning of cakes, stickiness in candy, and lower freezing temperatures in ice cream.

Exhibit 7.23 Relative Sweetness of Various Sugars as Compared to Sucrose

| | SUCROSE 100 | | |
LESS SWEET THAN SUCROSE		SWEETER THAN SUCROSE	
Glucose, Dextrose	74	Fructose	173
Sorbitol	60	Invert Sugar	130
Mannitol	50	(Glucose plus	
Galactose, Maltose	32	Fructose)	
Lactose	16		

Source: Freed, Myer, *Food Products Development,* February–March, 1970

Per Capita Consumption of
Caloric Sweeteners by Type

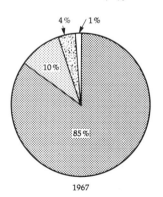

1967

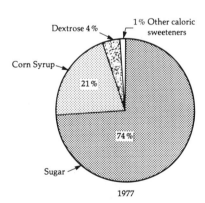

1977

Exhibit 7.24. The use of sweeteners other than sugar—especially those made from corn—has been increasing gradually over the years. (*Source: 1978 Handbook of Agricultural Charts.* U.S. Dept. of Agriculture, Agriculture Handbook No. 551, Washington, D.C., p. 54).

Summary   Carbohydrates, as our least expensive calorie source, are consumed in widely varying amounts throughout the world. All carbohydrates contain carbon, hydrogen, and oxygen in the same proportion as water and can be broken down into simple sugars termed *monosaccharides*. Glucose (blood sugar) is the most commonly occurring simple sugar. When two monosaccharides are linked together, they form a *disaccharide*, such as sucrose (table sugar).

Complex carbohydrates are termed *polysaccharides*, and are made up of many connected simple sugar units. Examples include starch, dextrin, glycogen, and fiber. Fiber is unique in that humans cannot effectively digest or break apart fiber chains.

The original source of carbohydrate is plants, and its chief bodily function is to supply energy. Concern has been expressed at the shift in American carbohydrate consumption from complex carbohydrate foods containing other nutrients to concentrated sugar foods with low nutrient density.

Carbohydrates as well as other nutrients go through processes of digestion, absorption, transportation, and metabolism in order to be utilized by the body. Most digestive action depends on enzymes to catalyze the breakdown of nutrients into simpler substances small enough to be absorbed into the body. When carbohydrates are fully broken down into monosaccharides, they can be absorbed through intestinal walls and transported to the liver, where all are converted to glucose.

Metabolism involves body processing of nutrients, and may be either *anabolic* (building processes) or *catabolic* (breaking down processes). The production of glycogen is an anabolic process, while the splitting of the molecule of glucose to release energy is a catabolic process.

Fiber, since it is undigestible, primarily performs the function of "scrubbing out" the digestive tract. *Dietary fiber* and *crude fiber* are not synonymous, and the variety of fiber types have differing effects on the body.

150

FATS 8

Highlights

Why we need fat

Consequences of consuming excess amounts and certain types of fats

Basic components of fat and the significance of polyunsaturated fatty acids

Process of hydrogenation

Lecithin, cholesterol, ketone bodies, and high- and low-density lipoproteins

Supermarket Nutrition: Choosing Fats and Oils

Fat is a food of the affluent people and cultures of the world. Economically deprived people are less likely to consume fat-rich foods such as meat and dairy products and more likely to consume low-fat plant foods such as grains and vegetables. Consider this contrast: in affluent America, the average person may get 40 to 45 percent of his calories from fats, while in the Orient, the average person may get only 10 percent of his calories from fats.

This high-fat diet doesn't make Americans healthier, however. Excess fat in our diets can make us overweight and may contribute to the development of diseases such as coronary heart disease, diabetes, and cancer. Most recommendations for changes in the American diet to make it more healthful call for the reduction of fat consumption to 30 or 35 percent of calories.

With all the publicity about the hazards of our high-fat diet, we should not get the idea that fat is something we can get along without, however. We need fat because it performs important functions in our bodies, but we don't need as much fat as most of us ingest.

WHY WE NEED FAT

Fats are a concentrated source of energy that make it possible for plants and animals, and people, to store energy compactly and efficiently (see Exhibit 8.1). A gram of pure fat will provide 9 calories, compared to 4 calories per gram of carbohydrate or protein, and 7 calories per gram of alcohol. This means that fats are two and a quarter times higher in caloric density than carbohydrates or protein. For people who need compact or concentrated sources of energy, the high caloric density of fats is an advantage. But for those who need to reduce the caloric content of their diets, it is a disadvantage.

When we have a surplus of energy foods—carbohydrate, protein, or fat—our bodies convert the surplus to fat for storage. This stored fat serves some useful purposes. It provides a reserve supply of energy to draw on in an emergency, for example, during illness or famine, and it

Exhibit 8.1   Functions of Fats

Supply Energy
Store Energy
Give Satiety Value
Carry Fat-Soluble Vitamins
Supply Essential Fatty Acids
Perform Metabolic Functions
Cushion Body Organs
Keep Body Warm

helps cushion body organs, such as kidneys, from shock. Having a layer of fat over our bones makes us look more appealing and serves as insulation against cold.

153
Kinds of
Fats
and
Their
Composition

Because fats are digested more slowly than other nutrients, they tend to slow down the digestion process. Thus a meal high in fat has high satiety value: it makes us feel satisfied longer than a meal having little fat.

The fats we eat carry with them other essential nutrients: most particularly the fat-soluble vitamins A, D, E, and K. Fat itself contains an essential fatty acid, *linoleic acid,* which our bodies must have and must obtain from food because we cannot synthesize it. Two other fatty acids, *linolenic* and *arachidonic,* are also necessary, but can be made in the body from other fats. We need linoleic acid for growth and well-being, but the amount needed is so small—2 percent of total calories—and the distribution so widespread that deficiencies are almost unknown. In human infants deprived of linoleic acid, growth is impaired and a scaly eczema results.

Metabolically, fats work with other nutrients to perform vital functions in every body cell. They are involved in enzyme reactions, in the structure of cell membranes, in the synthesis and regulation of hormones such as *sterols,* and hormone-like substances called *prostaglandins,* in blood vessel and tissue structure, in the transmission of nerve impulses, and in memory storage.

In the body, fats may combine with other substances to form compounds such as *glycolipids* (carbohydrate plus fat), *lipoproteins* (fat plus protein), and *phospholipids* (phosphate plus fat). They also form *cholesterol* and *7-dehydrocholesterol,* which are needed for the formation of vitamin D.

But few of us eat fat for these reasons! We eat it because it makes food taste better. Without fat foods would be dry, tasteless, and unappealing. Fat is a part of many of the products added to foods for flavor—butter, margarine, salad dressing, coffee creamers, whipped toppings—as well as an intrinsic ingredient in many ordinary foods such as peanut butter, cheese, and meat. No wonder the average American consumes 100 to 150 grams of fat a day (see Exhibit 8.2)! Because 60 percent of it is hidden within foods, we may not even realize we're eating it.

KINDS OF FATS AND THEIR COMPOSITION

Our foods contain many different kinds of fats, having different flavors, different melting points, and different compositions. The building blocks of fats (called *lipids* by scientists) are fatty acids. They are attached to a substance called *glycerol,* which is an organic alcohol. Simple fats are named according to the number of molecules of fatty acids attached to one molecule of glycerol: *monoglycerides,* one fatty acid; *di-*

CONSUMPTION OF FOOD ENERGY, PROTEIN, FAT, AND CARBOHYDRATE

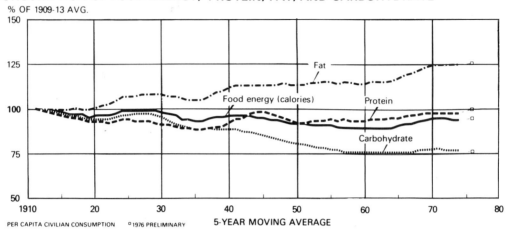

% OF 1909-13 AVG.

PER CAPITA CIVILIAN CONSUMPTION ◻1976 PRELIMINARY **5-YEAR MOVING AVERAGE**

Exhibit 8.2. (*Source: 1977 Handbook of Agricultural Charts.* U.S. Dept. of Agriculture, Handbook No. 524, Washington, D.C., p. 52).

glycerides, two fatty acids; and *triglycerides,* three fatty acids, as illustrated in Exhibit 8.3. About 98 percent of the fats in foods are triglycerides; this is the most common form of fat in the body as well. Monoglycerides and diglycerides may be used as food additives (you will see them listed on labels) to stabilize and emulsify the fats. They are also formed in the body as breakdown products of triglycerides during the digestive process.

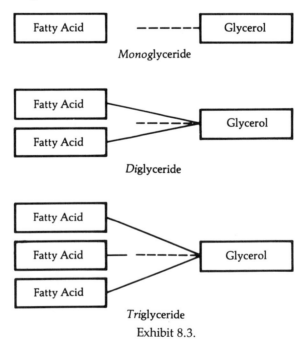

Exhibit 8.3.

154

155
Kinds of
Fats
and
Their
Composition

Fatty acids are made up of carbon, hydrogen, and a small amount of oxygen. There are 12 common fatty acids and they vary in the amount of carbon and hydrogen which they contain. A fatty acid with a small number of carbon atoms (4 to 6) is called a short-chain fatty acid; one with many carbon atoms (more than 12) is a long-chain fatty acid; and those in between, with 8 to 12 carbon atoms, are medium-chain fatty acids. The length of the carbon chain can affect digestibility. For example, infants are better able to digest short- or medium-chain fatty acids than long-chain fatty acids.

The terms *saturated* and *unsaturated* are used to describe the hydrogen component of fats. When a fatty acid has all the hydrogen atoms attached to it that it can hold, it is called a *saturated* fatty acid. When a fatty acid is capable of holding more hydrogen, it is called *unsaturated*. If an unsaturated fatty acid can hold more hydrogen at only one place on its carbon chain it is called *monounsaturated,* and if it can hold more hydrogen at more than one place on its carbon chain it is *polyunsaturated.* A fat that has a high proportion of saturated fatty acid is called a *saturated fat;* one with a high proportion of polyunsaturated fatty acids is called a *polyunsaturated fat.*

A saturated fat is usually solid at room temperature and it usually comes from animals. It will contain a large proportion of saturated fatty acids, such as *myristic* and *palmistic* acids. Some examples of saturated fats are beef, lamb, and pork (lard) fat, milk fat or butter, and coconut and palm oil. Note that the last two are exceptions: they are derived from plants.

The most common monounsaturated fatty acid is oleic acid. Oils high in monounsaturated fatty acids are olive oil and peanut oil.

Polyunsaturated fats are usually liquid at room temperature and usually come from plants. They are high in polyunsaturated fatty acids (often referred to as PUFA) such as linoleic and linolenic acids (both from plants) and arachidonic acids (from animals). Some examples of polyunsaturated fats are safflower, soy, corn, and cottonseed oil. Some animal foods that are exceptions to the "usually from plants" rule and are relatively high in polyunsaturated fats are poultry and fish. Exhibit 8.4 illustrates the relative amount of polyunsaturated fats in some common foods.

Polyunsaturated fats can become saturated in a process called *hydrogenation,* in which hydrogen gas is bubbled through the liquid oil, changing it to a solid:

Liquid				Solid
Polyunsaturated	+	Hydrogen	=	Saturated
Oil				Fat

This is the process used to make vegetable shortening or margarine from vegetable oils. If the polyunsaturated fatty acids are only partially hydrogenated they will still be able to hold more hydrogen and will be less solid than the fully hydrogenated fats.

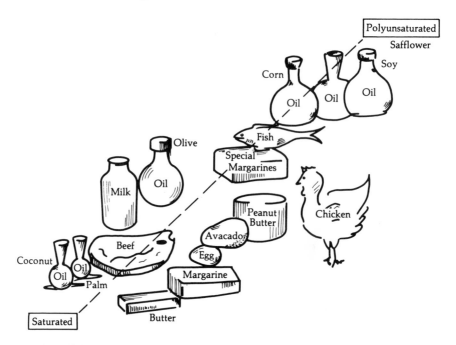

Exhibit 8.4.   Degrees of polyunsaturation of some common fats.

Research evidence indicates that saturated fats may cause our bodies to form cholesterol and raise the level of cholesterol in the blood. Polyunsaturated fats, on the other hand, appear to have the opposite effect and lower blood cholesterol. Monounsaturated fats are believed to have a neutral effect on blood cholesterol. High-blood cholesterol levels are believed to be related to the development of atherosclerosis and coronary heart disease (Chapter 19). This belief has led to the recommendation by some authorities that our diets should have a ratio of unsaturated fats to saturated fats of 2 to 1, or that polyunsaturated, monounsaturated, and saturated fats each supply about one-third of the total fat in the diet (see Dietary Goals, Chapter 18). To meet this recommendation, most Americans would have to reduce their use of meats and whole-milk dairy products and increase their intake of poultry, fish, and vegetable oils. (Suggestions for reducing animal fat intake can be found in Chapter 19.)

PHOSPHOLIPIDS AND STEROLS

Two other fatlike substances obtained from food that we also can synthesize in our bodies are *phospholipids* and *sterols*. Phospholipids are a combination of fats plus phosphate, and some forms also contain nitrogen. They are one of the fatty substances found in the blood. *Lecithin* is the best known example of a phospholipid. It is synthesized by both plants and animals and is found in foods such as egg yolk and soybeans. Often lecithin is added to foods, such as salad dressings, as an emulsifier.

Many nutritional claims have been made about the value of lecithin and it is widely sold as a health food supplement. To date no scientific evidence has developed to support these claims except for some research that showed it may help prevent gallstones in people who are at higher than normal risk of developing them.[1] Lecithin does not have the ability to remove fats from the blood or body, as claimed by those who sell it as a remedy for heart disease or an aid to weight reduction. Instead, lecithin must be counted as a contributor of calories (110 per tablespoon). We can synthesize all the lecithin we need in our own bodies, and therefore it is not considered an essential nutrient.

Cholesterol is the best known of the sterols, which are complex alcohols. It is synthesized in the body and is found in all animal foods. Two other common sterols, which are found in plants, are *ergosterol* and *sitosterol*. Cholesterol is an essential constituent of the cell membrane of every cell. It is needed for the formation of vitamin D, steroid hormones, and bile acids needed for the digestion of fats. Since we can synthesize all the cholesterol we need, we do not have to obtain it from food.

The controversy over the relationship between dietary cholesterol, blood cholesterol levels, and coronary heart disease is discussed in Chapter 19.

DIGESTION OF FATS

Contrary to the belief that "fat is hard to digest," food fat is easily and completely digested by the normal person. Fat digestion may be less complete in conditions where food moves rapidly through the intestines, for example, if a person has diarrhea or uses laxatives, or where the production of bile or fat-splitting enzymes, called *lipases*, is inhibited, for example, in liver disease.

Digestion of fats does not begin until they reach the stomach. However, chewing disperses fats into smaller particles and the solid fats are warmed by the body and become liquid as they move from the mouth to the stomach (Exhibit 8.5). In the stomach, only fat in the emulsified form is acted upon by gastric lipase, the enzyme which splits fat. An emulsified fat is dispersed in tiny particles having a large amount of surface area that can be acted upon. The emulsified fats are split into diglycerides, monoglycerides, fatty acids, and some glycerol.

[1] R. Tompkins, "Nutritional Management of Gallstones." *Nutrition and the M.D.*, Vol. 2, No. 9, July, 1976, p. 2.

Exhibit 8.5   Digestion of Fats

SITE	SUBSTRATE	ENZYME	AGENT	DIGESTION PRODUCT
Mouth and esophagus	Lipids	—	Body heat	Softer lipids
Stomach	Emulsified lipids	Gastric Lipase	—	Some Diglycerides, monoglycerides, fatty acids and glycerol
Stomach	Nonemulsified lipids	—	Body heat	Fluid fats
Small intestines	Nonemulsified lipids	—	Bile	Emulsified lipids
	Emulsified lipids	Intestinal & pancreatic lipases	—	Monoglycerides, a few diglycerides, free fatty acids and glycerol

The main digestion of fats takes place in the small intestine. Bile and pancreatic juice mix with the food (*chyme*) as it moves through the duodenum. The bile emulsifies the nonemulsified fats so that they can be acted upon by the pancreatic and intestinal lipases. These enzymes split the triglycerides into diglycerides, monoglycerides, and finally into free fatty acids and glycerol. See Exhibit 8.6 for a summary of this digestive action.

ABSORPTION AND TRANSPORT OF FATS

Fats are insoluble in water. This characteristic is important because it means that they must be combined with a water-soluble substance, usually protein (as *lipoproteins*), to be transported in the blood and lymph systems.

Up to 95 percent of dietary fats are absorbed. The remainder are excreted in the feces. During digestion, the fats are attached to bile salt, which makes them water soluble. As they are absorbed throughout the intestinal walls, the bile salts split off and stay behind.

The absorbed fats move in two paths. About one-third of the fats, those with fatty acid chains of 12 carbons or less, are absorbed through the intestinal wall directly into the portal vein. They are carried in the blood, attached to the blood protein *albumin*, to the liver. In the liver they are used or released into the blood in the form of lipoproteins for use by other tissues.

The other two-thirds of the fats, monoglycerides and diglycerides and fatty acid chains of 14 carbons or more, are resynthesized in the intestinal walls into new triglycerides. They are made soluble by being joined to proteins and phospholipids into complex substances called *chylomicrons* and very low-density lipoproteins. These are released in the lymph system and are transported to the subclavian vein, where

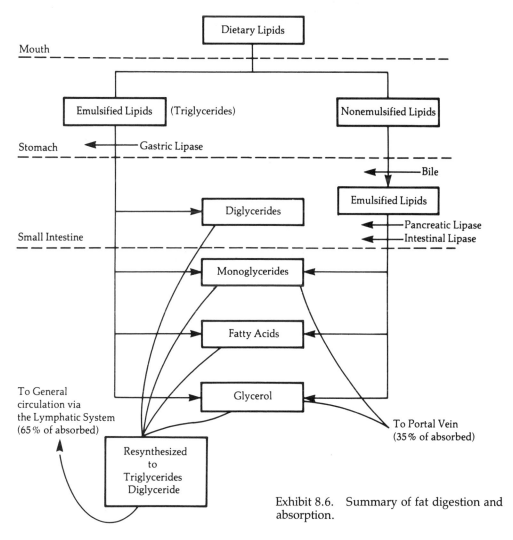

Exhibit 8.6. Summary of fat digestion and absorption.

they enter the blood and finally go to the liver. The liver forms the chylomicrons into new lipoproteins for transport in the blood to the body cells.

METABOLISM OF FATS

The liver is the key organ in regulating fat metabolism, although adipose tissue also plays a role. The liver removes lipoproteins from circulation, breaks down triglycerides and reforms them into new triglycerides, and synthesizes various types of lipoproteins and releases them for circulation in the blood.

The most active form of fats in the blood is the small amount of free fatty acids that are always present and bound to plasma albumin. The other fatty substances in the blood, triglycerides, phospholipids, and cholesterol, are combined with protein into large water-soluble lipoprotein molecules.

Lipoproteins come in two basic types: high density (HDL), having more protein than fat, and low density, having more fat than protein. The low-density lipoproteins are subdivided into two types: low density (LDL) and very low density (VLDL). The VLDL are high in triglycerides; the LDL have few triglycerides and are high in cholesterol and phospholipids. It appears that the LDL and VLDL carry triglyceride and cholesterol from the liver and the small intestines to the peripheral tissues where they are used. HDL seems to collect cholesterol from the tissues and carry it to the liver for excretion. The link between these different forms of lipoproteins and coronary heart disease is discussed in Chapter 19.

The adipose tissue is made up of fat storage cells. Fats are stored in adipose tissue primarily as triglycerides. When energy is needed by the body, triglycerides are broken down (*hydrolyzed*) in fat cells into free fatty acids. The fatty acids enter the blood, are attached to plasma albumin, and are transported to body cells.

In the cells, breakdown of fatty acids takes place in the portion of the cell called the *mitochondria*. In a series of complex chemical reactions involving numerous enzymes and coenzymes, the long carbon chains of the fatty acids are broken down into two-carbon fragments, and many intermediate compounds are formed. Eventually, hydrogen is split off and oxidized into water, carbon is split off and oxidized into carbon dioxide, and energy is released.

Exhibit 8.7 gives a highly simplified picture of fat digestion and metabolism. Throughout digestion, absorption, and metabolism of fats, hormones are involved in triggering and controlling the body responses.

The glycerol portion of triglycerides follows a different path as it is metabolized. It is transformed in the *cytoplasm* portion of the cell into an intermediate compound that can be used to make glucose, or can be oxidized to carbon dioxide and water for energy.

Both fats and carbohydrates are made of the same three elements: carbon, hydrogen, and oxygen. But fats supply greater amounts of energy than carbohydrates when they are metabolized because they contain proportionately less oxygen and more hydrogen and, therefore, have greater potential for oxidation.

If insufficient carbohydrate is present, for example, as a result of uncontrolled diabetes or an extremely low-carbohydrate diet, fat metabolism will increase to supply the energy needs of the body. This results in the intermediate products of fat metabolism, acids called *ketone bodies*, accumulating faster than the body can handle them. When ketones accumulate in the blood, the kidney draws water from the cells to try to remove them. This causes weight loss (illusionary—not real loss of fat)

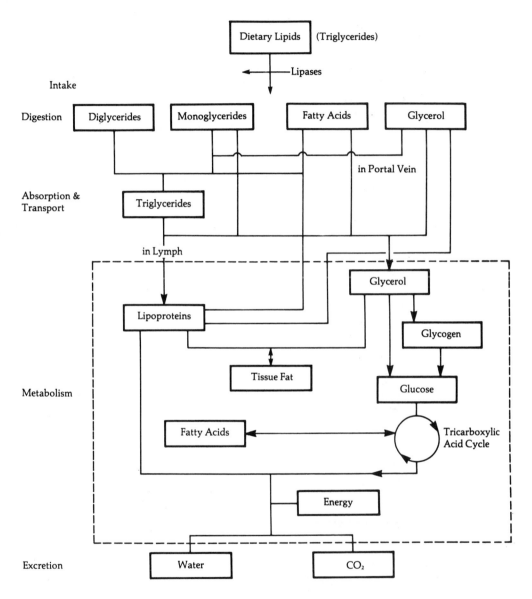

Exhibit 8.7. Summary of fat digestion and metabolism.

161

due to loss of water from the tissues. It can also lead to ketosis, or acidosis with severe dehydration, which could cause circulatory failure, kidney failure, or coma if not corrected.

SUPERMARKET NUTRITION: CHOOSING FATS AND OILS

The consumption of fats in the United States has been increasing steadily over the years, and the proportion of fat from animal sources has been decreasing while the amount from vegetable sources has been increasing, as illustrated in Exhibits 8.8 and 8.9. Keep in mind that these statistics, gathered by the U.S. Department of Agriculture, are based on foods purchased, not on actual consumption by consumers. Therefore, they could be too high for many people who carefully trim away the fat on meat and poultry products, drain fat from cooked bacon and ground beef, remove fat from meat drippings before making gravy, and generally do not eat all the fat they buy.

In terms of energy content, weight for weight all pure fats are alike and provide about 225 calories per ounce. But when fats are measured by volume, rather than by weight, there are calorie differences between solid fats and liquid oils, since a liquid measure of oil weighs slightly more than a solid measure of fat. Another reason for caloric differences between fats is the presence of such other ingredients as water or the incorporation of air through whipping.

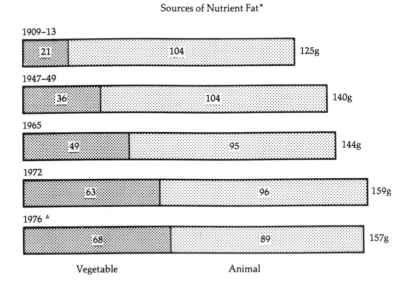

Sources of Nutrient Fat*

1909–13 21 104 125g
1947–49 36 104 140g
1965 49 95 144g
1972 63 96 159g
1976 ᐃ 68 89 157g

Vegetable   Animal

*Grams Per Capita Per Day.   ᐃPreliminary

Exhibit 8.8. (*Source: 1976 Handbook of Agricultural Charts. U.S. Dept. of Agriculture, Agriculture Handbook No. 504, Washington, D.C., p. 68*).

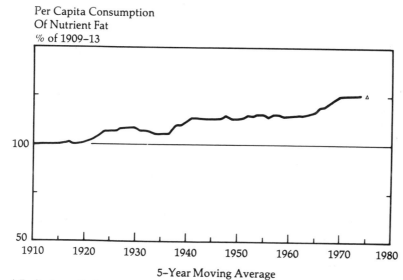

Per Capita Consumption
Of Nutrient Fat
% of 1909–13

5–Year Moving Average

△ Preliminary Estimate.

Exhibit 8.9. (*Source: 1976 Handbook of Agricultural Charts.* U.S. Dept. of Agriculture, Agriculture Handbook No. 504, Washington, D.C.)

Thus, butter and margarine, which are not pure fat because they contain 16 to 20 percent water, have fewer calories than oil or shortening. The calorie content of margarine may be further reduced through the addition of more water. This product is sold under the name of "imitation margarine" and is promoted as a lower calorie product for dieters. While it is true that imitation margarine is lower in calories, it is not as good a nutrition value because you are paying for the extra water and receive less fat for your money. (One label suggests that if imitation margarine is used for frying, this high-priced water should be allowed to cook away before the food is added!)

Both butter and margarine may be whipped with air and sold as "whipped" butter or margarine. The air increases their volume so they have fewer calories per volume measure, although calories per ounce are not changed. Exhibit 8.10 shows a comparison of the calorie value of commonly used fats.

Switching from butter to margarine or from hardened margarine to soft margarine does not save calories. Calories are only saved by using products with less fat, such as the imitation or whipped products. Saturated and polyunsaturated fats are also no different in calories. The difference between saturated and polyunsaturated fats and their believed effect on blood cholesterol levels is discussed in Chapter 19. Persons on cholesterol control diets are usually told to switch from butter and hardened margarine, which are high in saturated fats, to the more polyunsaturated soft margarine. However, not all soft margarines are

Exhibit 8.10   Comparison of the Calorie Value of Commonly Used Fats

FAT	CALORIES PER TABLESPOON	CALORIES PER OUNCE
Vegetable oil (any type)	120	240 (fl oz)
Vegetable shortening	111	250
Lard	117	255
Butter	102	203
Margarine (soft and hard)	102	203
Imitation margarine	55	102
Whipped butter or margarine	70	203

alike in the amount of polyunsaturated fats that they contain. Two differences in ingredients are involved: the kind of oil used and the degree of hydrogenation.

As we learned earlier in this chapter, hydrogenation causes liquid polyunsaturated oil to become more saturated and more firm. Margarines that contain a high percentage of *hydrogenated* vegetable oil, with this ingredient listed *first* on the label, will be more saturated than those that have liquid oil as the major ingredient. Those whose labels list partially hydrogenated oil first will probably fall in between these two polyunsaturated fat levels.

Using the Exhibit 8.12, which rates fats and oils by their level of polyunsaturation, you can see that margarines that contain highly saturated fats such as palm oil, coconut oil, and lard will not be as high in

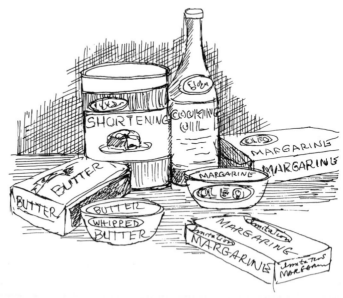

Exhibit 8.11.   Calorie differences between these products exist because some are nearly pure fat while others contain water or air, which increases their weight or volume but dilutes their calorie content.

Exhibit 8.12.   Fats and Fatty Acids in Selected Foods

Food	Total fat	Fatty acids [1]			
		Total saturated	Total monoun-saturated	Total polyun-saturated	Lino-leic
	Percent	*Percent*	*Percent*	*Percent*	*Percent*
Salad and cooking oils:					
Safflower	100	9	12	74	73
Sunflower	100	10	21	64	64
Corn	100	13	25	58	57
Soybean, unhydrogenated	100	14	24	57	50
Cottonseed	100	26	19	51	50
Sesame	100	15	40	40	40
Soybean, hydrogenated [2]	100	15	43	37	32
Peanut	100	17	47	31	31
Palm	100	48	38	9	9
Olive	100	14	72	9	8
Coconut	100	86	6	2	2
Vegetable fats—shortening, household	100	25	44	26	23
Table spreads:					
Margarine, first ingredient on label:					
Safflower (liquid)—tub	80	13	16	48	48
Corn oil (liquid)—tub	80	14	30	32	27
Corn oil (liquid)—stick	80	15	36	24	23
Soybean oil (hydrogenated)—stick	80	15	46	14	10
Butter	81	50	23	3	2
Animal fats:					
Chicken	100	32	45	18	17
Lard	100	40	44	12	10
Beef tallow	100	48	42	4	4
Fish, raw:					
Salmon, sockeye	9	2	2	5	1
Tuna, albacore	8	2	2	3	[3] < .5
Mackerel, Atlantic	10	2	4	2	[3] < .5
Herring, Atlantic	6	2	2	1	[3] < .5
Nuts:					
Walnuts, English	63	7	10	42	35
Walnuts, black	60	5	11	41	37
Brazil	68	17	22	25	25
Pecan	71	6	43	18	17
Peanut butter	52	10	24	15	15
Peanuts	48	9	24	13	13
Egg yolk	33	10	13	4	4
Avocado	15	2	9	2	2

[1] Total is not expected to equal "total fat".
[2] Common salad and cooking oil for commercial and household use.
[3] Less than.

polyunsaturated fats as those that are made of oils such as safflower, soy, corn, or cottonseed. In recent years palm oil has become a very popular ingredient for margarine due to its relatively low cost and bland flavor. This development has led to a number of brands of soft margarine becoming more saturated.

Some margarine manufacturers provide information about the proportion of saturated and polyunsaturated fats on the label. This is a voluntary option under the nutrition-labeling regulations.

Persons on cholesterol control diets also are advised to substitute vegetable oil for lard or vegetable shortening for cooking to reduce the amount of saturated fat in their diets. If this is done, it is important to use oils that rate high in polyunsaturates. If vegetable shortenings are used instead, label reading, as recommended for soft margarine, can help identify those that appear to contain the largest amount of polyunsaturated fat.

Vitamin A is naturally present in butter and is added to margarine in the form of carotene at a level prescribed by the Food and Drug Administration. Vitamin D also may be added to these two fats, and if it is, it will be listed on the label.

Vegetable oils are good sources of vitamin E, which in addition to serving as a nutrient also acts as a natural antioxidant to help prevent the fat from turning rancid. Fats high in polyunsaturates are more susceptible to oxidation than saturated fats. Since rancid fat has undesirable flavors and odors and also may contain potentially harmful substances, synthetic antioxidants are added to most vegetable oils and shortenings to prevent oxidation and extend shelf life. The question of the safety of these additives is discussed in Chapter 24.

Fat is ubiquitous in the American diet. It not only is a visible or, more likely, hidden natural constituent of foods such as meat, nuts and seeds, and dairy products, but also is a prominent part of many products that make our foods taste better, like salad dressing, sour cream, coffee creamers, and whipped toppings (see Exhibit 8.13). Fat also is a key ingredient used in the preparation of many foods, cakes, cookies, pastries, corn and potato chips, and many other snack foods and instant meals.

The consumer who is trying to reduce fat intake and cut calorie consumption needs to read labels diligently to identify the presence of fat and to estimate how prominent an ingredient it is in the product when there is no nutrition label giving the quantity of fat in grams and its percentage calorie contribution. Unless the label provides this information, it is nearly impossible for a consumer to determine whether the fat used in a product is saturated or polyunsaturated because the kind of fat used may not be stated specifically.

The most important thing for consumers to remember is that, no matter what type of fat is used, it will be a rich source of calories since it has two and one quarter times as many calories per unit as sugars,

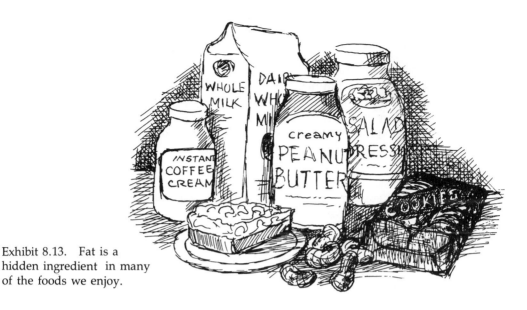

Exhibit 8.13. Fat is a hidden ingredient in many of the foods we enjoy.

starches, or protein. Persons on weight control diets will make their biggest calorie savings by cutting down on fats; in doing so they will also save money, since high-fat foods are, in general, also the highest priced foods.

Summary

Fats are the most concentrated source of energy of all the nutrients. They also serve the body by cushioning vital organs; insulating against cold; carrying fat-soluble vitamins; working in tandem with other nutrients in a variety of functions; and providing an essential fatty acid, *linoleic acid.* Since they are digested rather slowly, they add satiety value to meals.

The most common form of fat is termed a *triglyceride,* and is made up of *glycerol* to which three *fatty acids* are attached. Fatty acids are chains of carbon, hydrogen, and a small amount of oxygen. *Saturated* fatty acids contain all the hydrogen the chain can hold; *monounsaturated* and *polyunsaturated* fatty acids can hold more hydrogen.

Fats containing a relatively large amount of saturated fatty acids are usually obtained from animals and are solid at room temperature. Exceptions are the two plant oils coconut and palm. Polyunsaturated fatty acids predominate in plant oils such as corn, soy, and safflower. Poultry and fish are relatively high in unsaturated fatty acids.

Hydrogenation is the process of adding hydrogen to liquid oil, which saturates and solidifies it; this process is used in the production of margarine. Because of the possible relationship between saturated

167

fats and atherosclerosis, heart disease, and other disorders, many authorities recommend cutting back on highly saturated fatty foods.

Lecithin, a phospholipid, and *cholesterol,* a sterol, are also fatty type materials found in foods and synthesized by our bodies. Digestion of fats requires that bile emulsify and disperse them in tiny droplets to be acted upon by fat-splitting enzymes. Most fatty substances in the blood combine with protein for easier transportation to other sites in the body. Termed *lipoproteins,* these combinations are of two basic types: high density (HDL) and low density (LDL).

Fats can go through several metabolic pathways; when releasing energy, they are split into carbon dioxide and water. When insufficient carbohydrate is present, *ketone bodies* may form during fat metabolism and produce toxicity.

PROTEINS 9

Highlights

Composition and synthesis of proteins
The nitrogen cycle
Need for amino acids
Protein intake, quality, and rating system
Food sources and beneficial protein combinations
Dangers of unbalanced high-protein diets
Protein digestion, absorption, and metabolism
Supermarket Nutrition: Choosing Foods in the Meat Group
Supermarket Nutrition: Choosing a No-Meat Diet

Proteins are literally the "stuff of life." They make up three-fourths of the body. The cells of muscles, connective tissue, bones, brain, blood, skin, hair, and nails, as well as hormones and enzymes, all have protein as their basic structural material. Thus, while recognizing that all nutrients are essential to life, we must consider proteins the most essential. As such, they are appropriately named, for the word protein comes from the Greek *proteios,* meaning primary, or holding first place.

Learning to understand proteins is a major challenge to scientists because of the complexity of the substances that form proteins and the almost infinite number of ways that they can be combined. For many years, scientists have been studying the chemistry of proteins—how they are structured, synthesized, and used in the body—and they are still a long way from having a total understanding.

Some of the most important scientific discoveries of this century have been related to the proteins DNA (*deoxyribonucleic acid*) and RNA (*ribonucleic acid*) and how they carry the blueprint for the formation of each body protein from the cell nucleus to the manufacturing site for protein within the cell.

WHAT ARE PROTEINS?

Proteins are the largest and most complex of the organic molecules consisting, in some cases, of hundreds of smaller units, called *amino acids,* linked together.

The connecting links between proteins are like the universal couplings used on railroad cars. Just as a large number of many different kinds of railroad cars can be coupled together to make up a train, so can any number of different amino acids be linked together to make a protein (see Exhibit 9.1). And just as trains can be uncoupled to make them shorter, so can amino acids be uncoupled to make smaller protein units. Unlike trains, however, amino acids may be linked together in more

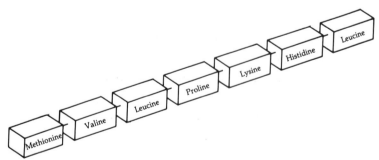

Exhibit 9.1.   A protein molecule is made up of various amino acids just as a freight train is made up of different freight cars coupled with a universal linkage.

than just straight chains. They may form spheres or globules, or the chains may form folded, sheetlike arrangements, for example.

Like carbohydrates and fats, proteins contain carbon, hydrogen, and oxygen. But they always contain nitrogen as well (and sometimes other elements such as sulfur, phosphorous, iron, or iodine). The nitrogen that makes protein different from fats and carbohydrates is the most common element on earth, making up about 80 percent of the air we breathe. But animals, including humans, are unable to capture this free nitrogen and turn it into protein. We must get our nitrogen from plants.

Plants are able to take up free nitrogen from the soil and combine it with carbon, hydrogen, and oxygen to form protein. Bacteria play an important role also. They break down nitrogen-containing substances in the soil to release the free nitrogen for plant use. A special type of bacteria, called *nitrogen fixing*, which grow in nodules on the roots of leguminous plants (beans, peas, alfalfa), are able to capture the free nitrogen in the air and make it available to those plants for protein manufacture. This is the reason why legumes, of all the plants, are the richest source of protein. Bacteria also help certain animals called ruminants—cattle, sheep, and goats—form protein from urea in their rumen (first "stomach"). The wastes from animals, plus decayed plants and animals that are returned to the soil, are a source of nitrogen for the growth of new plants. This nitrogen cycle, so vital to life, is pictured in Exhibit 9.2.

When carbon, hydrogen, oxygen, and nitrogen combine to form amino acids, the basic protein units, they always have two special combinations of elements: a *free carboxyl group*, consisting of one atom of carbon, two atoms of oxygen, and one atom of hydrogen (CO–OH); and a *free amino group*, which has one atom of nitrogen and two atoms of hydrogen (NH_2).

When two amino acids are coupled together, the free amino group of one combines with the free carboxyl group of the other, releasing one molecule of water (H_2O) as they form what is called a *peptide link* (Exhibit 9.3). A peptide link has one atom each of carbon, oxygen, nitrogen, and hydrogen (CO–NH). This peptide link is the universal coupling between all amino acids, and it is the linkage that must be split when proteins are broken down, for example, in digestion. This breakdown process is called *hydrolysis*, a splitting with water, because the water molecule must be added back at each peptide link.

Amino acid chains are called *peptides*. When two amino acids are combined, the substance is called a *dipeptide;* three amino acids linked together are a *tripeptide;* and many acids linked together are a *polypeptide*.

When a protein is made up of only amino acids, it is called a *simple protein* (although it could be a very complex compound). If amino acids are united with other compounds, such as fats (lipoproteins), carbohydrates (glycoproteins), phosphates (nucleoproteins), etc., they are called *conjugated proteins*.

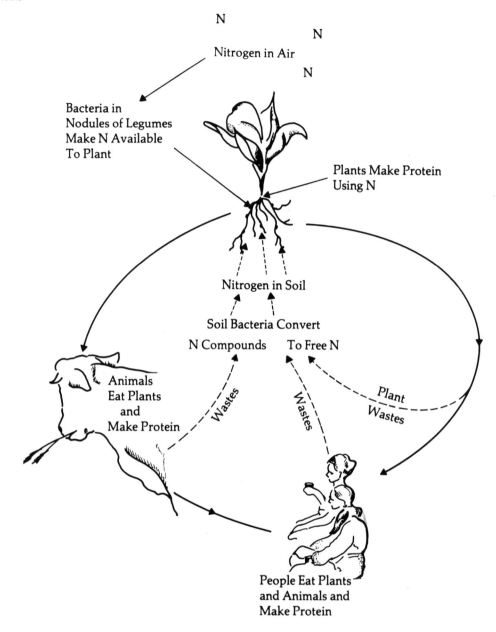

N

N

Nitrogen in Air

N

Bacteria in
Nodules of Legumes
Make N Available
To Plant

Plants Make Protein
Using N

Nitrogen in Soil

Soil Bacteria Convert

N Compounds   To Free N

Animals
Eat Plants
and
Make Protein

Wastes

Wastes

Plant
Wastes

People Eat Plants
and Animals and
Make Protein

Exhibit 9.2.   The nitrogen cycle.

CO–OH		NH		CO–NH		H_2O
Carboxyl Group	+	Amino Group	⟶ ⟵	Peptide Link	+	Water

Exhibit 9.3.

WHY WE NEED PROTEINS

Building and repairing body tissue is the most important function of proteins (see Exhibit 9.4). As mentioned earlier, proteins form the basis of every body cell. Thus it is obvious that the greatest need for protein is during periods when cells are growing rapidly: during infancy, childhood, adolescence, and pregnancy. During lactation, a woman needs extra protein to produce milk. Infants and children need the most protein in proportion to their size. The lack of protein in early childhood can lead to the deficiency disease *kwashiorkor* and eventual death. The lack of both protein and calories can result in another possibly fatal deficiency disease, *marasmus*.

In addition to supplying raw material for the formation of new tissues, including those that keep growing, such as hair, skin, and nails, protein also is needed to replace tissue that is lost, either through stress, caused by burns, hemorrhage, and illness, or through natural daily degradation. Our bodies, once formed, are not static, but are constantly being degraded and rebuilt. The turnover rate varies in different parts of the body. Some tissue, such as the lining of the intestine, renews itself every one to three days. Blood cells regenerate every 120 days. Liver cells have a high turnover rate too, but muscles renew themselves much more slowly, while the turnover of brain cells is negligible. This degradation of body tissue is one source of protein that we can reuse.

Another function of protein is to maintain two important balances in the body: water balance and acid-base balance, or pH.[1] For example, in maintaining water balance, proteins in the blood (plasma proteins) that are too large to pass through cell walls maintain the osmotic pressure needed to draw fluid back out of cells (water which forms from the oxidation of glucose, for example) and into the bloodstream. If plasma protein levels are low, fluid may accumulate in cells, and low-protein

Exhibit 9.4   Functions of Protein

Form Body Tissue
Provide Energy
Maintain Water Balance
Maintain Acid-Base Balance

---

[1] pH is the chemical symbol used to indicate the acidity or alkalinity of a solution. A pH 7.0 is neutral. Below 7.0 a solution is acid; above 7.0 it is alkaline

173

edema (swelling) results. Starving people, especially children, are often seen to have this type of retention of extra water in their tissues.

The pH of body tissues is just slightly alkaline (pH 7.4). Proteins are able to function as either acids or alkalines to maintain this pH because they have amino groups that are alkaline and carboxyl groups that are acidic. So they can unite with either acids or bases (*alkalies*) as needed to reduce excess acidity or alkalinity in body fluids.

In addition to forming major body tissues, proteins are also needed in smaller amounts to make the enzymes and hormones that regulate all body processes, as well as the antibodies that are needed to fight infections. When the protein intake is low, fewer antibodies are produced, and a person is more vulnerable to attack by infectious organisms. One amino acid, *tryptophan*, is a *precursor* (a form that precedes) of the B vitamin niacin, and another amino acid, *methionine*, can help reduce the need for two other B vitamins.

Any extra protein available in the body after its essential functions are satisfied is used as a source of energy. The calorie yield of protein is similar to that of carbohydrate—4 calories per gram. If we are getting enough energy from other sources, the excess protein is converted to fat for energy storage.

On the other hand, if we are not getting all the energy we need in our food from carbohydrate and fat sources, then we will use protein in our food to meet our energy needs, rather than our protein needs. This is because the growth and maintenance of tissue has a lower priority than our need for energy. If body fat stores are depleted and our diet lacks sufficient energy, we will draw protein from our body tissue to supply energy to keep our body processes functioning. Obviously, this is not a healthful condition!

HOW MUCH PROTEIN DO WE NEED ?

This question is not easily answered because there are many complications involved in determining protein needs. Variables include sex, body size, age and stage of growth, state of health (we may need more if we're recovering from surgery or a serious illness, for example), the composition of our diet, and other factors related to the digestibility and quality of protein food.

The Recommended Dietary Allowances for protein (see Exhibit 9.5) are based on studies, called nitrogen balance studies, of the minimum amount of nitrogen needed to maintain nitrogen equilibrium, that is, when intake of nitrogen equals loss of nitrogen in feces, urine, sweat,

CATEGORY	AGE (YEARS)	PROTEIN (g)
Infants	0.0–0.5	kg X 2.2
	0.5–1.0	kg X 2.0
Children	1–3	23
	4–6	30
	7–10	34
Males	11–14	45
	15–18	56
	19–22	56
	23–50	56
	51–75	56
Females	11–14	46
	15–18	46
	19–22	44
	23–50	44
	51–75	44
Pregnancy		+30
Lactation		+20

Source: *Recommended Dietary Allowances*, Ninth Edition (revised 1979). National Academy of Sciences, Washington, D.C.

hair, skin, nails, and other body secretions. This loss in an average adult male is thought to be about 33 grams per day. To this figure is added an extra amount to allow a liberal margin for individual variability and as insurance in times of stress.

Protein allowances for infants are based on the amount of protein in milk that will provide for optimal growth. Likewise, allowances for children and adolescents are calculated on information relating to growth rates and body composition. Protein needs during pregnancy are based on calculations of the protein in the fetus and additional maternal tissue; needs during lactation are based on the protein quantity in milk. All of these allowances are continually under review as new information becomes available.

Apparently there is a wide range of protein intake to which adults can adapt from a very low level of 25 to 35 grams per day to a high of 300 grams (if sufficient water is available). While there is little evidence that protein eaten in amounts above the recommended allowances has beneficial effects, neither is there evidence that intakes two and three times the RDA are harmful.

One simple way to quickly, but very roughly, estimate protein needs is to divide weight in pounds by three. Thus, if you weigh 150 pounds and divide this by 3, your estimated daily protein need is 50 grams. A somewhat more precise method is to multiply your weight in kilograms by 0.8 to find the grams of protein you need each day.

VARIABLES IN PROTEIN COMPOSITION AND QUALITY

Our need for protein is twofold: we have a general need for the nitrogen it contains, which can be supplied by any digestible form of protein, and a more critical need for specific amino acids, called *essential amino acids*. Scientists have identified 20 to 22 different amino acids in foods (see Exhibit 9.6). Of these, eight, and possibly nine, are called essential amino acids because we must get them from our food since our bodies cannot make them in sufficient quantities for our needs.

Exhibit 9.6   Amino Acids in Foods

ESSENTIAL AMINO ACIDS	SEMIESSENTIAL AMINO ACIDS	NONESSENTIAL AINO ACIDS
Isoleucine	Cystine	Alanine
Leucine	Tyrosine	Arginine
Lysine		Aspartic acid
Methionine		Cysteine
Phenylalanine		Glycine
Threonine		Glutamic acid
Tryptophan		Hydroxylysine
Valine		Hydroxyproline
Histidine		Proline
		Serine

Formerly it was thought that the ninth essential amino acid, histidine, was needed only by children, but recent evidence shows that it also may be essential to adults.[2] Infant rats need a tenth amino acid, arginine, but scientists do not agree on whether human infants also need arginine.

The so-called nonessential amino acids are necessary in the body but are not rated as essential because our bodies can synthesize them from foods if sufficient nitrogen is present. Two amino acids, cystine and tyrosine, are rated as "semiessential." This is because when cys-

[2] M. Crim and H. Munro, "Protein," in Nutrition Reviews' *Present Knowledge of Nutrition*, 4th edition. New York and Washington: The Nutrition Foundation, Inc., 1976, pp. 43–54.

tine is present in the diet it reduces the requirement for methionine, and tyrosine reduces the need for phenylalanine.

The protein value received from foods differs in quality and quantity, depending on several factors:

1. *The amount of protein the food contains.* Concentrated foods such as cheese and soybeans, having 30 percent protein, obviously are better sources than foods such as grains, which have 10 percent protein, or the green leaves of plants, which have only 1 to 3 percent protein.

2. *How effectively our body can use the protein.* This depends on the digestibility of the food and the biological value of the protein. Plant proteins are less digestible (60 to 70 percent) than animal protein (97 percent), and, in addition, they do not have as high a biological value. The biological value is the percentage of the absorbed nitrogen from a food that is retained by the body and is estimated from measurement of nitrogen intake and losses.

Scientists have developed techniques for measuring the amount of nitrogen in a food and comparing it with our use of the nitrogen. From this type of study they rate proteins by NPU, *net protein utilization.* A list of some protein foods with NPU is shown in Exhibit 9.7. Because eggs are closest to providing the perfect combination of amino acids for man, they are given an NPU rating of 100 and all other foods are compared with them.

Another rating of a food's protein value is PER, *protein effectiveness rating.* This is based on measurements of the growth rate of rats when

Exhibit 9.7   NPU and Limiting Amino Acids of Some Foods

FOOD	NPU (%)	LIMITING AMINO ACID
Egg	100	—
Rice	57	Lysine
Corn meal	55	Tryptophan
White flour	52	Lysine
Peanut flour	48	Methionine
Wheat gluten	37	Lysine
Soy flour	56	Methionine
Sesame seed	56	Lysine
Sunflower seed	65	Lysine
Cottonseed meal	66	Methionine
Peas	44	Methionine
Cow's milk	75	—
Beef muscle	80	—
Pork tenderloin	84	—
Fish	83	Tryptophan

Source: "Plant Proteins and Their Utilization." Cooperative Extension Service, The Ohio State University, Columbus, OH, 1970, p. 4.
* FAO Nutrition Meetings Report Series No. 37, p. 48, 1965.

they are fed different proteins. PER is the rating system that the Food and Drug Administration has adopted in setting the U.S. RDA for protein, but it is not considered the best rating method by many nutrition scientists.[3]

3. *Amino acid composition of foods.* This is the key factor in determining protein food's biological value and NPU. The more closely the amino acids in a food match our own utilization pattern, the better we can use them. Those foods having all of the essential amino acids in sufficient amounts for our needs are called *complete proteins.* Complete proteins are those we get from animal foods: eggs, milk, meat, fish, and poultry.

Foods in which one or more of the essential amino acids are present in amounts insufficient for our needs are called *less complete proteins.* (The less accurate term, *incomplete proteins,* formerly used for these proteins is being phased out.) These are the proteins we obtain from plants—legumes (beans, peas, lentils), nuts, grains, vegetables. It is inaccurate to say these foods supply incomplete proteins because one or more of the essential amino acids are not totally lacking in them. Rather, the amino acids are present in such limited amounts that we would have to eat very large quantities of that food to get enough to support growth. The lacking amino acids are called *limiting amino acids.* Exhibit 9.7 shows some limiting amino acids in plant foods.

4. *Total amount of protein in the diet.* The more adequate our protein intake, the less efficiently we utilize the protein. Generally, when a mixed diet containing high-quality protein is eaten, we utilize protein at only 65 to 70 percent efficiency.

5. *The calorie content of our diet.* When our energy consumption is low, the efficiency of our protein utilization decreases. This is because our bodies give priority to supplying energy needs.

6. *The balance of amino acids.* An oversupply of a single amino acid, exceeding certain levels, can severely depress the utilization of other dietary amino acids and can result in growth failure. This amino acid toxicity resulting from an imbalance of amino acids is most evident at low levels of protein intake.

SATISFYING OUR PROTEIN NEEDS

When eating foods to satisfy protein needs, it is important to keep some critical protein factors in mind. Most importantly, we need to remember that essential amino acids are not made in sufficient amounts in the body and must be obtained from foods. In addition, all of the

[3] M. Crim and H. Munro, "Protein," in Nutrition Reviews' *Present Knowledge of Nutrition,* 4th edition. New York and Washington: The Nutrition Foundation, Inc., 1976, p. 51.

essential amino acids must be present at the same time, or within a very short time, for our bodies to synthesize protein.

If one or more essential amino acids are present in only limited amounts, our ability to utilize the other amino acids in synthesizing body protein is limited accordingly. This concept, called the *law of the minimum,* is illustrated in Exhibit 9.8, which compares the body pool of essential amino acids to a barrel with one or two short staves. Just as the barrel holds liquid only to the level of the shortest stave, so our bodies can use amino acids only to the level of the most limited essential amino acid.

Because amino acids are not stored anywhere in the body for use as needed as are fats and carbohydrates, our reserves are depleted in just a few hours. However, the amino acid pool available to tissues comes not only from dietary (*exogenous*) sources, but also from the normal tissue breakdown (*endogenous source*). As far as body metabolism is concerned, the amino acids from these two sources are indistinguishable. Thus, the body itself forms a reserve pool of protein. On a protein-free diet, or a starvation diet, we will catabolize our own body tissue to

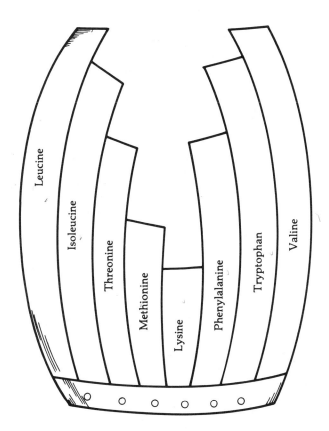

Exhibit 9.8.   The law of the minimum.

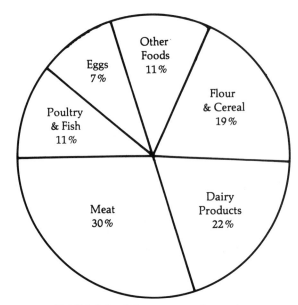

Exhibit 9.9. Diet sources of protein.

fulfill ongoing protein needs and maintain vital body functions. We can maintain vital functions for 30 to 50 days of total starvation, or until about one-fourth of our body protein is depleted.

The simplest way to be sure of getting all of the essential amino acids is to include some form of animal protein in each meal (see Exhibit 9.9). If plant foods are used as the chief source of protein, including a

Exhibit 9.10.   Limiting and Abundant Amino Acids in Some Common Plant Foods

	Lysine	Methionine	Tryptophan	Threonine
Legumes—Dry Beans and Peas	+ +	− −		
Soybeans	+ +	− −		+ +
Peanuts, Peanut Butter	+ +	− −		
Wheat Wheat Germ	− −	+ +		
Rice	− −			− −
Corn	− −		− −	
Sunflower Seeds, Sesame Seeds	− −	+ +	+ +	+ +

Limiting and abundant amino acids in some common plant foods.

− − = Limiting Amino Acid   + + = High Amount of Amino Acid

small amount of animal protein along with them will ensure an adequate supply of all the essential amino acids. Thus, with a peanut butter sandwich we might have a glass of milk or some cottage cheese; to our breakfast cereal we add milk; to our rice or beans we add some meat or cheese or fish. Many of our meals do include just this kind of combination.

If a meal has no animal foods, we need to eat a combination of plant foods so that the amino acids that are limited in one food are supplied in another. Exhibit 9.10 shows the limiting amino acids in popular plant proteins as well as those that are found abundantly in these foods. Using this chart, it's easy to see how plant proteins complement one another and how they should be combined.

For example, legumes, which are low in methionine and tryptophan, go well with sesame and sunflower seeds, which are good sources of these amino acids and at the same time are low in lysine that legumes supply in large amounts. Some typical combinations of plant proteins are: rice and beans, whole wheat with peanut butter, corn with beans, and soybeans with sunflower seeds. Using animal foods such as eggs, milk, or cheese simplifies the problem of supplying the limiting amino acids in plant proteins.

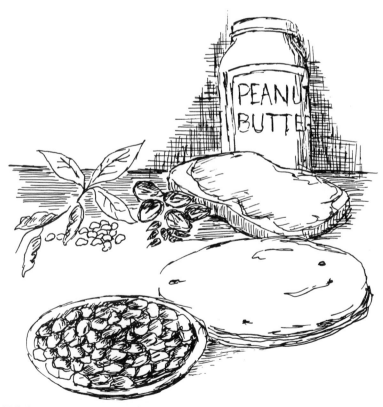

Exhibit 9.11. Some good combinations of complementary plant proteins.

Vegetarians, especially those who eat no animal foods at all, must plan their meals carefully so as to be sure to include complementary plant proteins in every meal. More information about vegetarian diets can be found at the end of this chapter.

In the average American diet, 60 to 70 percent of our protein needs are supplied from animal foods. Protein malnutrition in the U.S. is very rare, and most people, even those with low incomes, obtain a great deal more protein than they need. Even if inflated prices for animal foods causes us to use less of these foods, we can still get enough protein to satisfy our needs.

For example, see Exhibit 9.12, which illustrates the possible protein intake of an average American man eating an average American diet.

Exhibit 9.12

	GRAMS PROTEIN
2 eggs	14
4 servings bread, cereal	12
2 slices cheese	10
5-oz serving of meat	35
½ cup peas	8
1 baked potato	4
2 cups milk	18
½ cup ice cream	3
4 tablespoons peanuts	10
TOTAL	114

If his protein requirement is 55 grams (PER equal to milk protein), this man is getting twice as much protein as he needs. Even if he reduced intake to one egg, three ounces of meat, and one slice of cheese and eliminated the peanuts and ice cream, he would still be getting plenty of protein (75 grams). In thinking about satisfying protein needs, many people fail to take into account the amount received from foods other than meat, such as bread, milk, cheese, vegetables, and nuts.

Exhibit 9.13 shows the amount of protein provided by some of the common foods in the American diet.

While evidence is lacking that high-protein diets in themselves are harmful, diets that are out of balance, that is, excessively low in carbohydrate and high in protein can bring about potentially harmful metabolic changes, resulting from the production of ketones and uric acid. In addition, a high protein diet places a burden on the liver and kidneys to excrete the excess nitrogen. While a normal liver and good kidneys are believed capable of handling this load, organs that are not functioning adequately could become stressed or incapable of excreting the nitrogen

Exhibit 9.13   Protein in Some Common Foods

FOOD	AMOUNT	COMPLETE PROTEIN (GRAMS)	LESS COMPLETE PROTEIN (GRAMS)
Lean meat	3 oz	22	
Chicken, ½ breast, or 1 leg		23	
Fish	3 oz	28	
Egg	1 large	7	
Milk	8 oz	9	
Cheese, cheddar	1 oz	7	
Cheese, cottage	4 oz (½ cup)	16	
Dry beans, peas cooked	1 cup		14
Peanut butter	2 T		8
Sunflower seeds	¼ cup		9
Bread	1 slice		2–3
Oatmeal, cooked	⅔ cup		2–3
Rice, cooked	1 cup		4
Spaghetti	1 cup		5
Breakfast cereal, flake-type	1 oz or 1 cup		2
Breakfast cereal with added soy or dry milk	1 oz or ⅔ cup		5
Potato, cooked	1 medium		3–4
Peas, cooked	½ cup		4–5
Spinach, cooked	1 cup		1
Sweet corn	1 ear or ½ cup		2–3
Carrots	1 medium		0.8
Banana	1 medium		1.3

overload. Infants in particular are not equipped to excrete large amounts of nitrogen (Chapter 14).

Some scientists theorize that we would be healthier if we used less animal protein in our diets. One reason for this conclusion is that animal proteins, particularly beef, pork, and lamb, are associated with relatively large amounts of animal fat, which are both high in calories and high in saturated fatty acids. Animal protein foods also contain cholesterol. These factors are believed to be related to the development of coronary heart disease (Chapter 19). An excess of calories from the fat and protein in a high-meat diet also could be a contributing cause of obesity.

One theory about cancer of the colon holds that a high animal-protein diet could be a causative factor (Chapter 19). Another theory relating to osteoporosis, the loss in bone density in older people, suggests that one cause may be the unbalanced ratio of phosphorous to calcium resulting from the long-term consumption of a high-meat, low-milk diet. (Meat is high in phosphorous, while milk is our chief source of calcium.)

THE DIGESTION AND ABSORPTION OF PROTEINS

The digestion of proteins does not begin until the food reaches the stomach. There is no digestive action on them in the mouth except for the mechanical shearing of some of the larger molecules by chewing. In the stomach, hydrochloric acid and *pepsin* and the protein-splitting enzyme *protease* attack specific linkages on the ends of the protein chains, reducing them to shorter chains called *polypeptides* and *peptones*. Pepsin is present in the stomach in an inactive form, *pepsinogen,* which is converted to its active form by the hydrochloric acid (see Exhibit 9.14).

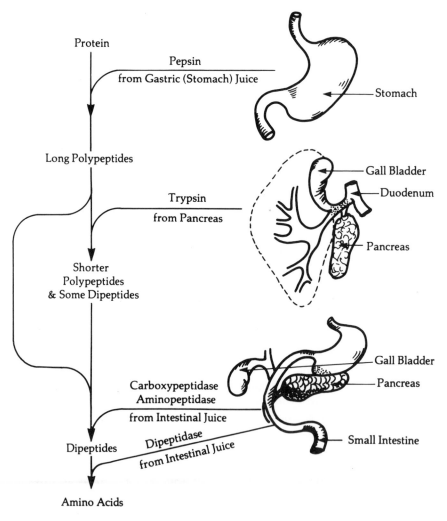

Exhibit 9.14.   Systematic breakdown of proteins to amino acids.

In the duodenum, the acid is neutralized and the food mixture becomes slightly alkaline. Here the pancreatic juice contains a strong *proteolytic* (protein-splitting) enzyme, *trypsin*, or *pancreatic protease*. Trypsin attacks the polypeptide chains selectively at the carboxyl groups. This reduces the length of peptides to two-amino-acid (*dipeptide*) and three-amino-acid (*tripeptide*) chains.

As the dipeptides and tripeptides travel down into the small intestine they are showered with juices secreted by the intestinal wall that contain *carboxypeptidases, aminopeptidases,* and *dipeptidases.* The carboxypeptidase starts chewing at the carboxyl end of the peptide linkage, and the aminopeptidase acts similarly on the amino group of the peptide linkage. Finally, the entire polypeptide or tripeptide chains are reduced to dipeptides, as shown in Exhibit 9.14. Now *dipeptidase,* a specific enzyme for acting upon dipeptides, goes into action, cleaving the linkage between the remaining two amino acids. The action of dipeptidase may take place either outside or inside the lumen (hollow part) of the small intestine.

The amino acids thus formed may be absorbed either by active transport or by a simple diffusion process across the intestinal wall and into the bloodstream. The blood carries them, via the portal vein, to the liver, which acts as a temporary amino-acid-holding tank. From the liver, the amino acids are carried to the fluid surrounding the cells in various parts of the body. By a special transport mechanism they enter the cells, where they are used for repair of old cells or for the formation of new proteins as the need may be.

Occasionally some individuals are unable to digest proteins into their component amino acids. As a result, larger protein fragments may get absorbed into the system and cause an allergic reaction. This generally is the reason why some people are allergic to specific foods such as milk, egg, or chocolate. (Information on allergies and their prevention or treatment can be found in Chapter 15 in the sections discussing nutrition for infants and children.)

METABOLISM OF PROTEINS

Because proteins are in a dynamic state of equilibrium, that is, constantly interchanging nitrogen from one part of the body to the other, there is continuous traffic of essential and nonessential amino acids to and from the common pool in the liver. The amino acids are taken up by the individual cells that use them in the synthesis of specific proteins. As pointed out earlier, all the amino acids for a specific protein must be present simultaneously in the cell for its synthesis; otherwise the protein is not formed and the amino acids are released back into the common pool.

Because each cell cannot necessarily synthesize all of the essential amino acids, it draws them from the common pool as needed. This pool is being continuously renewed from (1) dietary amino acids, (2) degradation of body protein, and (3) the synthesis of nonessential amino acids in the individual cells. The latter process is called *transamination* because amino groups are transferred from amino acids to nonnitrogenous substances to form different amino acids.

Amino acids not needed by the body cells for new synthesis or for repair work are released back into circulation to be channeled into either the glucose or fatty-acid metabolic cycles. However, before entering the nonnitrogenous metabolic cycles of glucose or fatty acids, they are *deaminated*. This means that the amino group (NH_2) is removed from the amino acid. The amino group is converted to urea and eliminated by the kidneys in the urine.

The remaining nonnitrogenous segment can either be used to form glucose for immediate energy use, be converted to glycogen for future energy use, be used to form fatty acids for immediate energy use, or be converted to triglycerides for storage as fat for future energy needs. The amino acids which, after deamination, enter the carbohydrate cycle are called *glucogenic* amino acids, and the ones that are metabolized as fatty acids are referred to as *ketogenic* amino acids.

This brief description is a highly simplified version of a very complex process, which is mediated by hormones and catalyzed by enzymes and coenzymes. As with fat and carbohydrate metabolism, the liver is the key organ in regulating protein metabolism.

SUPERMARKET NUTRITION: CHOOSING FOODS IN THE MEAT GROUP

A better name for this group would be the "protein group" since it includes many foods other than meat, such as eggs, poultry, fish, legumes (dried beans and peas), peanuts and peanut butter, and other nuts and seeds. While protein is the most important nutrient we get from this group, these foods also are a major supplier of other key nutrients, such as iron, B vitamins, and fat. In addition, the plant protein foods are a source of fiber.

In the American diet, the animal foods in this group supply nearly 50 percent of our total protein intake, as is illustrated in Exhibit 9.15. Foods in the "plant foods" category in the graph would include the plant protein foods of this group along with other fruits and vegetables.

The protein content of the foods in this group ranges from 6 to 18 percent in cooked legumes and nuts to 15 to 20 percent in lean meat, poultry, and fish. In general, the flesh of meat, fish, and poultry, and

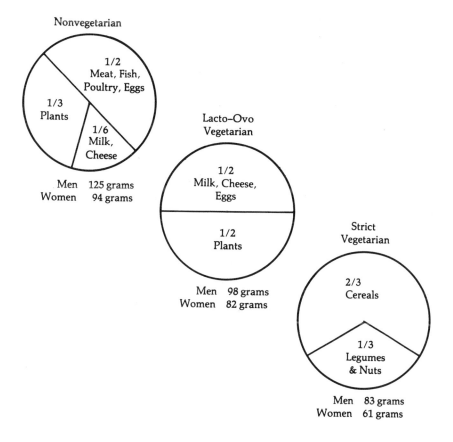

Exhibit 9.15. Protein sources in the average American diet.

eggs are similar in protein composition, supplying sufficient amounts of all the essential amino acids, while plant proteins are less complete and have limiting amounts of one or more essential amino acids. The differences in amino acid content and protein efficiency of plant and animal proteins is discussed on page 178. The most important fact to remember is that including a small amount of animal protein in the same meal with plant protein will enable a person to make more effective use of the amino acids in the plant protein.

Foods in this group have a high satiety value due to their fat and protein content. Both of these nutrients take longer to digest than carbohydrate, and fat tends to slow down the passage of food through the stomach. The proteins and fats from animal foods are almost completely (97 percent) digested. The plant protein foods are less completely digested because of their fiber content. Only a small portion of fiber is broken down in the human digestive tract (see Chapter 7).

In the average diet, foods in the meat group supply about 40 percent of our iron, 30 percent of our thiamin, 25 percent of our riboflavin, and 60 percent of our niacin. Other minerals and vitamins found in significant amounts in the meat group are other B vitamins—B_6, B_{12}, and folic acid (organ meats and legumes are the best sources of folic acid)—and the minerals phosphorous, potassium, sodium, magnesium, copper, and other trace minerals such as colbalt, manganese, and zinc. This group is also a source of about 55 percent of the fat in the American diet.

Nutrients not found in this group in any appreciable amounts are calcium (except if bones, for example from canned fish, are eaten) and vitamins C, A, and D. Exceptions are egg yolks, which contain vitamin A, liver, which stores these vitamins, and the fat of certain fish, which may contain vitamin D. Carbohydrate is not found in the animal foods in this group, except for small amounts of glycogen. The plant protein foods contain both starch and fiber.

Iron content is highly variable in this food group with organ meats such as liver, heart, and kidney being rich sources of iron, the nonred flesh of poultry and fish (except for oysters) being relatively low in iron, and red meats having average amounts. Cooked dry beans and peas and peanuts provide iron in comparable amounts to meat. However, the iron from plant foods is in a less available form and therefore less of it is absorbed by the body (see Chapter 11).

Exhibit 9.16 shows comparisons in nutrients and calories between ground beef, liver, frankfurters, fish, chicken, and cooked dry beans. Note that frankfurters are higher in calories than the other meats and lower in the other nutrients. This is because their fat content is high (up to 30 percent is allowed), and they may contain up to 10 percent water. The fat is homogenized and does not drip out much when frankfurters are cooked. Note also that liver is low in calories, because of the small amount of fat it contains, and rich in all of the B vitamins as well as vitamins A and C and protein and iron. Pork, which is not included in the exhibit, is particularly high in thiamin.

Two Variables: Fat and Water

Fat and water are the two major variables in animal foods, with most raw products having 50 to 60 percent water. Some of the water leaches out during cooking, carrying some of the water-soluble nutrients with it.

Fat may be distributed among the muscle fibers (called marbling) or deposited as an exterior covering. The deposited fat can be trimmed and discarded to cut down on fat and calorie consumption. But the fat intermingled with the fibers is not removable, except for that which melts and drips out during cooking. It is the fat that adds flavor to meat and makes it seem more juicy, but it has little or no effect on tenderness.

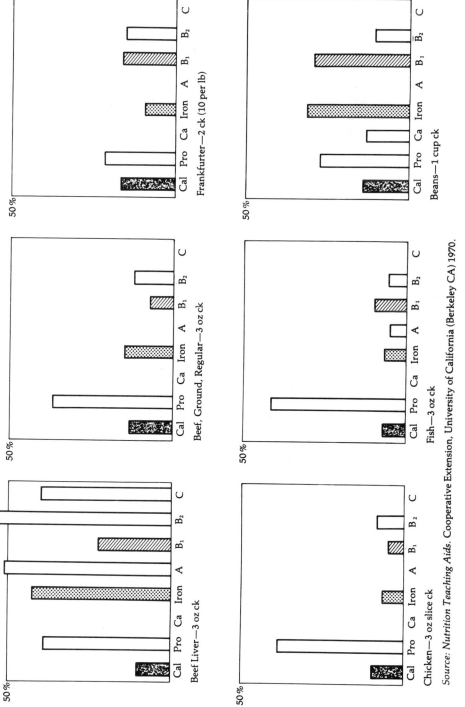

Exhibit 9.16.   Comparison of nutrients in some popular protein foods: percent of daily adult requirement.

Source: Nutrition Teaching Aids. Cooperative Extension, University of California (Berkeley CA) 1970.

189

In general, because the flesh of poultry has less intermingled fat than the flesh of beef, pork, or lamb, poultry is lower in fat, proportionately higher in protein, and lower in calories than other meats. White poultry meat has less fat than dark meat and somewhat fewer calories, but also smaller amounts of iron.

The meat cuts vary in the amount of fat by:

Age. The younger animals, such as lamb and veal, have less fat.

Breed Hogs genetically are fatter than other animals, but new breeds on the market are almost as low in fat as some beef animals.

Grade. Top grade beef animals are "finished" by grain feeding, which results in higher fat content; lower grade animals often are simply grass fed.

Location of the cut on the animal. The flank and hind leg, or "round," in beef have less fat within the meat than the shoulder or loin, for example.

For a comparison of the fat and calorie content of some popular meat cuts see Exhibit 9.17.

With fish, the fat and water content varies by species. The lean varieties have much less fat than meat and many fewer calories. Calories in the leanest species, such as crab and scallops, may be just 100 or less per three and one-half-ounce serving, compared to 220 for the same amount of lean beef. Calories for other fish range from 130 to 200 per serving. This explains why fish is so prominent in weight control diets!

Exhibit 9.17   Calories in Cooked Meats

| | | CALORIES | |
| | | FAT NOT | |
AMOUNT		REMOVED	LEAN ONLY
3 oz	Hamburger patty, broiled	250	190
3 oz	Beef chuck, pot-roasted	250	180
3 oz	Beef rib, roasted	290	210
3 oz	Beef round, roasted	220	160

Most fish and shellfish fall into the low-fat, high-protein group. These products have less than 5 percent fat and more than 15 percent protein. Included in this group are tuna, halibut, cod, flounder, haddock, ocean perch, whiting, crab, scallops, shrimp, and lobster. The fat content of many fish in this class is closer to zero than to 5 percent. Oysters and clams have a fat content of less than 5 percent and a protein content of less than 15 percent, with water being the other major component.

Medium-fat, high-protein fish are those with 5 to 15 percent fat and more than 15 percent protein. Included in this group are anchovies, herring, mackerel, salmon, and sardines. Only a few fish are in the high-fat, low-protein group—those that contain more than 15 percent fat and less than 15 percent protein. Fish in this category include certain kinds of lake trout and, during particular seasons, herring, mackerel, and sardines.

Cooking Method Adds or Subtracts Fat

The method of preparation has an important effect on the fat and calorie content of foods in the meat group. In broiling and roasting, fat drips out during cooking, whereas in frying, especially if a breaded coating is added, fat may be absorbed. Much fat can be drained off ground beef when it's cooked in crumbled form for casseroles and other dishes. However, when ingredients such as bread or cracker crumbs are added to ground beef that is made into meat loaf or meat balls, they absorb and hold fat. In stews and other meat dishes where gravies are included, the fat content increases greatly unless all of the fat is removed before the gravy is thickened. Creamed fish and poultry dishes also have greatly increased amounts of fat and calories. Exhibit 9.17 shows how fat and calorie amounts might vary.

Saturated Versus Polyunsaturated Fats

While the protein value of animal foods is similar, there are notable differences in the degree of saturation of their fats. (See Chapter 8 for a discussion of saturated and polyunsaturated fats.) The fat of beef, pork, and lamb contains 44 to 54 percent of the saturated fatty acids palmitic and stearic, 41 to 48 percent of the monounsaturated fatty acid oleic, and only 2 to 10 percent of the polyunsaturated fatty acid linoleic. Beef is higher in saturated fats than pork or lamb.

In contrast, the approximate fatty acid content of poultry fat is: 33 percent saturated, 39 percent monounsaturated, and 22 percent polyunsaturated. For fish fat is: 40 percent saturated, 40 percent monounsaturated, and 15 to 20 percent polyunsaturated, although this varies by species.

All animal foods contain cholesterol, and fish, meat, and poultry flesh are similar in cholesterol content. Exceptions are organ meats, such as liver; certain shellfish, particularly shrimp; and egg yolks—all of which are high in cholesterol. See Exhibit 9.18 for a comparison of the amount of cholesterol in some common foods. The controversy about the consumption of saturated fats, cholesterol, and the recommendation that egg yolk use be reduced as a method of preventing coronary heart disease is discussed in Chapter 19.

Exhibit 9.18.   Cholesterol Content of Common Measures of
Selected Foods (in ascending order)

Food	Amount	Cholesterol
		Milligrams
Milk, skim, fluid or reconstituted dry	1 cup	5
Cottage cheese, uncreamed	½ cup	7
Lard	1 tablespoon	12
Cream, light table	1 fluid ounce	20
Cottage cheese, creamed	½ cup	24
Cream, half and half	¼ cup	26
Ice cream, regular, approximately 10% fat	½ cup	27
Cheese, cheddar	1 ounce	28
Milk, whole	1 cup	34
Butter	1 tablespoon	35
Oysters, salmon	3 ounces, cooked	40
Clams, halibut, tuna	3 ounces, cooked	55
Chicken, turkey, light meat	3 ounces, cooked	67
Beef, pork, lobster, chicken, turkey, dark meat	3 ounces, cooked	75
Lamb, veal, crab	3 ounces, cooked	85
Shrimp	3 ounces, cooked	130
Heart, beef	3 ounces, cooked	230
Egg	1 yolk or 1 egg	250
Liver, beef, calf, hog, lamb	3 ounces, cooked	370
Kidney	3 ounces, cooked	680
Brains	3 ounces, raw	more than 1700

[1] Source: "Cholesterol Content of Foods," R. M. Feeley, P. E. Criner, and B. K. Watt. J. Am. Diet. Assoc. 61:134, 1972.

The plant protein foods in this group do not contain cholesterol. Foods from the legume family, except peanuts and soybeans, have very little fat—less than 1 percent. Soybeans, however, have about 20 percent fat, of which 55 percent is polyunsaturated linoleic acid. Peanuts and other nuts and seeds contain nearly 50 percent fat, with the degree of polyunsaturation variable by species. Peanut oil, for example, has less polyunsaturated fat (30 percent) than sunflower seed oil (70 percent).

Nuts and seeds, particularly sunflower seeds, are popular snack foods, and in recent years soynuts also have gained some popularity. The oil content of nuts and seeds makes them very high in calories. However, in addition to their relatively large amount of protein (20 to 30 percent), they also are rich sources of such important nutrients as iron and B vitamins. Peanuts are notable for their high niacin content, and sunflower seeds and soynuts for their high iron content. Exhibit 9.19 shows a comparison of the calories and nutrients in peanuts, sunflower seeds, and soynuts. Note the higher protein value and lower calorie content of soynuts.

Dry-roasted nuts have become popular with calorie-conscious consumers because many people believe these nuts to be lower in calories. However, the difference in calories between dry-roasted and regular oil-roasted nuts is too small to make a difference, just 6 calories per ounce. It is not the roasting process but the fat hidden inside the nuts that contributes most to the caloric level!

Some years ago researchers developed a peanut that does have fewer calories because some of the fat is removed. These partially defatted peanuts, even though they have a "peanutty" flavor and crunchy texture, have not received widespread distribution and use.

Exhibit 9.19   Comparison of Some Key Nutrients in Peanuts, Soybeans (or Soynuts) and Sunflower Seeds

100 GRAMS (3.3 OZ)	PEANUTS	SOYBEANS (OR SOY NUTS)	SUNFLOWER SEEDS
Calories	585	403	560
Protein—Grams	26	34	24
Fat—Grams	50	18	47
Iron—Milligrams	2.1	8.4	7.1
Niacin—Milligrams	17.2	2.2	5.4
Riboflavin—Milligrams	.13	.31	.23
Thiamin—Milligrams	.32	1.10	1.96

Source: B. Watt and A. Merrill, *Composition of Foods, Raw, Processed, Prepared.* U.S. Department of Agriculture, Agriculture Handbook No. 8, 1963, Washington, D.C., pp. 43, 58, 61.

Ways to Save Money on Protein Foods

The animal foods in this group are the most costly of all foods to produce since animals are used as "middlemen" to process the foods they are fed into food for people. It is much more efficient for people to eat food directly. For example, an acre of land that could yield 500 pounds of protein from soybeans would give only 50 pounds of protein if used to grow feed for beef cattle.

The price of feed grains has a direct influence on the price of meat. Chickens are the most efficient protein producers, while beef cattle are the least efficient (see Exhibit 9.20). This is an important reason why chickens and eggs are usually such good buys compared to other meats. This is also why people in less developed countries are encouraged to raise chickens and eggs for food.

As our nation has become more affluent, our consumption of meat, particularly beef and poultry, has increased considerably, as illustrated in Exhibit 9.21. The heavy consumption of meat in the United States often is criticized as being wasteful of grain resources. Agricultural economists, however, point out that grazing animals produce food from lands that could not be utilized for growing other crops because they are too hilly, rocky, or infertile. When grain prices go up, more cattle go to market without being "finished" on grain.

Exhibit 9.20 Protein Feed Required to Make a Pound of Protein

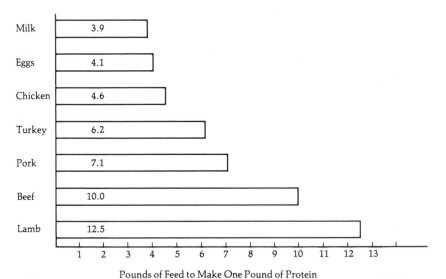

Pounds of Feed to Make One Pound of Protein

Source: Peng, A., Plant Proteins and Their Utilization. The Ohio State University, Cooperative Extension Service, Bulletin No. 524, 1970, p. 5.

Inflation has caused the price of meat to more than double in ten years. Consequently, many American families have found it necessary to look for ways to reduce their spending for foods in the protein group.

Eat Less. Since most Americans get more protein than they need, an economical way to improve our diets is to reduce our consumption of foods in this group by eating smaller portions and increase our consumption of breads, cereals, vegetables, and fruits. This change would result in diets lower in saturated fat and calories and higher in starch, fiber, calcium, and vitamins A and C. It was recommended as a Dietary Goal by the U.S. Senate Select Committee on Nutrition and Human Needs (see Chapter 18).

The usual recommendation is that we have two servings of foods from the protein group each day. But what is a serving? Generally a

Meat Consumption Per Person

	1975	1976	1977	1978[1]
	Pounds			
Total per capita				
meat consumption	182.4	194.7	193.0	187.0
Beef	120.1	129.3	125.9	120.3
Veal	4.2	4.0	3.9	3.0
Lamb and mutton	2.0	1.9	1.7	1.6
Pork	56.1	59.5	61.5	62.1

[1] Forecast.

Data published currently in *Livestock and Meat Situation* (ESCS).

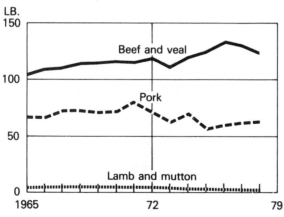

Pounds in carcass-weight basis. 1978 forecast.

Exhibit 9.21. In the last 50 years, beef has become increasingly popular, while the use of pork and lamb has dropped. (*Source: 1978 Handbook of Agricultural Charts.* U.S. Dept. of Agriculture, Agriculture Handbook No. 551, Washington, D.C., p. 81).

COUNT AS A SERVING 2 OR 3 OUNCES OF COOKED LEAN MEAT, POULTRY OR FISH — — SUCH AS

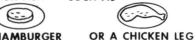

A HAMBURGER   OR A CHICKEN LEG   OR A FISH

ALSO-2 EGGS ◯ ◯

OR 1 CUP ▱ COOKED DRY BEANS OR PEAS

OR 4 TABLESPOONS ∬∬ PEANUT BUTTER

serving of meat is one which provides two to three ounces of lean meat: a medium-size hamburger patty (¼-pound cooked hamburger yields about three ounces), half a chicken breast or one leg, one pork chop (cut three to a pound), a piece of fish or meat with bone and fat removed measuring 2½ by 2½ by inches, two eggs, one cup cooked dry beans or peas, or four tablespoons peanut butter (Exhibit 9.22). In comparison, a T-bone steak, ½ inch thick, would supply six to eight ounces of protein.

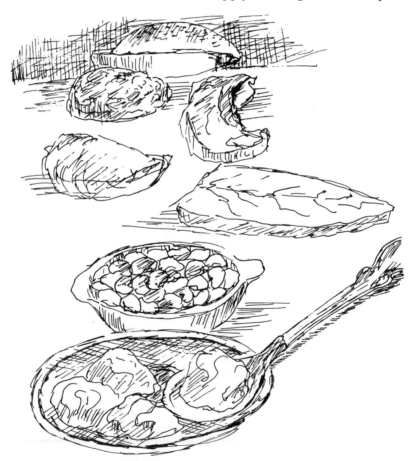

Exhibit 9.22. Since most Americans eat more protein foods than they need, one way to save money is to eat smaller portions.

Use Less Popular Cuts. The less tender meats, those from the parts of the animal that get the most exercise, such as the leg, rump, and shoulder, sell for a lower price per pound than the more tender higher priced cuts from the back, but they are just as nutritious. They do require longer, slower cooking to tenderize them, however. The least popular, least expensive cuts are the organ meats, such as liver, heart, and kidney, and they are the most nutritious part of the animal.

Consider the Amount of Waste. Some meat cuts that seem inexpensive because they have a relatively low price per pound actually cost more than other cuts selling for a higher price per pound because they have such a high proportion of waste, that is, bone and fat (see Exhibit 9.23). To determine which cuts give the most meat for the money, calculate the cost per serving by dividing the price per pound by the number of servings per pound. To be a better value, a cut yielding only two servings per pound would have to sell for less than half as much as a cut yielding four servings per pound.

Buy Larger Cuts and Bone-in Cuts. Boneless cuts and smaller convenient size portions almost always cost more than larger cuts. Do your own meat cutting to get more meat for your money.

Use Meat Extenders. Breads, cereals, rice, cracker crumbs, and dry milk make meat go farther. Because the protein in the meat complements the protein in the cereal products, the body will use the less complete plant protein more efficiently.

Exhibit 9.23. How Much Meat to Buy: Proportion of Lean to Waste

AMOUNT OF WASTE	SERVINGS PER POUND	EXAMPLES OF MEAT CUTS
No bone, little fat	4 to 5	Liver, kidney, boneless steaks and roasts, lean ground beef, stew meat, boneless ham.
Little bone, little fat	3 to 4	Round steak, ham steak, sirloin tip roast, leg of lamb, regular (25–30% fat) ground beef, pork sausage.
Medium bone, medium fat	2 to 3	All bone-in steaks and chops of beef, pork, and lamb; shoulder or chuck roasts, rump roasts, whole ham or ham butt.
Much bone, much fat	1 to 2	Short ribs, spareribs, beef and ham shanks, neck, brisket, breast, bacon.

COST OF ⅓ OF A DAY'S PROTEIN, MEATS AND MEAT ALTERNATIVES
AVG. RETAIL PRICES IN U.S. CITIES

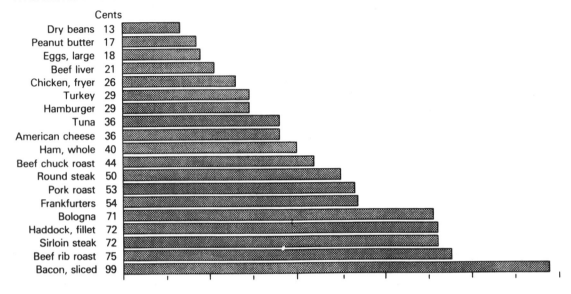

Cents

Dry beans	13
Peanut butter	17
Eggs, large	18
Beef liver	21
Chicken, fryer	26
Turkey	29
Hamburger	29
Tuna	36
American cheese	36
Ham, whole	40
Beef chuck roast	44
Round steak	50
Pork roast	53
Frankfurters	54
Bologna	71
Haddock, fillet	72
Sirloin steak	72
Beef rib roast	75
Bacon, sliced	99

Based on ⅓ of recommended dietary allowance for 20-year old man; costs for June 1978.

Exhibit 9.24.   While prices of these foods change considerably, especially during times of inflation, the relative cost of various products has remained similar over the years. (*Source: 1978 Handbook of Agricultural Charts.* U.S. Dept. of Agriculture, Agriculture Handbook No. 551, Washington, D.C., p. 49).

PER CAPITA CONSUMPTION OF SELECTED LIVESTOCK PRODUCTS

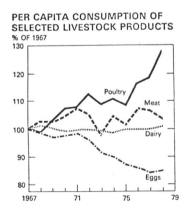

Exhibit 9.25.   Egg consumption in the United States has dropped dramatically in the past ten years, while poultry consumption has increased. (*Source: 1978 Handbook of Agricultural Charts.* U.S. Dept. of Agriculture, Agriculture Handbook No. 551, Washington, D.C., p. 55)

Use More of the Less Expensive Protein Foods in Place of Beef and Pork. Exhibit 9.24 shows a comparison of the cost of one-third of a day's protein from the different types of foods in the protein group (plus cheese). Eggs, poultry, some kinds of fish, beans, and peanut butter are all economical sources of protein.

Eggs as a Protein Source

Of all the protein foods, eggs are the most nearly perfect in terms of amino acid content for human needs. Egg protein is the yardstick against which all other protein foods are measured. The protein-to-fat ratio (that is, the amount of protein you get in proportion to fat) is higher in eggs than in meat. Egg yolks are a good source of biologically available iron and vitamin A as well as the B vitamins thiamin and riboflavin.

While their water content is higher than that of most other protein foods (74 percent), eggs have very little waste. Other advantages are their ease of preparation, their versatility, and the important contribution they make as an ingredient that provides protein structure in many foods.

Even though eggs are one of our best protein buys, Americans are eating fewer and fewer of them (see Exhibit 9.25). The reason appears to be related to their cholesterol content and the publicity about the controversy over the relationship between egg consumption and blood cholesterol (see Chapter 19). False notions that people have about eggs—for example, that brown-shelled eggs are more nutritious than white (they aren't, the color varies with breed of hen) or that fertilized eggs are superior to unfertilized (laboratory analysis shows no significant biochemical differences)—may cause some people to pay higher prices for eggs supplying no better nutrition than they would get from ordinary eggs.

For those people who need to restrict their cholesterol intake, imitation egg products are available to take the place of eggs. In these products the cholesterol-containing yolk has been replaced with milk protein (sodium caseinate) and vegetable oil. Minerals and vitamins are usually added. A comparison of the nutritive value of two brands of egg substitutes with a large egg is shown in Exhibit 9.26. Note that brand number 1 is much lower in calories than an egg because it has much less fat and somewhat less protein. Note also that sodium and potassium content is higher in the egg substitutes than in the egg.

Imitation Meats

The rising cost of producing animal protein and an increasing interest in vegetarian and cholesterol control diets have stimulated the research and development of imitation meat products. Called *meat analogs,* these products are made from protein derived from plants, usually

Exhibit 9.26   Nutritive Value of Egg Substitutes

	SECOND NATURE®	EGG BEATERS®	LARGE EGG*
Amount equivalent to 1 large egg	3 T (47 g)	¼ cup (60 g)	1 (50 g)
Protein, g	4.7	6.6	6.5
Fats, g	1.6	7.5	5.6
polyunsaturated, g	0.8	4.0	0.5
monosaturated, g	0.6	—	2.5
saturated, g	0.3	1.2	2.0
Carbohydrate, g	less than 1	—	0.5
Cholesterol, mg	—	less than 1	275.0
Sodium, mg	79.0	109.0	61.0
Potassium, mg	143.0	128.0	77.0
Calcium, mg	30.0	49.0	27.0
Phosphorus, mg	40.0	43.0	103.0
Iron, mg	1.1	1.1	1.3
Vitamin A, IU	803.0	810.0	590.0
Vitamin D, IU	23.0	26.0	—
Thiamin, mg	0.05	0.08	0.05
Riboflavin, mg	0.14	0.26	0.15
Niacin, mg	0.05	—	0.05
Calories	35.00	100.00	82.00

Source: B. Watt and A. Merrill, *Composition of Foods: Raw, Processed, and Prepared.* U.S. Department of Agriculture, Agricultural Handbook No. 8, Washington, D.C., 1963, p. 30.

soybeans or wheat. Another type of product is the meat extender, a form of soy protein added to ground meat to make it go farther.

Meat analogs synthesized from soy and wheat protein will not have as high a level of all the amino acids found in meat unless those which are lacking are added. Soy protein lacks methionine, for example, and wheat lacks lysine. Vitamin B_{12} also is lacking in the analogs unless it is added since this vitamin is found only in animal foods. The iron in these plant products is thought to be less available than that in meat, but the level of B-vitamins (other than B_{12}) is nearly comparable to meat.

Many different soy products are being used as meat replacements (see Exhibit 9.27). They include:

Soy flour. Made from dry soybeans; contains 40 percent protein.

Defatted soy flour. Soy flour with fat removed; contains 50 percent protein.

Textured soy protein. Defatted soy flour that is textured by an extrusion process.

Soy protein concentrate. Hard to digest carbohydrates are filtered out; contains 70 percent protein.

Soy protein isolate. More carbohydrates removed; contains 90 percent protein.

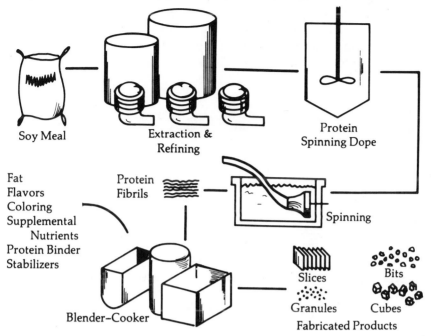

Soy Meal

Extraction & Refining

Protein Spinning Dope

Fat
Flavors
Coloring
Supplemental
Nutrients
Protein Binder
Stabilizers

Protein Fibrils

Spinning

Blender–Cooker

Slices

Bits

Granules

Cubes

Fabricated Products

Process Used to Make Textured Soy Products.

Exhibit 9.27. (*Source: Soybeans as a Protein Source.* University of California, Division of Agricultural Sciences, Leaflet 2762, 1975)

Spun fibers. With 95 to 98 percent protein—made from the soy protein isolate, which is dissolved in an alkaline substance, then "spun" into threads by a spinning machine much like the type used to make nylon fibers. An acid solution then congeals the fibers into pale gold threads of nearly pure protein. The threads are tasteless, odorless, and resemble taffy in texture. They can be woven into analogs to which flavors, colors, fats, and other nutrients (such as iron, niacin, thiamin, riboflavin, and methionine and other amino acids) are added. The resulting product can be made to resemble chicken, turkey, pork sausage, ham, hot dogs, fish, steak, ground beef, or just about any kind of meat. This process is considerably more costly so that the usual imitation meat product is made instead with the less costly, less refined forms of soy protein, such as defatted soy flour or soy protein concentrate.

You might expect that the meat substitutes would cost less than real meat since soybeans can be grown much more cheaply than animals. But while meat extenders generally have been less costly than meat, many analogs cost as much or more than meat because they continue to be specialty items and are not mass-produced or widely consumed. Consumer acceptance, which depends on eating quality, has been less enthusiastic than anticipated. The marketing and promotion has been based, not on the analogs' cost, but on the fact that they contain no cholesterol and no animal fat (polyunsaturated fats are usually added). Their high-sodium content has been a deterrent to their use by some people who are on special diets for the control of high blood pressure or coronary heart disease.

SUPERMARKET NUTRITION: CHOOSING A NO-MEAT DIET

Man is usually considered to be an omnivorous animal, thriving optimally on a mixed diet of both plant and animal foods. However, vegetarian diets based primarily on plant foods date back to ancient civilizations and continue to be followed in many parts of the world. In the past 15 to 20 years, plant food diets have gained in popularity in the United States, especially among the youth counterculture groups.

An estimated third of the world's people subsist on a vegetarian type diet, not from choice, but from necessity. The costly-to-produce animal foods are simply not available or are too scarce and expensive for the majority of people to use except on rare occasions. Some other reasons why people choose vegetarian diets include:

1. Religious beliefs that recommend against or prohibit meat eating.

2. Reverence for life, or belief in nonviolence, and a repugnance for killing living creatures to eat them.

3. Ecological concern that raising animals for food is a wasteful use of land resources.

4. Health beliefs that are based on the idea that a person can enjoy better health by eating only plant foods.

Broadly defined, vegetarians are people who eat no meat. However, there are several kinds of vegetarians:

1. *Total* or *strict vegetarians*, popularly called *vegans*, who eat only plant foods. Their diets include fruits, vegetables, legumes, cereal grains, honey, molasses, and plant oils. They get about two-thirds of their proteins from cereals and one-third from legumes and nuts.

2. *Ovo-vegetarians*, who use eggs along with plant foods.

3. *Lacto-vegetarians*, who use dairy products plus plant foods.

4. *Lacto-ovo-vegetarians*, who use both eggs and dairy products plus plant foods. About half of their protein comes from milk, cheese, and eggs, and the other half from plants. With careful planning, this group is most likely of all the vegetarians to have a nutritionally adequate diet.

Vegetarian diets, especially those having no animal foods at all, involve some nutritional risks, but they also have some advantages (see

Exhibit 9.28   Vegetarian Diets: Potential Benefits and Risks

ADVANTAGES	DISADVANTAGES
Low in fat and cholesterol	May lack sufficient amounts of all essential amino acids
Low in calories	May lack vitamin B_{12}
High in fiber	May lack sufficient calcium
Less expensive	May lack sufficient iron
	High in phytates, which may tie up trace elements

Exhibit 9.29). Because these diets have few or no animal foods they tend to be low in fat, and particularly low in saturated fat. There is some evidence that persons following vegetarian diets have lower blood cholesterol levels and reduced risk of coronary heart disease.

The vegetarian diet not only is lower in fat but also is higher in fiber than the typical mixed diet. This means fewer calories. Because of this, the typical strict vegetarian is likely to be 10 to 20 pounds underweight. (Very few vegetarians are overweight.) Because high-priced animal foods are omitted and lower priced legumes and cereals are used for protein instead, the vegetarian diet tends to be more economical.

However, the more limited the vegetarian diet is in animal foods, the higher the risk of nutritional deficiency. Potential nutritional risks include:

1. Insufficient protein, or an insufficient amount of all of the essential amino acids needed to build body tissue. (The differences in amino acid content of plant and animal foods is discussed earlier in this chapter.)

2. Lack of vitamin B_{12}. Since this vitamin is found, with a few minor exceptions, only in animal foods, the strict vegetarian is in danger of eventually developing a vitamin B_{12} deficiency. An additional problem is that pectin, found in large amounts in many fruits and some vegetables, can cause depletion of vitamin B_{12} in the body. Cellulose, another fibrous component of plants, also can deplete B_{12} when consumed at high levels.

3. Insufficient calcium intake may result when no dairy products are consumed. The calcium found in green leafy vegetables may be rendered unavailable by the presence of oxalic acid in these foods.

4. Iron deficiency may also result from a diet lacking in animal foods and red meats in particular. Iron from plant foods (nonheme iron) is less available to the body than iron from animal foods (heme iron).

5. Phytates or phytic acid, a component of the fibrous portion of whole grains, interferes with the absorption not only of iron but also of

other minerals, including zinc and copper. A diet high in whole-grain cereals could potentially result in a deficiency of these trace minerals.

6. Because energy-rich fats are low in vegetarian diets, the sheer volume of food needed to meet energy needs may be more than the average person, particularly if he is a child, can consume.

It is obvious that attaining a nutritionally balanced vegetarian diet is a challenge. It requires careful planning and close attention to including a variety of plant foods in every meal.

Most important is combining different sources of plant protein in order to have a full complement of adequate amounts of all of the essential amino acids. The amino acids need to be present together in the same meal. If even just one amino acid is present only in very small amounts, the body's ability to utilize the other amino acids in building body protein is limited.

Understanding this fact is vital for planning a strict vegetarian diet that supplies adequate protein. The vegetarian must know which amino acids are limited in the various plant foods and plan to combine plant foods, in the same meal, so that amino acids that are limited in one food are compensated for in another food.

Refer to Exhibit 9.11 and the discussion earlier in this chapter for information on combining complementary plant proteins to ensure an adequate supply of all the essential amino acids.

The use of fortified soybean milk, which has vitamin B_{12} and calcium added, is recommended for the strict vegetarian. The use of dark green vegetables, dried fruits, soybeans, and nuts can provide additional calcium as well as iron and other trace minerals. The use of increased amounts of breads, cereals, fruits, and vegetables is necessary to meet the strict vegetarian's calorie needs (see Exhibit 9.29). The sample menu plan for a strict vegetarian is shown in Exhibit 9.30. The nutrient evaluation of it shows that it is reasonably well balanced except for its calorie content. An improvement might be made by adding at least two cups of fortified soy milk and reducing the quantity of other foods eaten (for example, eat just one cup of pea soup for lunch and fewer nuts).

A vegetarian diet for a growing child must be planned with particular care to ensure an adequate supply of all essential amino acids, calcium, iron, folic acid, vitamin B_{12}, and all other nutrients to meet the child's growth requirements. A varied, well-planned lacto-ovo-vegetarian diet (Exhibit 9.31) will be adequate, but generally other vegetarian diets, especially those having no animal foods whatsoever, cannot be counted upon to optimally fulfill the child's nutrient needs.

To sum up, it is easier to get the nutrients we need from a mixed diet of plant and animal foods. However, good nutrition is possible for adults on an all-plant diet if the person has knowledge of food composition and uses skill in applying that knowledge to food selection.

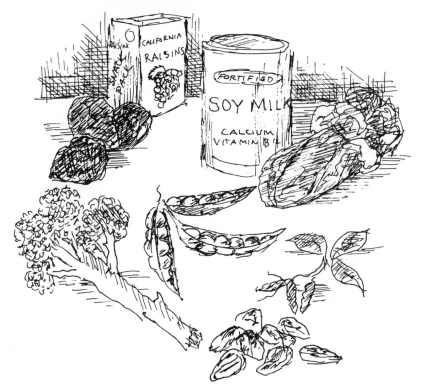

Exhibit 9.29.   Foods to emphasize in a vegetarian diet.

Summary

Proteins, comprising three-fourths of the body, are the largest and most complex of the nutrients. They are made up of basic units termed *amino acids,* which are linked together in a variety of unique forms. Proteins contain nitrogen in addition to carbon, hydrogen, oxygen, and sometimes other elements. The nitrogen, which differentiates proteins from other nutrients, is obtained originally by plants from the soil and from the air by the action of *nitrogen-fixing bacteria.*

Amino acids are coupled together by peptide linkages; hence a two- or three-amino acid fragment is termed a *dipeptide* or *tripeptide,* while a group of many amino acids linked together is termed a *polypeptide.* Proteins may be either *simple,* containing only amino acids, or *conjugated,* united with other compounds.

Protein's major function is building and maintaining body tissue, a continuous process due to the dynamic equilibrium state in which the body exists. Other functions include maintenance of water and acid-base balance; formation of enzymes, hormones, and antibodies; vitamin interaction; and production of energy at four calories per gram. When utilized as a source of energy, protein then becomes unavailable for other functions.

EARLY MORNING

Orange	1 medium
Bulgur	1 cup
with brewer's yeast	1 tablespoon
Toasted wheat-soy bread	1 slice
with honey	1 tablespoon

MID-MORNING SNACK

Shelled almonds	¼ cup

MIDDAY MEAL

Split pea soup	2 cups
Peanut butter sandwich:	
Peanut butter	2 tablespoons
Whole wheat bread	2 slices
Honey	1 tablespoon
Fruit-sunflower seed salad:	
Apple	½ medium
Banana	½ medium
Sunflower seeds	¼ cup
Lettuce	1 leaf

SNACK

Peach	1 medium

EVENING MEAL

Soybeans	1 cup
Brown rice cooked	1 cup
fried in oil	2 tablespoons
with chestnuts	2 tablespoons
with sesame seeds	2 tablespoons
Collards	1 cup
Pear	1 medium

EVENING SNACK

Raisins	¼ cup

Source: "Shopper's Guide." 1974 Yearbook of Agriculture, U.S. Department of Agriculture, Washington, D.C. 1974, p. 16.

We need protein both for its nitrogen and for the eight or nine essential amino acids our bodies cannot manufacture. The value of the protein we obtain from various foods depends on the amount of protein present, how effectively our body can use that protein, amino acid composition, total protein and calorie content of our diet, and amino acid balance.

Body protein can be built only if all essential amino acids are present at the same time. By including some form of animal protein in each meal, one insures a source of essential amino acids. If a meal has no animal foods, a variety of plant proteins can be eaten that will complement one another. Most Americans obtain several times as much protein

Exhibit 9.31   Meal Plan for an Ovo-Lacto-Vegetarian Diet

207
Summary

EARLY MORNING MEAL
Pineapple juice
Wheat flakes with milk
Doughnut (enriched)
Coffee

MID-MORNING
Peach

MIDDAY MEAL
Hard-cooked eggs—cream sauce
Whole-wheat bread—butter or margarine
Brussels sprouts
Molasses cookies   Milk

EVENING MEAL
Vegetarian baked beans
Green pepper stuffed with rice and tomato sauce
Tossed green salad   French dressing
Raisin pie
Milk

Nutritional Foundation of This Day's Food

MILK GROUP 2 CUPS	FRUIT-VEG. GROUP 4 SERVINGS	MEAT OR ALTERNATE 2 SERVINGS	BREAD-CEREAL— 4 SERVINGS (ENRICHED OR WHOLE GRAIN)
1 cup as beverage ½ cup with cereal ½ cup in cream sauce	1 serving— pineapple juice 1 serving—peach 1 serving— brussels sprouts 1 serving—green pepper	1 serving—2 eggs 1 serving— vegetarian baked beans	1 serving—wheat flakes 1 serving— doughnut 1 serving— whole-wheat bread 1 serving—rice

Foods That Provide Additional Nutrients and Food Energy to Meet Individual
Needs

FROM THE 4 FOOD GROUPS	FROM OTHER FOODS
Milk as beverage and in coffee Remaining ingredients in cream sauce Molasses cookies—enriched Tomato sauce Tossed green salad Raisin pie	Butter or margarine with bread Sugar in coffee French dressing

Source: "Shopper's Guide." 1974 Yearbook of Agriculture, U.S. Department of Argiculture, Washington, D.C. 1974, p. 15.

as they actually need. Animal proteins tend to be high in both calories and saturated fat; therefore, extremely high animal protein diets may contribute to obesity and coronary heart disease. There are additional dangers associated with unbalanced high-protein diets.

Proteins are broken down into peptide fragments and eventually into amino acids during the digestive process. Allergic reactions may be experienced by people whose digestive system allows larger protein fragments to be absorbed. Many metabolic pathways are available to amino acids once they are absorbed. Deaminated amino acids that enter the carbohydrate cycle are termed *glucogenic,* while those metabolized as fatty acids are termed *ketogenic.* The liver plays a key role in protein metabolism.

OUR NEED FOR WATER 10

Highlights

Significance of water as a solvent and carrier of nutrients and
other substances

How water is obtained and lost

Intracellular and extracellular water retention

Water as a coolant

Water, an inorganic compound, is classed as a nutrient because it is essential to life. However, it is not a source of energy like fats and carbohydrates, nor does it build or repair body tissue as does protein. Instead, it functions primarily as a solvent and transport vehicle for nutrients, wastes, and body substances.

While we can live without food for weeks, or until we deplete our stored carbohydrate and fat and a large portion of our body protein, we cannot survive without water for more than a few days (and we cannot live without oxygen for more than a few minutes). Water makes up between 55 and 65 percent of our body weight (up to 70 to 75 percent in infants). The loss of just 10 percent of body water results in serious consequences, and we will not survive if we lose 20 to 22 percent of it. The turnover of water used in the body is high: about 6 percent of the total is taken in and excreted every day.

We get our water from three sources:

1. The liquids we drink
2. The foods we eat, which contain varying amounts of water—from 5 percent in very dry foods such as crackers to 90 percent in juicy fruits
3. Our bodies, which produce water from the metabolism of carbohydrates, fats, and proteins.

We lose water through three mechanisms:

1. Evaporation of water from the skin
2. Respiration of water vapor from the lungs
3. Elimination of water in urine and feces.

This water cycle is illustrated in Exhibit 10.1.

Usually our intake of water and our excretion of water is finely balanced and averages between 2 to 2.5 liters in and out per day. If water losses are greater than intake, for example, in hot weather, during strenuous exercise, or as a result of vomiting or diarrhea, we become thirsty and will drink liquid to compensate. If we don't drink enough to displace the lost water, our thirst will trigger hormone action that will cause the kidneys to conserve water by making the urine more concentrated. If we consume more water than we need, our kidneys will excrete more-diluted urine.

LOCATION AND FUNCTIONS OF WATER

Water is found in the body in two places, within cells (*intracellular*) and outside of cells (*extracellular*). Maintenance of the balance of intracellular and extracellular water is very important. If too much water re-

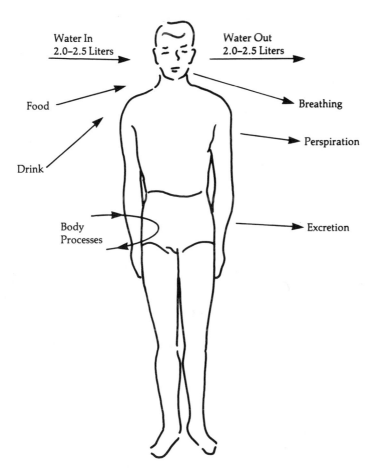

Water In
2.0–2.5 Liters

Water Out
2.0–2.5 Liters

Food

Drink

Breathing

Perspiration

Body
Processes

Excretion

Exhibit 10.1.   The water cycle: In the normal person under normal circumstances, water input and water output are maintained in balance.

mains in the cells, they swell, and the condition is called *edema*. On the other hand, if cells pump out too much water, they dehydrate and may collapse, bringing on symptoms of dehydration such as weakness, dizziness, and eventually collapse of the cardiovascular system.

The water moves in and out of cells through the cell membranes, which are semipermeable, by a process called *osmosis*.[1] Osmosis is the movement of water through a semipermeable membrane from a solution of lower concentration to a solution of higher concentration. The dissolved substances in the water, particularly the minerals sodium, potassium, and chloride (called *electrolytes*) and some sulfate, carbonate, phosphate, and proteins, create the osmotic pressure which regulates this movement of water into and out of cells.

[1]A semipermeable membrane allows some substances but not others to penetrate it.

SOLVENT AND CARRIER OF:
　　Nutrients and oxygen into cells
　　Wastes and other substances out of cells
　　Blood cells, hormones, antibodies
LUBRICANT:
　　For joint movement
CUSHION:
　　For body organs
SUPPORT:
　　For body cells
REGULATOR:
　　Of body temperature

In this movement, water carries nutrients and oxygen into the cells and carries out wastes and substances needed elsewhere in the body. Thus, water functions as the chief transport vehicle in the body. It is able to do this effectively because it is a solvent for almost all the essential nutrients and other substances the body produces and uses.

The extracellular water, which makes up about 15 to 20 percent of body weight, is found in a number of different places in the body where it performs different functions (see Exhibit 10.2):

1. In the blood, water is a major constituent of plasma and has a vital solvent-transport function carrying blood cells, nutrients, wastes, and other substances, and additionally, it maintains normal blood volume.

2. In the lymph system, water provides a solvent transport medium for nutrients, hormones, antibodies, etc.

3. In saliva, mucous, and the gastrointestinal tract, water functions as a lubricant as well as a transport medium and as a necessary compound for hydrolysis (splitting with water) of fats, carbohydrates, and proteins during digestion.

4. In the synovial fluid of bone ends, water serves as a lubricant for the movement of joints.

5. In the cerebrospinal fluid, which covers the surface of the brain, the spinal cord, and the pleural fluid, which covers the lungs, water serves as a cushion, protecting these delicate organs from striking against the bony cage in which they are held; water in the amniotic sac in the uterus has the same cushioning effect for the fetus.

6. In the interstitial (between cells) fluid, water bathes the cells and is held in readiness for movement into cells with nutrients, as needed.

Within cells, water has the important function of maintaining cell structure. As mentioned earlier, in situations where water is lacking, dehydrated cells will collapse.

Another vital function of water is regulation of body temperature. Through the evaporation of water from the skin, the body can regulate its temperature within reasonable limits of the normal range. Thus, when the outside temperature is high, we perspire more freely to help cool our bodies. And when we exercise and produce body heat, we perspire profusely to reduce body temperature and keep our bodies from overheating. Replacement of water lost during exercise is vitally important for this purpose and is discussed in greater detail in the section on teenage athletes in Chapter 16.

The consequences of failure to keep our bodies from overheating may be heat exhaustion and heat stroke. Heat exhaustion from water depletion, if extreme, can result in coma and death and is characterized by pronounced thirst, fatigue, muscle cramps, rapid heart rate, giddiness, and infrequent urination. Heat stroke is caused by the failure of the body to regulate its temperature by sweating.

The loss of water through perspiration or excretion is associated with a loss of the salt from the body. The use of salt on foods in extra amounts as well as drinking plenty of water is advised in situations where persons work or exercise in a hot environment and perspire profusely for extended periods of time. Salt-depletion heat exhaustion, brought on by the replacement of water lost during prolonged periods of sweating, accompanied by inadequate replacement of salt, is characterized by fatigue, nausea, vomiting, giddiness, exhaustion, fainting, rapid pulse, low blood pressure, difficulty breathing, and heat cramps, but not usually a high temperature.

Summary

From this brief review you can see that water is indeed essential. It is the solvent and transporter of nutrients, wastes, and many compounds produced and used in the body. It serves as a shock absorber, a lubricant, a coolant, and a chemical reactant, and functions both within and outside body cells. We obtain it from the water we drink and the foods we eat and drink, as well as from chemical reactions within the body. We lose it through excretion of urine and feces, perspiration, and expiration. Excessive losses or inceases in the body water are obviously not compatible with a healthy existence.

MINERAL ELEMENTS 11

Highlights

Inorganic nutrients as a whole and individually

Macro and micro elements

Interrelationships and toxicity

Action of mineral elements on the body, requirements and
deficiency effects, and sources

Supermarket Nutrition: Choosing Foods From the Milk Group

Mineral elements are inorganic substances that are essential components of both plant and animal tissues and that, by definition, are neither vegetable nor animal.[1] Like vitamins, mineral elements are needed in the body in small amounts and their prime function is regulating body processes (see Exhibit 11.1).

If a human body is cremated, the organic (carbon-containing) elements will be burned and the remaining material, equivalent to about a five-pound bag of sugar, is mineral or ash. Minerals, all together, make up about four percent of our body. About half of this is calcium, one-fourth is phosphorus, and the remainder is small amounts of other minerals (see Exhibit 11.2).

Exhibit 11.1   Recommended Daily Dietary Allowances, Minerals

| | AGE (YEARS) | MINERALS | | | | | |
		CALCIUM (MG)	PHOSPHO-RUS (MG)	MAGNE-SIUM (MG)	IRON (MG)	ZINC (MG)	IODINE (μG)
Infants	0.0–0.5	360	240	50	10	3	40
	0.5–1.0	540	360	70	15	5	50
Children	1–3	800	800	150	15	10	70
	4–6	800	800	200	10	10	90
	7–10	800	800	250	10	10	120
Males	11–14	1200	1200	350	18	15	150
	15–18	1200	1200	400	18	15	150
	19–22	800	800	350	10	15	150
	23–50	800	800	350	10	15	150
	51+	800	800	350	10	15	150
Females	11–14	1200	1200	300	18	15	150
	15–18	1200	1200	300	18	15	150
	19–22	800	800	300	18	15	150
	23–50	800	800	300	18	15	150
	51+	800	800	300	10	15	150
Pregnant		+400	+400	+150	*	+ 5	+ 25
Lactating		+400	+400	+150	*	+10	+ 50

Source: Recommended Dietary Allowances, Ninth Edition (revised 1979). National Academy of Sciences, Washington, D.C.

* The increased requirement during pregnancy cannot be met by the iron content of habitual American diets nor by the existing iron stores of many women; therefore the use of 30–60 mg of supplemental iron is recommended. Iron needs during lactation are not substantially different from those of nonpregnant women, but continued supplementation of the mother for 2–3 months after parturition is advisable in order to replenish stores depleted by pregnancy.

[1]Although technically the word *minerals* refers specifically to metals, the terms *mineral* and *element* are usually used interchangeably to describe this group of substances, some of which are metals and others of which are gases or other types of inorganic materials.

MACRO-ELEMENTS	MICROELEMENTS
Sodium	Iron
Calcium	Manganese
Phosphorus	Copper
Potassium	Iodine
Sulfur	Zinc
Chlorine	Fluorine
Magnesium	Chromium
	Cobalt
	Selenium
	Molybdenum

Human beings normally do not eat minerals in their pure or elemental forms, but rather as components of other nutrient substances, either of organic or inorganic origin, such as *calcium carbonate*, a mineral found in water.

Scientists divide the essential elements into two general categories, depending on the amount needed (see Exhibit 11.2). *Macroelements* are those that are present in relatively large amounts in the body and are needed in relatively large amounts in the diet—more than 100 milligrams. One Spanish peanut weighs about 500 milligrams; so to get an idea of what 100 milligrams looks like, visualize one-fifth of a peanut.

Microelements or trace elements are those needed in very minute amounts. For example, the Recommended Dietary Allowance for iron for adult females is 18 milligrams (about 1/25th of a Spanish peanut), and the amount needed of some other minerals is measured in *micromilligrams.* Each micromilligram, or microgram, is 1/1000th of a milligram.

Different minerals often work together as a team or in combination with vitamins, fats, proteins, or carbohydrates. But some minerals are antagonistic: an excess of one can nullify the effects of another. In addition, excess amounts of essential minerals often can be toxic. Thus, it is important that we obtain minerals in our diets in properly balanced amounts.

The many functions of minerals in the body might be grouped together in two categories: building and regulating. Building functions affect the growth and maintenance of the skeleton, teeth, blood, and all soft tissues. Regulating functions include the stimulation of chemical reactions that affect heartbeat, blood clotting, and nerve responses; maintenance of internal pressure of body fluids; regulation of acid-base balance; and the transport of oxygen from lungs to tissues and carbon dioxide from tissues to lungs.

In many instances, minerals function as integral parts of the enzymes, coenzymes, and hormones that are catalysts for metabolic reactions such as transmission of nerve impulses, muscle contractions, and so forth. As we consider the functions of the various elements, we will learn what roles they play in some of these essential functions.

Information about elements is presented here in a condensed, simplified form for easy comprehension. The references cited at the end of the book contain more detailed explanations of their functions in the body.

MACROELEMENTS

Sodium

Forms and Location. Sodium's most common form is as salt (*sodium chloride*). It is found, for the most part, in the body in blood plasma and fluids outside of cells (*extracellular fluids*).

Functions/Mode of Action.

1. Exerts osmotic pressure in fluids to help maintain normal water balance (see Chapter 10).

2. Helps the kidney maintain the acidity of the blood within normal limits and thereby helps maintain the body's acid-base balance.

3. Along with potassium, helps in the relaxing of a contracted muscle by involvement in neuromuscular transmission of nerve impulses. This function is especially important in maintaining the constant beat of the heart.

4. Facilitates absorption of various nutrients, including glucose, from the intestines.

Requirements and Deficiency Effects. Requirements are variable, depending on climate, amount of exercise, and other factors. If necessary, the body can adapt to low levels of sodium intake. A safe, low intake level is thought to be about 2.5 grams per day under average climatic and exercise conditions. Most people in the United States get five to ten times this amount. Deficiency symptoms, therefore, are rarely seen. In severe deficiency, cardiac arrest, convulsions, and generalized collapse could occur. See Chapter 10 for effects of salt-depletion heat exhaustion.

Sources. Ordinary table salt is our most common source. See Exhibit 19.6 for a list of sodium-containing foods. More information about the possible relationship between high-sodium diets and high blood pressure is presented in Chapter 19.

Form and Location. Potassium is found throughout the body, for the most part in cells (*intracellular fluid*) and as a nearly constant component of lean body tissue. Its common form is *potassium chloride.*

Functions/Mode of Action.

1. Functions on inside of cells, as sodium functions outside, exerting osmotic pressure to help maintain normal water balance.
2. Helps the kidney control the acid-base balance of the body.
3. With sodium, plays important role in transmission of nerve impulses from nerves to muscles across the neuromuscular transmission systems. This is particularly important in maintaining regular heart beat.

Requirements and Deficiency Effects. Healthy adults need about 2.5 grams of potassium per day, but our bodies apparently can cope with a wide range of intakes.[2] Potassium is a nearly constant component of lean body tissue (muscles, connective tissue, etc.). Need increases during periods of growth, including pregnancy, and also when we need to rebuild body tissue, for example after an injury, surgery, or a period of deprivation, including a strenuous low-protein diet. Some potassium is lost in sweating, and much is lost in diarrhea or from the use of diuretics, which are used, for example, to treat high blood pressure. A deficiency can cause irregular heart beats, muscle weakness, and poor intestinal tone. Death has resulted from serious potassium deficiency caused by excessive use of diuretics—for example, in a weight loss diet.

Sources. Potassium is abundant in almost all foods, both plant and animal. Especially high in potassium are fish, meat, legumes, potatoes, tomatoes, bananas, citrus fruit, dried fruit, spinach, carrots, broccoli, and milk.

Chlorine

Form and Location. Chlorine is the gas that forms the chloride part of table salt, *sodium chloride* (NaCl). It is found throughout the body, both within cells and outside of cells, in cerebrospinal fluid, the gastrointestinal tract, blood, and as part of the hydrochloric acid (HCl) in the stomach.

---

[2]National Academy of Sciences, National Research Council, Food and Nutrition Board, *Recommended Dietary Allowances,* eighth edition. Washington, D,C., 1974, p. 90.

Functions in the Body.

1. As part of hydrochloric acid (HCl), is important in maintaining the acid pH of the stomach needed in the digestion process. HCl is needed for absorption of vitamin B_{12} and iron and also helps to keep microorganisms in food from multiplying in the body.

2. Within cells is bound to potassium as potassium chloride; outside of cells, to sodium as sodium chloride. With these two minerals, chlorine plays a role in maintaining the osmotic pressure and water balance.

3. Its movement between the plasma and red blood cells, termed the *chloride shift,* is instrumental in maintaining the acid-base balance in the blood as it transports carbon dioxide to the lungs.

4. Chlorine also is important for maintaining acid-base balance of other body fluids—cerebrospinal, interstitial, and lymphatic.

Requirements and Deficiency Effects. Obtaining enough chlorine usually is no problem since people ingest it when eating salt. A person on a low-salt diet may become deficient in chlorine and need to obtain it from another source. When sodium is lost from the body, for example in sweat, chlorine normally is lost too. Thus a deficiency could result from salt-depletion heat exhaustion. Extended vomiting and loss of stomach acid also could deplete chlorine supply.

Sources. Table salt generally supplies all the chlorine needed. The mineral also is found in meat, milk, and eggs.

Calcium

Form and Location. In food, calcium is combined with organic substances or in the form of inorganic salts such as calcium carbonate. In the body, 99 percent of the calcium is in bones and teeth. The remainder is found mostly in blood and extracellular tissues, with very little present in organs and soft tissues.

Functions/Mode of Action.

1. In combination with phosphorus (*calcium phosphate*), calcium forms amorphous (noncrystalline) and crystalline mineral substances that are deposited in the protein matrix, or soft collagen, of bones and teeth, making them hard and strong. This process is called *mineralization;* when calcium and phosphorus are removed from bones, the process is termed *demineralization.* Mineralization and demineralization—or remodeling—of bones goes on throughout life. Bones are remodeled by the formation of new cells on the outside and the reabsorption of old cells on the inside. Up through the fourth decade of life, bones grow in total mass; thereafter, there is more absorption and less calcium laid down, and bones become more porous.

2. In blood plasma, is an essential for blood clotting. It functions as a catalyst for various chemical reactions in the clotting process.*

3. Is needed for nerve stimulation, muscle contraction, and good muscle tone. Most important is its role in the contraction and relaxation of the heart muscle.

4. Is needed for the intracellular cement substances and various membranes and influences the permeability of cells.

5. Activates a number of enzymes, for example, those involved in digestion of fatty acids.

6. Combines with vitamin B_{12} to assist in its absorption.

Requirements and Deficiency Effects. Calcium needs are variable and depend on a number of factors that affect ability to absorb calcium (Exhibit 11.3). These include the phosphorus, fluorine, vitamin D, lactose, protein, and fiber content of the diet and the hormone production in the body.

The ideal ratio of calcium to phosphorus in the diet is one to one, except in infancy, when the ratio should be closer to two to one. Excess phosphorous can cause an acceleration in the rate of bone resorption and thereby increase the need for calcium. Fluorine is believed to help prevent withdrawal of calcium from the bones, especially in older or immobilized people. Because vitamin D enhances the calcification of bones, when it is present in adequate amounts, people can function with less calcium. *Lactose* (milk sugar) increases the absorption of calcium by 15 to 20 percent, which is one reason why milk is such a good food source of calcium. High-protein diets, on the other hand, appear to interfere with the absorption of calcium and may increase need. A diet high in fiber from cereals such as bran and vegetables is likely to be high in *phytic* and *oxalic acid,* which bind calcium so we are unable to absorb it.

Because of these variables and because data for calculating calcium requirements are not available, scientists do not know the optimum level of calcium intake. The Recommended Dietary Allowance (Exhibit 11.1) is higher than the Food and Agricultural Organization and the World Health Organization recommendation of 400 to 500 milligrams per day. The RDA for children ages 1 to 10 is the same as that for adults, while the recommendation is higher for teenagers during their growth spurt and for pregnant and lactating women. There is some evidence that after menopause women may need more calcium to prevent osteoporosis because of changes in their hormone balances.[3]

---

*A catalyst is a substance that brings about a chemical reaction without being changed itself.

[3]M. Winick, "Nutritional Disorders of American Women." *Nutrition Today,* September-October, November-December, 1975, pp. 26-28.

Exhibit 11.3 Factors That Affect Calcium Absorption

ENHANCE	IMPEDE
Adequate vitamin D	Excess protein
Lactose	Excess phosphorus
Adequate fluorine	High-fiber intake

In children, calcium deficiency, especially when accompanied by protein and vitamin D deficiency, can result in stunted growth, poor quality bones and teeth (teeth soft and prone to decay, for example), and malformation of bones (rickets). Many of these defects cannot be repaired in later life.

Calcium deficiency may not show up as any specific symptom in adults. If a diet is deficient in calcium, the body will rob the bones for the calcium needed for other functions, and an adult can lose 40 percent of bone mass before evidence is apparent even on an X-ray. *Osteoporosis,* gradual demineralization of bones, in older people, especially women, may be the long-term result of a diet deficient in calcium.

Our bodies have a very good mechanism for regulating the calcium in the blood to keep it constant. When the calcium level in the blood gets low, *parathyroid* hormone is secreted, which causes more bone to be reabsorbed. When the calcium level goes up, a hormone secreted by the thyroid gland, *calcitonin,* causes calcium to be quickly deposited in the bone. Apparently the body makes a permanent adjustment to calcium intake. When a person consumes large amounts of calcium regularly, his body absorbs less; and on a regular low intake of calcium, absorption becomes more efficient.

Sources. Milk and cheese are the richest sources of calcium; most other foods contribute just small amounts (see Exhibit 11.4). Other sources are green leafy vegetables, except those high in oxalic acid; dried beans and peas; canned fish such as sardines, mackerel, and salmon if the bones are eaten; oysters; and rhubarb.

Phosphorus

Form and Location. A universal cell component, phosphorus is available in all plant and animal food. Therefore, a dietary deficiency does not occur. A greater problem may be getting too much phosphorus in proportion to calcium, resulting in loss of calcium from bones. Like calcium, phosphorus is found in foods as phosphate in combination with organic substances or as inorganic salts. Before it can be absorbed, it must be converted to a soluble form. We absorb more phosphorus (50 to 70 percent) from food than calcium (20 to 40 percent). A deficiency of vitamin D can reduce absorption of phosphorus.

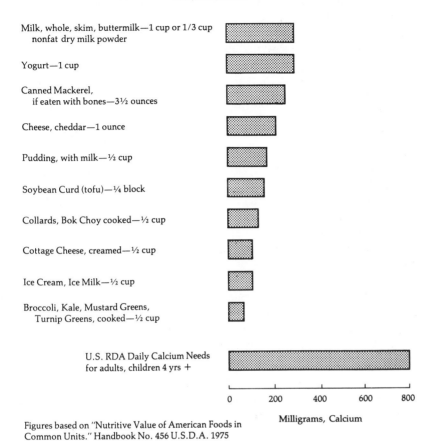

Figures based on "Nutritive Value of American Foods in Common Units." Handbook No. 456 U.S.D.A. 1975

Exhibit 11.4. (*Source: M. Hall, S. Burrill, EFNEP teaching aid* University of California, Cooperative Extension)

Functions/Mode of Action.

1. Works hand-in-hand with calcium in mineralization of bones and teeth (see Chapter 15).

2. In the form of inorganic phosphates, is an important buffer in body fluids to neutralize acidity.

3. In the form of organic phosphate, is a key component of many compounds having vital metabolic functions, including:

a. Nucleic acids—ribonucleic acid (RNA) and deoxyribonucleic acid (DNA)—which regulate protein synthesis in cells and carry the genetic code.

b. Phospholipids needed to promote emulsification and transport of fats and fatty acids. They are also constituents of cell membranes, regulating movement of dissolved substances in and out of cells.

c. Adenosine mono-, di-, and triphosphates (AMP, ADP, ATP), which store and control the release of energy.

d. Niacin-containing coenzymes and the active form of thiamin needed in energy metabolism.

e. In addition, enzymes involved in many body processes are made from proteins that contain phosphate.

Requirements and Deficiency Effects. Because the ideal ratio of calcium to phosphorus after infancy is believed to be one to one, the Recommended Dietary Allowances for phosphorus (Exhibit 11.1) are set at the same levels as those of calcium. The efficiency of phosphate absorption varies with the source of the phosphorus and with the ratio of calcium to phosphorus in the diet.

While dietary phosphorus deficiency has not been observed, a depletion of this mineral can occur as a result of a vitamin D deficiency or a person taking nonabsorbable antacids, such as *aluminum hydroxide* or *calcium carbonate*, which keep phosphorus from being absorbed. Symptoms of deficiency are weakness, loss of appetite, general feeling of ill health, and pain in the bones. Vitamin D supplements or discontinuance of the antacids and provision of adequate phosphorus in the diet can eliminate the symptoms. Other reasons for phosphorus deficiency are genetic abnormalities that block vitamin D metabolism, liver disease, and use of other drugs such as phenobarbital and anticonvulsants.

Sources. All plant and animal foods supply phosphorus. It is especially plentiful in meat, poultry, fish, eggs, cheese, milk, and whole-grain cereals. Phosphorus tends to be found in the seeds of plants, while calcium is found in the green leaves.

Magnesium

Forms and Location. Magnesium is another mineral found in all body tissue, especially in bones. It is closely related to calcium and zinc and, like calcium, is present in food in the form of somewhat insoluble salts or as a part of organic compounds. The magnesium salts are poorly absorbed and appear to follow the same route in the body as calcium salts do in absorption. Because of this, a high intake of calcium will interfere with magnesium absorption and vice versa. Excess supplies appear to be stored in the bones rather than excreted.

Other factors that affect magnesium absorption include total intake, the time food remains in the intestines (fiber in the diet can shorten this time), rate of water absorption, and the amounts of lactose and phosphate in the diet.

Functions/Mode of Action.

1. Catalyzes a large number of enzyme functions involved in energy transfer and release—for example, the conversion of ATP to ADP and the reverse.

2. Involved in protein synthesis and is essential for maintenance of RNA and DNA structure.

3. Plays an important role in maintaining the electrical potential in nerves and muscles needed for conducting nerve impulses to muscles to trigger their contraction and relaxation.

4. Promotes the activity of other biological agents, such as the release of the hormone *thyroxin* from the thyroid gland and the retention of calcium in tooth enamel.

Requirements and Deficiency Effects. Recommended Dietary Allowances for magnesium (Exhibit 11.1) are based on studies of the needs of adult males. The RDA for infants is based on the magnesium content of human milk. Allowances for other groups are only estimates.

Magnesium deficiency can be a complication of kwashiorkor and occurs frequently in alcoholics. Diabetics, surgical patients with restricted diets, and people who use diuretics for a long time also may develop magnesium deficiency. Apparently the body can adjust to wide variations in magnesium intake as it can for sodium intake. Dietary deficiency of magnesium for the average person is thought to be rare since magnesium is widely distributed in food.

Deficiency of magnesium causes neuromuscular problems—hyperexcitability with tremor and convulsions—which are sometimes accompanied by behavioral disturbances, delirium, and depression. Other symptoms are loss of appetite, nausea, and apathy. Calcification of soft tissue and low levels of calcium and phosphate in the blood also result from magnesium deficiency.

Sources. Plant foods, especially seeds, are the best sources of magnesium, while animal foods are poor or fair sources. Whole grains are a rich source, but milling removes much of the magnesium and enrichment does not replace it. Other good sources are milk, nuts, dried beans, and other vegetables. Since magnesium is a constituent of chlorophyl, green plants, especially leaves, are good sources. Coffee and cocoa also supply significant amounts.

Sulfur

Forms and Location. Sulfur is an element that does not receive much attention from nutrition scientists, and its complete function has not been established. It is a component of several essential amino acids—methionine, cystine, and cystein—as well as of the B vitamins thiamin and biotin. Mucopolysaccharides found in cartilage, tendons, skin, bones, and heart valves contain sulfur. Sulfur combined with fat (*sulfolipid*) is found in large amounts in the liver, kidneys, salivary glands, and the white cells of the brain. *Insulin* and *heparin*, an anticoagulant, are other body compounds that contain sulfur.

Functions/Mode of Action.

1. Sulfur compounds are involved in many oxidation-reduction reactions in the body. One important compound in these reactions, *glutathione,* is found in high concentration in red blood cells.

2. The metabolism of sulfur compounds results in the formation of sulfuric acid, which reacts with and detoxifies substances such as phenols, cresols, and steroid sex hormones.

Requirements and Sources. No Recommended Dietary Allowances for sulfur have been set. A diet that supplies enough of the sulfur-containing amino acids is believed to adequately meet the body's sulfur needs. These amino acids are found especially in meat, milk, eggs, and legumes. Sulfur is an easily recognized (from flavor and odor) constituent of the cabbage-family vegetables—cabbage, cauliflower, broccoli, and brussel sprouts. It is responsible for the "rotten egg" odor (*hydrogen sulfide* gas) produced when these vegetables are rotting and when eggs deteriorate and the sulfurous odor when these foods are cooked.

MICROMINERALS OR TRACE ELEMENTS

Iron

Forms and Location. Iron is the best known of the trace elements and the one that is the most likely to be lacking in our diet. It has received much attention from nutrition researchers. Iron is found in both organic and inorganic forms, and human bodies can use either form. In fact, we can absorb pure elemental iron, for example, that which might get into food from an iron cooking utensil. Absorption of iron is relatively poor: usually we absorb only about 10 percent of our intake. The less oxidized compounds of iron, the *ferrous* forms, are more readily absorbed than the oxidized, *ferric* forms. Vitamin C taken with iron improves its absorption because it protects ferrous iron from oxidation.

The organic iron that is part of hemoglobin, called *heme* iron, is in the ferrous form and is absorbed much better (up to 35 percent absorbed) than is the *nonheme* iron (less than 10 percent absorbed). We use nonheme iron from plants more efficiently if some heme iron from animals is present at the same time. Thus, meat in a meal significantly increases our absorption of nonheme iron. The reason for this is not known. In general, we absorb iron best when we eat a mixed diet.

In the body, 65 to 70 percent of the total iron is in the *hemoglobin* (an iron-protein) in red blood cells. Other "working forms" of iron in the body are *myoglobin* (an iron-protein similar to hemoglobin) in muscles and enzymes in every cell. A plasma protein, *transferrin,* holds iron and delivers it to tissues as needed. The storage forms of iron are *ferritin* and *hemosiderin,* which are retained in liver, spleen, bone marrow, and muscles and which are recycled in the body as needed for hemoglobin manufacture. Ferritin has a great capacity to store iron and holds about 20 percent of all the iron in the body.

Functions/Mode of Action.

1. Is a structural component of hemoglobin in red blood cells necessary for transport of oxygen from lungs to tissues and carbon dioxide from tissues to lungs. Hemoglobin also has a mild buffering function in maintaining the pH of the blood.

2. Is a component of *myoglobin* in muscles, essential for transfer of oxygen from hemoglobin to muscle cells.

3. Is an important part of enzymes needed in the oxidation reactions to release energy in the cells.

Requirements and Deficiency Effects. A unique feature of iron is that we lose very little of it and continually reuse it. An average man loses only about 0.9 milligrams per day, while a woman during menstrual years loses an average of 1.5 milligrams. Because red blood cells must be remade every 120 days, about 20 milligrams of iron a day are needed for this purpose.

Recommended Dietary Allowances (Exhibit 11.1) are based on the daily need for replacement iron and on the general assumption that only about 10 percent of dietary iron is absorbed. When iron stores decrease and iron needs increase, people are able to absorb more iron.

An ordinary mixed diet provides 5 to 6 milligrams of iron per 1,000 calories. Thus, men can easily meet their iron needs on an average diet, but many women and teenage girls who consume fewer than 1,800 calories a day will obtain only 10 to 12 milligrams of iron—less than the recommended amount. Other groups at risk of iron deficiency are infants and preschool children, adolescents, and pregnant women.

Iron-deficiency anemia results from inadequate iron intake. In iron-deficiency anemia, the red blood cells are small and contain less hemoglobin. This means their capacity to carry oxygen is reduced and less energy can be released. A person may have anemia with no symptoms or show signs of fatigue, listlessness, lack of energy, and inability to perform at peak proficiency both physically and mentally. Severe anemia can lead to an overworked heart.

Faulty digestion, increased infections, reduction in iron-containing enzymes, cellular damage, and low iron stores are additional outcomes of an iron-deficient condition.

Any condition that causes blood loss, such as hemorrage, or gastrointestinal bleeding, such as ulcers, can increase iron needs and result in iron deficiency. People with a genetic defect in which they lack transferrin in blood plasma have severe iron-deficiency anemia.

Excess iron is toxic, and supplemental iron should not be taken in amounts greater than the RDA. An iron overload of 100 milligrams a day for an extended time can result in deposition of iron in the liver, pancreas, spleen, and heart—a condition called *siderosis*. Deposition in the heart can cause heart failure; in the pancreas it may destroy the cells where insulin is produced.

Hemachromatosis is a condition in which an individual absorbs iron very efficiently—two to four milligrams a day instead of just one—and this can result in the problems listed above. A concern for people with

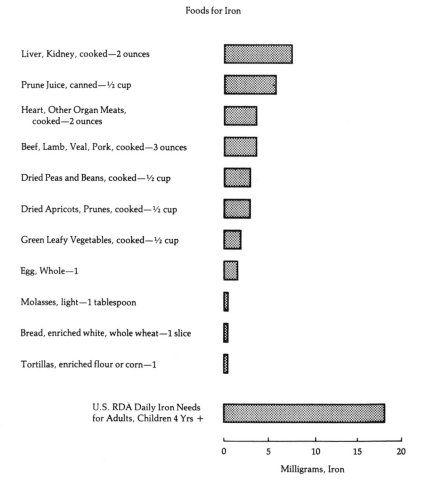

Foods for Iron

Liver, Kidney, cooked—2 ounces	
Prune Juice, canned—½ cup	
Heart, Other Organ Meats, cooked—2 ounces	
Beef, Lamb, Veal, Pork, cooked—3 ounces	
Dried Peas and Beans, cooked—½ cup	
Dried Apricots, Prunes, cooked—½ cup	
Green Leafy Vegetables, cooked—½ cup	
Egg, Whole—1	
Molasses, light—1 tablespoon	
Bread, enriched white, whole wheat—1 slice	
Tortillas, enriched flour or corn—1	
U.S. RDA Daily Iron Needs for Adults, Children 4 Yrs +	

0   5   10   15   20

Milligrams, Iron

Figures based on "Nutritive Value of American Food in Common Units." Handbook No. 456 U.S.D.A. 1975.

Exhibit 11.5. (*Source:* M. Hall, S. Burrill, EFNEP teaching aid, University of California, Cooperative Extension)

hemachromatosis led the Food and Drug Administration to recommend against increasing the amount of iron added to cereals and breads in the enrichment program.

Sources. Few foods are really rich sources of iron and these are foods that many people eat rarely or not at all: liver, heart, and oysters (see Exhibits 11.5 and 11.6). Red meats are good sources, but fish and poultry have much less iron. Refinement of cereal grains removes much of their iron, but most is added back in the enrichment process. Phytates in whole grains interfere with iron availability. Green leafy vegetables contain iron but are not good sources because the iron is not very available.

Many foods have small amounts of iron. Therefore, people have to work at getting enough iron in their diets all day long. A comparison of two menus (Exhibit 11.7) shows how low intake of iron can be improved by a few changes in each meal.

Exhibit 11.6 Sources of Iron

EXCELLENT	VERY GOOD	GOOD	FAIR
Liver (pork esp. high)	Shrimp	Egg	Potato
Heart	Sardines	Fish	Mushrooms
Oysters	Prunes	Asparagus	Sauerkraut
Clams	Apricots	Broccoli	Winter squash
Lean meat	Bran	Collards	Sweet potato
Chili con carne	Wheat germ	Tomato juice	Molasses
Dry beans and peas	Raisins	Dates	Whole wheat or enriched bread
Prune juice	Peanuts	Pickles	Chocolate
	Liver sausage	Bran flakes	Peanut butter
		Oatmeal	
		Enriched rice and pasta	

Copper

Forms and Location. We ingest copper in our diets in both organic and inorganic forms and can absorb elemental copper, for example, from food cooked in copper utensils. If we could nibble on a copper penny, there would be enough copper in it to supply our needs for three years.

Copper is present in all body cells but is concentrated in the blood and muscles. High concentrations also are found in the brain, liver, heart, and kidneys. At birth an infant has a high concentration of copper in the liver.

Exhibit 11.7   Comparison of the Iron Supplied by Two Menus

AMOUNT	FOOD	MILLIGRAMS IRON*	AMOUNT	FOOD	MILLIGRAMS IRON*
1/2 cup	Orange juice	0.1	1/2 cup	Tomato juice	1.1
1 cup	Corn flakes	0.8	1 cup	Oat flakes, fortified	2.4
1 cup	Milk	0.1	1 cup	Milk	0.1
Total for breakfast		1.0	Total for breakfast		3.6
1	Peanut butter sandwich		1	Peanut butter sandwich	
2 slices	Bread, white enriched	0.6	2 slices	Bread, white enriched	0.6
2 tablespoons	Peanut butter	1.2	2 tablespoons	Peanut butter	1.2
1 medium	Carrot	0.5	1 medium	Carrot	0.5
1 medium	Apple	0.4	4	Dried apricots	1.0
4	Sugar cookies	.6	4	Oatmeal raisin cookies	1.4
Total for lunch		3.3	Total for lunch		4.7
3 ounces	Fish, breaded	1.1	3 ounces	Fish, breaded	1.1
1 medium	Potato, baked	1.1	1 medium	Potato, baked	1.1
1/2 cup	Green beans	0.4	1/2 cup	Green peas	1.5
1 wedge	Iceberg lettuce	0.4	1 cup	Romaine lettuce	0.8
1/2 cup	Jello	0	1/2 cup	Chocolate pudding	0.4
Total for dinner		3.0	Total for dinner		4.9
8 ounces	Yogurt, fruit flavored	0.2	1 cup	Milk with 2 tablespoons molasses	2.5
20	Pretzel sticks	trace	1/4 cup	Sunflower seeds	2.2
Total for snacks		0.2	Total for snacks		4.7
TOTAL FOR DAY		7.5	TOTAL FOR DAY		17.9
PERCENT OF U.S. RDA		40%	PERCENT OF U.S. RDA		100%

*Source: C. Adams, Nutritive Value of American Foods in Common Units. Agriculture Handbook N. 456, U.S. Department of Agriculture, Washington, D.C., 1975.

Functions/Mode of Action.

1. Is needed in enzymes that are involved in the storage and release of iron to form hemoglobin. Thus, utilization of iron in the body is dependent on copper.

2. Has a key role in connective tissue metabolism and is needed in formation of elastin and collagen of the aorta.

3. Is part of enzymes involved in metabolism of glucose for energy release.

4. Is needed in formation of phospholipids in the nerve walls.

Requirements and Deficiency Effects. No Recommended Dietary Allowances have been established for copper, but a suggested range is 2–3 milligrams for adults. Severe copper deficiency is rare in man, suggesting that intakes are adequate. A typical adult man consumes 2 to 5 milligrams of copper per day and absorbs 0.6 to 1.6 milligrams.[4] Deficiencies in children generally have been seen as a result of kwashiorkor or other complications such as a defect in the copper-carrying protein in the blood, chronic diarrhea, or poor absorption. Some cases of anemia in children, resulting from intestinal malfunction or a high milk diet, require copper as well as iron to cure them. Copper deficiencies are also seen in premature infants fed exclusively on modified cow's milk for two to three months.[5] Infants with copper deficiency have anemia and low levels of copper in their blood and other tissues, plus bone demineralization and other blood disorders.

Sources. We obtain sufficient copper from a varied diet; in fact, it's difficult to get too little. Copper may be added to some foods during processing, for example, to milk, which might be passed across copper rollers; but it also is removed during processing. For example, when grain is milled, one-fourth of the copper is lost. On the other hand, in whole grains phytates bind copper and prevent its absorption.

Good sources of copper are nuts, dried beans and peas, some shellfish, organ meats such as liver, dried fruits, and cocoa. Copper content of vegetables depends on the copper content of the soil. Cow's milk is a poor source of copper, but human milk has enough to fulfill the requirements of an infant.

Iodine

Forms and Location. We use iodine in both inorganic and organic forms. Inorganic iodine usually is present as iodide. In addition, we also may absorb iodine through the skin if it is applied there. Most of the

[4]B. O'Dell, "Copper," in Nutrition Reviews' *Present Knowledge in Nutrition,* fourth edition. New York, Washington, D.C.: The Nutrition Foundation, Inc., 1976, p. 304.
[5]National Academy of Sciences, National Research Council, Food and Nutrition Board, *Recommended Dietary Allowances,* eighth edition. Washington, D.C., 1974, p. 95.

iodine in the body is in the thyroid gland and the remainder circulates in the blood. Iodine is another of the nonmetal elements with biological effects.

Function/Mode of Action. Iodine is a part of the thyroid hormones, *thyroxine* and *triiodothyroxine,* which regulate basal metabolism. Thyroid hormones also increase growth up to a certain level, but beyond this level they will break down body protein. Use of thyroid hormones in weight control programs is not considered wise because of this effect.

Requirements and Deficiency Effects. Only trace amounts, or micrograms, of this mineral are required. Infants need 40 to 50 micrograms per day, and children approximately 100 micrograms. Adults probably need 100 to 150 micrograms. The Recommended Dietary Allowances (Exhibit 11.1) provide for approximately double the minimum amount thought to be necessary to supply body needs.

An iodine deficiency causes goiter as the thyroid gland enlarges to try to make more thyroid hormones. Iodine deficiency during the first three months of pregnancy or prior to pregnancy can result in the birth of a child, called a *cretin,* who is dwarfed and mentally deficient. World-wide, two to five percent of children are believed to be retarded due to the lack of iodine.[6]

Excess iodine is toxic. An intake of 25 to 30 times the recommended levels over a long time can cause high levels of thyroxin, thyroid enlargement, impaired glucose tolerance, and heart failure. Persons having naturally overactive thyroid glands (*hyperthyroidism* or *Graves disease*) have protruding eyeballs and other symptoms of excess thyroid hormones.

Iodine toxicity has been observed in persons who overzealously eat large amounts of kelp (one popular weight control diet featured the use of kelp) or dried seaweed concentrate as a supposed "health food."

Sources. Iodine is found in minute amounts in seafood, kelp, and dried seaweed and in milk, cheese, and eggs when animals have been fed iodine-rich foods. Most vegetables are low in iodine, and the level depends on the iodine level in the soil. In the days before iodized salt and mass food distribution, the northern section of the United States was known as the *goiter belt* because the lack of iodine in the soil led to diets low in iodine.

Because of the unreliable distribution of iodine in foods, the addition of potassium iodide to table salt was initiated to prevent iodine deficiency. This supplementation is optional, and both iodized and noniodized forms of salt are available to consumers. Regular use of iodized salt is recommended, except in the case of persons with defective iodine-regulatory systems, because it will ensure an adequate supply of iodine for most people. Most food processors and food service establish-

[6]R. Cullen and S. Oace, "Iodine: Current Status." *Journal of Nutrition Education,* Vol. 8, No. 3, July-September, 1976, pp. 101-2.

ments do not use iodized salt, however; thus a person who eats all meals out might not get enough iodine.

Some foods, for example cabbage, contain *goitrogens*, which interfere with the body's use of iodine. On a normal mixed diet they are not of concern, but they have been known to cause iodine deficiency if they are consumed two or three times every day as a staple in the diet.

Zinc

Forms and Location. Organic compounds of zinc are found in both plants and animals. In the body, the highest concentrations of zinc are in the eye and spermatozoa, as well as the liver, bones, skin, hair, nails, and blood (especially in red blood cells).

Functions/Mode of Action.

1. Is an essential component of or cofactor with many enzymes that are responsible for such key functions as:
   a. Transport and transfer of carbon dioxide by red blood cells
   b. Metabolism and digestion of proteins
   c. Formation of RNA and DNA

2. Is cofactor with the hormone *insulin*, which regulates blood glucose levels, and of reproductive hormones.
3. Is a component of hair, nails, connective tissue, and blood and is needed to heal wounds.

Requirements and Deficiency Effects. The human requirement for zinc is well defined. An intake of 3 milligrams of zinc a day under 6 months of age and 5 milligrams from 7 to 12 months is sufficient. Adult intakes are 15 milligrams a day.

The Recommended Dietary Allowances (Exhibit 11.1) are based on the assumption that a varied diet of both animal and plant foods is consumed. We absorb only about half of the zinc in foods. Animal foods are higher in zinc than plant foods, and the zinc they contain is better utilized. In fact, deficiencies of zinc have been seen when diets are composed mainly of cereal grains because the phytates and fiber in whole grains interfere with the absorption of zinc. Actual intake of zinc in the United States is short of the RDA, and this is a matter of concern to some nutritionists. Some children have been found to have just a marginally adequate intake.[7] Pregnant women and women using oral contraceptives need more zinc.

Because of the critical role of zinc in many metabolic processes, all body systems are adversely affected by a deficiency. Deficiency can cause impaired growth of all tissue, impaired wound-healing, retarded maturation of sex organs, anemia, loss of taste, smell, and appetite, hair

[7]H. Sandstead, "Zinc," in Nutrition Reviews' *Present Knowledge in Nutrition*, fourth edition. New York, Washington: The Nutrition Foundation, Inc., 1976, pp. 290-95.

loss, growth failure in children, mental depression, and congenital malformations.

Dietary deficiency of zinc is rarely seen in the United States, but it has been observed in the Middle East where the soil is very deficient in zinc and a high cereal diet is consumed. Low levels of zinc in the blood have been observed in people having a number of conditions, particularly alcoholism and alcoholic liver disease, chronic kidney disease, chronic infections, tuberculosis, and other conditions that result in protein deprivation.

Sources. While all plants and animals contain zinc, the animal foods are better sources because their zinc is more available to us. Foods such as meat, fish, egg yolk, and milk are the best sources, and oysters are especially high in zinc. Good plant sources are peanuts, dried peas and beans, and whole-grain cereals.

Manganese

Forms and Location. Although their names are much alike and both are found in every living cell, manganese and magnesium are not at all alike in their action in the body. Manganese, while acting in every cell, is especially high in the pituitary gland, lactating mammary glands, liver, pancreas, kidney, intestinal wall, and bones.

Functions/Mode of Action. Manganese has many metabolic functions—as a catalyst, cofactor, or component of many enzymes—but scientists do not know exactly how it functions. Some of the activities of manganese include:

1. Synthesis of such complex carbohydrates as mucopolysaccharides
2. Utilization of glucose
3. Synthesis of fats and cholesterol
4. Development of the pancreas
5. Contraction of muscles
6. Formation of normal bone structure
7. Development of normal reproduction function

Requirements and Deficiency Effects. No Recommended Dietary Allowances have been set for manganese and no human deficiencies have been observed. Scientists estimate that the average adult needs 2.5 to 5 milligrams a day, and this is the amount found in normal diets. Only about 30 to 50 percent of manganese in food is absorbed. In animals deficient in manganese, many effects have been observed, such as slowed growth, crippling deformities, and interference with reproduction.

Sources. Manganese is found in all plant foods, but animal foods are not especially good sources. Nuts, grains, vegetables, and fruits all contain manganese. Refining grain causes a considerable loss, which is not replaced in the enrichment process.

Fluorine

Forms and Location. Fluorine, like chlorine, is a gas that is found as fluoride in foods and water in organic and inorganic forms. We absorb only soluble inorganic fluorides—not insoluble salts or organic fluoride. The soluble fluoride in drinking water is almost completely absorbed.

The highest concentration of fluorine in the body is in calcified tissues—bones, cementum, dentine, and enamel of teeth—but it is widely distributed in tiny amounts in soft tissues throughout the body. Once fluorine is incorporated in our bones, it stays there. Therefore, as we get older, the fluorine concentration in our bones increases.

Functions/Mode of Action. Unlike most other minerals, fluorine has no known metabolic functions although it does seem to activate or inhibit certain enzymes. Its presence in bones and teeth has a strengthening effect. If it is incorporated in the teeth when they are being calcified (infancy and childhood), it makes them more decay resistant (see Chapter 15). In addition, its presence in dental plaque is believed to inhibit the bacterial enzymes that form acids and break down tooth enamel.

Fluorine also is incorporated in our bones and may function in some way in the maintenance of bone structure, preventing calcium withdrawal and senile osteoporosis. This function has yet to be proven conclusively.

Because fluorine's essential role in the body is not established—technically, we can survive without it—scientists question whether it should be considered a true nutrient. The general scientific opinion today is that it is not an essential nutrient, but that it is needed for optimal health, especially of teeth.

Requirements and Deficiency Effects. No Recommended Dietary Allowances have been established for fluorine. The range of intake for people in this country is .03 to 3.1 milligrams per day. Most of what we take in is excreted: 80 percent in the case of children and 98 percent in the case of adults.

Sources. The average diet does not supply enough fluorine. The few good sources are tea, fish with bones, such as sardines, and bonemeal. In a few places in the country, the water supply is naturally high in fluorine (1.2 to 4 parts per million), and in these places children have been found to have very decay-resistant teeth. As a result of these findings, the idea of adding fluoride to water supplies as a way to improve fluorine intake was developed. Numerous studies have shown that fluoridation of drinking water at a rate of about one part per million is a safe, effective, inexpensive way to reduce the incidence of tooth decay. It may also be an aid to maintenance of strong bones in older adults.

However, fluorine is very toxic at not very high levels. For example, an intake of 6 to 10 parts per million will cause animals to develop deformed teeth and bones. At a level of 2.8 parts per million, mottling or staining of teeth will occur. (These mottled teeth, though unattractive, are very decay resistant.)

Concern about the toxicity of fluorine has caused many people to believe that fluoridation of public drinking water is a hazardous practice that should not be allowed. Vociferous protests by those who oppose fluoridation have resulted in this practice being discontinued or not initiated in many major population centers in the United States.

See Chapter 15 for the current recommendations for fluoride supplementation in infants and children.

MINOR TRACE ELEMENTS

The following elements are minor in the sense that at present scientists don't know very much about them, how they function, or why we need them. Perhaps in the years to come all of them, plus many others, will be considered to be as vital as the other minerals we have discussed.

Cobalt

Our only need for this mineral is believed to be in its organic form as part of vitamin B_{12}. Cobalt is present in almost all foods, and a deficiency in humans has not been observed.

Molybdenum

This mineral is a component of some essential enzymes. No Recommended Dietary Allowance has been set and no deficiencies have been observed in humans. Our need for molybdenum is minute and molybdenum is widely distributed in small amounts in many foods.

Selenium

In recent years, this element has become a fad nutrient, probably because it has an action similar to another fad nutrient, vitamin E. Totally unproven claims have been made about selenium's ability to cure illnesses such as cancer and heart disease, and to prevent such things as sexual dysfunction and aging.[8]

Selenium originally was thought to reduce the need for vitamin E because it too is an antioxidant. Now scientists think that it may be the other way around: the need for vitamin E may be to reduce the need for selenium! A selenium-containing enzyme is believed to protect the cell membrane and hemoglobin from oxidative changes and breakdown.

People in the United States who get a varied diet of both plant and animal foods probably get more than enough selenium to meet their needs, and no Recommended Dietary Allowance has been set. However, the quantity available from plant foods is dependent on the amount in the soil. In addition, quite a bit may be lost during milling of grain, food preparation, and processing.

Selenium is toxic, a fact discovered when grazing animals were poisoned by eating plants grown in soil having a high selenium level. On the other hand, selenium can help reduce the toxicity of other minerals, such as mercury. Because of selenium's toxicity, selenium supplements are not considered safe. They are also considered unnecessary because of selenium's wide availability in food. More information is needed about how selenium functions in the human body before any recommendations regarding the need for it are made.

Other Elements

These include those that have been found to be essential to some animals and that are being studied for their potential need by humans including chromium, silicon, nickel, vanadium, and tin. For example, recent studies suggest that chromium deficiency may be a causal factor in coronary artery disease and atherosclerosis.*

The entire field of trace elements is undergoing intense investigation at present and will certainly become more important to students of nutrition in the future.

SUPERMARKET NUTRITION: CHOOSING FOODS FROM THE MILK GROUP

Milk and such foods made from milk as cheese, yogurt, and ice cream make up one of the Four Food Groups primarily because they supply such large amounts of one key nutrient—calcium. The other ma-

---

[8]"Are Selenium Supplements Needed by the General Public?" *Journal of the American Dietetic Association*, Vol. 70, March, 1977, p. 249.

*H. A. Schroeder, "The Role of Trace Elements in Cardiovascular Diseases," in T. Labuza ed., *The Nutrition Crisis*, St. Paul, MN: West Publishing Co., 1975, pp. 374–92.

jor nutrients we get from milk, protein and riboflavin, are relatively easy to obtain from other foods, but the only other fairly good sources of calcium are green leafy vegetables and dried beans and peas (legumes). So when we don't use milk, it is very difficult to get enough calcium in our diets.

The recommended two-cup serving of milk per day for an adult will supply over 70 percent of our RDA for this nutrient, while four cups of milk will supply over 95 percent of a teenage boy's need for calcium. Milk's contribution of riboflavin is important too: two cups will supply about half of an adult's riboflavin needs, while four cups will supply all of a teenage boy's needs. Two cups of milk also supply about one-fourth of an adult's protein needs, and four cups will fulfill over half of a teenage boy's protein needs.

The milk proteins, casein and lactalbumin, are second only to egg protein in their growth-promoting ability. They supplement less complete proteins, for example those in cereals, better than other proteins. For this reason, milk-plus-cereal or milk-plus-toast make good breakfast combinations. The amino acid *tryptophan,* found in abundant amounts in milk, is thought to be important in the formation of neurotransmitters in the brain and also is believed to be an aid to inducing sleepiness that is more effective than sleeping pills. Thus, the long-recommended sleep-inducing remedy of a glass of warm milk may have some basis in fact.

Some other nutrients found in milk are lactose (milk sugar), fat, vitamins A and E, which are dissolved in the fat, and the minerals phosphorus and sodium. Phosphorus works with calcium in building bones and teeth and is present in a good ratio. Milk has small but worthwhile amounts of all of the B vitamins, including B_{12}, but very little vitamin C and iron. The iron is well assimilated, however. Not much vitamin D is found naturally in milk, but often it is added.

Kinds of Milks

Whole milk is about 87 percent water, 3.5 percent butterfat, 3.5 percent protein, and 6 percent lactose. Usually it is pasteurized and homogenized. Homogenization has no effect on nutritional value. It is simply a mechanical process, using centrifugal force, which breaks up the fat globules so they will not separate and rise to the top as cream.

Pasteurization is a brief heat treatment (161°F for 15 seconds) used to destroy bacteria, such as salmonella, that could cause disease. Pasteurization does not adversely affect the nutrients milk is important for, although it does reduce thiamin and vitamin C levels. Since milk is not considered a useful source of these vitamins, this change is not considered nutritionally important.

When butterfat is removed from whole milk to make nonfat or skim milk, the fat-soluble vitamins A and E are removed with it, and the calorie content is reduced approximately one-half, from 160 calories per cup to 85. The remaining nonfat milk is still just as rich as whole milk in calcium, protein, riboflavin, and other nutrients not dissolved in the fat. Because of this, people who are trying to reduce their calorie intake or their consumption of saturated fats are encouraged to use non-fat milk instead of whole milk. (See Exhibit 11.8 for information on fat content and calories in milk and dairy products.)

For those who don't like the taste of nonfat milk, a third type of milk—low-fat milk—is a popular choice. Standards for low-fat milk vary by state. In some states it contains two percent butterfat and has about 120 calories per cup; in other places it contains one percent butterfat and has 100 calories per cup. Another variable is the addition of extra amounts of milk solids, which increase the nutrients and calorie count about 15 per cup. The nutrition label will explain the fat and calorie content; the ingredient list will note if extra milk solids have been added.

Vitamin A may be added to nonfat and low-fat milks to bring the level back up to that of whole milk. Vitamin D also may be added to all forms of milk. This is an easy way of assuring that growing children and pregnant and lactating women get enough of this essential nutrient. In some states, the addition of vitamins A and D to milk is mandatory; in other states it is voluntary. If it's voluntary in your state, you will need to read labels to find out if these nutrients are added to the brand of milk you buy. The Food and Drug Administration limits the amounts: 2,000 IU of vitamin A and 400 IU of vitamin D per quart.

When all of the water, as well as the fat, is removed from milk by

Exhibit 11.8   Fat Content and Calories in Milk and Dairy Products

	PERCENTAGE FAT	CALORIES PER CUP
Whole milk	3.3	150
Low-fat (2%) milk		
No milk solids added	2.0	120
Milk solids added		125
Low-fat (1%) milk	1.0	
No milk solids added		100
Milk solids added		105
Nonfat (skim) milk		
No milk solids added	Trace	85
Milk solids added		90
Buttermilk	Trace	100
Chocolate milk	3.3	210
Chocolate drink (low-fat milk)	2.0	180
Plain yogurt (low-fat)	2.0	145
Flavored yogurt (low-fat)	2.0	230

Source: Nutritive Value of Foods. U.S. Department of Agriculture, Home and Garden Bulletin No. 72, Washington, D.C. 1977, p. 5–7.

dehydration, the remaining product is known as nonfat dry milk. The dry milk solids retain the essential nutrients—protein, calcium, and riboflavin—and when they are reconstituted with the same amount of water that was removed, the resulting milk is comparable in nutritional value to fresh nonfat milk.

Another form of milk is evaporated milk, which is usually sterilized in cans and has approximately half of the water removed. Undiluted evaporated milk contains about twice the amount of all the nutrients of whole milk and it is easily reconstituted by adding an equal amount of water. Evaporated milk also may be made from nonfat milk and will then contain half the calories of whole evaporated milk. Do not confuse evaporated milk with sweetened condensed milk, which is evaporated milk with a large amount of added sugar. The sugar helps to preserve it but also adds many calories.

Fermented Milks

Whole, low-fat, and nonfat milk all may be fermented or cultured to make buttermilk or yogurt. Lactic acid-producing bacteria are added to fresh pasteurized milk and allowed to grow at a lukewarm temperature. As the bacteria grow, they produce lactic acid from the lactose. The acid causes the milk protein to coagulate, or thicken, producing a sour, thick milk. Sometimes lactic acid may be added directly to milk instead of culturing the milk with bacteria.

Buttermilk normally is made from nonfat milk and is less thick than yogurt, which is usually made from low-fat or whole milk. Both buttermilk and yogurt have approximately the same nutritive value and calories as the milk from which they are made.

Extensive claims have been made about the miraculous nutritional value of yogurt, but the facts do not support these claims. Yogurt is simply another form of milk and is as nutritious as milk. Today the most popular yogurt is the flavored type, in which fruits, sugar, and other flavorings are added, doubling the calories and diluting the milk nutrients.

Acidophilus milk is a less common form of fermented milk. It is made by culturing milk with acidophilus bacteria. Because it has a softer and more finely divided curd than regular milk, it is sometimes used in special diets. Recently a new form of nonfermented acidophilus milk, called *sweet acidophilus,* was introduced. In this milk no fermentation takes place and its supposed benefit is due to the addition of the acidophilus bacteria to the intestines. Actual evidence of this beneficial effect is lacking, however.

Since the dairy industry traditionally prices milk on the basis of its butterfat content rather than nonfat milk solids, the higher the butterfat, the higher the price. So the products with the least amount of fat and calories usually give us the most food value for our money. Nonfat dry milk gives the best nutritional value of all.

Overuse of Milk

Occasionally a young child, usually a finicky eater, will drink so much milk that he does not have "room" for other important foods. This could lead to iron-deficiency anemia due to an insufficient intake of iron-rich foods such as meats and vegetables.

Infrequently, adults who drink unusually large amounts of milk, for example to help soothe an ulcer, are found to have problems from the ingestion of too much calcium. High cholesterol levels may also be related to overuse of high-fat, whole milk products by susceptible individuals.

People who lack the enzyme lactase, which is needed to digest lactose, may be able to drink just small amounts of milk. Often they can tolerate fermented dairy products such as yogurt and ripened cheese, because fermentation reduces the amount of lactose in these foods. (See Chapter 15 for more on lactose intolerance.)

A question mothers often ask is, "Will adding chocolate flavoring to milk reduce the availability of calcium?" Researchers have found that while the oxalic acid in chocolate does have the ability to bind some of the calcium in a form that is unusable in the body, the degree to which this happens is too small to significantly reduce the calcium content of the milk. Chocolate-flavored milk does have added amounts of sugar, however, and a significantly higher caloric value. So its constant use in place of unflavored milk might be considered undesirable.

Other Ways to Get Milk

Not everyone likes to drink milk, but many other forms of it can be included in the diet in order to provide a plentiful supply of calcium (see Exhibit 11.9). Exhibit 11.10 shows the amount of various types of milk-containing foods that need to be eaten to obtain as much calcium as is available from an eight-ounce serving of milk.

Milk can be included in many foods, such as soups, cereal cooked with milk, creamed or scalloped vegetables, puddings, custard, etc. Nonfat dry milk can be added to such foods as ground beef used in patties, meatballs, and meatloaf; homemade cookies, breads, and tortillas; and mashed potatoes.

Eating cheese is a popular way of adding milk to the diet and some forms of cheese have more calcium than others. Exhibit 11.10 shows that a person receives as much calcium by eating a 1½-ounce piece of processed American cheese as he does from drinking a glass of milk, but needs to eat 1⅓ cups (about 11 ounces) of cottage cheese to get this

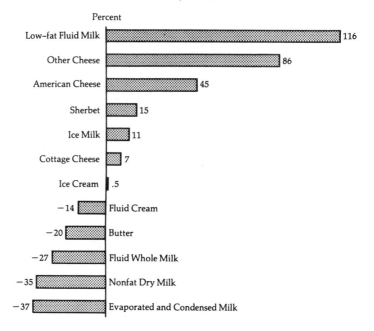

Changes in Per Capita Dairy
Product Sales, 1966–76

Percent

Low–fat Fluid Milk	116
Other Cheese	86
American Cheese	45
Sherbet	15
Ice Milk	11
Cottage Cheese	7
Ice Cream	.5
−14	Fluid Cream
−20	Butter
−27	Fluid Whole Milk
−35	Nonfat Dry Milk
−37	Evaporated and Condensed Milk

Exhibit 11.9.   Use of low-fat milk and easy-to-serve cheese products has been increasing greatly, while the use of other products has been declining. (*Source: 1977 Handbook of Agricultural Charts.* U.S. Dept. of Agriculture, Handbook No. 524, Washington, D.C., p. 79)

much calcium. This is because when cottage cheese is made, much of the calcium is lost in the whey (the liquid that separates from the coagulated protein curds).

Cheese is of two basic types: ripened, or fermented, and unripened, or fresh. A comparison of their calories, protein, fat, and calcium values is shown in Exhibit 11.11.

Fresh, unripened cheese has a short keeping time compared to ripened cheese. The two main types are cottage cheese and cream cheese. Cottage cheese is made from nonfat milk. After the curds (protein) have separated from the whey (liquid), a small amount of cream may be added to the curds to moisten them. Thus, there are three types of cottage cheese: nonfat cottage cheese—the dry curds—which tends to be dry and somewhat unpalatable; low-fat cottage cheese with about 2 percent fat; and creamed cottage cheese with 4 percent fat. Cream cheese, in contrast, because it is made from cream, has about 37 percent fat and is much higher in calories than cottage cheese. A good substitute for cream cheese is neufchatel cheese, which has about 20 percent fat.

Most ripened cheeses, such as cheddar, brick, and roquefort, are made from whole milk, although a few are made from low-fat milk (some types of mozzarella and ricotta) or skim milk (mysost and sapsota).

These Milk Products and Other Foods Containing Milk Give About as Much Calcium as 1 Cup of Fresh Whole Milk . . . or 1 Cup Milk Made From Nonfat Dry Milk.

243
Supermarket
Nutrition

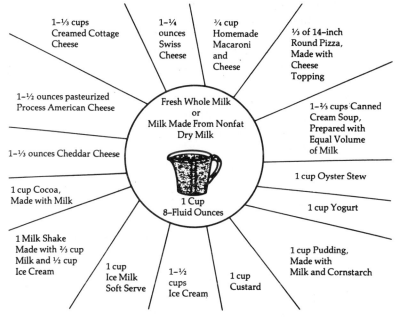

Exhibit 11.10. Calcium equivalents for one cup of fresh whole milk. (*Source:* Smart Shopper Recipe, U.S. Dept. of Agriculture, Consumer and Marketing Service, Washington, D.C.)

Exhibit 11.11 Comparison of Some Popular Forms of Cheese

	CALORIES PER OUNCE	PERCENTAGE OF FAT	PROTEIN PER OUNCE	CALCIUM PER OUNCE
Ripened Cheese				
Cheddar	115	35%	7 g	204 mg
Processed	105	30	6	174
Processed cheese food	95	24	6	163
Processed cheese spread	82	21	5	159
Unripened cheese				
Cream cheese	100	37	2	23
Cottage cheese, creamed	30	4	3.5	17
Cottage cheese, low-fat, 2%	25	2	3.9	19

Source: B. Watt, A. Merrill, *Composition of Foods: Raw, Processed Prepared.* Agriculture Handbook No. 8, U.S. Department of Agriculture, Washington, D.C. 1963, p. 81.

Ripened cheeses are very concentrated sources of protein, fat, and calories, but they are also very rich in calcium. Fermentation, usually by bacterial action and sometimes by molds or yeasts, is what gives ripened cheeses their distinctive flavor and extends their keeping time (compared to unripened cheese) considerably. Processed cheese is a blend of cheddar cheese that has been melted together and pasteurized. It keeps well and melts without becoming stringy, but usually is more bland in flavor than unprocessed cheese.

Cheese food and cheese spreads have added amounts of water, nonfat milk, or whey solids and may also have added flavors. Although a less concentrated source of cheese, these products are lower in fat and calories than other cheese sources and represent a good value because of the nutritious nonfat milk and whey solids that are added to them.

Saturated Fat in Milk and Imitation Milk Products

Nearly 65 percent of butterfat is saturated, while 30 percent is polyunsaturated. Because of this, people who have been advised to reduce saturated fat intake as a way to reduce or control the blood cholesterol level usually are told to avoid butterfat. For them, the nonfat products (nonfat milk, cottage cheese, ice milk) are recommended. As we saw earlier, the nonfat products cost less and are considerabley lower in calories, yet still provide all of the important milk nutrients.

In recent years, a number of milklike products (milk, cream, sour cream, ice cream) have been introduced and promoted on the basis of being "better for your health" because they contain no butterfat, no cholesterol, or no milk. The names of these products vary, depending on state regulations. The federal government defines them as *filled milk* products if the butterfat has been removed and replaced by some other form of fat and *imitation* if they are not made from milk. But in some states, California, for example, the term *imitation* is used to refer to filled milk products and *nondairy* is used for those not made from milk.

When the butterfat is removed and replaced by an equal amount of another type of fat, the calorie content is not reduced. The ratio of saturated to polyunsaturated fat may change depending on the type of fat used in place of butterfat. But most often, this fat is coconut oil, because it gives the best flavor and is low in cost, and it is more saturated than butterfat. If soybean oil is used and it is not hydrogenated, then saturated fat content will be reduced and the polyunsaturated fat content increased. So be wary when these products are promoted on the basis of having no milk or "no animal fat." Read the ingredient list on the label and find out what kind of fat replaces the butterfat; read the nutrition label to see if the ratio of saturated to polyunsaturated fat is listed.

Exhibit 11.12 shows the differences in fat and calorie content between ice cream, ice milk, imitation ice cream and ice milk, and the so-

Exhibit 11.12 Fat and Calorie Content of Popular Forms of Frozen Desserts

	KIND OF FAT	PERCENTAGE OF FAT	CALORIES PER ½ CUP
Ice cream	Butterfat	11.0%	135
Imitation ice cream	Vegetable fat	11.0	135
Ice milk	Butterfat	4.3	93
Imitation ice milk	Vegetable fat	4.3	93
Soft-serve ice milk	Butterfat	2.6	112
Sherbet	Butterfat	2.0	135

Source: Nutritive Value of Foods. U.S. Department of Agriculture, Home and Garden Bulletin No. 72, Washington, D.C. 1977, p. 7.

called dietetic ice cream. The amount of milk solids in ice cream and ice milk is established by government regulations. Because there are no such regulations for the imitation products that are made with vegetable fats, they may or may not give you as much protein, calcium, and riboflavin as the "real thing." For the person concerned about reducing saturated fat and calories, the lower fat, ice milk products are generally the best choice.

The nondairy products, such as coffee whiteners, and sour-cream and whipped-cream products, are promoted on the basis of having no milk. Since milk is nutritious, this is not a valid reason for buying them, except for persons who are allergic to milk components, such as protein or lactose. Some promotions are also misleading because the products often contain milk-derived ingredients, such as lactose and sodium caseinate, and the person who is allergic to milk may not be able to tolerate the nondairy products either. The nutritional value of these pseudo-dairy products depends on their ingredients. Most contain some kind of fat and sugar and some form of protein, usually either from soybeans or milk. Their caloric value may be as high as or higher than the product being imitated, but the consumer often thinks the caloric value is lower. The fat is often highly saturated coconut oil.

Reading ingredient lists and nutrient labels, if they are provided, is the best way to determine the product's content. See the sample label in Exhibit 11.13.

Summary

The inorganic substances known as mineral elements function in the body basically by *building* or *regulating*. They are needed in relatively small amounts, and an excess can be antagonistic or even toxic. Minerals often work in teams, activating enzymes, coenzymes, and hormones, or forming essential combinations such as bone crystals. *Macroelements* are

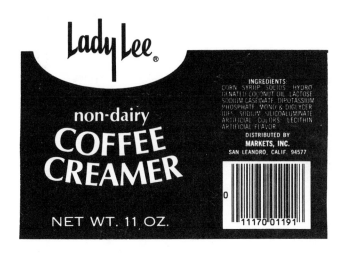

INGREDIENTS:
CORN SYRUP SOLIDS, HYDRO
GENATED COCONUT OIL, LACTOSE
SODIUM CASEINATE, DIPOTASSIUM
PHOSPHATE, MONO & DIGLYCER
IDES, SODIUM SILICOALUMINATE
ARTIFICIAL COLORS, LECITHIN
ARTIFICIAL FLAVOR

DISTRIBUTED BY
MARKETS, INC.
SAN LEANDRO, CALIF. 94577

Exhibit 11.13.   This typical label from a nondairy coffee creamer shows that the name is misleading, since it contains two milk-derived ingredients, lactose and caseinate. Hydrogenated coconut oil is a highly saturated fat.

those minerals present in relatively larger amounts in the body, while *microelements* are those we need in very small amounts.

Individual minerals are summarized in this chapter by form and location, function or mode of action, requirements and deficiency effects, and food sources. The forefront of nutrition today is in mineral research, as there are many elements about which we know very little.

VITAMINS 12

Highlights

Array of vitamins needed for good health

Origins, forms, and food sources of vitamins

Recommended amounts and conditions of hypervitaminosis

Effects of vitamin deficiency

Functions of vitamins in the body

Supermarket Nutrition: Choosing foods in the fruit and vegetable group

V*itamin* is a common household word, probably because of the large amount of publicity vitamins have received over the years in advertisements and in news reports about their ability (often unproven) to prevent colds, retard aging, and "keep us fit." In fact, to many people, nutrition means vitamins, and when asked to define a balanced diet, the average person often answers "getting enough vitamins."

Thus, most people not only know vitamins are essential but tend to overrate their value. At the same time, very few people understand what vitamins actually are and how they function in the body.

Like the macronutrients—fats, carbohydrates, and proteins—vitamins are complex organic compounds needed for growth, maintenance, and regulation of metabolic processes. However, unlike the macronutrients, vitamins are needed in just minute amounts (thus—*micronutrients*) and often do not undergo any digestive process—they are simply absorbed "as is" in the intestine.

As organic compounds, vitamins are found naturally only in living things. The original sources of most vitamins are plants, which synthesize them. Subsequently, animals eat the plants as a source of vitamins. Humans, in turn, get vitamins from both plants and animals. Some vitamins also are synthesized by microorganisms.

Many vitamins function as *coenzymes* and are necessary adjuncts to enzymes in catalyzing specific metabolic processes in the body. However, unlike enzymes, vitamins are consumed in their functions and must be obtained regularly from dietary sources, since they are not produced in any appreciable amount in the body.

Vitamins are divided into two groups: those that are fat soluble (A, D, E, and K) and those that are water soluble (C, niacin, thiamin, riboflavin, folic acid, pantothenic acid, pyridoxine, B_{12}, and biotin). All of the water-soluble vitamins, except vitamin C, are classified as B vitamins. Fat-soluble vitamins are stored in body fat, and a daily intake of them is less crucial than is a daily intake of water-soluble vitamins, which are not stored in the body.

Because water-soluble vitamins are usually excreted if excess amounts are eaten, they are less likely to have toxic effects when ingested in large amounts, although some toxic reactions have been observed when very large amounts are taken over a period of time (see Chapter 20). Those vitamins that are stored in body fat, especially vitamins A and D, can build up to toxic levels with serious and potentially fatal results. A reaction to an excess of vitamins is termed *hypervitaminosis*.

While most nutrition scientists believe that ingesting vitamins in amounts greatly above our needs is unwise, some have advocated use of super-size doses of vitamins (*megadoses*) to prevent or cure certain conditions. This controversial use of vitamins as drugs is discussed in Chapter 20, as is the question of the need to supplement our diets with vitamin pills. Some of the vitamins are quite unstable and are destroyed by such factors as heat, oxidation, and light.

Many of the vitamins were discovered as a result of researchers trying to find the cause for certain diseases, such as scurvy, beriberi, and pellagra. Because of this research and the generally good quality of the American diet, these deficiency diseases are rarely seen in the United States today.

Much complex information about vitamins and their functions has been accumulated and is continuing to be developed by nutrition scientists. To simplify and expedite comprehension of this information, it is presented in abbreviated, semitabular form. A more in-depth discussion of the individual vitamins is available in the references listed at the end of the book.

THE FAT-SOLUBLE VITAMINS

Vitamin A

Forms and Sources. Retinol is the name of preformed vitamin A, which is found in animal foods. Provitamin A in the form of carotene and other carotenoids is commonly found in plant foods (see Exhibit 12.1). The average American diet provides about half of total vitamin A intake as retinol and half as carotene (see Exhibit 12.2).

In the body, provitamin A is converted to retinol. Individuals vary in their ability to make this conversion: on the average, carotene conversion and absorption ranges from 25 to 50 percent. Cooking weakens the cell walls of vegetables and makes carotene absorption more efficient. The presence of fat in the diet promotes vitamin A absorption and use in the body.

In fruits and vegetables, such colors as yellow, orange, and green are often, but not always, clues that the yellow-orange colored carotene is present. (The green chlorophyl may mask a yellow or orange color in green vegetables.) Food value tables list an overall value for vitamin A, or vitamin A activity, that includes preformed vitamin A plus provitamin A.

Recommended Amounts and Toxicity. For many years requirements for vitamin A were expressed as *International Units* (IU). However, the Food and Nutrition Board of the National Research Council has recommended that a more accurate term, *retinol equivalents* (RE), be used. The Board also recommends that the vitamin A value in foods be expressed as RE, taking into account the difference in biological activity of preformed vitamin A and provitamin A. Beginning in 1974, the Recommended Dietary Allowances (Exhibit 12.3) were given in both IU and RE, but most food value charts continue to use IU.

Vegetables and Fruits for Vitamin A

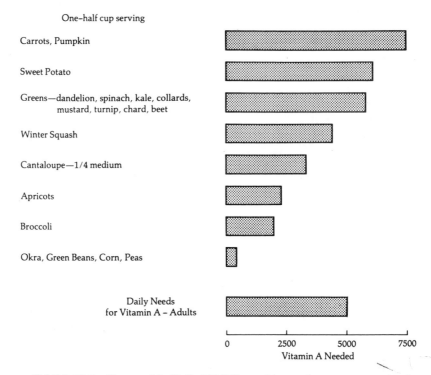

One–half cup serving

Carrots, Pumpkin

Sweet Potato

Greens—dandelion, spinach, kale, collards,
    mustard, turnip, chard, beet

Winter Squash

Cantaloupe—1/4 medium

Apricots

Broccoli

Okra, Green Beans, Corn, Peas

Daily Needs
for Vitamin A – Adults

0   2500   5000   7500

Vitamin A Needed

Exhibit 12.1 (*Source:* M. Hall, EFNEP teaching aid, University of
California, Cooperative Extension)

The RDA for vitamin A are based on the RE needed to maintain
adequate blood concentrations and prevent deficiency symptoms, with
added amounts for individual variation and a wide margin of safety.
The RDA for infants is based on the average vitamin A content of human
milk. Recommended Dietary Allowances for children and adolescents
are interpolated from infant and adult allowances.

Most of the vitamin A is stored in the liver and excess intakes are
toxic. A prolonged daily intake of more than 50,000 IU of vitamin A by
adults and 18,500 IU by children can lead to symptoms such as dry and
itching skin, swelling over long bones, headache, nausea, diarrhea, and
eventual loss of calcium from the bone. Mental aberrations from swelling of the brain also have been observed in conjunction with a high
vitamin A intake. The excess use of carotene has not been found to be
toxic but may lead to a development of yellow skin.[1]

[1]J. Hathcock, "Nutrition: Toxicology and Pharmacology," in Nutrition Reviews'
Present Knowledge in Nutrition, fourth edition. New York, Washington: The Nutrition
Foundation, Inc., 1976, p. 505.

Exhibit 12.2   Vitamin A: Sources, Functions, and Deficiency Effects

EXCELLENT SOURCES	GOOD SOURCES	FAIR SOURCES
Liver	Tomato and tomato juice	Orange and orange juice
Carrots	Peach	Cheese
Collards	Watermelon	Milk, whole
Broccoli	Butter	Egg yolk
Peppers	Margarine	Corn
Spinach (and other greens)		Prunes
Squash (winter)		
Sweet Potato		
Apricots		
Cantaloupe		
Pumpkin		

FUNCTIONS IN THE BODY	DEFICIENCY EFFECTS
1. Enables eye to adjust to changes in light—from bright to dark—by restoring a chemical, *rhodopsin*, in the retina from another chemical, *retinene*.	1. *Night blindness*, inability to see in a dim light.
2. Helps maintain the structural integrity and functional effectiveness of the epithelial (outer) cells of skin, cornea, and intestinal mucosa. Needed for formation of *mucopolysaccharide*, a normal carbohydrate found in mucous. If vitamin A is not present, keratin replaces mucopolysaccharide and makes the skin rough and dry. Mucopolysaccharide is needed in tears to keep the cornea of the eye healthy. In the intestines, healthy mucous membrane is needed to keep infectious bacteria from entering the body.	2. *Keratinization*, or formation of a horny layer of skin; in severe deficiency, cracking of skin. *Xerophthalmia*, an eye disease in which the cornea becomes opaque; may lead to blindness. Decreased resistance to infections. Impaired wound healing.
3. Maintains many physiological processes needed for growth, especially bone growth and tooth formation. Needed in the liver for carbohydrate metabolism and synthesis of glycogen for energy storage and for fat metabolism, especially of cholesterol. Needed in adrenal gland for formation of the hormone *cortisone*.	3. Faulty and limited bone growth in children; possible compression of spinal cord and brain resulting in pinched nerves and neurological problems. Defective formation of tooth enamel; less resistance to tooth decay.

Vitamin D

Forms and Sources. Vitamin D is found in two forms: *ergocalciferol* (vitamin D_2), primarily a synthetic form of vitamin D made by the irradiation of *ergosterol* from plants and fungi; and *cholecalciferol* (vitamin D_3), a naturally occurring form in animals, primarily found in fish livers, in cod liver and halibut liver, for example. Minimal amounts of cholecalciferol are present in fish, egg yolks, liver milk, butter, and cheese.

Exhibit 12.3   Recommended Daily Dietary Allowances,[a] Vitamins

	AGE (YEARS)	FAT-SOLUBLE VITAMINS			WATER-SOLUBLE VITAMINS							
		VITAMIN A (μg R.E.)[b]	VITAMIN D (μg)[c]	VITAMIN E (mg α T.E.)[d]	VITAMIN C (mg)	THIAMIN (mg)	RIBOFLAVIN (mg)	NIACIN (mg N.E.)[e]	VITAMIN B_6 (mg)	FOLACIN[f] (μg)	VITAMIN B_{12} (μg)
Infants	0.0–0.5	420	10	3	35	0.3	0.4	6	0.3	30	0.5[g]
	0.5–1.0	400	10	4	35	0.5	0.6	8	0.6	45	1.5
Children	1–3	400	10	5	45	0.7	0.8	9	0.9	100	2.0
	4–6	500	10	6	45	0.9	1.0	11	1.3	200	2.5
	7–10	700	10	7	45	1.2	1.4	16	1.6	300	3.0
Males	11–14	1000	10	8	50	1.4	1.6	18	1.8	400	3.0
	15–18	1000	10	10	60	1.4	1.7	18	2.0	400	3.0
	19–22	1000	7.5	10	60	1.5	1.7	19	2.2	400	3.0
	23–50	1000	5	10	60	1.4	1.6	18	2.2	400	3.0
	51+	1000	5	10	60	1.2	1.4	16	2.2	400	3.0
Females	11–14	800	10	8	50	1.1	1.3	15	1.8	400	3.0
	15–18	800	10	8	60	1.1	1.3	14	2.0	400	3.0
	19–22	800	7.5	8	60	1.1	1.3	14	2.0	400	3.0
	23–50	800	5	8	60	1.0	1.2	13	2.0	400	3.0
	51+	800	5	8	60	1.0	1.2	13	2.0	400	3.0
Pregnant		+200	+5	+2	+20	+0.4	+0.3	+2	+0.6	+400	+1.0
Lactating		+400	+5	+3	+40	+0.5	+0.5	+5	+0.5	+100	+1.0

Source: Recommended Dietary Allowances, Ninth Edition (revised 1979). National Academy of Sciences, Washington, D.C.

[a] The allowances are intended to provide for individual variations among most normal persons as they live in the United States under usual environmental stresses. Diets should be based on a variety of common foods in order to provide other nutrients for which human requirements have been less well defined.

[b] Retinol equivalents. 1 Retinol equivalent = 1 μg Retinol or 6 μg β-carotene.

[c] As cholecalciferol. 10 μg cholecaciferol = 400 I.U. vitamin D.

[d] α tocopherol equivalents. 1 mg d-α-tocopherol = 1 α T.E. See text for variation in allowances and calculation of vitamin E activity of the diet as α tocopherol equivalents.

[e] 1 NE (niacin equivalent) is equal to 1 mg of niacin or 60 mg of dietary tryptophan.

[f] The folacin allowances refer to dietary sources as determined by *Lectobacillus casai* assay after treatment with enzymes ("conjugases") to make polyglutamyl forms of the vitamin available to the test organism.

[g] The RDA for vitamin B_{12} in infants is based on average concentration of the vitamin in human milk. The allowances after weaning are based on energy intake (as recommended by the American Academy of Pediatrics) and consideration of other factors such as intestinal absorption.

Most of the milk that is sold is fortified by the addition of a concentrate of vitamin D_2 or D_3. Cholecalciferol is synthesized from 7-dehydrocholesterol when direct sunlight (ultraviolet rays) shines on human skin.

Vitamin D is of little use to the human body until it has been chemically altered twice: first in the liver and then in the kidney (see Exhibit 12.4 for functions and deficiency effects). Each time, the body attaches an oxygen-hydrogen pair—once at the first position on the molecule, once at the 25th position. The final product is the biologically active form *1, 25, dihydroxy vitamin D*. This active form is considered to be a steroid hormone and is known to be up to 50 times more powerful than the parent vitamin D, which is considered a *prohormone,* in curing bone deficiencies.

Recommended Amounts and Toxicity. RDA, formerly expressed as International Units (IU), are now given as micrograms of cholecalciferol. Ten micrograms cholecalciferol equal 400 IU Vitamin D. Exact human requirements are not known. The Recommended Dietary Allowance for infants is based on a level thought to promote an adequate growth rate and optimal calcium absorption. Less is known about the need for this vitamin by older children and adults. It is thought that adults who get some vitamin D from a mixed diet and are exposed to some sunlight will form sufficient vitamin D to satisfy their needs. Supplementation during pregnancy and lactation is advised.

Exhibit 12.4   Vitamin D: Functions and Deficiency Effects

FUNCTIONS IN THE BODY	DEFICIENCY EFFECTS
1. Promotes absorption of calcium and phosphorus in intestine. Stimulates calcium and phosphorus mobilization from the bone, thereby contributing these minerals to the blood pool so they are present in sufficient amounts for proper bone calcification. 2. Enhances levels of phosphates in the body by helping with the reabsorption of phosphates from the kidney to the bloodstream. This, too, is important in normal bone calcification. 3. Maintains normal level of the enzyme *alkaline phosphate,* which is needed for release of phosphorus from compounds so it is available for bone formation. 4. Needed for formation of the enzyme *adenosine triphosphatase,* which is believed to be necessary for collagen formation in bone (part of bone matrix). 5. Plays a role, not clearly understood, in regulation of amino acid levels in the blood (by protecting them from loss in the kidney) and the level of citric acid in bones and tissues.	1. Reduces levels of calcium and phosphorus in blood. This, together with lack of the enzyme alkaline phosphatase (also under influence of vitamin D), results in serious defects in calcification of bones. When this occurs in growing children, they develop *rickets.* Symptoms include soft long bones which bend (bowed legs), excessive cartilage at growing ends of bones, hard nodules in front of chest, flattening of back of skull, and a narrow, distorted chest. Adults develop *osteomalacia,* which is defective calcification of bones as they are continually being remodeled. Weight-bearing bones such as the pelvis become deformed; pelvic bones and back become tender and painful. Susceptibility to tooth decay results when insufficient supplies of vitamin D are available during periods of tooth development (prenatal, infancy, early childhood).

Vitamin D is stored in body fat and excessive intakes are dangerous, especially to infants and young children. Intake of vitamin D at levels four to five times greater than the RDA for prolonged periods has resulted in *hypercalcemia* (excess calcium in the blood) and growth failure in infants; and in kidney stones, calcium deposits in various organs including the kidney, and hypertension in infants and adults. Symptoms of excess dosage include a loss of appetite and body weight, excessive thirst, vomiting, and irritability.

Vitamin E

Forms and Sources. Four forms of vitamin E have been identified: *alpha-, beta-, gamma-,* and *delta-tocopherol.* But usually only the alpha form is mentioned since it accounts for about 80 percent of the total activity of vitamin E. Tocopherols are alcohols and are antioxidants. Another four compounds called *tocotrienols* (*alpha, beta, gamma,* and *delta*) have some degree of vitamin E activity. All eight forms are found in food.

Since vitamin E is fat soluble, it is found in many fat-containing foods such as vegetable oils, plant seeds, nuts, eggs, milk, and liver (see Exhibit 12.5).

Recommended Amounts and Toxicity. RDA for Vitamin E, stated as milligrams of alpha tocopherol equivalents (αTE) (see Exhibit 12.3), have been set rather arbitrarily. They are believed to be adequate since there has been little evidence of deficiency of this nutrient in the United States, except in premature infants and persons having a defect in their ability to absorb fat.[2] Vitamin E is stored in tissues throughout the body and is consumed slowly. This, along with vitamin E's common availability in food, may explain why deficiencies are not seen.

Large doses of vitamin E have been recommended to prevent or cure various conditions without scientific evidence to support this use. Concern exists that these large doses could be harmful since the vitamin is fat soluble and cumulative effects are hypothetically possible. However, to date there is no documented evidence that vitamin E is toxic, even in large doses.

Vitamin K

Forms and Sources. Like other fat-soluble vitamins, vitamin K is a group of substances rather than a single entity. Vitiman K_1, named *phytylmenaquinone,* is found in plants; vitamin K_2, referred to as *multiprenylmenaquinone,* is produced by bacteria. In addition to the natural forms

[2]J. Bieri, "Vitamin E," in Nutrition Reviews' *Present Knowledge in Nutrition,* fourth edition. New York, Washington, D.C.: The Nutrition Foundation, Inc., 1976, pp. 98-99.

Exhibit 12.5   Vitamin E: Sources, Functions, and Deficiency Effects

EXCELLENT SOURCES	GOOD SOURCES	FAIR SOURCES
Vegetable oils	Liver	Egg yolk
Shortening	Butter	Whole milk
Whole wheat	Codfish	Dry beans
Margarine	Green leafy vegetables	Meat
Wheat germ	Human milk	Fish
Nuts		Poultry
Sunflower seeds		Bread
		Cereal grains

FUNCTIONS IN THE BODY	DEFICIENCY EFFECTS
1. Protects red blood cells from destruction, or *hemolysis,* by preventing the oxidation of the cell membrane.	1. Premature infants have *hemolytic anemia* and symptoms of irritability and edema.
2. By consuming oxygen for its own oxidation, serves as an antioxidant–protector of other biological materials such as vitamins C and A, essential fatty acids, and possibly tissues such as lungs.	2. Increased amounts of vitamin E are needed when a diet is high in polyunsaturated fatty acids, which tend to oxidize in the body and release *free radicals*—which are considered harmful although their exact effect in the body is not completely understood.
3. Needed in cell respiration, for final biochemical changes by which energy is released from glucose and fatty acids.	
4. Found to be needed, in experimental animals, for normal reproduction. Some unproven theories and myths about the powers of vitamin E to improve sexual performance, prevent aging, etc., are discussed in Chapter 20.	
5. In rats, vitamin E deficiency may result in permanent sterility in males and failure to conceive in females. This effect has never been observed in humans, however, probably because our diets are not deficient in this nutrient.	

of vitamin K, other forms have been synthesized. One, called *menadione* (vitamin K_3), has about twice as much biological activity as the natural forms.

Because vitamin K_2 is synthesized in our body by intestinal bacteria, food sources of vitamin K are not usually needed by healthy people. The vitamin is not found to any great extent in animal foods, but is found in dark green vegetables, such as spinach and kale, as well as in cabbage, cauliflower, peas, and cereals (see Exhibit 12.6).

Recommended Amounts and Toxicity. Dietary deficiency of this nutrient is rare since it is synthesized by bacteria in the intestines, and no Recommended Dietary Allowances have been established for it.

Exhibit 12.6   Vitamin K: Functions and Deficiency Effects

FUNCTIONS IN THE BODY	DEFICIENCY EFFECTS
Essential to blood coagulation. Is required for the formation of four protein substances needed in blood coagulation, known as *K-dependent clotting factors*. The one present in the highest concentration in blood plasma is *prothrombin*. Prothrombin is converted to *thrombin*, which then converts *fibrinogen* in the blood to *fibrin*, the key substance in blood clotting.	Hemorrhaging results when blood does not clot. For this reason, vitamin K has been called the *antihemorrhagic factor*. Problems of hemorrhaging due to lack of vitamin K have been seen in some newborn infants (see Chapter 6) and in older people who are taking anticoagulation drugs such as *coumarin*. Persons undergoing antibiotic treatment may have a temporary lack of vitamin K since antibiotics depress the intestinal bacteria that form this nutrient. Persons with diseases in which there is chronic diarrhea or poor absorption also may lack vitamin K.

Vitamin K does not appear to have side effects if used in large amounts, but excessive doses of the synthetic form of vitamin K (*menadione*) have produced hemolytic anemia in the rat and are toxic to newborn infants at levels above 5 milligrams.[3] The toxic effect seems to be one of excessive breakdown of red blood cells.

THE WATER-SOLUBLE VITAMINS

Vitamin C

Forms and Sources. Ascorbic acid, the chemical name of vitamin C, is a shortened form of *antiscorbutic (scurvy-preventing)* factor. A relatively simple organic acid, vitamin C, having six carbon atoms in each molecule, is structurally similar to the single, six-carbon sugars such as glucose. It is the least stable of all the vitamins, being easily oxidized to *dehydroascorbic acid.* (*Dehydro* means minus hydrogen: in oxidation, the ascorbic acid loses two hydrogen atoms per molecule.) Both ascorbic acid and dehydroascorbic acid are found in foods. Dehydroascorbic acid has less biological activity—about 80 percent of that of ascorbic acid—but may be converted back to ascorbic acid in the body by the addition of hydrogen, which is a *reduction* process and opposite to the *oxidation* process.

[3]National Academy of Sciences, Food and Nutrition Board, National Research Council, *Recommended Dietary Allowances,* ninth edition. Washington, D.C., 1979, p. 62.

The oxidation-reduction reaction between ascorbic acid and dehydroascorbic acid is reversible in both plants and animals. However, if dehydroascorbic acid is further oxidized, it no longer has vitamin C activity, and this reaction is not reversible. Thus, foods with ascorbic acid or dehydroascorbic acid will fulfull our vitamin C needs, but foods in which so much oxidation has taken place that dehydroascorbic acid has been lost will be poor sources of vitamin C. See Chapter 22 for more information on ways vitamin C is lost in food and how it can be retained.

Fruits and vegetables are our principal sources of vitamin C (see Exhibits 12.7 and 12.8). But keep in mind that vitamin C levels in foods are highly dependent on how the foods have been handled.

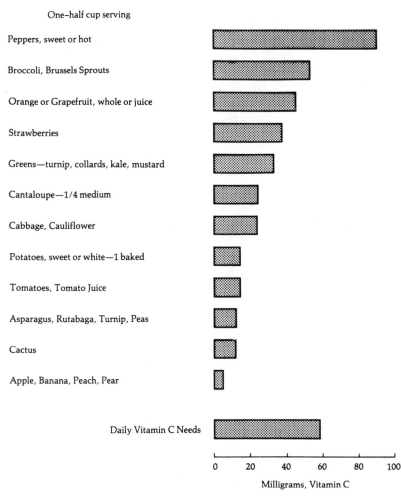

Exhibit 12.7. (*Source:* M. Hall, EFNEP teaching aid, University of California, Cooperative Extension)

Exhibit 12.8 Vitamin C: Sources, Functions, and Deficiency Effects

Excellent Sources	Good Sources	Fair Sources
Chili peppers	Asparagus	Sauerkraut
Green peppers	Radishes	Peas
Parsley	Tomatoes and tomato juice	Cucumbers
Broccoli	Potatoes (white)	Celery
Brussel sprouts	Sweet potatoes	Iceberg lettuce
Kale	Romaine lettuce	Carrots
Cauliflower	Honeydew melons	Bean sprouts
Spinach	Pineapples	Blueberries
Cabbage	Liver	Avocadoes
Collards		Nectarines
Strawberries		Boysenberries
Papaya		Bananas
Oranges and orange juice		Peaches
Lemons		
Grapefruits and grapefruit juice		
Guavas		
Cantaloupes		
Tangerines		
Watermelons		

Functions in the Body	Deficiency Effects
1. Essential for formation of *collagen*, a protein that is an important component of the intracellular material needed to keep tissues firmly bound together. Collagen is needed in healing wounds and in providing tensile strength to new tissue. Sometimes it's referred to as the *cementing substance* between cells.	1. Scurvy results from an acute lack of vitamin C. Symptoms include fatigue, poor appetite, bleeding and swollen gums, and sometimes loose teeth, hemorrhages (some under the skin), rough skin, and pains in joints. In young children, symptoms of latent scurvy are failure to grow properly, weakness, restlessness, irritability, swollen joints, and tenderness in leg muscles. Delayed wound healing.
2. Needed for formation of the bone matrix and tooth dentine. This is related to its function in formation of collagen. When collagen formation is limited, bone matrix and tooth dentine are limited in their capacity to hold calcium and phosphorus.	2. Teeth that are subject to decay or breaking. Failure to grow properly in children.
3. Helps maintain normal elasticity and strength of blood vessels and capillaries.	3. Hemorrhages of small blood vessels under the skin.
4. Influences formation of *hemoglobin*, the absorption of iron from the intestine, and the deposition of iron in the liver. By acting as a reducing agent, vitamin C converts food iron from the ferric to the ferrous form, which is the only form that the body can absorb.	4. Iron-deficiency anemia could be related to lack of vitamin C, if there is also a low level of iron intake.
5. Functions in some way, not yet understood, in protecting the body against infections and bacterial toxins. It is thought that infections somehow reduce the level of vitamin C in the tissues and body fluids.	5. Infants with scurvy have lowered resistance to infections. Guinea pigs show less resistance and greater injury from infection on limited vitamin C.
6. Takes part in a number of metabolic reactions involving amino acids, such as *tyrosine* and *tryptophan*, and the vitamin *folacin*. Believed to be involved in secretions of adrenal hormones, including *thyroxin* and *adrenaline*. Has a sparing effect in several vitamins, including A, B, and E.	6. Less resistance to stress and other metabolic disorders related to these functions.

Vitamin C also is added to many foods, particularly fruit drinks and juices. Juices such as apple, cranberry, and pineapple with vitamin C added all could be considered excellent sources of the vitamin.

Recommended Amounts and Toxicity. The minimum requirement of vitamin C needed to prevent scurvy is thought to be 10 milligrams per day.[4] The Recommended Dietary Allowances (Exhibit 12.3) are set high enough to allow a wide margin for individual variation and loss of this nutrient from foods. Thus, these allowances are believed to be adequate for healthy people.

The controversial issue of whether much larger amounts of vitamin C (as much as 100 times more than the RDA) should be taken as a way to prevent the common cold is discussed in the section on Nutrients as Drugs in Chapter 20. Most nutrition scientists believe that taking large amounts of vitamin C has no extra benefits, except to alleviate a deficiency or during periods of unusual physical stress such as recovery from an illness or surgery.

Because vitamin C is water soluble, excess amounts taken above our needs are generally excreted in the urine. Therefore, toxic effects have not been observed when amounts moderately above the RDA are used. However, when huge amounts are used, several grams per day, for example, toxic effects may develop.

Thiamin (Vitamin B_1)

Forms and Sources. Thiamin as it is found in food is a crystalline substance made up of carbon, hydrogen, oxygen, nitrogen, and sulfur. It is second to vitamin C in its instability, but is more stable in dry form than when dissolved in water. Synthetic thiamin is usually produced in more stable forms as one of its salts, such as *thiamin hydrochloride* or *thiamin mononitrate.*

The enzyme *thiaminase,* which is found in some raw fish and is formed by bacteria in plant foods, splits thiamin into two parts, making it unavailable to the body. A thiamin deficiency has been observed in animals fed large amounts of raw fish. Heating destroys this enzyme, so cooking fish before eating it is recommended.

Protein-rich foods as a group are the best sources of this nutrient (see Exhibit 12.9). Pork has much more thiamin than beef or lamb. Whole grains are also a good source, but refined cereals lack thiamin unless they have been enriched, since it is found mainly in the bran and germ.

[4]National Academy of Sciences, Food and Nutrition Board, National Research Council, *Recommended Dietary Allowances,* ninth edition. Washington, D.C., 1979, p. 64.

Exhibit 12.9 Thiamin (Vitamin B₁): Sources, Functions, and Deficiency Effects

Excellent Sources	Good Sources	Fair Sources
Sunflower seeds	Whole wheat flour	Beef
Sesame seeds	Oatmeal	Fish
Peanuts	Enriched cereals	Poultry
Soybeans	Peas	Eggs
Wheat germ	Enriched pasta	Enriched or whole-grain
Liver	Lamb	bread
Kidney	Enriched or brown rice	Potatoes
Pork		Collards
		Oranges and orange juice

Functions in the Body	Deficiency Effects
1. Forms the coenzyme *thiamin pyrophosphate*, which functions as a *cocarboxylase* in the metabolism of glucose in the tissues. A cocarboxylase is a substance needed to split apart carbon compounds. When there is insufficient cocarboxylase to metabolize glucose, intermediate metabolic compounds accumulate. These cause symptoms associated with thiamin deficiency. Reduction in release of energy also results. Because of its coenzyme activity, helps promote appetite and better functioning of digestive tract. Also promotes effective functioning of the nervous system. 2. Thiamin pyrophosphate has a significant role in converting *glucose* (a six-carbon sugar) to *ribose* (a five-carbon sugar), which is an essential building block of DNA and RNA in the cell nucleus.	1. The deficiency disease *beriberi* results from lack of thiamin. Symptoms of beriberi include loss of appetite, nausea, vomiting, irritability, mental depression, leg cramping, and difficulty walking. Functioning of the heart may be impaired, causing defective blood pumping and accumulation of fluids (*edema*) in different parts of the body, such as the feet and legs. A serious deficiency can be life threatening because of the involvement of the heart and nervous system. A less serious deficiency may cause poor appetite, less than optimal growth in children, weight loss, depression, irritability, inability to concentrate, and fatigue.

Recommended Amounts and Toxicity. Since thiamin is needed in energy metabolism, the Recommended Dietary Allowances (Exhibit 12.3) are based on individual calorie requirements, allowing 0.5 milligrams per 1,000 calories.[5] Persons who consume fewer than 2,000 calories per day, especially older adults, usually should not reduce thiamin consumption below 1 milligram per day, however. Alcoholics have an increased requirement for thiamin, since it is needed in the metabolism of alcohol; yet their intake is often inadequate due to limited food consumption.

There is no evidence that thiamin intake above the recommended amounts is beneficial to healthy people, nor is there evidence that excess amounts are toxic.

[5]National Academy of Sciences, Food and Nutrition Board, National Research Council, *Recommended Dietary Allowances*, ninth edition. Washington, D.C., 1979, p. 67.

Exhibit 12.10 Riboflavin (Vitamin B_2): Sources, Function, and Deficiency Effects

Excellent Sources	Good Sources	Fair Sources
Liver	Meat	Whole-grain cereals
Milk	Poultry	Enriched cereals
Cheese	Fish	Enriched pasta
Heart	Eggs	
Kidney	Broccoli	
Wheat germ	Collards	
Yeast	Spinach	
	Squash	
	Dry beans and peas	
	Nuts	

Function in the Body	Deficiency Effects
Is an essential component of a group of coenzymes called flavoproteins. Flavoproteins, such as *flavomononucleotide* and *flavoadenine dinucleotide*, are very important in numerous oxidation-reduction processes in cells for releasing energy from fats, carbohydrates, and proteins.	Symptoms usually build up over a period of time and include lesions around the mouth and nose, hair loss, and a scaly condition of the skin. Other effects are failure to grow in children, sensitivity to light, and eventual development of opacity (cloudiness) of the cornea of the eye, which could lead to blindness.

Riboflavin (Vitamin B_2)

Forms and Sources. A unique feature of riboflavin is that it has an orange-yellow color and adds a greenish fluorescence to foods. In its reduced form (hydrogen added) it becomes colorless; and when it's reoxidized (hydrogen removed) it turns orange-yellow again. It is more sensitive to light than most nutrients and is somewhat unstable, depending on conditions. Cooking and drying of foods can increase the availability of riboflavin.

Riboflavin is widely distributed in foods from both plant and animal sources, but one of our major dietary sources is milk and milk products (see Exhibit 12.10). Riboflavin may be found in a free form or in the form of enzymes called *flavoproteins* and several coenzymes. Before we can absorb it, it must be *phosphorylated* (combined with phosphorus) in the intestines.

Recommended Amounts and Toxicity. Because life-threatening deficiencies of this nutrient have not been reported, it is believed that it may be synthesized in the body by intestinal bacteria, thereby reducing the amount we need to get from food. Recommended Dietary Allowances (Exhibit 12.3) are calculated on the basis of calorie consumption of the individual at 0.6 milligrams per calorie regardless of age. There is no evidence that the requirement increases as energy consumption goes up. Nor is there evidence that this nutrient has toxic effects if used in large amounts. Excesses are excreted in the urine.

Niacin

Forms and Sources. The early name for niacin was *nicotinic acid.* Another form, *nicotinamide,* was found later to have similar action. In 1971 the term niacin was adopted for both substances so the vitamin would not be confused with the nicotine in tobacco.

Niacin is found in foods in both its free and combined forms. The body forms a small amount of niacin from tryptophan, and niacin can be synthesized in the intestine by bacteria. When therapeutic doses of niacin are given, the amide form is usually used because the acid form may cause dizziness and skin reactions such as red rash, flushing, and a feeling of heat.

Niacin is found in animal foods, usually in the form of nicotinamide, and in plant foods, usually in the form of nicotinic acid (see Ex-

Exhibit 12.11   Niacin: Sources, Functions, and Deficiency Effects

Excellent Sources	Good Sources	Fair Sources
Yeast	Meat	Enriched and whole-grain
Peanuts	Nuts	bread
Liver	Wheat germ	Enriched and whole-grain
Chicken		cereal
Fish		Enriched pasta
Soybeans		Broccoli
Sesame seeds		Collards
Sunflower seeds		Peas
		Potatoes
		Tomatoes
		Bananas

Functions in the Body	Deficiency Effects
1. Important constituent of two coenzymes, *nicotinamide adenine dinucleotide* (NAD) and *nicotinamide adenine dinucleotide phosphate* (NADP), both of which are involved in oxidation-reduction reactions for releasing energy in the cells. 2. NAD serves as a coenzyme in the process of synthesizing fatty acid from glucose.	1. Vital chemical processes are hampered when these two coenzymes are not present in sufficient amounts. This could cause injury to tissues throughout the body. Those most likely to show damage are skin, gastrointestinal tract, and nerve tissue. The disease that results from long-term lack of niacin is *pellagra.* Symptoms of pellagra include diarrhea, dermatitis (dry, scaly, cracking skin—especially where exposed to sunlight), and dementia (the "three Ds"). Mental aberrations include poor memory (especially of recent events), anxiety, insomnia, irritability, and depression. In advanced stages there are delirium, hallucinations, disorientation, and stupor. Symptoms of a less acute lack of niacin are a sore mouth and tongue, weakness, and failure of children to grow properly.

hibit 12.11). In addition, foods containing tryptophan are a source of some niacin in the body. The *niacin equivalent* of foods is calculated by considering both the niacin and tryptophan content. The RDA are expressed as mg of niacin equivalent (NE), but only niacin content is given in food value tables.

In general, foods that contain thiamin and riboflavin, particularly protein foods, also are good sources of niacin. Because milk and eggs are low in niacin, but have proteins high in tryptophan, their contribution to the body's pool of niacin may be higher than that reflected in food value tables. In cereals, much of the niacin is in "bound" form, which may not be available to us.

Recommended Amounts and Toxicity. Recommended Dietary Allowances for adults (Exhibit 12.3) are estimated on the basis of the calorie content of the diet—6.6 milligrams per 1,000 calories and not less than 13 milligrams for persons who consume diets of less than 2,000 calories. There are no data on which to base the niacin requirements of children from infancy through adolescence or for pregnant and lactating women, so the allowances might be considered to be informed guesses. The long-term effects of using large doses of niacin (see Chapter 20) are not known.

Folacin   blood

Forms and Sources. The name folacin is a general term that includes *folic acid* and several other related compounds that have the biologic activity of folic acid. Up to 25 percent of total food folacin is in a free form. The remainder is found in food as *polyglutamates,* which require the action of an intestinal enzyme, *conjugese,* to free the folic acid for its metabolic activity. Scientists do not know exactly how much of the folacin in food is actually absorbed for folic acid activity. (See Exhibit 12.12 for information on the sources of folacin.)

Once folic acid is absorbed it must be converted to its coenzyme form *tetrohydrofolic acid* by a series of reduction (hydrogen-added) reactions. The coenzyme form is also widely distributed in food.

Because there are a number of different forms of this vitamin found in nature, in both animal and plant foods, scientists have not yet developed complete information about folacin sources. In addition, the vitamin can be quite unstable in some foods. For example, 70 percent of it may be lost from green leafy vegetables held in a warm temperature for several days.

Recommended Amounts and Toxicity. Recommended Dietary Allowances (Exhibit 12.3) are based on the amount of folic acid needed to overcome a lack of red blood cells in deficient individuals, with adjustments based on the estimated amount available from a varied diet and allowances for individual differences. Needs are considerably higher during pregnancy. For infants the RDA is based on the amount of folic acid in human milk. Written statements from physicians are required for

Exhibit 12.12   Folacin: Sources, Functions, and Deficiency Effects

Excellent Sources	Good Sources	Fair Sources
Liver	Cabbage	Squash
Yeast	Cauliflower	Tomatoes and tomato juice
Green leafy vegetables	Kale	Beef
(beet greens, mustard	Spinach	Peanuts
greens)	Peas	Other nuts
Soybeans	Chick peas	Whole wheat bread
Fresh asparagus	Bran flakes	Brown rice
Oranges and orange juice	Wheat germ	Cottage cheese
Broccoli	Wheat bran	

Functions in the Body	Deficiency Effects
1. Folacin coenzymes perform a transfer function, carrying single carbon units needed for building *purines* and *pyrimidines.* These compounds are then used for building nucleic acids, which are vitally important in the composition of the cell nucleus.	1. Major deficiency effect is *macrocytic anemia,* in which red blood cells are fewer in number, larger in size, and have less hemoglobin than normal. Young red blood cells, called *megoloblasts,* which are being formed in bone marrow, fail to mature. Reduction in number of white blood cells also results.
2. Folacin coenzymes are also essential for the breakdown of many, possibly all, amino acids.	2. Such amino acids as *histidine* are not efficiently utilized, and a residue appears in the urine.
3. Coenzymes supply carbon and hydrogen atoms for synthesis of methyl groups needed in metabolism. Other nutrients also have this function.	3. Some general symptoms of folic acid deficiency include weakness, fatigue, poor growth in children, a smooth red tongue, gastrointestinal disturbances, and diarrhea. The latter two are caused by lack of maturation of epithelial cells in the intestine.

prescriptions of more than 0.1 milligrams of folacin a day, not because of any known toxic effect of folacin but because a high intake will mask symptoms of *pernicious anemia,* a more serious problem that requires treatment with vitamin B_{12}.

Vitamin B_{12}

Forms and Sources. Vitamin B_{12} is not a single compound, but a group of complex compounds, called *corrinoids* or *cobalamins,* which contain nitrogen, cobalt, and phosphorous. They are large, red-colored molecules, so complex that they have not yet been synthesized in the laboratory. All forms of the vitamin found in food are believed to have about equal biological activity, and all originate from the growth of bacteria and fungi. Neither plants nor animals can synthesize this nutrient. Vitamin B_{12} is produced commercially for use in supplements by growing, or culturing, the bacteria and fungi that are able to synthesize it. (See Exhibit 12.13 for information on the functions and deficiency effects of Vitamin B_{12}.)

The coenzyme form of vitamin B_{12} is the most common form found in food and it is somewhat unstable. We absorb only 30 to 70 percent of the B_{12} we consume, and persons having pernicious anemia are unable to absorb it at all. In the body, vitamin B_{12} is converted to its coenzyme form if it is not already in that form when eaten. Only animal foods supply vitamin B_{12}, plant foods have none, unless they have been contaminated with microorganisms or feces. Nor is there any vitamin B_{12} in yeast, the common source of other B vitamins. The best sources of vitamin B_{12} are liver and other organ meats, such as kidney and heart, and bivalves such as clams and oysters. Other good sources are meat from all animals, poultry, fish, eggs, shellfish, milk, and cheese.

Recommended Amounts and Toxicity. The Recommended Dietary Allowances for vitamin B_{12} (Exhibit 12.3) are based on studies that show the minimal amount needed to prevent blood changes, studies that show levels of B_{12} in healthy and deficient persons, and studies that correlate the turnover rate in the body. To this estimate is added an extra amount to allow for individual differences and a margin of error. A larger amount is recommended for pregnant and lactating women. Oral supplementation is recommended for strict vegetarians. Persons with pernicious anemia cannot absorb vitamin B_{12} taken orally and must receive injections for treatment to be effective.

Exhibit 12.13   Vitamin B_{12}: Functions and Deficiency Effects

Functions in the Body	Deficiency Effects
1. The coenzyme, combined with proteins, circulates in blood and is stored in the liver and kidneys. Its chief function is to aid in the formation of nucleic acids (DNA, RNA) and its action is similar to that of folacin. Is, therefore, essential for normal functioning of all body cells—especially in the gastrointestinal tract, bone marrow, and nervous system.	1. Deficiency not seen in normal persons, except in cases of vegetarians who eat no animal foods (see chapter 8). Symptoms include sore tongue, weakness, loss of weight, apathy, tingling sensation in extremities, and other mental or nervous abnormalities.
2. When B_{12} coenzyme is lacking in the blood, new red blood cells fail to develop normally in the bone marrow.	2. Pernicious anemia occurs in people with a metabolic defect that keeps them from absorbing B_{12}. They are said to lack an *intrinsic factor* needed in this process. Symptoms include megaloblastic anemia and low red-blood cell count, weakness and fatigue, smoothness of the tongue, sore and cracked lips and other mucous membranes, and decrease or total lack of hydrochloric acid in the stomach. The central nervous system is affected and the spinal cord degenerates.
3. Appears to be needed in folacin metabolism. May affect ability of the liver to store absorbed folacin through its effect on the synthesis of the amino acid methionine.	
4. Appears to play a role, along with pantothenic acid, in the formation of certain amino acids.	
	3. Symptoms of folacin deficiency may also occur when B_{12} is lacking in the diet.

Vitamin B_{12} supplements often are prescribed for treatment of various neurologic disorders. However, this is usually done for their placebo effect because scientists have found no evidence that B_{12} supplements actually are useful in treating neurologic disorders. Nor have scientists found evidence of any toxicity when this vitamin is used in large doses.

Pyridoxine (Vitamin B_6)

Forms and Sources. Pyridoxine and two closely related compounds, *pyridoxal* and *pyridoxamine,* make up what is known as the vitamin B_6 group. All three forms have about the same biological activity in the body. Pyridoxine is found largely in plant foods; pyridoxal and pyridoxamine are found mainly in animal foods. Of the three, pyridoxine is the most stable. Cooking and processing may destroy up to 50 percent of the vitamin B_6 activity in some foods, and milled cereals lose about 75 percent of their vitamin B_6 (see Chapter 22).

Exhibit 12.14 Pyridoxine (Vitamin B_6): Sources, Functions, and Deficiency Effects

EXCELLENT SOURCES	GOOD SOURCES	FAIR SOURCES
Yeast	Beef	Green pepper
Sunflower seeds	Pork	Dried fruit
Liver	Lamb	Spinach
Wheat germ	Poultry	Sweet potato
Wheat bran	Fish	Broccoli
Avocado	Nuts	Cabbage
Banana	Peanuts	Cauliflower
	Whole grain	Potato
	brown rice	Tomato juice and tomato
		Bran flakes

FUNCTIONS IN THE BODY	DEFICIENCY EFFECTS
1. Combines with phosphate and functions as a coenzyme, usually as *pyridoxal phosphate,* in an exceptionally large number of different types of enzymes involved in various aspects of amino acid metabolism. In one way or another, vitamin B_6 is involved in the synthesis and catabolism of all amino acids. 2. Especially important is its involvement in a precursor of *heme,* the red blood cell protein. 3. Is an active agent in glucose metabolism and may also be involved in fatty acid metabolism. 4. Involved in regeneration and normal functioning of nerve tissue.	1. Characterized by a large number of abnormalities in amino acid and protein metabolism. Symptoms are similar to those seen in niacin and riboflavin deficiencies: poor growth; convulsions; anemia; decreased antibody formation; abdominal distress; vomiting; kidney, liver, and skin injuries; irritability; depression; and confusion.

In general, vitamin B_6 is found in foods high in other B vitamins—liver, meat, some vegetables, and whole grain cereals (see Exhibit 12.14).

Recommended Amounts and Toxicity. Requirements for this vitamin are related to protein intake, especially of the sulfur-containing amino acid, methionine. Estimates for the Recommended Dietary Allowances (Exhibit 12.3) are based on various studies of the metabolism of protein in the body. Little data are available for establishing the need for children and adolescents. Need is believed to increase with women who take oral contraceptives, with pregnancy, and with age. Some drugs are antagonists to pyridoxine (see Chapter 20). Several genetic conditions may cause abnormalities in B_6 metabolism, and B_6 supplements can relieve the symptoms. There are few data on the toxicity of B_6 in large doses. However, B_6 dependency was induced by feeding 200 milligrams to subjects for 33 days.[6]

Pantothenic Acid

Forms and Sources. This nutrient might be considered the most commonly occurring of all the vitamins for it is found in every cell of both plants and animals. It appears in several biologically active forms such as *coenzyme A* (CoA) and *acyl carrier protein* (ACP) as well as *pantothenic acid* (see Exhibit 12.15). Synthesized forms used as supplements are often stable salts such as sodium or calcium pantothenate.

Exhibit 12.15   Pantothenic Acid: Functions and Deficiency Effects

FUNCTIONS IN THE BODY	DEFICIENCY EFFECTS
1. As part of coenzyme A, is essential for many chemical reactions in the body, such as those involving the release of energy from carbohydrates, fats, and proteins. CoA also is needed to form many important compounds, including cholesterol, adrenal hormones, and acetycholine, which regulates nerve tissue. 2. Is a part of the enzyme *fatty acid synthetase*, which is needed for synthesizing fatty acids.	1. Not observed in man under normal conditions. When deficiency was induced in experimental studies, subjects developed symptoms such as fatigue, headaches, insomnia, personality changes, nausea, abdominal distress, vomiting, numbness and tingling of hands and feet, muscle cramps, impaired coordination, and some loss in ability to produce antibodies.

[6]National Academy of Sciences, Food and Nutrition Board, National Research Council, *Recommended Dietary Allowances*, ninth edition. Washington, D.C., 1979, p. 76.

Because of the widespread availability of pantothenic acid, dietary deficiencies are unlikely. Excellent sources are yeast, liver, eggs, wheat and rice germ, bran, peanuts, and peas. Good sources are meat, poultry, milk, whole grains, broccoli, and sweet potato. Most fruits and vegetables are fair sources. When grain is milled, pantothenic acid is lost and it is not replaced in the enrichment process. Some pantothenic acid is lost when food is processed—particularly during canning.

Recommended Amounts and Toxicity. The actual requirement for this vitamin is not known and dietary recommendations are only estimates. No official Recommended Dietary Allowances have been established.

Biotin

Forms and Sources. Biotin is widely distributed in nature in at least five forms that are active in the body. It is bound to protein in both foods and tissues, usually with the amino acid *lysine.* A large portion of biotin used in the body is synthesized by intestinal bacteria (see Exhibit 12.16). In addition, it is found in egg yolk, yeast, liver, cereals, legumes, and nuts. Egg white, however, contains a substance called *avidin* that binds biotin and makes it unavailable. Cooking destroys avidin and only the regular consumption of large amounts of raw egg whites could cause a deficiency of this nutrient.

Exhibit 12.16   Biotin: Functions and Deficiency Effects

FUNCTIONS IN THE BODY	DEFICIENCY EFFECTS
Is a component of an enzyme *acetyl CoA,* which is required in metabolic reactions where carbon dioxide is transferred to other molecules *(carboxylation reactions).* These reactions are important in the synthesis of fatty acids, in producing energy from glucose, and in forming several amino acids as well as nucleic acid and glycogen.	Deficiency unlikely. Only artificially induced deficiency (by feeding large amounts of raw egg white) has been observed.

Recommended Amounts and Toxicity. No Recommended Dietary Allowances have been set. Only small amounts of biotin need to be supplied by the diet because of the synthesis of this vitamin by intestinal microorganisms. In fact, studies show that three to six times as much is excreted as ingested, which is a reflection of the major contribution by microorganisms in the body.[7]

[7]National Academy of Sciences, Food and Nutrition Board, National Research Council, *Recommended Dietary Allowances,* ninth edition. Washington, D.C., 1979, p. 8.

The fruit and vegetable group might also be called the "vitamin C and A" group since these are the two most important nutrients we get from these foods. But fruits and vegetables do much more for us than supply large amounts of vitamins C and A. Their flavors, colors, and textures provide a contrast to foods of the other groups and add a lot to our eating pleasure. Additionally, these foods are a good source of fiber, acting as scrub brushes in our teeth and intestines. Fruits and vegetables also "fill in the gaps" with small but important amounts of other nutrients: iron, calcium, potassium, and many trace minerals; B vitamins and folic acid; carbohydrate in the form of both sugar and starch; and even small amounts of protein.

Because of the dilute nature of these foods, which contain 75 to 95 percent water plus some fiber, and their lack of fat, they are generally of high-nutrient density, that is, low in calories for the amount of nutrients they provide.

While fruits, except for rhubarb, are botanically a specific part of the plant (that part which contains the seeds), vegetables can be any part of the plant: root (carrots, beets), stem (asparagus, celery), tuber or underground stem (potato), leaf (spinach, lettuce, cabbage), flower (broccoli, cauliflower), fruit (tomato, squash, peppers), or seed (peas, corn) (see Exhibit 12.17). Whether we categorize the fruit of a plant as a fruit or vegetable in our diet seems to depend on how sweet it is: cantaloupe is eaten as fruit, for example, but squash is considered to be a vegetable and both are in the same family.

Many variables affect the nutritive value of fruits and vegetables: species and variety, part of plant eaten, growing conditions, stage of maturity when harvested, storage conditions, and preparation method. These factors are discussed in Chapter 21.

Nutrients in Different Parts of the Plant

Fruit. Cellulose forms the structural portion of the fruit and it is cemented together with pectin. The fruit usually is higher in sugar, and calories, than other parts of the plant, and sugar content increases with ripening, while acidity decreases. Some fruits have little starch, others, like bananas, have more. Provitamin A is found in fruits such as peaches, apricots, and cantaloupe that are yellow or orange; usually the brighter the color the higher the vitamin A content. Many fruits are excellent sources of vitamin C, including citrus, cantaloupe, papaya, guava, and strawberries. Fruits such as apples, peaches, pears, grapes, cranberries, and dried prunes and apricots have very little vitamin C.

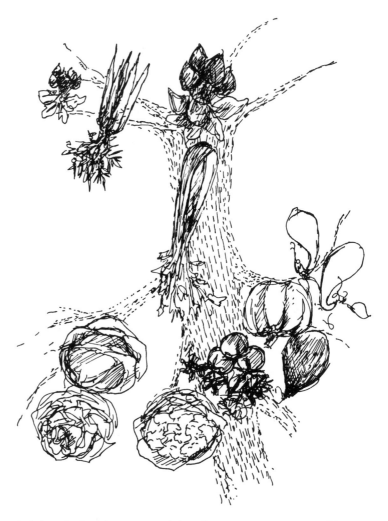

Exhibit 12.17   Many parts of the plant are eaten as vegetables.

The stone fruits and grapes are considered to be fairly good sources of iron.

Of the vegetables that are eaten as fruit, those in the pepper family, green and red pepper, and chili peppers, are outstanding sources of vitamin C as well as being rich in vitamin A. Tomatoes have only one-third to one-half as much vitamin C as oranges. The yellow or orange vegetables such as squash and pumpkin also are known for their vitamin A. The red coloring of tomato masks its orange-carotene color, and it too is rich in vitamin A. Tomatoes also make a worthwhile iron contribution.

Roots and Tubers. These vegetables serve as the storehouse of starch for the plant, and they tend to be higher in calories than stems and leaves. Sweet potatoes are particularly high in calories because of their high sugar content, and they are also an exceptionally rich source of vitamin A. Carrots are another root vegetable high in vitamin A. The red color of beets, unlike that of tomatoes, does not mask carotene and this vegetable is among the least nutritious of the roots and tubers. Potatoes and turnips, while having no vitamin A, are good sources of vitamin C. They also have worthwhile amounts of iron and B vitamins.

Flowers, Buds, and Stems. In this group, broccoli is one of the more nutritious vegetables with its large amounts of provitamin A and vitamin C, as well as some iron, calcium, and B vitamins. Celery, on the other hand, is so high in water and fiber that it's probably the lowest calorie food we eat, and its nutritional contribution is minimal. Green stalks of celery and asparagus will have notably more vitamin A than the white varieties. Cauliflower, because the leaves are tied over the tops of the heads while it matures to keep it white instead of green, has no vitamin A, although it is a fair source of vitamin C. This group is low in calories because these vegetables contain little starch.

Leaves. The most active part of the plant is the leaf, where, in the photosynthesis process, the plant cells, using chlorophyl, in the presence of sunlight, are producing sugar for plant growth from carbon dioxide and water. Many nutrients are concentrated in the leaves such as calcium, iron, vitamin C, and provitamin A. Darker green leaves have more vitamin A than lighter green ones. Oxalic acid is often present in leaves and it can interfere with the absorption of calcium in some instances. The amount of interference depends on the quantity of oxalic acid present. Exhibit 12.18 shows the variation in the effect of oxalic acid on calcium availability in the leaves of different types of plants. Leaves are high in fiber and water and have little or no carbohydrate and very few calories.

Exhibit 12.18   Calcium-to-Oxalate Ratio in Vegetables

FOOD	CALCIUM	OXALATE	CALCIUM-TO-OXALATE RATIO
Beet greens	0.12%	0.92 %	1:8
Spinach	0.12	0.89	1:7
Swiss chard leaves	0.13	0.66	1:5
Turnip greens	0.24	0.015	16:1
Kale	0.31	0.013	24:1
Mustard greens	0.24	0.008	30:1
Collard greens	0.36	0.009	40:1
Broccoli (leaves and flower buds)	0.21	0.005	42:1

Seeds. In the seed, the plant stores nutrients for the growth of the new plant, and, as a result, seed-type vegetables such as peas and corn have larger amounts of protein and starch and are higher in calories than most other vegetables. Many seeds also are good sources of iron, calcium, thiamin, and niacin. Green peas and yellow corn also supply vitamin A and small amounts of vitamin C.

Effect of Maturity and Storage Conditions on Nutrients

With fresh fruits and vegetables, top eating quality and top nutritional value go together. Produce that is wilted or spoiled will have less food value and excessive waste as well as poor flavor and texture (Exhibit 12.19). So buying fresh produce that has been marked down usually will not give us good nutritional value for our money.

Fruits and vegetables that are still immature generally will have less vitamin C and provitamin A than those that are ripened to the peak

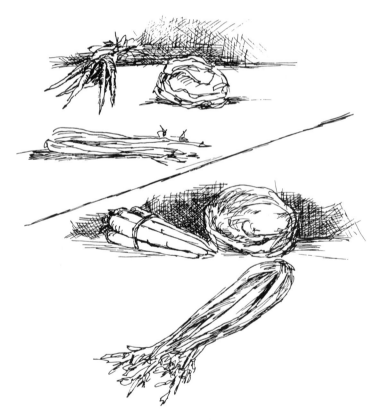

Exhibit 12.19. With fresh produce, top eating quality and top nutritional value go together. Wilted, spoiled produce will have less food value than fresh produce. Topless carrots have more nutrients than those with tops still on.

of eating quality. But overmaturity can result in a reduction of vitamin content. For example, an overmature, hard head of lettuce having a large proportion of white inner leaves, will have considerably less provitamin A than the less mature, darker green, looser-leafed head. The overmature, firm head of lettuce also will have a bitter taste. So avoiding the "hard heads" and choosing those with some give when squeezed gently will give us both better eating quality and more nutrition for our money.

Fresh vegetables and fruits that are stored under refrigeration and kept moist, except for potatoes and dry onions, will retain not only their flavor and eating quality but also their nutrients better than those that are held at room temperature. This is because fresh vegetables and fruits are still alive and continue to age after they have been picked. (More on this in Chapter 21). Cold temperatures retard this maturing process as well as help prevent spoilage. So, to get the besh nutrient value, shop at markets where produce is kept refrigerated, and at home store fresh produce in the refrigerator.

Retention of moisture is also important for keeping vegetables crisp. In most markets vegetables are sprayed with water occasionally and at home they should be stored in the refrigerator in plastic bags, covered containers, or crisper drawers. The wax coating used on cucumbers, apples, oranges, and other foods serves the purpose of holding in moisture as well as protecting the product from invasion by spoilage organisms. This wax is edible and not harmful.

Because fresh vegetables and fruits are still alive, tops left on vegetables such as carrots can withdraw nutrients from the part that we eat in order to continue growing. For this reason it is wise to buy "topless" carrots, which have had the tops removed in the field immediately after harvest, and washed carrots that are packages in plastic bags to hold in moisture.

The nutrient most likely to be lost during storage is vitamin C as it tends to oxidize when exposed to air. However, in some vegetables vitamin C is very stable. For example, cabbage held in cold storage showed no loss of vitamin C in one to two months. Sweet potatoes also retain nutrients well in storage. Unlike other vegetables, white potatoes retain vitamin C best when stored at 50 to 70 degrees. When potatoes are stored at temperatures below 50 degrees, the starch begins to change to sugar, producing a peculiar sweet flavor and more browning when potatoes are cooked. This change can be reversed by holding cold storage potatoes for a few days at a warmer temperature.

Ways to Get the Most Nutrients for Your Money

When making choices among fresh produce, consider first the relative nutrient value between foods. For example, dark-green Romaine lettuce is more nutritious than iceberg (head) lettuce; carrots are more nutritious than beets; oranges are more nutritious than apples; broccoli is more nutritious than cauliflower; and so on.

Also consider price per unit and the amount of waste in determining the cost per serving. Potatoes, for example, are nutritious, sell for a low price per pound, and have little or no waste, if you eat the skin. Asparagus, on the other hand, is high priced, has almost a third waste, and is less nutritious than many other vegetables. So potatoes are eaten often, and asparagus rarely, as a special flavor treat, if you are trying to get the most food value for your money.

To sum up, the best nutrition buys in the fresh produce department are:

1. Foods with a high nutrient value in proportion to their cost
2. Foods with the least amount of waste
3. Fruits and vegetables that are in season—as opposed to high-priced, out-of-season products—and those that are year-round good buys such as potatoes, carrots, and cabbage
4. Foods that are refrigerated and, in the case of crispy vegetables, kept moist, so they retain both nutrient value and eating quality
5. Foods that are mature—or will ripen at home, and are at the peak of eating quality as opposed to the immature and the overmature.

The question of whether fresh or processed fruits and vegetable are a better value nutritionally is discussed in Chapter 21. Processed fruits and vegetables do not necessarily cost more than fresh ones. When fruits and vegetables are in season, they may be considerably less

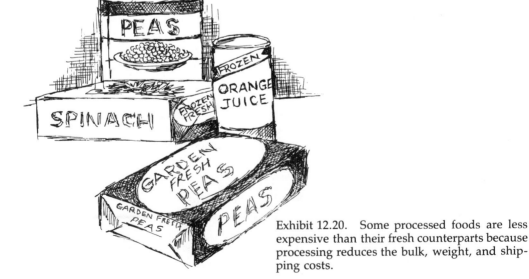

Exhibit 12.20. Some processed foods are less expensive than their fresh counterparts because processing reduces the bulk, weight, and shipping costs.

expensive if purchased fresh than if processed. But the rest of the year, processed forms may be less expensive. In addition, if processing reduces the bulk, weight, shipping, and storage costs, the canned or frozen product may be a year-round better value. Some examples are frozen spinach, frozen or canned peas, and frozen concentrated orange juice (Exhibit 12.20).

Another consideration in choosing between home-prepared products and processed products is quality and flavor. Most people think that fresh corn on the cob, fresh strawberries, fresh peaches, and freshly squeezed orange juice do taste better than their frozen or canned counterparts. U.S. Department of Agriculture statistics show that there has been a turnaround in vegetable eating in the United States, with people using more fresh products (see Exhibit 12.21). Since the 1940s the consumption of fresh vegetables had been giving ground to the consumption of processed ones, but after reaching a low of 96 pounds per person in 1972, this trend appears to have been checked, with the consumption of fresh vegetables rising to 100 pounds per person in 1976. One reason for this change has been the increased use of salads and salad vegetables.

When selecting processed fruits and vegetables, consider the following factors which affect cost and nutritive value.

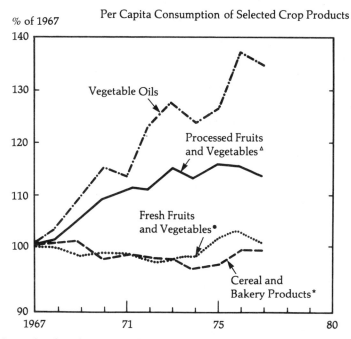

% of 1967 — Per Capita Consumption of Selected Crop Products

Items Combined in Terms of 1957–59 Retail Prices. ᐃ Including Potatoes and Sweet Potatoes. •Excludes Melons. *Grain components only.

Exhibit 12.21. (*Source: 1978 Handbook of Agricultural Charts.* U.S. Department of Agriculture, Washington, D.C.)

Reduced Price. Sometimes a surplus leads to special sales to induce consumers to buy more, and the products are a good value. But sometimes processed foods are marked down at the end of the season to move them before the new crop comes in. These canned or frozen foods will already be nearly a year old, and while perfectly safe, probably will have lost some nutritive value, particularly vitamin C, especially if the storage temperature of canned foods was warm, or if freezer temperature fluctuated. Eating quality depreciates with age as well. Before buying large amounts of this type of sale item, buy a sample first and check the quality.

Foods in dented cans are sometimes reduced in price for a quick sale. The food is safe as long as the can is intact and shows no sign of leaking. Check the extent of the damage to the cans and avoid buying those that are dented along the seam line or the upper or lower edge as these are the weakest parts of the can. Never buy or use food in cans that are bulging as this could be a sign of gas-producing microbial action inside the can with the hazard of food poisoning.

Grade. Lower grade fruits and vegetables will be lower priced but may be just as nutritious, although not as desirable for eating, as higher grade products. Usually store brands or no-name brands are 10 to 20 percent less expensive than advertised brands and could be nearly identical in quality and nutritional value.

Form and Packaging. Whole fruits and vegetables usually cost more than slices, chunks, or halves, but will be no more nutritious. Small or "mixed pieces" are even less expensive. Larger size cans or packages usually give more food for the money, but if your family is small, and you end up with leftovers, which must be stored and reheated, you will also have reduced food value. Large, "loose packs" of frozen fruits and vegetables are a better buy and are convenient because the amount needed can be removed without defrosting the entire package.

Specialty packs, foods packed with special sauces and flavors, etc, are more costly than plain varieties and have more calories too. However, these added sauces and flavors may make vegetables taste so much better that family members, particularly children, are more likely to eat them, and, for this reason, some people think they are worth the extra cost.

Calories in Fruits and Vegetables

Vegetables as a group are known as the dieter's friends because of their relatively small number of calories per serving. A comparison of the calories found in half-cup servings of some popular vegetables shows that many indeed are low in calories (see Exhibit 12.22).

As can be seen, the vegetables that are lowest in calories are the crispy, watery ones that are mostly water and fiber. Higher calorie vegetables are more starchy or sugary.

LESS THAN 10	10 TO 20	OVER 20	
Cabbage	Asparagus	Beets	(30)
Cauliflower	Broccoli	Potato	(55)
Celery	Green beans	Peas	(60)
Cucumber	Carrots	Winter squash	(65)
Lettuce	Spinach	Corn	(85)
Green pepper	Summer squash	Sweet potato	(120)
Parsley	Sauerkraut		
Bean sprouts	Tomatoes		

The calories listed in Exhibit 12.23 are those found in plain vegetables with no added flavorings or sauces. The "saucy calories" can add up fast, as can be seen from Exhibits 12.23 and 12.24.

Exhibit 12.23 Calories per Tablespoon of Selected Sauces, Flavorings, and Dressings

	CALORIES
Mayonnaise	100
Butter or margarine	100
Thousand Island dressing	80
Bleu cheese dressing	75
French dressing	65
Hollandaise sauce	50
Sour cream	30

Cooking method affects calories too. This is especially true of potatoes, which to begin with do not have as many calories as many people think. But adding fat to potatoes when they are cooked can greatly increase the calories. Exhibit 12.25 shows what happens with the caloric content of the same amount of potatoes—one-half cup cooked—when prepared by different methods.

Since potatoes are such a nutrition bargain, finding ways to prepare them that makes them taste good, but does not add so many calories, makes more sense than not eating them at all if you are watching your weight. For example, two tablespoons of cottage cheese added to a baked potato in place of sour cream adds up to just 80 calories; potato slices broiled using one teaspoon of oil total just 85 calories.

Because fruits have proportionately more sugar than vegetables, they generally have more calories per serving. But in many cases fruits are still considered to be high-nutrient-density foods because of the important amounts of vitamin C and provitamin A that they contain (see Exhibit 12.26).

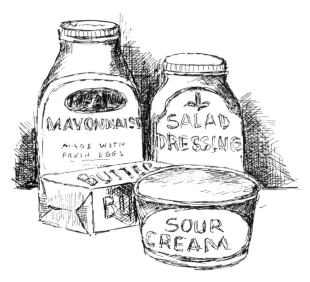

Exhibit 12.24.   Saucy calories add up fast!

Among the fruits, avocado is unique because of its oil content, 6 to 8 percent depending on variety, and it is the oil that makes avocados so high in calories compared to other fruits. Only 10 percent of the oil in avocados is polyunsaturated; 15 percent is saturated, and the remainder is monounsaturated.

When fruits are preserved by canning and freezing, sugar is usually used to prevent enzyme action and to help retain the texture of the fruit. This sugar adds calories as well as cost. So do methods of prepa-

Exhibit 12.25 Calories per Half-Cup Serving Cooked Potatoes Based on Preparation Method

PREPARATION METHOD	CALORIES
Plain boiled, no fat	55
Mashed, milk and butter added	100
Baked, with 2 tablespoons sour cream	110
or 1 tablespoon butter	150
Hash browned	175
French fried (10 pieces)	215
Pan fried, from raw	230
Potato chips (only 10, not ½ cup)	115

Exhibit 12.26   Calories Per Typical Serving of Popular Fruits

30–50 CALORIES	50–75 CALORIES	75–100 CALORIES	OVER 100
½ cup raw strawberries	½ fresh grapefruit	1 raw apple	5 large dried prunes (110)
1 fresh peach	1 medium orange	1 banana	¼ cup raisins (115)
1 fresh plum	3 fresh apricots	1 pear	¼ cup dates (120)
¼ cantaloupe	10 cherries		½ avocado (180)
½ cup fresh pineapple	2 in. × 8 in. slice watermelon		
10 raw grapes			

ration, as seen in Exhibit 12.27. Thus, both calories and money are saved by eating the plain instead of the sugared or fancy fruit.

Juices, Drinks, and Imitations

Fruit and vegetable juices are a popular and convenient substitute for eating the whole fruit. Some people have the idea that the juice is more nutritious than the whole fruit because nutrients have been "released" from the plant cells. However, the fact is that some nutrients and fiber are left behind in the pulp. So unless the entire fruit or vegetable is pulverized and consumed, which usually is not the case, the juice will not be as nutritious as the fruit or vegetable from which it was made. Juices usually are lower in fiber than the fruit itself, especially in the case of apples and other fruits where the peel normally is eaten.

The nutritive value of juice, of course, depends on the nutritional value of the fruit or vegetable from which it is made. Thus, some juices, notably apple, cranberry, and grape are appreciably lower in nutrient value than citrus and tomato juice, and their nutritional contribution is

Exhibit 12.27   Calories per Half-Cup Serving of Peaches Based on Processing and Preparation Methods

PROCESSING OR PREPARATION METHOD	CALORIES
Fresh, sliced	30
with 2 teaspoons sugar	60
Canned, water pack (diet)	50
Canned, light syrup	70
Canned, heavy syrup	95
Frozen, sugared	130
Peach pie, 4 in. slice	350

mainly the calories from their sugar content. Pineapple juice is in between these two groups—less nutritious than citrus juice, but more nutritious than apple or cranberry juice. Sometimes nutrients such as vitamin C are added to the less nutritious juices.

In addition to 100-percent juice products in fresh, canned, and frozen form, there are many drinks, aides, punches, and imitations that contain little or no actual fruit juice. Choose these carefully, as they can be high in calories and low in nutritional value (see Exhibit 12.28).

One type is the powdered juice substitute that contains no fruit juice at all. Ingredient lists tell you that it contains, as its first ingredient, sugar, followed by many flavoring substances such as citric acid, preservatives, and nutrients such as vitamins A and C. When mixed with water, these products may look, smell, and taste much like the real thing. However, they do not have the fiber and the many minerals and vitamins found in natural fruit juices.

Frozen juice substitutes also are popular. Ingredient labels show that these products contain more than one form of sugar as their most important ingredient, various forms of acid including citric, flavoring ingredients, by-products of the juice industry such as pulp and rind, and added nutrients. Because of the pulp and coloring, these products may look and taste so much like the real juice that some people who use them do not realize that they are imitation, even though the label does reveal this fact.

A third type of juice that is very popular is the diluted juice drink or drink that contains from 5 to 30 percent fruit juice, with water and sugar being the two most prominent ingredients. Usually the products

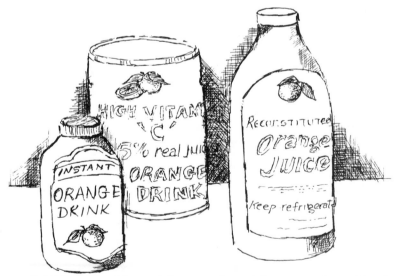

Exhibit 12.28. None of these products offers a good nutritional value compared to frozen orange juice concentrate.

that are called "drink," "punch," or some other name (without the word juice) have the tiniest amount of juice and those labeled (name of fruit) "juice drink" have more juice. The label, at least in the case of orange products, must state prominently the percentage of actual juice contained in the product. When these products are fortified with nutrients, most likely vitamin C, a complete nutrition statement must be included on the label. A comparison of the nutrients in some of the drink products, compared to those in 100-percent juice is shown in Exhibit 12.29.

This comparison shows that the drinks and juice drinks provide a large share of their calories from added sugar and that they are low-nutrient-density foods. They are more popular with children than fruit juice and are heavily advertised to children on television.

While these products often cost less per serving than fruit juice, they are a poorer nutrition value because of their dilution with sugar and water. Because of the great variation in the quantity of juice, sugar, and water in these products, the cost per serving in either cents or calories is not a valid basis for determining value.

When you buy the diluted products, where water is the first ingredient on the label, you pay a high price for water, compared to adding your own to concentrates or powders. A popular form of orange juice now found in refrigerated dairy cases of supermarkets is often mistaken for freshly squeezed orange juice, when actually it is made from frozen concentrate. Generally it costs about twice as much as orange juice mixed at home from frozen concentrate, and it may be more diluted or contain added sugar.

When buying high-sugar juice products, you pay a high price for sugar, compared to adding it. In addition, these high-sugar solutions can be a contributing cause of dental decay. Bathing the teeth in sugar-

Exhibit 12.29   Comparison of Sugar, Calories, and Vitamin C in Popular Drinks

8 OZ SERVING	PERCENTAGE FRUIT JUICE	NO. OF CALORIES	PERCENTAGE OF CALORIES FROM ADDED SUGAR	PERCENTAGE RDA VITAMIN C
Soft drink	0	110	100%	0
Powdered drink mix	0	100	100	15%*
Powdered breakfast or fruit drink	0	120	100	200*
Canned fruit drink	5–10	125	90–95	70*
Canned juice drink	35	125	65	70*
Frozen orange juice (reconstituted)	100	120	0	200
Frozen "imitation" orange juice	0	125	100	200
Frozen lemonade	12	100	93	30

* If added

water solutions is conducive to the growth of the bacteria that cause tooth decay. Also, it has been found that the imitation fruit punches and drinks contain carboxylic acids, which attack the calcium of teeth and increase the growth and appearance of cavities. Natural fruit juices contain carboxylic acids, too, but they also contain substances, which the imitations and juice drinks do not have, that protect teeth from these acids.

Learning to Like Vegetables

Many people, particularly children, consider vegetables something they eat because "they're good for you" rather than something they crave. Because of this, vegetables, more than other foods, need to look good and taste good, or many people will not eat them. The secret for preserving both the eating quality and nutritive value of vegetables is to not overcook them. They should be cooked just until crispy and tender, not overcooked to the mushy stage.

Often children prefer vegetables served raw because the flavors are milder. While cooking helps to release some nutrients from cells making

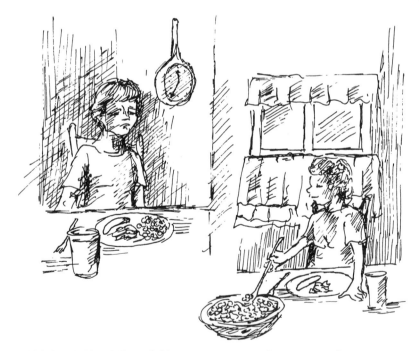

Exhibit 12.30.   When children are encouraged to try a small amount of each vegetable served, they are eventually likely to develop an appreciation for them.

them more available, it also destroys heat-sensitive nutrients such as vitamin C and B vitamins. So if raw vegetables are more acceptable, it is sensible to serve them, rather than trying to force people to eat cooked vegetables. Through learning to enjoy the flavor of a raw vegetable, a person may eventually learn to like the cooked form too.

A family rule that everyone taste a small amount of each food served, including vegetables, often results in children eventually learning to like a variety of vegetables (Exhibit 12.30). On the other hand, nagging and statements such as "eat it, it's good for you" are likely to cause children to develop an entrenched dislike for vegetables that they may never grow out of.

Summary

Originating mainly in plants, vitamins are complex organic compounds needed in extremely small amounts for growth, maintenance, and regulation. Often acting as *coenzymes*, they team with enzymes to catalyze metabolic processes. In this role, they are used up and need to be replenished since the body cannot effectively manufacture them. They usually are absorbed into the body "as is," rather than being broken down during digestion.

Vitamins are commonly looked upon either as *fat-soluble* (A, D, E, and K) or *water-soluble* (C and the B vitamins: niacin, thiamin, riboflavin, folic acid, pantothenic acid, pyridoxine, B_{12}, and biotin). Fat-soluble vitamins are more readily stored in the body; in fact, large excesses over a period of time can be toxic. Some vitamins are destroyed when exposed to heat, light, air, and other factors.

Individual vitamins are described in this chapter by forms, sources, bodily functions, deficiency effects, and recommended amounts.

Part IV

NUTRITION THROUGHOUT THE LIFE CYCLE

NUTRITION DURING PREGNANCY AND LACTATION 13

Highlights

Effects of poor nutrition, alcohol, and drugs
Weight gain during pregnancy
Causes and consequences of low birth weight
Nutritional requirements and use of dietary supplements
Special needs of the vegetarian mother
Beneficial effects of breast feeding
Dietary needs for lactation

The ages and stages of human development do not always have clear lines of demarcation: infancy tends to blend into early childhood, school age into teens, teens into maturity. And when does a middle-aged person become elderly? Then, too, each individual has his or her own rate of development. One person may seem old at 65 while another seems to be in the prime of life.

One thing is certain: We begin to age from the time we are conceived. And preparation for nutritional health in old age begins during our first years of life.

What a woman eats while she is pregnant has great effect on both her health and the growth and development of her baby. The unborn baby, quite obviously, is totally dependent on his mother for all his nutrients, which come from either the food she eats or her own body tissue. Other substances the mother ingests, such as drugs or alcohol, also may make their way to the fetus and can have undesirable effects.

At one time it was thought that the baby had first call on nutrients and would be sufficiently nourished no matter what the mother ate. But now we know this is not true. Poorly nourished mothers are less likely to give birth to healthy babies than are well-nourished mothers.

Several other notions about diet in pregnancy that were in vogue just a few years ago now have been disproven. One was that pregnant women should restrict weight gain as much as possible in order to have a smaller baby and an easier birth. Another was that sodium intake should be restricted to prevent water retention and toxemia. It is now believed that much harm may have been done by such practices.[1]

A problem in this vitally important area of nutrition is that not enough research has been done in recent years on the nutritional requirements in pregnancy. And, for obvious reasons, very little research is done on humans. Most of what we know is based on animal research, and how much of it can be applied directly to humans remains a question. As a result, many recommendations are based on limited data. Variables in social, economic, and psychological environments make it difficult to separate nutrition from other factors affecting the outcome of pregnancy.

IMPORTANCE OF DIET DURING PREGNANCY

Prenatal nutrition may affect an individual throughout life. For example, scientists have found that many children born to women who drink alcohol excessively while pregnant have a pattern of physical and

[1] D. B. Jelliffe, "Feeding Mother and Fetus—Diet in Pregnancy." *Nutrition and the M.D.*, Vol. 1, No. 9, July, 1975, p.2.

mental birth defects. The more severe problems are called the *fetal alcohol syndrome*. Growth deficiency is one of the most prominent symptoms and is related to the fact that heavy drinkers often have limited food intake. Other signs are small brain size, some degree of mental deficiency, and certain facial characteristics such as a low, broad nasal bridge, a long, convex upper lip, increased eye folds, small nails, and limited joint movement. Evidence to date shows that children with the fetal alcohol syndrome never catch up to normal growth and that their IQs do not improve with age.[2]

Animal studies of nutritional deprivation and reproduction show that fewer deprived animals become pregnant, that they have smaller litters, that individual babies are smaller, that there is an increase in mortality for both fetuses and mothers, and that often there are *permanent*, damaging effects that cannot be reversed even with excellent diets after birth.

No such parallel studies have been conducted with humans, but studies of babies and children in both affluent and impoverished societies give some evidence that effects of nutritional deprivation are similar in humans to those found in animals.[3]

The nutritional health of the mother *before* she becomes pregnant is thought to be nearly as important as her nutrition during pregnancy. The nutritional health of the mother and birth weight of the baby are closely related. Nutritionally deprived mothers tend to have low birth weight babies; that is, full-term babies whose weight is lower than normal (below 5 pounds 8 ounces) as well as premature babies. Birth weight has been found to be vitally important in determining the health of the individual throughout life. Low birth weight also is associated with increased rates of infection and illness and greater risk of death for the infant within the first 28 days of life.

A comprehensive study by the Committee on Maternal Nutrition of the National Research Council identified twelve reasons why a woman may give birth to a baby of less than normal (or healthy) weight: youth of the mother (under 17), frequent pregnancies, short stature, low prepregnancy weight for height, limited weight gain during pregnancy, poor nutritional status, smoking, drinking alcohol, chronic disease, certain infections, complications of pregnancy, and a history of prior reproductive loss (see Exhibit 13.1).[4]

[2]K. L. Jones and G. F. Chernoff, "The Fetal Alcohol Syndrome." *Pediatric Basics*. No. 19, 1977.

[3]R. M. Pitkin, "Nutrition in Pregnancy." *Dietetic Currents*, Vol. 4, No. 1, January-February, 1977, p. 1.

[4]Committee on Maternal Nutrition, Food and Nutrition Board, National Research Council, *Maternal Nutrition and the Course of Pregnancy*. Washington, D.C.: National Academy of Sciences, 1970. In R. E. Shank, "A Chink in Our Armor." *Nutrition Today*, Vol. 5, No. 2, Summer 1970, pp. 2-11.

Exhibit 13.1. Factors Related to a Poor Outcome of Pregnancy

Youth of mother (under 17)
Low prepregnancy weight
Low weight gain during pregnancy
Poor nutritional status
Frequent pregnancies
Short stature
Smoking
Drinking alcohol
Diseases that influence nutritional status
Complications of pregnancy
History of prior reproductive loss
Certain infections

Source: Committee on Maternal Nutrition, Food and Nutrition Board, National Research Council, *Maternal Nutrition and the Course of Pregnancy*. Washington, D.C.: National Academy of Sciences, 1970.

Of these, the scientists identified the two most likely causes of poor pregnancy outcome as poor nutrition and youth of the mother (see Exhibit 13.2). Girls younger than 17, who are pregnant before their own growth is completed, have greater nutritional requirements than do

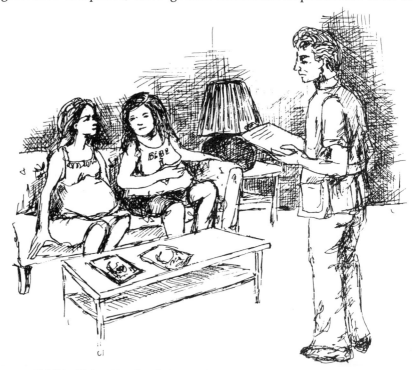

Exhibit 13.2.   Youth of the mother is one of the two most likely causes of poor pregnancy outcome. The other is poor nutrition.

adult women. For them, pregnancy creates a dual growth demand, that of the fetus and that of the girl's body. A further problem is the poor nutritional status and eating habits of many teenage girls, who so often follow fad weight diets in order to lose weight. Adolescent pregnancies have been associated with premature births, low birth weight babies, and infant deaths. Poor nutrition is also an important predisposing factor in toxemia of pregnancy. Improved nutritional status results in decreased rates of toxemia.

Low prepregnancy weight and insufficient weight gain during pregnancy, both symptoms of poor nutrition, are associated with low birth weight babies and other complications. Maternal height is another factor affecting the outcome of pregnancy. The smallest women are confronted with the largest hazards in pregnancy, with high rates of infant mortality, low birth weight, and difficult labor.

Excessive smoking, alcoholism, and drug addiction may diminish the amount of food a pregnant woman eats in addition to causing direct adverse effects on both her body and that of the infant.

WEIGHT GAIN DURING PREGNANCY

During pregnancy new tissue and fluid are formed: about 9 pounds for the baby and placenta and 15 pounds for the mother (see Exhibit 13.3). Of the mother's 15 pounds, the increased size of the uterus accounts for 2 pounds, increased blood volume and fluids for about 8½ pounds, and body changes for breast feeding for approximately 4½ pounds.[5] The total is 24 pounds, which is considered to be the average optimum weight gain during pregnancy. Most women gain 24 to 30 pounds while they are pregnant, but the exact amount a particular woman should gain depends upon her height and size, the size of her baby, and other variables; so no one weight gain is correct for every woman. The optimal weight gain for an overweight mother, for example, is only about half of that for a very thin mother.*

Even more important than how much weight is gained is the rate of gain: it should be smooth and progressive. As can be seen from Exhibit 13.4, the gain during the first three months, or trimester, is relatively small—just 1½ to 3 pounds. From then on weight should go up slowly and steadily about 14 ounces, or just under a pound, a week—or 10 to 11 pounds in both the second and third trimesters. A sudden,

[5]R. E. Shank, "A Chink in Our Armor." *Nutrition Today*, Vol. 5, No. 2, Summer, 1970, pp. 2-11.

*R. L. Naeye, "Weight Gain and the Outcome of Pregnancy." *American Journal of Obstetrics and Gynecology*, Sept. 1, 1979, Vol. 135, No. 1, pp. 3-9.

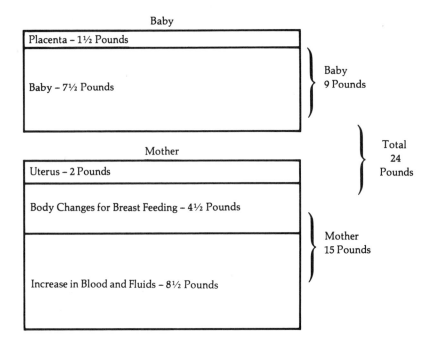

Baby

| Placenta – 1½ Pounds | } Baby 9 Pounds |
| Baby – 7½ Pounds | |

Mother

Uterus – 2 Pounds	} Mother 15 Pounds
Body Changes for Breast Feeding – 4½ Pounds	
Increase in Blood and Fluids – 8½ Pounds	

} Total 24 Pounds

Exhibit 13.3. Distribution of weight gain during pregnancy: just over one-third of the total weight gain is the baby. (*Source:* University of California, Cooperative Extension, *Nutrition for a Healthy Pregnancy*. Berkeley, CA: Cooperative Extension Service, University of California in cooperation with Maternal and Child Health, California Department of Health, 1976, p. 19.)

Exhibit 13.4. Rate of weight gain during pregnancy: the weight gain should be slow and steady. A fast weight gain may indicate problems. (*Source:* University of California, Cooperative Extension, *Nutrition for a Healthy Pregnancy*. Berkeley, CA: Cooperative Extension Service, University of California in cooperation with Maternal and Child Health, California Department of Health, 1976, p. 21.)

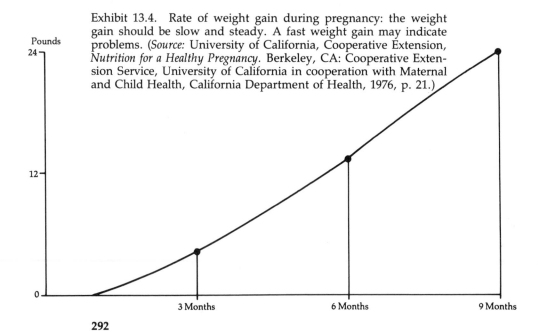

excessive weight gain can be a signal of a serious problem, that is, retention of water in the tissues, and should be closely monitored by a physician.

A steady weight gain of more than a pound a week is a clue that the woman is getting more calories than she needs. Since this could lead to postpregnancy overweight problems, she would be wise to control her calorie intake so her weight gain is within the norm of just under a pound a week.

A woman who is obese when she becomes pregnant should not attempt to lose weight during pregnancy. Neuropsychological abnormalities can occur in the infant if maternal fat stores are used for energy, as they are when calorie intake is less than needed. Moreover, reducing the calorie intake below needs will result in use of protein in the diet for energy, and this protein is needed for formation of new tissue. So an overweight woman should expect to gain weight within the normal range during pregnancy. However, she should guard against excessive weight gain, just as a person of normal weight should do.

A pregnant teenager particularly should not follow a weight control diet during pregnancy because her nutrient needs are so high and her risk of having a low birth weight baby already is so much greater than a mature woman's.

NUTRIENT NEEDS DURING PREGNANCY

The best nutritional preparation for pregnancy that a woman can have is to be well nourished from childhood and through adolescence. During pregnancy, the body becomes more efficient at using nutrients: fewer nutrients are lost; more are retained and absorbed. A woman who is accustomed to eating a diet of foods representing the Four Food Groups will need to make few changes in her eating habits during pregnancy.

She will, however, need more calories—usually about 300 more per day—to provide for the necessary weight gain. The added calories should come from nutritious foods, not low-nutrient-density, high-calorie extras such as fats and sugars, to supply the extra amounts of the other nutrients she needs.

Exhibit 13.5 shows the Recommended Dietary Allowances for nutrients during pregnancy and lactation. Nearly all the nutrients need to be increased. Those of greatest concern in addition to calories are: protein, for tissue and fluid formation; calcium, phosphorus, and vitamin D, for bone and tooth development; iron and folic acid, to prevent anemia; and B vitamins, to assure utilization of the added calories.

The routine use of vitamin and mineral supplements, with the possible exceptions of iron and folic acid, during pregnancy has now fallen

Exhibit 13.5   Recommended Daily Dietary Allowances

	For Pregnancy				For Lactation			
	AGE				AGE			
	11–14	15–18	19–22	23–50	11–14	15–18	19–22	23–50
Body size								
Weight kg	46	55	55	55	46	55	55	55
lb	101	110	120	120	101	110	120	120
Height cm	157	162	163	163	157	162	163	163
in	62	64	64	64	62	64	64	64
Nutrients								
Energy, kcal	2700	2400	2400	2300	2900	2600	2600	2500
Protein, gm	76	76	24	74	66	66	64	64
Vitamin A, RE[1]	1000	1000	1000	1000	1200	1200	1200	1200
Vitamin D, μg[2]	15	15	12.5	10	15	15	12.5	10
Vitamin E, activity[3]	10	10	10	10	11	11	11	11
Ascorbic Acid, mg	70	80	80	80	100	100	100	100
Folacin, μg	800	800	800	800	500	500	500	500
Niacin, mg equiv. NE[4]	17	16	16	15	20	19	19	18
Riboflavin, mg	1.6	1.6	1.6	1.5	1.8	1.8	1.8	1.7
Thiamin, mg	1.5	1.5	1.5	1.4	1.5	1.5	1.5	1.5
Vitamin B$_6$, mg	2.4	2.6	2.6	2.6	2.5	2.5	2.5	2.5
Vitamin B$_{12}$, μg	4.0	4.0	4.0	4.0	4.0	4.0	4.0	4.0
Calcium, mg	1600	1600	1200	1200	1600	1600	1200	1200
Phosphorus, mg	1600	1600	1200	1200	1600	1600	1200	1200
Iodine, μg	175	175	175	175	200	200	200	200
Iron, mg[5]	18+	18+	18+	18+	18	18	18	18
Magnesium, mg	450	450	450	450	450	450	450	450
Zinc, mg	20	20	20	20	25	25	25	25

Source: Recommended Dietary Allowances, Ninth Edition (revised 1979)! National Academy of Sciences, Washington, D.C.

[1] Retinol equivalents. 1 Retinol equivalent = 1 μg retinol or 6 μg β-carotene.

[2] α tocopherol equivalents. 1 mg d-α-tocopherol = 1 μT.E.

[3] As cholecalciferol. 10 μg cholecalciferol = 400 I.U. vitamin D.

[4] 1 NE (niacin equivalent) is equal to 1 μg of niacin or 60 μg of dietary tryptophan.

[5] This increased requirement for pregnancy cannot be met by ordinary diets; therefore, the use of supplemental iron is recommended.

into disfavor among many physicians, and the emphasis instead is on eating a wide variety of foods from the Four Food Groups. Vitamin and mineral supplements are potentially harmful if they give a false sense of security and the idea that a balanced diet is not needed when they are used. Also, high doses of any nutrient can be toxic during pregnancy. For example, large amounts of vitamin A are extremely toxic to the fetus and excess amounts of vitamin D impair fetal development. Several cases of scurvy in newborn infants have been found to be caused by large doses of vitamin C taken by the mother during pregnancy.[6] High doses of vitamin C have also been shown to cause spontaneous abortion in guinea pigs and rats.[7]

The needs for additional calcium, phosphorous, and vitamin D can be met by adding one and one-half to two cups of milk to the normal recommended amount of two cups for a mature female. Pregnant teenagers should add another cup. The additional milk will also supply a portion of the protein, B vitamins, and calories. Nonfat milk, with just half the calories of whole milk, is recommended for most women who need to avoid gaining too much weight. The milk should be supplemented with vitamin D (listed on the label) and, if nonfat milk is used, with vitamin A as well.

Women who don't like to drink milk will need to use other forms of dairy food such as cheese. (See Chapter 11 for more ways to add milk to the diet.)

A woman who is already eating the recommended two 3-ounce servings of protein foods per day will need to increase this amount only by one more serving to be sure to get enough protein. The proteins should supply the full range of essential amino acids in each meal. The easiest way to do this is to include some animal protein. However, the plant proteins can be adequate if eaten in the right combination to supply all the essential amino acids (see Chapter 9).

Iron and folic acid are the two nutrients most likely to be lacking during pregnancy, and if the mother's intake is insufficient, the fetus will tap the mother's own reserve. As a result, a number of women develop iron-deficiency anemia during pregnancy. Some also show symptoms of folic acid-deficiency anemia. Folic acid is an essential growth factor, and low folate stores in the mother have been shown in animal studies to severely affect fetal growth. In human studies, folate-deficient mothers were found to give birth to four times as many low birth weight infants as mothers with normal amounts of folic acid.[8]

[6]M. Winick, "Toxicity of Nutrients on the Human Fetus." *Nutrition and the M.D.*, Vol. 3, No. 4, February, 1977, pp. 1-2.

[7]J. N. Hathcock, "Nutrition: Toxicology and Pharmacology," in Nutrition Reviews' *Present Knowledge in Nutrition*, fourth edition. New York, Washington, D.C.: Nutrition Foundation, Inc., 1976, p. 506.

[8]Studies by English investigators reported in *Archives of Diseases in Childhood* (January, 1977) and discussed in "Influence of Folic Acid on Infant Birthweight and Growth." *Nutrition and the M.D.*, Vol. 3, No. 6, April, 1977, p. 1.

Even when a woman consumes liver or kidney once a week and several servings of iron and folic acid a day from dark, green, leafy vegetables and fruits, along with other foods containing these nutrients, she probably will not be able to get the amounts she needs from her foods—especially if she did not have good stores of them before pregnancy. For this reason, supplementation with iron salts, for example, with ferrous sulfate at the rate of 30 to 60 mg iron per day, is recommended during the second and third trimesters. A daily supplement of 400 to 800 micrograms of folic acid also is generally recommended. Since iron from vegetable sources appears to be less well absorbed than iron from animal sources (see Chapter 11), pregnant vegetarians need to be particularly concerned with getting enough iron.

The need for vitamin B increases in proportion to the calorie increase during pregnancy and usually can be met easily through increases in the consumption of milk and protein foods. Vegetarians who consume no animal foods need to be especially concerned about getting enough vitamin B_{12}. Recent animal studies have shown a relationship between maternal intake of B_{12} and birth weight. Rat pups whose mothers received more B_{12} experienced lower mortality rates and more resistance to infection during the first months of life than did those pups whose mothers had received less B_{12}.[9] It is believed that B_{12} concentration may be twice as high in the fetus as in the mother. Because vitamin B_6 concentration in fetal circulation is five times that of the mother, this B vitamin is very important in prenatal diets too. Good food sources of B vitamins include meat, legumes, wheat germ, whole-grain cereals, and leafy greens.

A pregnant woman who is trying to keep her calorie consumption within the optimal amount should not cut down on the four recommended servings from the bread and cereal group. She should use more of the whole-grain cereals and bran and wheat germ and less of the refined cereals and the high-sugar, high-fat, bakery products such as doughnuts, sweet rolls, cakes, cookies, and pie. Whole-grain cereals are important sources of iron, other trace elements, and B vitamins.

Constipation is often a problem during the latter months of pregnancy, and the fiber supplied by bran and whole grain cereals as well as by fresh vegetables and fruits, especially prunes, is important to help prevent this problem. Laxatives should be avoided.

Foods in the bread and cereal group also supply needed amounts of carbohydrates. A low-carbohydrate diet is hazardous during pregnancy because the ketosis (see Chapter 7) that may result impairs fetal development. A pregnant woman is subject to relative hypoglycemia (see Chapter 19), which is enhanced by inadequate calorie and carbohydrate intake. Carbohydrates should be eaten in small amounts

[9] "Vitamins and the Fetus: The Benefits of B_{12}." *Science News*, Vol. 103, April 7, 1973, p. 220.

throughout the day rather than in one or two high-carbohydrate meals to help prevent hypoglycemic symptoms.

A woman who suffers from nausea and vomiting during the early months of pregnancy may find that eating frequent, small meals and nibbling carbohydrate foods such as crackers whenever her stomach is empty, for example, when she wakes up in the morning, may help alleviate these symptoms.

Iodine is a very important mineral that needs to be present for both the mother and the developing infant to have normally functioning thyroid glands. If a pregnant woman uses iodized salt, she can meet her requirement for this mineral.

Sodium, from salt and other sources, is also essential during pregnancy, and its restriction could result in an excess burden on the kidney. If the diet supplies insufficient sodium, the kidney must extract it in order to recirculate it. Thus, the routine restriction of salt and sodium in the pregnant woman's diet is not considered to be wise, although such a restriction may be necessary under certain conditions.

PROPER DIET DURING PREGNANCY

The health of the mother and her baby depend on the kinds of foods she eats before and during pregnancy.

The Four Food Groups can be used as the basis for planning a diet during pregnancy, as shown in Exhibit 13.6. Add to it one more serving of foods from the meat group and one or two more servings of milk, being sure the milk is fortified with vitamin D and A if nonfat. Be sure to eat at least four servings of fruits and vegetables with one being a good source of vitamin C and one being a dark-green leafy vegetable.

Exhibit 13.6 Daily Food Guide

	NUMBER OF SERVINGS		
FOOD GROUP	NONPREG- NANT WOMAN	PREGNANT WOMAN	LACTATING WOMAN
Protein foods (animal and vegetable)	3	4	4
Milk and milk products	3	4	5
Grain products	3	3	3
Vitamin-C-rich fruits and vegetables	1	1	1
Leafy green vegetables	2	2	2
Other fruits and vegetables	1	1	1

Source: Nutrition During Pregnancy and Lactation. Maternal and Child Health Unit, California Dept. of Health, Sacramento, CA., 1975, p. 34.

Exhibit 13.7   Sample Meal Pattern

	NONPREGNANT WOMAN	PREGNANT WOMAN	LACTATING WOMAN
Breakfast:	1 svg. Vitamin C rich fruits and vegetables 1 svg. Grain products 1 svg. Milk and milk products	1 svg. Vitamin C rich fruits and vegetables 1 svg. Grain products 1 svg. Milk and milk products	1 svg. Vitamin C rich fruits and vegetables 1 svg. Grain products 1 svg. Milk and milk products
Morning Snack:	Optional	Optional	Optional
Lunch:	2 svgs. Grain products 1 svg. Protein foods 1 svg. Other fruits and vegetables 1 svg. Milk and milk products	2 svgs. Grain products 1 svg. Protein foods 1 svg. Other fruits and vegetables 1 svg. Milk and milk products	2 svgs. Grain products 1 svg. Protein foods 1 svg. Other fruits and vegetables 1 svg. Milk and milk products
Afternoon Snack:	1 svg. Protein foods ½ svg. Milk and milk products	1 svg. Protein foods ½ svg. Milk and milk products	1 svg. Protein foods 1 svg. Milk and milk products
Dinner:	1 svg. Protein foods 2 svgs. Leafy green vegetables	2 svgs. Protein foods 2 svgs. Leafy green vegetables 1 svg. Milk and milk products	2 svgs. Protein foods 2 svgs. Leafy green vegetables 1 svg. Milk and milk products
Evening Snack:	½ svg. Milk and milk products	½ svg. Milk and milk products	1 svg. Milk and milk products

Source: Nutrition During Pregnancy and Lactation. Maternal and Child Health Unit, California Dept. of Health, Sacramento, CA., 1975, p. 34.

Eat the recommended four servings from the bread and cereal group, using whole-grain cereals as much as possible (see Exhibit 13.7).

The pregnant woman should get enough calories to gain just about a pound a week during the second and third trimesters of pregnancy, or 25 to 30 pounds total. These calories should come from nutrient-rich foods, rather than foods high in calories and low in vitamins, minerals, and protein.

Supplements of minerals and vitamins, except for iron and folic acid, are not needed when the diet includes a variety of foods from the Four Food Groups.

Pregnant teenagers are at greater nutritional risk than mature women and have increased needs for all of the nutrients. It is especially important for them to increase milk consumption to five to six cups per day.

Caloric deprivation during pregnancy is especially serious. Dieting during pregnancy for weight loss or to keep from gaining weight is dangerous to both mother and baby and should be avoided.

The pregnant woman should avoid certain antibiotics, anticonvulsants in certain cases, laxatives, diuretics, digestive aids, diet pills, pep pills, sleeping pills or tranquilizers, aspirin, megadoses of vitamin and mineral supplements. In general, the effects of any drug or medication taken by a pregnant woman should be carefully weighed against the possible effects on the fetus. She should not eat raw meat (to avoid toxmoplasmosis, see Chapter 25) and should drink alcohol either in small amounts or not at all.

BENEFITS OF BREAST FEEDING

Mother's milk has many nutritional benefits for the infant, which we will discuss in the next section. A mother benefits from breast feeding her baby, too: she can derive a great sense of self-satisfaction and accomplishment from being able to feed her baby; she may enjoy a feeling of closeness with her youngster that sets the stage for a continuing warm mother-child relationship; nursing can give the mother a chance to relax and enjoy her baby; her uterus returns to normal size more quickly; nursing will help her lose some of the weight gained during pregnancy; and she will have an extraordinary appetite and be able to enjoy eating without gaining too much weight.

Besides, breast feeding is convenient. The mother's milk is readily available, free from outside contamination, always the right temperature, and takes no work to prepare. It costs less than many of the more costly types of ready-to-use formulas, but it is not without cost since the mother must eat more in order to be able to feed her baby adequately. Breast milk can be the infant's only food source for the first four to six months of life.

In spite of all these benefits, many mothers choose not to nurse their babies for a variety of reasons. They may have a physical ailment or disease that makes nursing unadvised; they may be employed and unable to be available for nursing at every feeding; they may lack confidence in their ability to nurse, perhaps trying it briefly and giving up; they may not have been given adequate encouragement by their doctor or husband; or perhaps they simply don't like the idea. Of all these reasons, the most unfortunate is lack of confidence.

Up to 85 to 90 percent of women can nurse their babies successfully if they are determined to do so and stick with it long enough to get the system operating. The frequent sucking of a hungry baby stimulates the breasts to produce milk and allow it to flow (the "let down" reaction) (see Exhibit 13.8). Tension and early overconcern by the mother that her baby is "not getting enough to eat" and premature resorting to supplemental feeding can be counterproductive and keep her from developing an adequate milk supply. Being overanxious and giving up too soon are the principal reasons why mothers who want to nurse are unsuccessful in nursing their babies.

In recent years more mothers have been choosing to breast feed and physicians have become more supportive. Groups such as the La

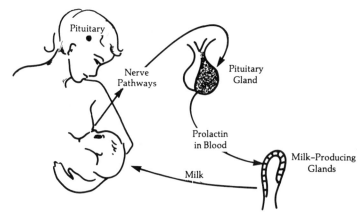

Exhibit 13.8. When the infant sucks, the mother's pituitary gland is stimulated to produce the hormone *prolactin*, which in turn stimulates the milk-producing glands in her breasts.

Leche League are available in many communities to supply information and support for new mothers and mothers-to-be who want to learn how to nurse their babies.

DIET DURING LACTATION

Milk production requires more nutrients—more calories, protein, minerals, and vitamins—than pregnancy, as you can see from Exhibit 13.9. The nursing mother produces, on the average, 20 to 30 ounces of milk per day, or nearly a quart. Since human milk averages 20 calories per ounce, this means that 20 ounces of milk have 400 calories and 30 ounces have 600 calories. It takes about 20 additional calories for the body to produce 100 calories of milk. So the total calorie cost of producing 20 ounces of milk is 480 (400+80); for 30 ounces of milk it is 720 (600+120).

The nursing mother also has high needs for protein, calcium, phosphorus, and vitamin D. But getting these nutrients will not be difficult because she will have a hearty appetite. She should continue to eat the same well-balanced diet, based on the Four Food Groups, that she ate in pregnancy and add to it more milk and more calories. (See Exhibit 13.6 for the optimum number of servings from each food group during pregnancy and lactation.) As during pregnancy, the calories should come from nutrient-rich foods.

Milk is the best food for protecting the mother's bones and teeth against a drain of calcium and phosphorus. She needs at least one cup more than in pregnancy, or a total of five cups a day. The milk should be fortified with vitamin D. The nursing mother also needs plenty of fluids—2 to 3 quarts a day—to provide the liquid for the breast milk.

Exhibit 13.9 Extra Calories Needed by Lactating Mother for Milk Production

AMOUNT OF MILK	CALORIES IN MILK	CALORIES TO PRODUCE MILK	TOTAL ADDITIONAL CALORIES NEEDED
1 oz	20	4	24
10 oz	200	40	240
20 oz	400	80	480
30 oz	600	120	720

Fruit juice might be used, in addition to milk and water, to add nutrients as well as fluid.

Because birth control hormones have the effect of reducing milk production, some other form of birth control is recommended during lactation. (Nursing itself acts to some extent to prevent conception, but it is not reliable!) Drugs such as barbituates, laxatives, aspirin, and birth control hormones can be transmitted through breast milk; so their use should be minimal. The specific drugs that should be omitted during nursing include any drug or chemical in large amounts, diuretics, atropine, reserpine, adrenal steroids, morphine and its derivatives, hallucinogens, anticoagulants, bromides, ergot, antithyroid drugs, antimetabolites, cathartics, and flagyl. The use of sulfa preparations is also not wise in the first two weeks of nursing because of the jaundice problem. As far as the contraceptives are concerned, it was felt until very recently that they should not be used; however, some of the newer ones, with very small amounts of active hormones, may be acceptable.

To sum up, lactation is the normal outcome of pregnancy and provides a simple way to feed an infant exactly what he needs. A diet based on the Four Food Groups with added amounts of milk and calories will provide the nutrients the mother needs for milk production.

Summary

Myths on the subject of pregnancy and lactation abound, and as research continues to be conducted, there is concern over potentially adverse consequences of certain practices. It has been found that babies do *not* have first call on the pool of nutrients available in the mother's body, and may indeed suffer from a mother's deficient diet. A weight gain of 25 to 30 pounds at the rate of just under a pound per week is now considered to be desirable, and the pregnant mother should not attempt to lose weight.

Low birth weight can result in irreversible damage to the child. Chief among its several causes is poor nutrition and youth of the mother, which generates a double nutritional demand. Alcohol consumption, smoking, and drug addiction can have direct adverse effects as well as causing lowered food intake with resulting nutritional deficiencies. Drugs and supplements of any kind should be taken with great care. Iron and folic acid are now believed to be the only nutritional supplements needed during pregnancy.

The greater nutritional needs of mother and developing baby may be met by increasing the consumption of high-nutrient-density foods to furnish approximately 300 additional calories daily. This may be accomplished easily by following the Four Food Group plan and eating an additional one to two servings from the milk and protein food groups. Calcium from the milk group is particularly important, as is the consumption of whole-grain breads or cereals for increased fiber. Iodized salt is recommended, and vegetarians may need to use a vitamin B_{12} supplement.

Breast feeding holds many advantages for the mother as well as the infant. Lactation increases the mother's calorie requirement by 400 to 800 calories daily and requires plenty of fluids. An increase in consumption of milk is particularly helpful, adding calories, fluid, and protection from calcium-phosphorous drain of the mother's bones and teeth. The nursing mother must also be careful about using drugs, which might be transmitted through breast milk to the infant.

INFANT NUTRITION 14

Highlights

Growth and developmental characteristics of infants
Effects of under- and overnutrition
Nutritional needs of infants
Comparison among breast milk, formula, and cow's milk
Anti-infective and anti-allergenic factors in human milk
Feeding and weaning patterns
Prevention and treatment of infant obesity
Special nutritional problems of the premature infant

The critical importance of nutrition to the individual's lifelong physical and mental health that began in the womb continues through the first year of life.

During the first year, the infant grows faster than at any other time during life. Malnourishment in infancy and early childhood can result in the individual's never reaching full growth potential. Crucial brain development takes place now, too, and deprivation of nutrients can mean less than optimal mental development. Satisfaction of the infant's nourishment needs also contributes to his emotional development in a most basic way.

In recent years researchers have developed a great deal of new information about infant nutritional needs and the benefits of breast feeding. Recommendations for feeding infants have changed drastically as a result, but not all of the recommendations have received general acceptance as yet.

DEVELOPMENTAL CHARACTERISTICS OF INFANTS

A newborn infant quite obviously is not a miniature adult or even a miniature child. Because there are many developmental differences between infants and young children, their nutritional needs are quite different.

To begin with, an infant is totally helpless and must depend on caretakers to supply all nourishment. His only way of making nutritional needs known is to cry. The infant learns that his world is a secure place when his need for food is satisfied. His emotional satisfaction is enhanced when he is cuddled close to his caretaker's warm body while he is being fed. This physical and psychological bonding during feeding, especially as seen in breast feeding, is now considered a very important phase of a child's emotional development.

The newborn baby has a strong sucking reflex for obtaining nourishment, but cannot chew or swallow solid foods. During the first year, an infant learns to move solid foods to the back of his throat with his tongue, instead of thrusting them forward, and he learns to chew (see Exhibit 14.1). When eye-hand coordination and small muscle control develop, he can learn to pick up foods with his fingers, or even with a spoon, and put them in his mouth and to drink from a cup instead of from a nipple.

Growth during infancy is tremendous (see Exhibit 14.2). The infant will double his birth weight in about 6 months and triple it by the end of the first year. His length will increase by about 50 percent and his blood volume will triple in the first year. His body composition will change from 75 to 80 percent water at birth to closer to the adult level of 55 to 60 percent by one year. His lean body mass will increase and his

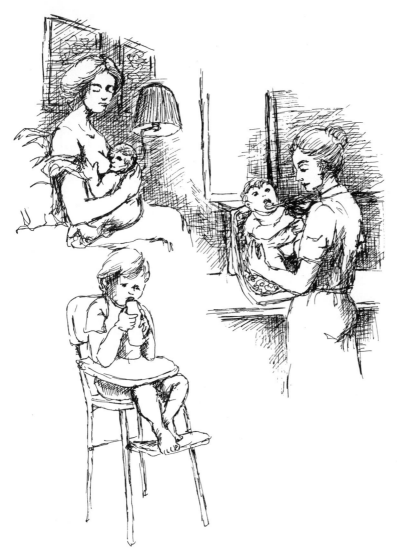

Exhibit 14.1. During the first year, a baby develops many eating skills.

body fat will accumulate rapidly during the first 12 months. His bones and teeth will grow and become more solidly calcified. His brain and nervous system will grow and develop. His gastrointestinal system, kidneys, liver, and other organs will mature and become more efficient at digesting and absorbing food.

Growth and development proceed in an orderly, predictable sequence, but at different rates in different children. They take place in

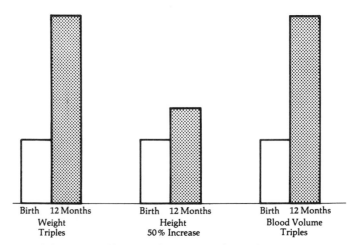

Exhibit 14.2. Changes during an infant's first year of life.

two ways: *hyperplasia,* an increase in cell number, and *hypertrophy,* an increase in cell size due to increased concentration of protein or fat. Each tissue or organ has a critical period of development, usually during hyperplasia, during which nutritional deprivation may cause irreversible adverse effects on that tissue or organ.

For example, the brain approaches adult size, weight, and cell number of age two. From the second trimester of pregnancy to 6 months of age is the *brain growth spurt* period when brain cells rapidly multiply and grow. This continues to a lesser extent until a child is 18 to 24 months old. Throughout its growth spurt the brain needs adequate nutrients.

Animal studies show that severe malnutrition during crucial brain growth periods can produce brain defects that cannot be rectified nutritionally.[1] However, animal studies cannot be directly extrapolated to humans. Human brains may not be as vulnerable as those of animals because they are so large and complex, and they may be preferentially allocated scarce nutrients. Human studies do show that severe malnutrition of long duration in infancy does significantly alter mental ability and human behavior, and that this effect is irreversible.[2] The effects of lesser, chronic undernutrition on brain development are harder to measure.

[1]National Institute of Child Health and Human Development Center for Research for Mothers and Children, "Malnutrition, Learning, and Behavior." U.S. Department of Health, Education, and Welfare, Public Health Service, National Institutes of Health, Publication No. (NIH) 76-1036. Washington, D.C.: U.S. Government Printing Office, 1976, p. 11.

[2]*Ibid.,* p. 12.

Since the infant's head size increases rapidly as the brain grows, one measurement doctors use to determine developmental progress is head circumference. Other routine measurements used are height and weight. Usually a physician will plot an infant's height and weight on a standard height-weight chart to determine growth progress and compare it with norms for age and sex. The skinfold thickness measurement, which is helpful in measuring body fat and pinpointing under- and overnutrition, is rarely used in infants.

EFFECTS OF UNDER- AND OVERNUTRITION ON DEVELOPMENT

Undernutrition early in life can result in some permanent impairment of physical growth. Infants who do not get enough to eat, because of either illness or deprivation, over a significant period of time tend to be shorter as well as underweight. Undernutrition will slow the bone growth and delay calcification. The deposition of fat and growth of lean body mass also will be retarded. The undernourished infant will have a smaller reserve, and is more susceptible to illness. Moreover, any serious illness may be more life-threatening for the undernourished infant than for other infants.

After a debilitating illness or deprivation, an undernourished infant, given a good diet, first will gain weight rapidly. Then his height will increase rapidly. But this "catch-up" growth may never be enough to allow the infant to reach full genetic potential in stature as an adult. Much is yet unknown about the ability of undergrown children to catch up.

Overnourished infants who become obese, on the other hand, tend to have advanced skeletal ages and will be taller as well as heavier than normal-weight infants. However, fat babies are not healthy babies either, as they are more prone to severe lower respiratory infections.[3]

One unresolved question is whether infantile obesity causes adult obesity. One theory, which is highly controversial, is that obesity frequently begins in infancy or childhood and that there are one or more critical periods during development when overnutrition can cause an abnormal increase in fat cell numbers.[4] Once the fat cells are formed, they never disappear.

According to this theory, many obese adults have an excess number of fat cells formed in infancy which led to major problems controlling

[3]C. G. Neumann, "Obesity in Infancy—Prevention and Management." *Nutrition and the M.D.*, Vol. 1, No. 9, July, 1975, p. 1.

[4]J. L. Knittle, "Obesity in Childhood: A Problem in Adipose Tissue Cellular Development." *Journal of Pediatrics*, Vol. 81, 1972, p. 1048.

their weight. (More on this in Chapter 5.) Those who believe this theory emphasize the need to change infant feeding practices in order to prevent adult obesity.

Other researchers have shown that the diagnosis of infant obesity due to an excess number of fat cells is unreliable and that most fat babies become lean during childhood.[5] They also claim that obese people who were obese in infancy are only a small portion of the total number of obese adults.

Many experts believe that genetic factors are more important than infant obesity in determining adult obesity: the obese youngster with one or two obese parents is the one who is likely to become an obese adult.[6] Whatever its cause, the adult obesity problem seems more likely to arise if the infant does not lose baby fat by school age.

While there are many unresolved questions regarding the long-term effects of under- and overnutrition in infancy, there is general agreement that a normal-weight or slightly thin baby is the healthiest and that the goal of infant feeding practices should be to attain and maintain this optimum weight level.

NUTRITIONAL NEEDS OF INFANTS

Usually the caloric needs of infants, shown in Exhibit 14.3, are calculated on the basis of their weight in kilograms:

0–6 mo—115 calories/kg body wt = 400–700 calories/day
6–10 mo—105 calories/kg body wt = 1,000 calories/day

Considering that a dieting adult female may use a 1,000-calorie-a-day diet, it is easy to appreciate how high the infant's energy needs are in proportion to his size.

If the infant's energy needs are not met, protein will be used for energy and there will be little or no increase in his lean body mass. Excess calories result in increased fat deposition and will lead to overweight and obesity. Height and weight measurements, compared to the norm for the infant's age and sex, are the guidelines used to determine if the caloric intake is optimal.

[5]T. Sveger, "Does Overnutrition or Obesity During the First Year Affect Weight at Age Four?" *Acta Paediatr Scand*, Vol. 67, 1978, pp. 465-67. Also R. Jung, M. Gurr, M. Robinson, W. James, "Does Adipocyte Hypercellularity in Obesity Exist?" *British Medical Journal*, Vol. 2, July, 1978, pp. 319-21.

[6]Marginal Comments, "The Origins of Obesity." *American Journal of Diseases of Children*, Vol. 130, May, 1976, pp. 465-67.

NUTRIENT	UNIT	ALLOWANCE	
		0 TO 6 MO. OLD	6 MO. TO 12 MO. OLD
Food energy	cal	kg wt × 115 cal.	kg × 105
Protein	g	kg wt × 2.2 g	kg × 2.0
Fat-soluble vitamins			
Vitamin A	μg R.E.[1]	.420	.400
Vitamin E	mg & T.E.[2]	3	4
Vitamin D	μg[3]	10	10
Water-soluble vitamins			
Ascorbic acid	mg	35	35
Folacin	μg	30	45
Niacin	mg equi N.E.[4]	6	8
Riboflavin	mg	0.4	0.6
Thiamin	mg	0.3	0.5
Vitamin B_6	mg	0.3	0.6
Vitamin B_{12}	g	0.5[5]	1.5
Minerals			
Calcium	mg	360	540
Phosphorus	mg	240	360
Iodine	μg	40	50
Iron	mg	10	15
Magnesium	mg	50	70
Zinc	mg	3	5

Source: Recommended Dietary Allowances, Ninth Edition (revised 1979). National Academy of Sciences, Washington, D.C.

[1] Retinol equivalents. 1 retinol equivalent = 1 μg retinol or 6 μg β-carotene.

[2] α tocopherol equivalents. 1 μg d-α-tocopherol = 1 μT.E.

[3] As cholecalciferol. 10 μg cholecalciferol = 400 I.U. vitamin D.

[4] 1 NE (niacin equivalent) is equal to 1 μg of naicin or 60 μg of dietary tryptophan.

[5] The RDA for vitamin B_{12} in infants is based on average concentration of the vitamin in human milk. The allowances after weaning are based on energy intake (as recommended by the American Academy of Pediatrics) and consideration of other factors such as intestinal absorption; see text.

Protein

Because rapid growth requires sufficient protein, protein is the infant's second most important nutritional need. The infant needs all of the eight essential amino acids required by adults plus histidine. Protein malnutrition will result in a reduction in bone growth as well as retardation in the development of lean body mass. The current recommendations for the infant's protein requirements are:

> 0–6 mo—2.2 g/kg body weight or 1.6 g/100 calories
> 6–12 mo—2.0 g/kg body weight or 1.4 g/100 calories

Thus, at a calorie intake of 500 per day, an infant needs about 8 grams of protein; at 1,000 calories per day, he needs double this amount, or 16 grams. However, because new findings indicate that the protein level in human milk is lower than originally thought, the RDA for protein for infants will need to be recalculated.[7] Excess protein will be used for energy and may contribute to an obesity problem, but it can also overburden the infant's immature kidneys with potentially serious results.

The residues of protein digestion—nitrogen, hydrogen, and phosphorus—along with minerals such as sodium and potassium are called the *renal* (kidney) *solute* (dissolved-substances) *load*, which the kidneys must extract. An infant's immature kidneys are less able than a mature adult's to handle an excess renal solute load, and serious complications, such as life-threatening dehydration, can result from doing so. For this reason, overfeeding protein can be as harmful to an infant as lack of protein. Overconcentrated formulas and undiluted evaporated milk are particularly hazardous because of the high renal solute load they cause.

Fat

Fat is an important, concentrated source of energy for the infant, who has a small capacity for food. It is a source of the essential fatty acid linoleic acid. The lack of linoleic acid has been shown to result in poor growth and a severe skin rash. Fat also carries the fat-soluble vitamins A, D, E, and K. The infant's fat digestion mechanism is poorly developed, for example, production of bile salts is low, and the unsaturated fats are easier for the infant to digest. The triglycerides of medium-chain fatty acids are absorbed more readily.

Sometimes nonfat (skim) or low-fat (2 percent) milk are given to infants instead of formula with the goal of reducing saturated fat or calories in their diets. This recommendation must be questioned. Because of their lack of fat, these milks do not provide enough energy or linoleic acid. If an infant drinks enough of them to satisfy calorie needs, the renal solute load is too high.

Carbohydrates

No specific recommendation is made for the amount of carbohydrate needed by an infant. However, carbohydrate is important to provide energy and to maintain the level of glucose in the blood. Galactose, a monosaccharide (single sugar) is formed, along with glucose, from the breakdown of *lactose* (milk sugar), and plays a unique role in forming

---

[7]D. B. Jelliffe, "Protein in Cow's Milk." *Nutrition and the M.D.*, Vol. 3, No. 4, February, 1977, p. 2.

myelin in brain tissue and the *glycoproteins* of collagen (connective tissue). Both of these substances are formed during the immediate newborn period. Lactose is the only sugar that forms galactose. Both human and cow's milk contain lactose, but sometimes other sugars are substituted for lactose in infant formulas.

The young infant does not have the enzyme *amylase*, which is needed for the digestion of starch; thus there is no reason to add cereal to his diet before this enzyme is present—at about three to six months.

Water

Water is even more essential to the infant's survival than food. An infant has a large surface area in proportion to size and consequently loses a greater amount of water through evaporation than an adult (60 percent of his intake compared to 40 or 50 percent for adults). Since the infant's immature kidneys do not function as efficiently as an older child's, he needs more water to process wastes. For these reasons and because of his small size, an infant will succumb more rapidly than an adult to the ravaging effects of dehydration.

Normally the amount of water an infant receives in breast milk or properly diluted formulas is adequate. A baby given whole cow's milk with its higher renal solute load needs to be offered additional amounts of water. During times of stress and illness when milk intake is low, during periods of diarrhea or vomiting when water loss is great, and during very hot weather when body evaporation is high, an infant should be offered additional amounts of water and should be closely watched for signs of dehydration.

Minerals

Infants need all of the minerals required by adults. The recommended allowances are listed in Exhibit 14.4 and a discussion of their specific functions can be found in Chapter 11.

Iron is the nutrient most likely to be insufficient in the infant's diet. Because of this, iron-deficiency anemia is the most common nutritional disorder among infants between the ages of 6 and 24 months. A newborn infant has iron stores established before birth that he uses during the first few months of life. From then on he must get iron from his food. Since cow's milk has little available iron, formula-fed infants need an iron-fortified formula or an iron supplement. The use of iron-fortified cereals and other iron-rich foods after 6 months of age also helps to add iron to the diet.

For the breast-fed infant, nutrition researchers are not in agreement about the need for iron supplementation. Human milk has more iron than cow's milk, and this iron is known to be much more available:

49 percent is absorbed from breast milk compared to 4 percent from fortified formulas and cereals. The lower protein and phosphorous and higher lactose and vitamin C levels are thought to be factors in the absorption of iron from breast milk. Studies have shown that full-term infants who are fed only breast milk until they triple their birth weight are not likely to develop iron-deficiency anemia unless iron stores at birth are low. However, many authorities recommend that breast-fed infants be given an iron supplement from the age of 3 to 4 months as a precautionary measure because the level of iron stores at birth is unknown.[8] Usually the supplement given is ferrous sulfate, which is the most readily absorbed form of iron.

Since excess iron can be harmful, the total of added iron in formula, cereal and other foods, and supplements should be monitored so it is not greatly above the recommended amounts of 10 milligrams a day for infants 0 to 6 months of age, and 15 milligrams a day for infants 6 to 12 months old.

Fluorine, the mineral that helps in the development of caries-resistant teeth, is not present in either breast milk or cow's milk in adequate amounts. Even if a mother drinks fluoridated water, her breast milk may not have the optimal amount of this nutrient; so supplementation is often recommended for breast-fed infants as well as for formula-fed infants. The most recent recommendations vary according to the fluoridation of water in a particular area (see Exhibit 14.3).

Zinc's importance in infant nutrition, especially for optimal growth, has just been recognized in recent years. Although human milk contains less zinc than cow's milk, it appears that human milk contains a compound, called a *ligand,* not found in cow's milk that is capable of binding zinc so it is more available to the infant.[9] One study showed that the zinc-binding ligand was absent in the infant's intestines at the time of birth and develops during the early part of life.[10]

Calcium and phosphorus are essential for the growth and development of the infant's bones and teeth, and their absorption rate is much higher during this time of rapid growth. Breast milk contains the optimum ratio of calcium to phosphorus for infants, which is 2 to 1. An oversupply of phosphorus contributes to the renal solute load.

[8]Committee on Nutrition, American Academy of Pediatrics, "Iron Supplementation for Infants." *Pediatrics,* Vol. 58, 1976, p. 765. Also J. A. McMillan, S. A. Landow, and F. A. Oski, "Iron Sufficiency in Breast-fed Infants and Availability of Iron from Human Milk." *Pediatrics,* Vol. 58, 1976, p. 686.

[9]J. P. Wing, "Human Versus Cow's Milk in Infant Nutrition and Health: Update, 1977." *Current Problems in Pediatrics,* Vol. 8, No. 1, November, 1977, p. 11.

[10]Research conducted by L. S. Hurley and coworkers at University of California at Davis and reported in *From Your Home Advisor,* May, 1977, p. 2.

Exhibit 14.4 Fluoride Supplements: Dosage Per Day, Based on Fluoride
in Water Supply

AGE OF CHILD	FLUORIDE IN WATER LESS THAN 0.3 PPM*	FLUORIDE IN WATER 0.3 TO 0.7 PPM	FLUORIDE IN WATER MORE THAN 0.7 PPM
Birth - 2 yrs.	0.25 milligrams	0	0
2 to 3 yrs.	0.50 milligrams	0.25 milligrams	0
3 to 12 yrs.	1.00 milligrams	0.50 milligrams	0

Source: Council on Dental Therapeutics: "Prescribing Fluoride Supplements" in "Dosage
Recommendations for Dietary Fluoride Supplements." *American Journal of Diseases of Children,* Vol. 133, July, 1979, pp. 683–84.

* parts per million.

Vitamins

The infant's need for vitamins is listed in Exhibit 14.4. Infant formulas are required by the Food and Drug Administration to contain at least the minimum levels of vitamins needed by infants. The vitamin content of breast milk varies somewhat with the mother's diet. In general, milk from a well-nourished mother provides acceptable levels of all the vitamins but D and K.

Vitamin D, which works together with calcium and phosphorus in mineralization of bones and teeth, may be obtained in sufficient amounts if an infant is regularly exposed to sunshine. Infant formulas are fortified with vitamin D. If whole milk is given to infants instead of formula, it is important that vitamin D-fortified milk is used.

Recent changes in methods for measuring vitamin D in milk show that human milk contains far more vitamin D than had been supposed. It is now known that vitamin D concentration in mature milk is about the same as the concentration in vitamin D-fortified milk formulas. However, there is some uncertainty about how well the infant can use the newly discovered form of vitamin D in human milk. So some authorities continue to recommend the use of vitamin D supplements for breast-fed infants as a precautionary measure. Excess vitamin D is extremely toxic to infants, and overdoses should be carefully avoided.

Vitamin K is needed for the synthesis of several blood-clotting factors. It is formed in the intestines by bacteria, but a newborn infant, who is born with a sterile intestinal tract, will not have enough vitamin K during the first few weeks of life. Commonly, infants are given a prophylactic dose of vitamin K intramuscularly at birth to improve their blood clotting time in case of hemorrhage. Because breast milk has only one-fourth as much vitamin K as cow's milk, breast-fed babies risk vitamin K deficiency in early life.

Vitamin E is found in human milk in much larger amounts than it is in cow's milk. *Colostrum,* the first milk a mother produces, is particularly rich in vitamin E. The requirement for this vitamin depends on the degree of saturation of fats in the diet. The higher the level of unsaturated fats, the greater the need for vitamin E. Infant formulas that contain more polyunsaturated fats have been fortified with higher levels of vitamin E for this reason. Iron added to the formula increases the requirement for vitamin E also. The combination of high unsaturated fatty acids and iron in a formula can produce a deficiency of vitamin E and hemolytic anemia especially in premature infants.

Since both breast milk and infant formulas provide adequate amounts of all of the other vitamins, routine supplementation with vitamins, other than those discussed above, is generally considered unnecessary, but it is still a very common practice. When other foods, such as cereals, vegetables, fruit, and meats, are added to the infant's diet, the vitamin intake will increase even more. An infant fed whole milk instead of formula or breast milk should be given a vitamin C-rich food such as orange juice if he is not receiving a vitamin supplement, since cow's milk is low in this vitamin.

WHAT KIND OF MILK IS BEST FOR BABIES?

Human milk is best for human babies. This fact has been known for a long time, but in the past 5 to 10 years research has uncovered striking new reasons why this is true.[11] In tandem with this, the percentage of U.S. women who breast feed their babies has been increasing dramatically—up to 50 percent in some areas of the country.

Pediatricians are becoming more emphatic about recommending breast feeding as a preferred alternative to bottle feeding for the first year of an infant's life, and The American Academy of Pediatrics in 1978 published this statement: "Full-term infants should be breast fed except if there are specific contraindications or when breast feeding is unsuccessful."[12]

When breast feeding is not feasible, commercially prepared infant formulas are recommended as a better choice than homogenized whole milk. The switch from breast milk or formula to whole milk before the

[11]D. B. Jelliffe and E. F. P. Jelliffe, "Breast Is Best: Modern Meanings." *The New England Journal of Medicine,* Vol. 297, No. 17, October 27, 1977, pp. 912-15.

[12]"Breast Feeding." *American Academy of Pediatrics,* Vol. 62, No. 4, October, 1978, pp. 591-601.

end of the infant's first year of life is now being discouraged by pediatric leaders.

Milks are highly complex mixtures that differ greatly from one mammal to another. Thus, cow's milk and human milk are different in many respects. Through the years, food technologists have made modifications to cow's milk to produce infant formulas that more closely resemble human milk. Until recently it was thought that the modern formulas and human milk were really much the same. But evidence now shows that the two milks are dissimilar in many important ways. The major differences between human milk, homogenized cow's milk, and infant formulas are listed in Exhibit 14.5.

Exhibit 14.5   Comparison of Composition of Three Milks

Milk	Nutrients
	PROTEIN
Human	Low level: recent evidence shows only 0.8 to 0.9 percent protein. (Previous estimates were up to 1.1 percent.) Free amino acids provide 20 percent of nitrogen-containing compounds. Has more nucleotides (factors that enable the body to make protein). High in lactalbumin (60 percent) and low in casein (40 percent). Forms soft, flocculent curds that are easy to digest. Amino acid combination uniquely suited to metabolic peculiarities of newborn infant, whose liver is inefficient in converting methionine to cystine and in metabolizing tyrosine. High in amino acids cystine and taurine. (Taurine is important in other animals in transmission of nerve impulses, particularly in the retina of the eye.) Low in renal solutes. Nonallergenic.
Cow	Comparatively high: 3.5 percent (5 grams protein per 100 calories). High in casein (80 percent), which forms tough, not easily digested curds. Low in free amino acids, nucleotides, and amino acids cystine and taurine; high in amino acids tyrosine and phenylalanine. High in renal solutes. May be highly allergenic.
Formula cow's milk base	Moderate in protein: 1.7 percent (2.3 grams per 100 calories). Heated and acidified so protein forms a more digestible curd. Amino acid content same as cow's milk (addition of taurine is being investigated). Has few free amino acids and nucleotides. Moderate in renal solutes. Potential for protein overload if not properly diluted. May be allergenic.
	FAT
Human	Good source of linoleic acid. High in cholesterol (varies with mother's diet). Contains lipase, which makes free fatty acids more available. Cholesterol may be needed for forming nerve tissue or bile salts.
Cow	Low in linoleic acid. Contains cholesterol.
Formula	Vegetable oils (soy, corn, safflower) used in place of butterfat. High in polyunsaturated fats and low in cholesterol. Linoleic acid is two to three times that of human milk—consequences unknown.

Exhibit 14.5   (Cont'd)

	SUGAR
Human	High in lactose: 6.8 percent. Lactose provides galactose, which is needed for brain development. Is less sweet. Aids in protein and calcium utilization and iron absorption.
Cow	Lower in lactose: 4.9 percent.
Formula	Has about the same amount of lactose as human milk. Some brands may have other forms of sugar.
	MINERALS
Human	Optimum ratio of calcium to phosphorus (2:1). Has one-third as much sodium and potassium as cow's milk (right for infant's needs) and reduced renal solute load. Iron is in more usable form—49 percent is absorbed—and iron-deficiency anemia is uncommon. Lacks fluorine. Zinc is more available because of zinc-binding ligands.
Cow	Has four times more calcium, six times more phosphorus. Has too much phosphorus in proportion to calcium. Also high in sodium and potassium. High renal solute load. Lacks iron—iron- deficiency anemia common. Has more zinc, but it may be less available. Has more fluorine.
Formula	Level of sodium and potassium reduced to be more like human milk. Calcium to phosphorus ratio same as cow's milk. Renal solute load variable, depending on brand. May be iron fortified, but only 4 percent of iron is absorbed.
	VITAMINS
Human	Vitamin D may be insufficient. Richer in vitamin E, lacks vitamin K, and has sufficient vitamin C and A to meet infant's needs. B vitamins vary with diet—may be low in B_{12} if mother eats strict vegetarian diet and has no supplement.
Cow	Needs to be vitamin D fortified. Little vitamin C.
Formula	Fortified with vitamins to meet minimum requirements. May not have enough vitamin E if iron fortified.
	PROCESSING, ADDITIVES, CONTAMINANTS
Human	No processing—served direct from source to child—so no bacterial contamination. May contain drugs taken by mother and chemicals absorbed by mother from environment.
Cow	Pathogens destroyed in pasteurized milk. May be contaminated during preparation or storage. May contain drugs administered to cows and chemicals absorbed in cows from environment.
Formula	Heat treated, boiled, dehydrated. Contains emulsifiers, thickening agents, pH adjusters, antioxidants.

Anti-Infective, Anti-Allergenic Factors in Human Milk

The conclusion that researchers have reached is that the composition of human milk is uniquely suited to the needs of the growing infant. In addition, human milk contains factors that protect the infant against infection during the time in his life when he is most vulnerable. These anti-infective properties of breast milk are clearly more necessary in environments where sanitation and health practices are less adequate than they are in the average American home.

Human milk is rich in a wide range of anti-infective factors that no formula can imitate. The "first milk," or colostrum, is especially high in the protective factors. These include *immunoglobulins,* which form antibodies. These immunoglobulins generally are not absorbed in the infant's intestinal tract but act by protecting the mucous membranes of the tract against bacterial invasion. This protection lasts until the infant's own immunity system has matured.

Antibodies to many types of microorganisms have been found in human milk. They include antibodies to bacteria that cause tetanus, whooping cough, pneumonia, and diptheria; antibodies to salmonella and staphylococci bacteria; and antibodies to polio virus and influenza virus.

Other protective substances in addition to immunoglobulins in human milk include the heat-stable "anti-staph factor"; *lysozyme,* which may contribute to the development of desirable bacteria in the intestine; *lactoferrin,* which inhibits unfriendly bacteria; the *bifidus factor,* which promotes the growth of the friendly bacteria *Lactobacillus bifidus* in the intestines, which in turn inhibits the growth of dangerous organisms; and many white cells (like those found in the blood), which make antibodies against certain bacteria or viruses or destroy them directly. Recently a new antiviral substance was found in milk, and the search still goes on.

These protective factors in human milk assure an infant of better health during the first year of life. Breast-fed infants are less prone to suffer from gastrointestinal illness and diarrhea; they have fewer and milder episodes; and they are also less likely to have respiratory illness.

Since human milk does not contain proteins that cause allergies in human infants, breast feeding may delay or even eliminate allergic reactions to milk. From 1 to 7 percent of all infants may be sensitive to cow's milk protein—the commonest food allergen in infancy. The most dangerous time for developing this allergy is in the first three months of life, when the infant's immature intestinal wall is relatively "open" to the absorption of foreign protein molecules such as those found in cow's milk. The immunoglobulins in human milk, on the other hand, protect the intestines against invasion by proteins that cause allergies.

Another major reason for favoring breast feeding over bottle feeding is that it helps prevent infant obesity. Breast-fed babies are seldom overweight. The fat, protein, sugar, and calorie levels in human milk are adjusted to their needs and the infants are in charge of regulating the supply. More sucking causes the formation of the milk-producing hormone *prolactin* and produces more milk; less sucking results in less prolactin and less milk being produced. There's no partly full bottle in sight for the mother to urge the baby to finish. The "empty bottle" syndrome is often the forerunner of the "clean plate" syndrome in which the parent tries to take over regulating the child's food intake rather than letting the child develop his own sense of satiety.

Mothers who breast feed tend to spend more time feeding and holding their babies. Even though an infant is closely held while being fed a bottle (and often this is not the case), the quality of the interchange

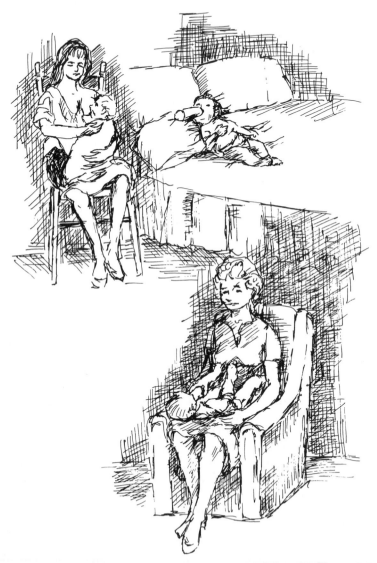

Exhibit 14.6. Breast feeding requires a closeness between mother and infant; with bottle feeding, a mother may choose not to hold her baby.

between the mother and baby is different. Breast feeding provides the baby with more sensory stimulation—smell, taste, feel, and even the sound of the mother's heartbeat (see Exhibit 14.6). Very young babies are thought to be able to distinguish their own mother from other mothers by the odor of her breast milk.

For all of these reasons, breast feeding is the preferred method for providing the infant with optimum nutrition and emotional satisfaction. Bottle feeding with modern infant formulas is a satisfactory second choice that can also promote healthy infant development. The use of homogenized whole cow's milk during the first year is not considered desirable. Nonfat or skim milk are potentially harmful and should not be used in infant feeding during the first year.

The fact that several generations of children have been bottle fed cow's milk and formulas and have grown up to be healthy and well developed physically and mentally is evidence that these milks are satisfactory substitutes for breast milk. However, there are those who point out that long-term effects of infant feeding practices in obesity, heart disease, high blood pressure, and other adult conditions are not fully known.

FEEDING PATTERNS: WHEN AND WHAT?

For the first four to six months of life, an infant needs no foods other than breast milk or infant formula. Recent research shows that there are no advantages and some disadvantages when solid foods are introduced too early and that an infant will be better off nutritionally if he's not given solid foods until he is developmentally ready.[13]

Early introduction of solid foods and/or substituting whole cow's milk for breast milk or formula can result in the infant getting too many calories; too much protein, sodium, and phosphorus, which overburden his kidneys; and not enough iron and zinc. Whole milk also can cause gastrointestinal bleeding, blood loss, and anemia in some infants.

Although an infant usually can tolerate solid foods at a very young age, they may cause him to gain weight too rapidly or develop allergies to foods such as milk protein, eggs, and gluten (wheat protein). The notion that adding solid foods will help an infant sleep through the night has been shown to be untrue. If the solid foods cause an infant to reduce the amount of milk that he drinks, he may not get enough of the essential nutrients in milk.

[13]P. Pipes, "When Should Semisolid Foods be Fed to Infants?" *Journal of Nutrition Education*, Vol. 9, No. 2, April-June, 1977, pp. 57-59.

Readiness for Solid Foods

After four to six months of age, however, the infant needs foods other than milk for both nutritional and developmental reasons.

The infant's feeding behavior can be used as a guide to when solids should be introduced (see Exhibit 14.7). When an infant changes his tongue movement from up and down to back and forth and is able to move food from the front of his tongue to the back of his throat, rather than thrust it forward, he is showing readiness to be fed mushy solids, such as cereal diluted with milk, from a spoon. When the infant learns to chew at about six to seven months, he needs solids, such as toast or crackers, that will give him practice chewing.

If solid foods are withheld when an infant is developmentally ready for them, he may have more difficulty accepting them when they are offered later, and learning to chew may be retarded.

To postpone or monitor any allergic reaction, especially when there is a family history of allergies, some authorities recommend that solid foods be introduced one at a time at weekly intervals so the cause of any reaction can be pinpointed. The first solid food offered might be rice cereal, followed by a different cereal each week. After cereals, other foods such as strained vegetables (carrots, squash, beans, and peas) can be added. Because meats and liver often are not well accepted by infants, their introduction might be postponed until last. Starchy dinners

Exhibit 14.7. Foods for an Infant

AVERAGE AGE	DEVELOPMENTAL STAGE	APPROPRIATE FOODS
Birth to 4–6 mo	Sucks and swallows liquids. Tongue moves from side to side. Cannot swallow solids.	Breast milk or infant formula
4–6 mo	Moves tongue back and forth. Can move food to back of throat to swallow.	Mushy solids—cereal diluted with milk, strained vegetables, strained fruits, strained meats, liver
6–7 mo	Begins to learn to chew.	Toast, crackers Chopped vegetables, fruit, meat
8–10 mo	Grasps objects with fingers and puts in mouth.	Bite-sized cubes of cooked vegetables, tender meats, like chicken liver; soft raw fruit, like banana
10–12 mo	Holds spoon. Can move food to mouth.	Foods easy to eat with spoon—cooked cereals, vegetables, fruits
9–12 mo	Drinks from cup. Ready to be weaned from breast or bottle.	Whole milk

with meat may be preferred by an infant to strained meats, but they are high in starch and low in protein so may be a less desirable choice. Puddings and desserts should be avoided or used sparingly because they are high in sugar calories and could encourage the development of a heightened desire for sweet foods.[14]

Many babies are offered strained fruits at the same time as cereals and before most of the other foods. This may not be the wisest choice of foods at this time because of the fruits' high calorie count, sweet taste, and general lack of important nutrients. When an infant begins to learn to chew, foods with coarser textures, such as chopped instead of strained vegetables and meats, should be fed so that he learns to accept these textures.

Table foods eaten by the rest of the family may not be a good choice for infants if they have been seasoned with salt, sugar, or other condiments. The infant's foods should be bland in flavor and unsalted to avoid a sodium overload. Home-cooked foods can be used for infants instead of commercially prepared baby foods if salt and seasonings are not added. They can be mashed, strained, or chopped depending on the food and the baby's ability to chew. Care should be taken to cook foods for maximum nutrient retention (see Chapter 22) and to keep them clean and free from bacterial contamination (see Chapter 25).

Once an infant learns to grasp objects with his fingers, he will enjoy feeding himself bite-size finger foods such as cubes of cooked vegetables or tender meats (like chicken liver), slices of banana, or cubes of melon. When he can hold a spoon and move it to his mouth, he's ready to practice feeding himself and should be given the chance to do so. This is a time for great patience on the part of the caretaker!

To sum up, no nutritional or developmental advantage will be gained by introducing solid foods prior to the time when an infant is developmentally ready for them at four to six months of age. Overfeeding and excessive weight gain are the major hazards when solid foods are added to the infant's regular milk intake. Underfeeding milk is a serious nutritional hazard if solids cause a reduction in the amount of milk an infant consumes. When an infant is developmentally ready for solid foods, it is important they they be added to his diet.

Weaning Time

At some time between nine and twelve months of age, an infant will show signs of being developmentally ready for weaning: (1) he will learn to drink from a cup; (2) he will be eating a variety of food; and (3) he will begin to lose interest in nursing or become impatient with it—he may even bite or chew on the nipple rather than suck. At this point the mother knows he's ready to give up nursing!

[14]"Faulty Infant Nutrition: Iatrogenic and Maternal Factors." *Nutrition and the M.D.*, Vol. 2, No. 8, June, 1976, p. 2.

Usually these signs develop over a period of time and allow for a gradual discontinuation of breast or bottle feeding, perhaps by deleting one feeding at a time. An occasional strong-minded infant will take matters into his own hands and simply refuse to nurse. Some infants, on the other hand, become emotionally attached to sucking, especially if they are put to bed with a bottle or allowed to use nursing as a method of falling asleep. They may be willing to nurse long past the time when they are developmentally ready to stop.

There are two schools of thought on whether children should be breast or bottle fed after this time. One group, including some mothers who are strong advocates of breast feeding through the second and even third year, claims that some children have an emotional need for the closeness and security that nursing offers. In their view, the long-nursed youngster will become more independent by having his dependency needs met when it is natural for him to be dependent.

The other group believes that missing the opportunity to wean a child when he is developmentally ready for it results in an undesirable emotional attachment to breast (and mother) or bottle, which becomes difficult to overcome.

Aside from the emotional-developmental issue, two serious consequences can result when babies are not weaned when they are ready for it. In some children, milk may remain their chief source of food, to the exclusion of other foods needed to supply nutrients, such as iron and other trace elements, B vitamins, and vitamin C.

The other problem is the development of dental caries. Prolonged bottle feeding, past the usual weaning stage, and especially when the young child is put to bed with a bottle and allowed to suck for an extended period of time, has been identified as the cause of a particular pattern of tooth decay known as *nursing-bottle caries* or the *baby-bottle syndrome*. As the child sucks, his tongue protects his lower front teeth, while the upper teeth, especially the four in front, are bathed in the sugar-containing milk or liquid. Bacterial action on the sugar produces acid which decalcifies the teeth, as described in Chapter 15. Eventually decay may girdle the teeth around the gum line and, if not corrected, can result in loss of the four upper front teeth.

The lactose in cow's and human milk is fermentable in the mouth just as are other sugars such as sucrose and fructose. Juices such as apple juice, which are sometimes given to a child in a bottle in place of milk, add the further tooth-eroding factor of acid. If the caretaker adds table sugar to the milk to make it more enticing to the child, this compounds the problem.

Some researchers have linked cases of this type of tooth decay with frequent, at will, breast feeding when carried on into the second and third year. However, other researchers have disputed this finding.[15]

[15]L. A. Kotlow, "Breast Feeding: A Cause of Dental Caries in Children." *Journal of Dentistry for Children,* Vop. 44, May-June, 1977, pp. 192-193.

Weaning from breast or bottle when a child is developmentally ready and avoiding the practice of putting him to bed with a bottle can prevent this serious tooth decay problem in young children.

PREVENTING AND TREATING OBESITY

There is general agreement among health professionals that an obese infant is at risk and that preventing obesity is far easier than curing it. To prevent obesity, inappropriate feeding that leads to excess energy intake, i.e., bottle feeding with a "drink every drop" philosophy and early introduction of solid foods, should be avoided. Breast feeding alone, with solid foods added at 4 to 6 months of age, appears to be the best way to avoid infant obesity.

Once an infant becomes obese, treatment is difficult and is not aimed at weight reduction but at slowing the rate of gain. The goal should be to hold weight gain at a stable level while the baby grows in length so he slowly grows out of obesity. Severe calorie restrictions must be avoided, as they can reduce the lean body mass, inhibit growth, and deplete energy reserves needed to handle stress. Calorie intake should not be reduced below 90 to 100 calories per kilogram of body weight per day. Nonfat milk should not be substituted for formula even when an infant is overweight. Instead, the volume of milk, if over 30 ounces, should be reduced and water substituted. Solid foods with large amounts of starch and sugar, such as strained dinners and puddings and desserts, should be avoided.

The mother also needs to learn that not all of her baby's cries are hunger cries, to distinguish between cries, and not to feed her baby every time he cries. She also can encourage physical activity by dressing her young baby during his awake times in a way that allows free movement of arms and legs and, as he grows, giving him opportunities to be physically active.

PREMATURE INFANTS: A SPECIAL NUTRITIONAL PROBLEM

Preterm babies have special nutritional needs because of their immature development (see Exhibit 14.8). They are unable to absorb fat normally because of a smaller secretion of bile acids; lipase also may be low. Because they have a low production of enzymes needed for protein digestion, they may not absorb protein. Amylase, the enzyme needed for starch digestion, is very low, and lactase, the enzyme for splitting lactose, also may be in short supply. Their immature gastrointestinal tract causes many problems:

Exhibit 14.8. Nutrition-Related Developmental Problems of Premature Infants

Impaired fat and protein absorption
Insufficient enzymes for lactose and starch digestion
Weak or undeveloped sucking reflex
Impaired gastrointestinal action
Reduced intestinal resistance to foreign proteins
Small capacity for food
Increased need for vitamin E
Low iron stores

(1) Inadequate motility may result in delayed gastric emptying time and poor bowel motility

(2) Weak sucking and poor coordination of sucking and swallowing with breathing may make feeding difficult. The very young can't suck at all and need to be fed by some other method

(3) Incomplete development of the sphincter between the stomach and esophogus may result in much vomiting

(4) Foreign proteins are more able to pass through the intestinal walls, resulting in decreased ability to fight infections and more likelihood of developing allergies

(5) Capacity for food is small. They may consume only one-third as much milk—and nutrients—as full-term infants.

The smaller the infant, the greater the rate of growth and the greater the need for energy, protein, vitamin E, and the minerals sodium, calcium, phosphorus, copper, and iron. Yet because the infant has such a small capacity for food and decreased ability to absorb fats, both human milk and formulas for full-term infants may not be adequate for some low birth weight infants. Special formulas for premature infants, with 40 to 50 percent of calories from vegetable oils, appear to provide for improved fat absorption. However, a hemolytic form of anemia in premature infants with vitamin E deficiency has been associated with high levels of polyunsaturated fats in these formulas and the presence of iron fortification. Since premature infants have a greater need for vitamin E than full-term infants, some authorities recommend that they not be given an iron-fortified formula during the first two months of life. However, the premature infant's iron stores at birth are low, are rapidly depleted, and will become insufficient after two to three months instead of four to six months. So, both breast-fed and bottle-fed infants need to be monitored for signs of anemia, and iron supplements need to be given when necessary.

Protein levels must be carefully adjusted for premature infants. Authorities are not in agreement as to what the optimum level is. If protein is too low, weight gain is poor and edema may result; if it is too high, the infant may be lethargic, unable to handle the high renal solute load, and have other adverse physical reactions that could lead to decreased intellectual development in early childhood.

Human milk is thought by some authorities to fall short in protein, calcium, phosphorus, and sodium, and they recommend the use of the special premature infant formula instead.[16]

But human milk has other properties—high digestibility and anti-infective factors—that make it the preferred food according to some authorities.[17]

Its fat, for example, can be absorbed even in the absence of bile acids and lipase. Studies show that premature infants fed human milk didn't gain as much or as rapidly at first as those fed formula. The formula babies did not lose as much at birth, but they had more edema, which is what was thought to have accounted for their greater weight gains. From then on the weight gain was found to be equal on both milks. If human milk is used, authorities recommend that the infant should be monitored for nutritional deficiency and supplements given when needed.[18]

Summary

The first year of life is a period of tremendously fast growth and brain development. It is important that infant feeding meet both nutritional and emotional needs. Developmentally, a baby must learn in this period to coordinate the tongue to swallow solids, to drink from a cup, and to pick up and transfer foods to the mouth. Growth takes place by *hyperplasia,* an increase in the number of cells, and *hypertrophy,* an increase in the size of cells. Each organ undergoes a critical period of development during which nutritional deficiencies can have irreversible adverse effects.

Neither undernourishment nor overnourishment is desirable for babies. Preventing infant obesity is far easier than curing it. The drink-every-drop approach to bottle feeding should be avoided, as should solid foods that are high in starch or sugar. Physical activity should be encouraged. Treatment of infant obesity is aimed at slowing the rate of gain, rather than reducing the child's weight.

Infants have very high energy needs for their size. High quality protein is the second most important nutritional requirement; but since an infant's kidneys are immature, excessive protein intake can cause dehydration and serious complications. Nonfat milk is not recommended for infants, since it does not supply enough energy or the es-

---

[16]L. J. Filer, "Feeding Low Birth Weight Infants." *Infant Nutrition, Part 2.* Bloomfield, N. J.: Health Learning Systems, Inc., 1977, pp. 18-22.

[17]Ibid.

[18]S. J. Foman, R. G. Strauss, "Nutrient Deficiencies in Breast-Fed Infants." *The New England Journal of Medicine,* Vol. 299, No. 7, April 17, 1978, pp. 355-56.

sential fatty acid, linoleic acid. The most critical need for infants is water, obtained in milk and juices as a supplement.

Infants need the same array of vitamins and minerals as adults, and are particularly prone to iron-deficiency anemia. Supplements must be used with care, especially vitamins A and D, which are toxic if given in doses that are too large.

The composition of human milk is ideally suited to the needs of the growing baby. In addition, breast milk helps protect the infant against infection and allergies. After four to six months of age, the child needs to have solid foods introduced for both nutritional and developmental reasons. Weaning usually occurs around nine to twelve months of age, and prolonged bottle feeding, especially in bed, may cause dental caries.

Premature infants may have immature gastrointestinal tracts and poor sucking-breathing coordination. Great care must be taken to meet their nutrition needs.

NUTRITION DURING CHILDHOOD 15

Highlights

Goals of childhood nutrition

Developmental characteristics and common food-related problems

Building children's interest in various foods

Inappropriate foods for children

Dental disease, food allergies, metabolic disorders, and hyperactivity in children

In contrast to the burst of new research information developed in the past ten years about infant nutrition, much less research has been done recently in childhood nutrition. Principal activities have been to study groups of children to determine their nutritional and health status; to identify nutritional deficiencies that are most commonly seen in children; and to recommend changes in nutrition education, television food advertising directed to children, and school lunch programs to help overcome identified problems.

NUTRITION FOR PRESCHOOL CHILDREN

During early childhood, a child is learning food habits that may have lifelong effects. At this time, the parents' role in determining what foods are available for the child predominates. As the child moves into elementary school, he becomes more emancipated from his parents and has more opportunities to make food choices. Early learning experiences at home will play a strong part in his ability to choose foods wisely as he moves out of the realm of parental control.

Nutritional Requirements

Children need the same basic nutrients as teenagers and adults, but they need them in different amounts depending on their age. The recommended dietary allowances for children of different ages are listed in Exhibit 15.1. The Four Food Groups can easily be adapted to the needs of young children simply by adjusting the number of servings and the amounts needed.

Studies show that iron is the nutrient most likely to be low in the diets of preschool and school-age children. An important cause of iron-deficiency anemia in young children who are otherwise well nourished from the calorie-protein standpoint has been found to be excess milk consumption, which results in the exclusion of iron-containing foods. Another cause is a dislike for vegetables, especially green leafy ones, and other foods that are good sources of iron, such as liver and prunes. If fruits and vegetables are shunned, the youngster also may not be getting enough vitamins A, C, and folic acid. Among the vitamins, C has been identified as the one most likely to be lacking.[1]

While protein is essential during the growth years, studies show

[1]Center for Disease Control, U.S. Department of Health, Education, and Welfare, *Ten State Nutrition Survey, 1968-70*, DHEW Publication No. (HSM) 72-8133. *V-Dietary*. Washington, D.C., 1972.

Exhibit 15.1   Recommended Daily Dietary Allowances for Children

NUTRIENT	UNIT	CHILD, 1–3 YEARS	CHILD, 4–6 YEARS	CHILD, 7–10 YEARS
Food energy	cal	1300	1700	2400
Protein	g	23	30	34
Fat-soluble vitamins				
Vitamin A	μg R.E.[1]	400	500	700
Vitamin E	mg & T.E.[2]	5	6	7
Vitamin D	μg[3]	10	10	10
Water-soluble vitamins				
Ascorbic acid	mg	45	45	45
Folacin	μg	100	200	300
Niacin	mg equiv N.E.[4]	9	11	16
Riboflavin	mg	0.8	1.0	1.4
Thiamin	mg	0.7	0.9	1.2
Vitamin B_6	mg	0.9	1.	1.
Vitamin B_{12}	μg	2.0	2.5	3.0
Minerals				
Calcium	mg	800	800	800
Phosphorus	mg	800	800	800
Iodine	μg	70	90	120
Iron	mg	15	10	10
Magnesium	mg	150	200	250
Zinc	mg	10	10	10

Source: Recommended Dietary Allowances, Ninth edition (revised 1979). National Academy of Sciences, Washington, D.C.

[1] Retinol equivalents. 1 retinol equivalent = 1 μg retinol or 6 μg β-carotene.

[2] α tocopherol equivalents. 1 μg d-α-tocopherol = 1 μT.E.

[3] As cholecalciferol. 10 μg cholecalciferol = 400 I.U. vitamin D.

[4] 1 NE (niacin equivalent) is equal to 1 μg of naicin or 60 μg of dietary tryptophan.

that most American children get plenty of protein even when family incomes are low.[2]

Calcium, phosphorus, vitamin D, and riboflavin needs are easily satisfied if the child drinks one-half to one quart of milk a day depending on his age. If children who are allergic to cow's milk are given milk substitutes such as soy milk, these should be fortified with calcium and vitamin D.

The low-nutrient-density foods that are high in sugar and fat are no more appropriate for this age group than any other. While children have relatively high energy needs, especially when they are very active,

[2]G. Own, G. Lippmann, "Nutritional Status of Infants and Young Children, USA." *Pediatric Clinics of North America,* Vol. 24, No. 1. February, 1977, pp. 211-27.

they need to get their calories from foods that provide the other important nutrients as well. Thus, a glass of fruit juice is a better choice than
a soft drink. A graham cracker with peanut butter is a better snack than
a candy bar, although it too can contribute to tooth decay if allowed to
stick in the teeth.

Preschool Years: A Time for Learning

The second year of life is a time of transition from infancy to childhood. Internal organs have matured, growth slows, activity increases,
eating skills improve, and nutritional needs become similar to those of
older children. During preschool years, learning takes place at a rapid
pace, and food habits and eating behavior are developed during this
time.

Later, others outside the family influence the child's food habits—
his friends, teachers, television advertising. But parents get the first
crack at helping their child establish eating patterns that will allow him
to enjoy a wide variety of nutritious foods to help maintain optimum
health.

Wise parents keep this goal uppermost in their minds: helping a
child learn to enjoy food (Exhibit 15.2). If this goal is reached, other
important goals, such as the child eating enough of the right kinds of
food and liking a lot of different foods, probably will be reached too. But
if mealtime becomes a time for nagging and unpleasantness and eating
becomes a parent-child battle, then a child may become so balky and
fussy about food that the important nutritional goals cannot be met.

Growth Slows Down: Appetites Decrease. After the rapid growth spurt
in infancy, a young child grows much more slowly. More of his energy
intake is used for activities; much less is applied to growth. A dramatically decreased appetite is seen in most youngsters early in the second
year, because the child now needs to eat much less in proportion to his
size than he did in infancy. Scientists call this *physiologic anorexia* —loss
of appetite caused by a natural, physiological factor.

Often parents don't understand the reason for their young child's
decreased appetite and may become overanxious and begin trying to
coax the child to eat. This is a common cause of feeding problems that
begin during the second year and may go on throughout childhood.
Children often learn that refusing to eat makes parents anxious, and it
then becomes a "weapon" for influencing parental behavior (Exhibit
15.3).

Well-informed parents, on the other hand, recognize that the decreased appetite is normal and that the child himself is usually a fairly
good judge of how much food he needs. Exhibit 15.4 gives a guide to
child-size servings for two- to three-year-olds and three- to six-year-
olds. One rule of thumb for serving sizes is a teaspoon or bite of each
food for each year of age. Large servings can be overwhelming or repul-

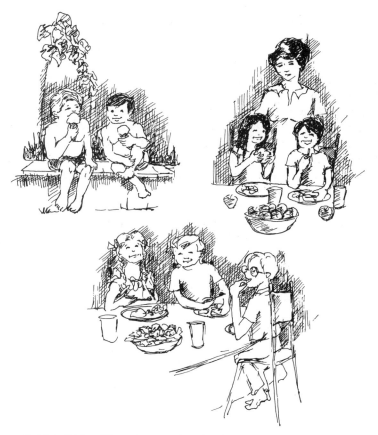

Exhibit 15.2.   The prime goal in feeding young children is to help them learn to enjoy food.

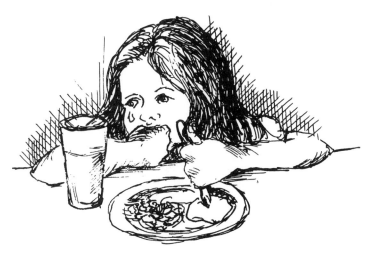

Exhibit 15.3.   Overanxious parents and too much coaxing may start feeding problems.

sive to a child; it's better to offer small servings and let the child ask for seconds.

Individual Differences. The serving sizes suggested in Exhibit 15.4 need to be adapted to each child's needs. Some children have hearty appetites and eat everything; some have small appetites and are picky eaters. Some children are very active and need more food than children who are less active. Some children have small capacities and need a little food often; others prefer fewer and larger meals. Many have temporary "runs" or "food jags" on certain foods, which they eat in preference to all others. Usually these jags soon wear off if parents are patient and don't make a fuss over them.

The best thing for parents to do is learn to accept their child as the individual he is and not try to mold him into some preconceived notion of what they think he should be. No child need be expected to like all foods, for example. Parents also need to recognize that appetites fluctuate and that trying to force-feed a child when he doesn't feel like eating is not only unlikely to succeed, but can intensify and make permanent the child's dislike for particular foods.

Need for Snacks. Young children who have a small capacity for food in addition to small appetites usually need more than three meals a day. They simply cannot eat enough at a meal to tide them over to the next meal and to give them all the food they need for growth and activities. Snacks can help a child avoid fatigue and thereby have a better appetite at mealtime. Having an established time for snacks, like mid-morning, mid-afternoon, bedtime, is better than allowing a child to nibble constantly.

Exhibit 15.4   Child-Size Servings

	SERVING SIZES FOR CHILDREN	
DAILY NEED	2–3 YEARS OLD	3–6 YEARS OLD
3 servings milk	4–6 oz.	6 oz.
2 servings		
Eggs	½ medium	1 medium
Meat, poultry, fish	1 to 2 oz.	2 oz.
3 servings		
Cereal	2 T cooked	¼ cup cooked
	⅓ cup ready to eat	½ cup ready to eat
Bread	¼ to ½ slice	½ to 1 slice
3 servings		
Vegetables	1 to 2 T. or oz.	2 to 4 T. or oz.
Fruit	¼ to ½ of whole fruit	½ of whole fruit
Juice	3–4 oz.	4 oz
	(⅓ to ½ cup)	(½ cup)

This is the time to establish good snacking habits. Nutritious foods should be available for snacks so that the child can become accustomed to eating these foods instead of candy, cookies, soft drinks, and other foods that are high in sugar and fat and low in other essential nutrients. Suggestions for nutritious snack foods for children can be found in Chapter 27.

Suspicion about New Foods. Few children have a spirit of adventure when it comes to food. Usually they are afraid to try a new food and may decide they don't like it without even tasting it. For most children it's wise to consider the introduction of each new food as a learning experience rather than a means of meeting nutritional needs. The person providing food needs to have a casual, relaxed attitude. Assume the child will like the food, but don't try to force him. Let him see you eat and enjoy the food. Remove uneaten food without comment. Serve it again. Don't worry. If he says he doesn't like it, don't impress this on his mind so that he remembers he has to dislike it the next time it's served.

Some families have a rule that everyone taste a small amount (a bite) of each food served. Children left to their own devices often develop a taste for new foods this way. In one study it was found that children who were expected to try at least a little of each vegetable and entree served developed a relatively open-minded, flexible approach to new foods in general.[3]

To arouse a child's interest in a new food, talk about it while it's being bought or prepared. Involve the child in the preparation if possible. Introduce just one new food at a time and in very small portions. Serve it along with a favorite food so it is associated with "something good."

Looks and "Feel" Are Important. Children like colorful, attractive food, just as adults do. Bright colors and mild flavors are appealing. Children also like a variety of textures, colors, and temperatures, but not extremes. Sometimes they are supersensitive to the feel of food in the mouth and may object to lumpy tapioca pudding, stringy green beans or peaches, scum on cocoa, seeds in berries, or gristle in meat. Again, it takes experience to learn to tolerate these things.

Imitation. Children tend to do as adults do, not as they say. So family members need to set a good example of eating and enjoying a variety of foods and keeping their dislikes to themselves. Youngsters often seem to be more likely to be influenced by their fathers' attitudes towards foods than their mothers'. Many times a child will eat foods at

[3]M. Walker, M. Hill, F. Millman, "Fruit and Vegetable Acceptance by Students." *Journal of the American Dietetic Association*, Vol. 62, No. 3, March, 1973.

nursery school or when eating with friends that he won't eat at home because he sees other children eating them (Exhibit 15.5).

Desire to be Independent. As he matures, a child is learning to be his own self and very likely will want to make his own food choices as a way of expressing his independence. He doesn't want to be told what and how much to eat and may rebel if a caretaker gets too adamant. He's also anxious to be able to do things for himself: feed himself, serve himself, pour his own milk, as well as "help Mommy" prepare and serve food and clean up afterwards. A wise parent or caretaker will do all he or she can to promote this independence. Offering as many choices as possible among desirable foods as well as letting a child determine how much he will eat is one way to help a child learn to make decisions and feel independent.

Poor Coordination. A young child's physical coordination is often not well developed and his attempts at feeding himself may be messy. Parents need to be understanding and not punitive about spills and messes at this age. A child enjoys finger foods such as raw vegetables and fruits in strips, wedges, or chunks; meat in bite-size pieces; and bread and sandwiches in quarters. Soup is easier to drink from a cup than to eat with a spoon. Mugs and small glasses that don't tip over easily will help a child learn to use eating utensils.

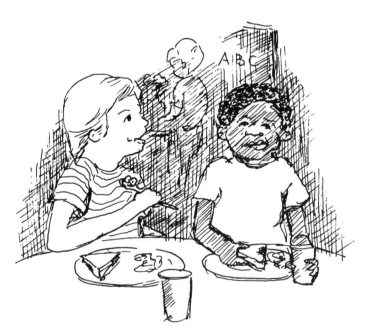

Exhibit 15.5.   A child who eats with other children often learns to like foods he doesn't eat at home.

Dawdling. A young child often is slow in eating because he is not adept at self-feeding and gets tired or because he is not very hungry. A helping hand (but not force-feeding) may be needed sometimes. And it is important to make eating as simple as possible for him. If dawdling is prolonged and frequent, it may help to set a time limit (for example, by setting a timer) for mealtime and then remove the food at the end of the time.

Fatigue. A child who has been playing hard may be too tired to eat. Perhaps he needs to eat sooner or have a chance for quiet play or relaxation before eating.

Need for Vitamin and Mineral Supplements. A young child who eats a reasonable variety of foods from the Four Food Groups normally does not need vitamin and mineral supplements. However, judicious use of supplements might be advised by a pediatrician in situations where a child's fussy eating is resulting in omission of entire food groups, such as fruits and vegetables, and is causing a parent to be anxious about the child's nutritional health.

Some Foods are Inappropriate for Young Preschool Children. Very young children developmentally are not ready for foods that older children may enjoy.

Rich, fatty foods, such as pie, fried eggs, and french-fried potatoes, often do not appeal to small children whose digestive systems may not be ready to handle excess fat.

Very coarse foods, such as bran, may be irritating to a young child's immature digestive tract.

Tough, stringy goods, particularly meats, may be too hard for a very young child to chew if he doesn't have all his teeth yet or has not

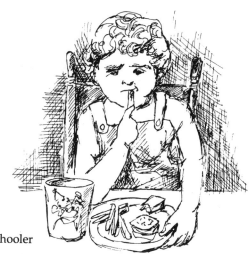

Exhibit 15.6. Finger foods are easy for a preschooler to eat, and also help him to feel independent.

learned to chew efficiently. He may prefer foods such as ground beef, liver, fish, or eggs until his chewing skills improve.

Crunchy, hard-to-chew foods, such as peanuts or popcorn, can be hazardous if a child swallows them whole and chokes on them or aspirates them into his lungs. Some raw vegetables such as carrots may fit in this category.

Highly spiced and strong-flavored foods, such as "cabbagey" vegetables, often are not enjoyed by young children because they have more taste buds than adults and are more sensitive to flavors.

"Mixtures" of foods, such as casseroles and stews, while appropriate for young children are sometimes not liked by them as well as the same foods served separately.

Foods containing caffeine, such as coffee, tea, and cola drinks, are not desirable for young children who are lively enough without being stimulated by caffeine.

NUTRITION FOR SCHOOL-AGE CHILDREN: A "BENIGN TIME"

Through the elementary school years children's growth is slow but fairly even, and energy needs and appetites increase gradually with increased size. Wide variations in quantities of food eaten can be seen among school-age children with exercise and activity level having a strong influence (see Exhibit 15.7). Very active children who participate in athletics will need more food than sedentary children. Sex differences in food needs also appear during these years, with boys gradually outdistancing girls.

A nutrition concern for this age group is balancing energy input with output. Growth needs plus high activity levels may result in a child being underweight. Thinness is often a characteristic of children of this age and is not a cause for concern when the child eats a varied and balanced diet. However, undernourished children have less stamina, become fatigued more readily, and have fewer nutritional reserves for resisting or fighting infectious diseases that are prevalent in school populations.

Sedentary children may become overweight and need to be encouraged to become more active as well as to reduce their food intake in order to avoid becoming obese. Psychological causes for overeating may also need attention. Some studies show that obesity in childhood is a key indicator of lifelong obesity. Children who are obese or slender at seven years of age seldom change their body form at later ages, according to one research finding.

Eating patterns may contribute to poor nutrition during this period. Surveys show that many children go to school with no breakfast or very little breakfast; some carry inadequate lunches or throw much of their lunch away rather than take the time to eat it. As a result, their

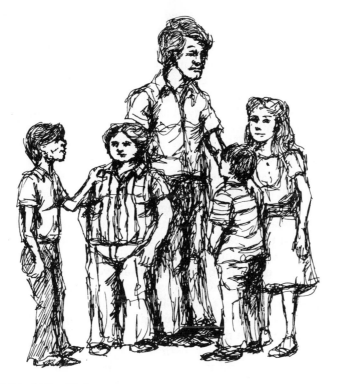

Exhibit 15.7.   Wide variations in weight, activity level, and food intake may be observed among school-age children.

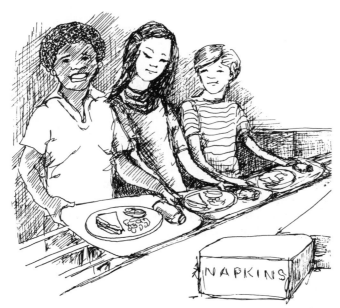

Exhibit 15.8.   A child's school performance may be related to the breakfasts and lunches the child eats regularly.

total day's nutrient intake is below their needs. Poor performance in school—restlessness, inattention, and inability to concentrate—may also be related to not eating well in the morning or at noon (Exhibit 15.8).

Another common eating pattern for this age group is substituting snacking for major meals or continuous snacking during the day. This pattern can be detrimental to nutritional health in several ways. If snacks are low-nutrient-density, high-sugar, high-fat foods, the child may be getting too many calories but too few essential nutrients, especially when snacks take the place of meals. In addition, frequent contact with sugary foods can lead to more tooth decay. Growing children do need snacks between meals but these should be foods that contribute nutrients as well as calories.

Food dislikes and fussy eating habits may carry over from preschool years, especially when parents continue to nag and remind the child that he's a fussy eater and thereby reinforce the child's image of himself as a fussy eater and make him feel that it's necessary to continue to live up to this expected behavior. But active, growing children who are allowed to make their own choices from a variety of nutritious foods may gradually grow out of food dislikes and improve their eating habits as their appetites increase. By about age 10, children's eating patterns often become more like those of adults.

In the later years of this growth period, the child should be storing nutrients such as iron and calcium in order to be prepared for the demands of the teenage growth spurt which comes next.

DENTAL DISEASE DURING CHILDHOOD

The most common chronic, nutrition-related disease among children in the United States is tooth decay (the scientific term is dental caries). It affects 98 percent of the people in the United States. The most cavity-prone ages are 5 to 8 and 12 to 16. Forty to 59 percent of 3 and 4 year olds have some decay. By age 6, when the first permanent teeth have erupted, more than a third of the children have at least one permanent tooth affected by decay. By 12 years of age, 90 percent of children have one or more decayed teeth, and the average is five teeth affected. By age 17, an estimated 98 percent have an average of 12 permanent teeth damaged by decay.[4]

Tooth decay is the result of several interacting factors: (1) susceptible teeth, (2) oral bacteria, and (3) food eaten.

[4]A. Nizel, "Preventing Dental Caries, Nutrition Factors," in The Pediatric Clinics of North America, Vol. 24, No. 1, *Symposium on Nutrition in Pediatrics.* Philadelphia, Pa.: W. B. Saunders Co., February 1977, pp. 141–55.

Susceptible Teeth

Different people have differing degrees of susceptibility to dental decay. Heredity and diet both play a role in the development of teeth and saliva. The arrangement and anatomy of the teeth also are involved: very crowded, crooked teeth or teeth with deep natural fissures are more difficult to brush and to keep free from decay-causing elements.

A child's tooth development begins during the early months of pregnancy. At about the fourth or fifth month of pregnancy mineralization of the primary teeth begins, and by 1 year of age it is completed. Permanent teeth begin to be mineralized at birth and are usually completely formed by 12 years of age. Third molars, wisdom teeth, may not be completely formed until 18 to 25 years of age.

Formation of teeth is primarily a one-way event. Once formed, they are not remodeled systematically, from the inside, as a result of dietary stress. The changes, demineralization and decay, take place due to action on the outside of the teeth. Damaged teeth cannot repair themselves.

Diet during the tooth formation years plays an important role in the development of decay-resistant, healthy teeth. As discussed elsewhere, protein, calcium, phosphorus, and vitamin D are all essential for tooth formation. Lack of vitamin A during this time also has been shown to be a factor in later susceptibility to decay.

The mineral fluorine, in the form of fluoride compounds, has been proven to be the one nutrient that exerts the greatest beneficial effect on resistance to decay. Studies show a close correlation between fluoride ingestion during tooth development and the absence of later decay. Fluorides are known to be deposited in the enamel as the teeth are being calcified, but it is not known why fluoride inhibits decay. Fluorides have the capacity to remineralize decalcified enamel but are less protective of teeth that have already erupted. This is why the presence of fluoride is so important during the years when teeth are forming.

Studies have consistently confirmed a 60 percent reduction in the incidence of tooth decay in children who consumed water with the beneficial amount of fluoride (0.7 to 1.2 parts per million depending on climate) compared with those whose water contains little or no fluoride. If a community water supply lacks fluoride, fluoridated water can be purchased as bottled water or fluoride supplements can be prescribed by a dentist or physician.

The amount and composition of saliva also influences the development of tooth decay. Saliva rinses the teeth, buffers and dilutes the acid produced by bacteria, and also has anti-bacterial, immunological, and remineralization properties that help protect the teeth. If the amount of saliva is reduced (for example, as a result of radiation treatment on salivary glands) or if its composition is abnormal, tooth decay is much more likely. Chewing on fibrous foods, such as celery, or sugarless gum stimulates a copious flow of saliva and increases the mechanical washing away of food debris.

Oral Bacteria

Decay begins with demineralization of the outer surface of the tooth by acids that are produced by bacteria that ferment carbohydrate foods in the mouth (see Exhibit 15.9). Dental plaque plays a prominent role in this process. Plaque is a sticky, gel-like substance that clings to the surface of the teeth. It contains, among other things, compounds called *polysaccharides,* which are formed from sucrose by oral bacteria, plus the bacteria themselves. Millions of bacteria are concentrated on specific sites on tooth surfaces in plaque. More than one kind of bacteria are involved, but the one thought to be the primary cause of decay is *Streptococcus mutans.* The bacteria ferment the carbohydrates in the mouth, produce acids, and the acids break down tooth enamel. The bacteria then invade the tooth, causing infection and further breakdown.

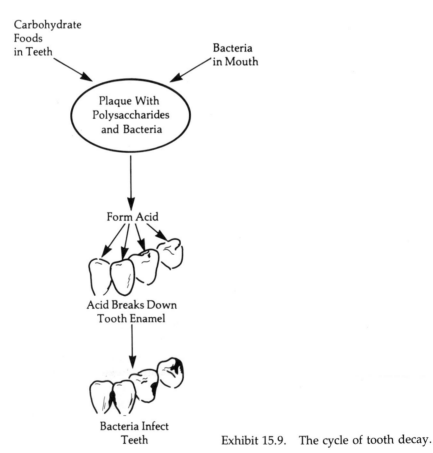

Exhibit 15.9.   The cycle of tooth decay.

Food Eaten

Food, particularly starches and sugars, must accumulate in the mouth in order for the acid-producing bacteria to have something to grow on. In animal experiments, when rats were fed a decay-producing diet by stomach tube, they developed no tooth decay since no foods were present in their mouths.

Sucrose, as found in ordinary sugar, stands out as the primary decay-producing food. But the form that it's in, the time that it stays in the mouth, and the frequency of the exposure are all important factors. Sticky sweets that cling to the teeth, such as caramels, are more decay-producing than foods that are quickly cleared. Liquids are less of a problem than solids since they don't require chewing. Liquids that contain sugar plus acids, such as lemonade and fruit drinks, are additionally harmful because these acids also attack tooth enamel. (See Exhibit 15.10 for a comparison of the decay-causing effects of popular foods.)

The most important factor of all is now believed to be the *frequency* of food consumption. It correlates more closely with the amount of tooth decay than does the total amount of sugar eaten. Each time oral bacteria are fed sugar they produce 20 to 30 minutes of acid. Thus, the snacking habit, especially of sweet foods, is believed to be an important reason for the increasing amount of tooth decay found in the United States.[5]

Foods that do not break down readily in the mouth, such as popcorn, nuts, and cheese are not decay causing and are thought to have a certain amount of antidecay activity. Other foods such as crackers, bread, and potato chips contain starches that cling to the teeth, are broken down by bacteria, and then cause decay. Marshmallows, dates, cookies, candy, sugared cereals (when eaten as a snack without milk), and bread and jelly are highly decay-causing because they are both sticky and high in sugar.

Exhibit 15.10   Comparison of Decay-Causing Effect of Popular Foods

HIGHLY DECAY-CAUSING	SOMEWHAT DECAY-CAUSING	ANTIDECAY ACTION
Candy—especially sticky candy such as caramels	Soft drinks	Popcorn
Marshmallows	Fruit drinks, ades, punch	Nuts
Dry fruit—raisins, dates	Lemonade	Cheese
Cookies	Graham crackers	Raw celery
Bread and Jelly	Potato chips	
Bread and Honey	Bread	
Graham crackers with peanut butter	Crackers	
Sugared cereals (eaten dry, without milk)	Nonsugared cereal (eaten dry, no milk)	

[5]D. P. DePaola and M. C. Alfano, "Diet and Oral Health." *Nutrition Today*, Vol. 12, No. 3, May-June, 1977, pp. 6-32.

None of these foods needs to be a problem, however, if they are eaten as part of a meal and the teeth are brushed afterwards. If brushing isn't possible, the next best thing is to rinse and swish the mouth with water and eat a "detergent food," such as celery or other raw vegetables, which acts as a natural toothbrush because it is high in fiber.

Many people have the idea that only white sugar—sucrose—causes tooth decay and that so-called natural sugars—molasses, honey, raw sugar or fruit sugars as in dried fruit—and milk sugar (lactose) will not cause decay. This notion has been disproven. Animal studies show that these natural sugars do not protect against decay and that when honey and raw sugar are substituted for white sugar there is extensive tooth decay.[6] Only complex carbohydrates such as the sugar-alcohol xylitol and non-nutrient sweeteners such as cyclamates and saccharine have been shown not to cause tooth decay. Phosphates may be able to counteract the effects of sugar when added to food, for example, to sugared cereals. In studies of two large groups of school children, tooth decay was reduced from 30 to 50 percent when children ate breakfast cereals containing phosphates. However, other researchers have been unable to duplicate these results.

Because of the close relationship between diet and tooth decay, dentists have become more active in providing their patients, and their patients' parents, with nutrition information. The American Dental Association recommends eating a balanced diet from the Four Food Groups, brushing and flossing teeth daily to remove food particles and plaque, and drinking fluoridated water or using a fluoride supplement to develop decay-resistant teeth (see Exhibit 15.11).

FOOD ALLERGIES

Foods are just one of many substances that can cause allergic reactions in children. A child is said to have an allergy when his body reacts abnormally to a substance in the environment that does not bother most people. Infants and children are more likely to develop food allergies than adults. The symptoms of a food allergy can range from gastrointestinal disturbances, such as nausea, vomiting, bloating, abdominal pain, gas, and diarrhea, to nasal inflammation, asthma, hives, eczema, headaches, and many other signs and symptoms.

Reactions may be acute or mild, immediate (within 4 hours), or delayed (up to 72 hours). Often the food causing the problem is difficult to pinpoint. The most frequent offenders are eggs, milk, and wheat, with corn, chocolate, nuts, fish and shellfish, and peas and peanuts being next (see Exhibit 15.12). Other common foods that may be troub-

---

[6]A. Nizel, "Preventing Dental Caries, Nutrition Factors," in The Pediatric Clinics of North America, Vol. 24, No. 1, *Symposium on Nutrition in Pediatrics*. Philadelphia: W. B. Saunders Co., 1977, pp. 141-55.

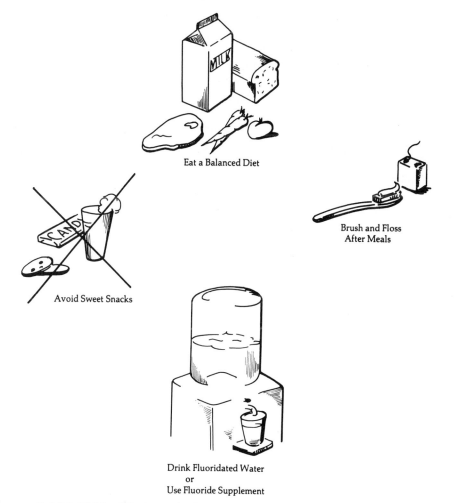

Eat a Balanced Diet

Brush and Floss
After Meals

Avoid Sweet Snacks

Drink Fluoridated Water
or
Use Fluoride Supplement

Exhibit 15.11.   Much tooth decay can be prevented by following these four steps.

Exhibit 15.12.   Foods that Frequently Cause Food Allergies in Young Children

Eggs
Milk   } Most frequent offenders
Wheat

Corn
Chocolate
Nuts, especially peanuts
Fish, shellfish
Peas

Grapefruit
Oranges
Strawberries
Tomatoes

lemakers are grapefruit, oranges, strawberries, and tomatoes. Food additives, colorings, and flavors also can cause allergic reactions in some children. Sometimes a child can tolerate a small amount of the food or can eat it only occasionally, but will react if he eats a large amount of it or eats it regularly. Sometimes a food can be tolerated, except at times of anxiety or stress or when other substances, such as pollens, are causing allergic reactions.

Genetic factors appear to be involved: children whose parents are allergic (not necessarily to food) are more at risk. When allergies run in the family, it is wise to follow the procedure suggested in Chapter 14 for gradually introducing new foods into the infant's or child's diet so problem foods can be identified promptly.

When allergies do develop, identifying their cause can be a long, involved, and sometimes frustrating process. Skin tests, which are used for identifying nonfood causes of allergies, are not very reliable for foods. Usually some form of an elimination diet is used. For example, an entire food group may be eliminated from the diet. If allergic symptoms clear up after a week or so, the foods may be added back, one at a time, allowing time for symptoms to reappear. If the symptoms don't disappear when a food group is eliminated, deleting another food group may be tried.

Another aid to identifying the cause of an allergy is for parents to keep a diet diary of all the foods a child eats, including snacks, and also include a log of symptoms—what they are and when they occur. Sometimes a cause and effect relationship can be seen from this record.

Once the cause of a child's food allergy is identified, how is it treated? To date the only really effective treatment is to eliminate the offending foods. In the case of foods such as wheat, milk, or eggs, avoiding them is extremely difficult as they are found as ingredients in so many common foods. Constant label reading is necessary, and often many ready-made foods must be avoided. Recipes for homemade foods must be remodeled to avoid the problem ingredients. In some cases another form of the food can be tolerated: for example, cooked fruits are less likely to cause problems than fresh fruits.

One hopeful aspect of childhood allergies is that sometimes the child will grow out of them after age five and eventually will be able to tolerate the problem foods.

METABOLIC DISORDERS

Food intolerances are sometimes caused by an inborn lack of digestive enzymes, which makes it impossible for a child to digest certain nutrients. The most common example of this condition, caused by a lack of the enzyme lactase, is *lactose intolerance.* Other examples are *phenyl-*

ketonuria (PKU), in which there is a lack of the enzyme needed to convert the amino acid phenylalanine to tyrosine; *galactosemia,* in which the enzyme for utilizing galactose and lactose is lacking; and *cystic fibrosis of the pancreas,* which involves a lack of pancreatic enzymes and poor absorption of food. All of these conditions except lactose intolerance are present at birth and result in an infant's "failure to thrive" and gain weight normally. Treatment generally involves elimination of the nonabsorbed nutrients from the diet.

Lactose Intolerance. This usually develops during childhood and adolescence and is seen infrequently in children under three years old. It occurs among many people of nonEuropean descent, including almost 100 percent of African black people, 75 percent of American black people, over 80 percent of Oriental people, and almost as many Mexican-Americans.[7] School children who refuse milk often may do so because of this condition.

Low lactase levels result in only partial digestion of the lactose of milk. The undigested lactose stays in the intestines, where it ferments and produces uncomfortable symptoms such as abdominal bloating, cramps, excess gas, and diarrhea.

Usually lactase is not totally lacking, and some children can tolerate the lactose in a single glass of milk without problems. The symptoms occur with larger intakes. Milk served at room temperature seems to be better tolerated than ice-cold milk.

All fluid milks contain about the same amount of lactose—12 grams per cup. Fermented milk products such as yogurt and buttermilk have about half as much lactose and often will cause no discomfort (see Exhibit 15.13). Most ordinary cheeses have almost no lactose because it is lost in the whey, so cheese can serve as a good source of calcium for children who can tolerate little milk. Calcium deficiency can result if all dairy products are avoided.

Because lactose and dried whey are added to many products, in cases where lactose intolerance is severe, food labels will need to be read to avoid these ingredients. They are often found in imitation or nondairy products; so care must be exercised when using one of these products.

A relatively inexpensive method for adding the enzyme lactase to milk to change lactose into glucose and galactose has been developed but has not been adopted by major milk producers.[8] The lactase enzyme additive is produced commercially for addition to milk by consumers. It is a powder that can simply be stirred into milk. After 24 hours the lactose is reduced by 70 percent in refrigerated milk; after several days it is reduced by 90 percent.

[7] F. J. Simoons, J. D. Johnson, N. Kretchmer, "Perspective on Milk Drinking and Malabsorption of Lactose." *Pediatrics,* Vol. 59, No. 1, January, 1977, pp. 98-109.

[8] F. H. Rosenberg, "Lactose Intolerance." *American Journal of Nursing,* Vol. 77, No. 5, May, 1977, pp. 123-24.

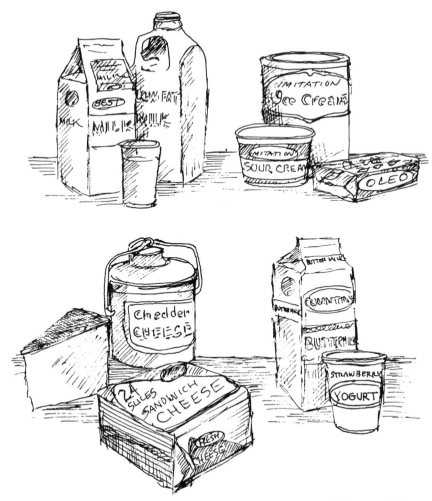

Exhibit 15.13.   Fermented dairy products, shown in the bottom half of this illustration, contain less lactose and are more readily tolerated by people who are lactose-intolerant.

HYPERACTIVITY

Hyperactive children have been the focus of much research attention in recent years. By some estimates, as many as 20 percent of school children were thought to be "hyperactive." However, other studies have shown that a much smaller number of children show real evidence of this disorder.[9] The real difficulty lies in the fact that hyperactivity is

[9]Institute of Food Technologists' Expert Panel on Food Safety and Nutrition and the Committee on Public Information, "Diet and Hyperactivity: Any Connection?" Chicago, IL: Institute of Food Technologists, April, 1976, p. 2.

not a pure disease or syndrome and there are no precise medical, neurological, or psychological methodologies to use in the diagnosis of hyperactivity.

The terms *hyperactive, hyperkinesis,* and *hyperkinetic behavior syndrome* have been used somewhat loosely to describe a symptom, or symptoms, rather than a disease. Generally these terms describe a child whose behavior patterns may include excess or undirected motor activity, a short attention span, poor powers of concentration, low frustration level, impulsiveness, distractibility, excitability, irritability, restlessness, aggressiveness, rejection of disciplinary measures, underachievement, and classroom disruption in school. The symptoms are difficult to measure and interpret objectively. Many children may have a short attention span and can be easily distracted without being overactive. Because of this, children with this type of problem are now categorized as having an "attentional deficit disorder."

A controversial theory, proposed by Dr. Benjamin Feingold, that hyperactivity in children is caused by certain chemicals in foods brought about great interest among parents and teachers in the idea of curing these symptoms through changes in children's diets.

Dr. Feingold, an allergist and emeritus director of the Laboratory of Medical Entomology of the Kaiser Foundation Research Institute of San Francisco, theorized that children diagnosed as hyperkinetic can be successfully treated with a diet that excludes all foods containing natural salicylates (including many fruits and nuts and two vegetables—tomatoes and cucumbers), all foods containing synthetic food colors or flavors (as found in many prepackaged foods and drinks), and some foods containing certain additives (BHT).

The treatment Dr. Feingold prescribed was an *exclusion diet* for the whole family, not just the hyperactive child. Fruits and vegetables containing natural salicylates and all foods containing artificial color and flavor and some additives were to be omitted. Feingold claimed to have such dramatic results in reducing hyperactivity among children he treated that his proposal received widespread attention from parents, educators, legislators, and consumer activists and much publicity in the mass media. His books, *Why Your Child Is Hyperactive* and *The Feingold Cookbook,* have become a popular layman's guide for treating hyperactivity through diet.

However, his theory was not generally accepted by nutrition scientists, who felt that it was based on a small number of case studies rather than on a scientifically controlled experiment. The observations of the children by parents and teachers were not objective, said the critics, and the rating of hyperactivity was subject to suggestibility: confident expectations generated in parents and children by Feingold could have affected both the syndrome and/or the parents' rating. Critics suggested that the diet prescribed for the whole family could have resulted in other changes, for example, in family dynamics, which may have provided the children with more attention.[10]

Scientists also were concerned because so many widely distributed and highly nutritious foods were being labeled as potentially harmful with so little evidence and because the Feingold diet might not meet long-term nutrient needs of children.

Because there was such widespread interest in the Feingold diet, several carefully controlled studies were conducted at prominent universities to test it. These studies were double blind—neither the researchers nor the parents or children knew which diet they were receiving at any given time—and included some objective as well as subjective determinations of the children's behavior.

In none of the studies conducted to date have researchers been able to detect the kind, frequency, or degree of changes in behavior related to artificial food colors described by Dr. Feingold. A small group of children may be adversely affected by food additives, and this question deserves further study, the researchers concluded. But the hypothesis that hyperactivity in children is *frequently* or *generally* the result of artificial food colors and flavors was not supported by the results of objectively conducted experiments using diets based on Dr. Feingold's guidelines.[11] However, research continues, and new information may develop on this subject in the years to come.

A University of California at Berkeley study that sampled 5,000 children and investigated those reported to be hyperactive showed that the severity of the problem is affected by the child's home and school environments.[12] Another study suggests that some hyperactive children may not metabolize sugars in the normal way. Since many of the artificially colored foods that children eat (candy, soft drinks, etc.) are high in sugar, this ingredient, rather than the food colors, may account for the changes in behavior observed by Feingold.

Summary

A most important goal of early childhood nutrition is helping the child to establish positive eating patterns and to learn to enjoy a wide variety of nutritious foods. The Four Food Groups can be adapted easily to the young child's needs by adjustment of numbers and amounts of servings. Iron is the nutrient commonly found to be lacking in the diet

[10]National Advisory Committee on Hyperkinesis and Food Additives, Report to the Nutrition Foundation. New York: Nutrition Foundation, 1975.

[11]National Advisory Committee on Hyperkinesis and Food Additives, Statement Summarizing Research Findings on the Issue of the Relationship between Food Additive-Free Diets and Hyperkinesis in Children. New York: The Nutrition Foundation, 1977.

[12]"A Major Study Refutes Widely Believed Claims about Hyperactivity in Children." University Bulletin, Vol. 27, No. 7, August 16, 1978. Berkeley, CA: University of California.

of children; this often occurs as the result of overconsumption of milk and dislike of vegetables.

During this time growth slows, appetite decreases, and food "jags" are common. Parents should not overreact to this *physiologic anorexia*, and should realize that the child himself is a fairly good judge of how much food he needs. Small servings of a variety of nutritious foods, with opportunity to ask for seconds, is recommended.

Each young child is unique, and many children have a small capacity in addition to a small appetite. This is the time to establish good snacking habits. Children are often suspicious of new foods, and a flexible "taste-a-small-amount" approach may help to overcome this suspicion. Children often respond well when allowed to participate in food preparation and when new foods are gradually introduced in small portions, served along with favorites. One must consider that children also respond to the appearance and texture of foods and that they are imitative, want to be independent, and may have poor coordination. Some foods are inappropriate for young preschool children, such as those that are hard to chew, highly spiced, or high in fat or fiber.

The middle school years are a benign time of fairly slow but even growth. Sedentary children may become overweight and need to be encouraged to become more active. Problems at this time center around skipping breakfast and substituting snacking for meals.

Dental disease is the most chronic nutrition-related disease among American children. Major contributors to this problem are frequency of food consumption; consumption of sticky, high-sugar foods; and lack of brushing. Substitution of honey, raw sugar, and other "natural sugars" does not reduce decay, but fluoridated water or a fluoride supplement does help to develop decay-resistant teeth.

Food allergies, difficult to pinpoint, may cause a variety of symptoms ranging from gastrointestinal disturbances to rashes and nasal congestion. Identification and treatment often involves the use of a diet diary and an elimination diet. Other food-intolerance disturbances include lactose intolerance, phenylketonuria (PKU), galactosemia, and cystic fibrosis. Hyperactive or hyperkinetic children tend to display excess motor activity and a short attention span. Causal and treatment theories are controversial and include the use of an exclusion diet.

NUTRITION DURING ADOLESCENCE 16

Highlights

Developmental changes and growth patterns
Teenage nutritional requirements and eating habits
Obesity and weight manipulation during adolescence
Relationship between diet and complexion problems
Nutritional needs of the young athlete

Adolescence is the time when children grow into mature men and women. They undergo profound, complex, interrelated changes that are physical, physiological, psychological, emotional, and social. In the process boys and girls become sexually mature, achieve the ability to reproduce, and develop the kind of physique they will have as adults.

The rapid physical growth rate in adolescence is second only to the prenatal and infancy period.[1] Nutrition is known to be very important during this rapid growth time, but its significance is not as clearly understood as the importance of nutrition during the prenatal and infant growth period. Research in adolescent nutrition has not been extensive and knowledge of adolescents' requirements for various nutrients is limited and incomplete. One reason for this is that other animal species used in nutrition research do not experience the growth spurt that humans do at this time.

PHASES OF DEVELOPMENT

The boundaries of adolescence are blurry. Adolescence starts with changes in hormonal activities and ends with the last stage of sex organ maturation and physical maturation. In this broad sense it covers over half the entire growth and development period and extends throughout the major part of the child's second ten years of life.

The ages at which children enter and complete this growth phase vary so widely that some researchers suggest that research and nutrient recommendations be made on the basis of developmental phases rather than age (see Exhibit 16.1).[2] Three distinct phases have been identified: prepuberty, puberty, and postpuberty.

Prepuberty is the first stage, when early and rather hidden changes associated with the beginning of altered endocrine activities start taking place at about the age of 8 for girls and 10 for boys.

Puberty is the middle period of adolescence, when the observable changes in sexual development and growth take place. This period tends to start at about ages 10 to 12 for girls and 12 to 14 for boys.

Postpuberty is a time for the finishing-off process of attaining adulthood, covering the last two to three years. Growth is completed, and the transition is made to adult maturity.

The growth and maturation during adolescence proceeds in a predictable order for each child. But the timing varies greatly among indi-

---

[1]J. I. McKigney and H. N. Munro, *Nutrient Requirements in Adolescence.* U.S. Department of Health, Education, and Welfare, Public Health Service, National Institutes of Health, DHEW Publication No. (NIH) 76-771. Washington, D.C., 1976.

[2]W. Daniel, Jr., "Nutrition and Adolescence." *Dietetic Currents*, Vol. 3, No. 4, July-August, 1976.

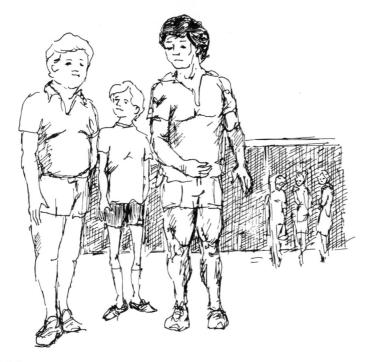

Exhibit 16.1. During puberty, boys of the same age may be very different in physical and sexual development.

viduals, with girls generally being about two years ahead of boys. Within any grade level of junior high students are some who are sexually immature and who still look like children, some who appear to have completed their sexual development and growth spurt, and others who are in the midst of change. Exhibit 16.2 shows the typical age groupings that will occur if boys and girls are grouped according to the timing of the growth spurt that takes place during puberty.

THE TEENAGE GROWTH SPURT AND NUTRIENT NEEDS

Because growth is so rapid, requirements for all nutrients increase greatly during this time (see Exhibit 16.3). The increase in body size is one of growth in both height and weight. Because bones grow rapidly and are progressively mineralized, the bone-forming nutrients calcium, phosphorus, vitamin D, and protein are vitally needed. Growth variability affects the need for calcium. Boys who grow tall very rapidly are most at risk of not getting enough calcium. Late-maturing girls who shun milk because of its calories are another group likely to lack calcium.

Muscle, or lean tissue, and fat tissue also increase rapidly and change in proportion for boys and girls. Girls gain proportionately more

Exhibit 16.2   Timing of Puberty Growth Spurts

TIME OF GROWTH SPURT	BOYS	GIRLS
Early	11–13	9–11
Moderate	13–14	11–12
Late	over 14	over 12

Exhibit 16.3.   The Adolescent Growth Spurt: Physical Changes and Special Nutrient Needs

CHANGES	NUTRIENTS NEEDED IN EXTRA LARGE AMOUNTS
Rapid bone growth	Calcium
	Phosphorus
Rapid increase in height	Vitamin D
Rapid increase in muscle tissue	Protein
Increase in blood volume and number of red blood cells	Iron
	Calories

fat than lean tissue and retain this ratio during the rest of growth. Boys, on the other hand, acquire more muscle and less fat. On the average, boys gain about twice the amount of lean tissue gained by girls.

Because boys generally experience greater growth of bone and muscle tissue, their need for protein, calcium, and other tissue-building nutrients, as well as calories, is much greater than that of girls. At the peak of their growth spurt, boys have the highest need for nutrients of any age group with the exception of pregnant and lactating women.

Growth studies have shown a close relationship between growth in height and protein intake during childhood and in specific periods such as adolescence. Protein tends to average 12 to 16 percent of total energy intake during adolescence, with 15 percent appearing to be optimal.

The increased rate of growth in height during adolescence also requires an increase in calories. If calories are restricted during rapid growth, the laying down of lean body mass and nitrogen retention is jeopardized, even when protein is adequate. For girls, calorie requirements peak just before they begin to menstruate, at about age 13, and then drop. Boys reach their maximum intake at about 16 years.

The difference between girls and boys in calorie needs at the peak of the growth spurt is considerable. Girls need approximately 2,400 calories, while boys need 3,000. However, adolescents who are participating in athletics or who are exceptionally active may have calorie needs well above these amounts.

Most at risk during this stage of growth are adolescent athletes from low-income families, who cannot afford the amount of food needed to supply the athletes with adequate calories for both growth and strenuous activity.

Another difference between boys and girls is in the growth and number of red blood cells. In boys, the number of red blood cells rises rapidly during the growth spurt, while in girls the number remains constant. Thus, during puberty boys have a high need for iron to form red blood cells. Girls too, however, have an increased need for iron as a result of blood loss once they begin to menstruate. After the growth spurt, the male's need for extra iron ends, while the female's need continues until menopause.

ARE ADOLESCENTS WELL NOURISHED?

The Ten-State Nutrition Survey showed that among the age groups studied, adolescents between the ages of 10 to 16 years of age had the highest prevalence of unsatisfactory nutritional status, with boys showing more evidence of poor nutrition than girls.[3] However, the overall nutritional status of all American teenagers is not really known because there has been no nationwide study of a statistically valid sampling of American youth. Yet many persons are convinced that teenagers must be on the brink of nutritional disaster because of their allegedly atrocious food habits or because of misinterpretation of dietary studies.[4]

Surveys usually show that some teenagers have food intakes that fail to meet the Recommended Dietary Allowances for essential nutrients (see Exhibit 16.4). But this does not mean they are suffering from malnutrition, especially since the RDA for this age group is based on estimates, not exact data.

The nutrient most often found to be lacking in diets of teenage boys and girls is iron, because the requirement is so high. Yet iron absorption is more efficient during times of increased need, and it is assumed that this happens during the teenage growth spurt. However, both boys and girls may develop iron-deficiency anemia if their diets do not supply enough of this mineral. (See Chapter 11 for ways to add iron to the diet.)

Folic acid requirements are high during growth and development as well, and may not be fulfilled when teenagers shun fruits and vegetables, the best sources of this nutrient.

Some studies have shown that vitamin A intakes are low with some teenagers; sometimes vitamin C intake is insufficient; and calcium

[3]"Highlights from the Ten-State Nutrition Survey." *Nutrition Today*, Vol. 7, No. 4, July-August, 1972, pp. 6-7.
[4]R. L. Huenemann, "A Review of Teenage Nutrition in the U.S." Talk sponsored by the U.S. Department of Agriculture, Agricultural Research Service, Washington, D.C., 1972.

Exhibit 16.4 Recommended Daily Dietary Allowances for Teenagers

NUTRIENT	UNIT	ALLOWANCE			
		TEENAGE BOY		TEENAGE GIRL	
		11–14 YR.	15–18 YR.	11–14 YR.	15–18 YR.
Food energy	cal	2700	2800	2200	2100
Protein	g	45	56	46	46
Fat-soluble vitamins					
Vitamin A	μg R.E.[1]	1000	1000	800	800
Vitamin E	mg & T.E.[2]	8	10	8	8
Vitamin D	μg^3	10	10	10	10
Water-soluble vitamins					
Ascorbic acid	mg	50	60	50	60
Folacin	μg	400	400	400	400
Niacin	mg equiv NE[4]	18	18	15	14
Riboflavin	mg	1.6	1.7	1.3	1.3
Thiamin	mg	1.4	1.4	1.1	1.1
Vitamin B_6	mg	1.8	2.0	1.8	2.0
Vitamin B_{12}	μg	3.0	3.0	3.0	3.0
Minerals					
Calcium	mg	1200	1200	1200	1200
Phosphorus	mg	1200	1200	1200	1200
Iodine	μg	150	150	150	150
Iron	mg	18	18	18	18
Magnesium	mg	350	400	300	300
Zinc	mg	15	15	15	15

Source: Recommended Dietary Allowances, Ninth Edition (revised 1979). National Academy of Sciences, Washington, D.C.

[1] Retinol equivalents. 1 retinol equivalent = 1 μg retinol or 6 μg β-carotene.

[2] α tocopherol equivalents. 1 μg d-α-tocoperol = 1 μT.E.

[3] As cholecalciferol. 10 μg cholecalciferol = 400 I.U. vitamin D.

[4] 1 NE (niacin equivalent) is equal to 1 μg of naicin or 60 μg of dietary tryptophan.

and riboflavin may be low when teenagers do not drink milk. But generalizations are risky because of the many variations in teenage eating practices.

The most common nutritional problems seen in this age group are tooth decay, anemia, and obesity. Of particular concern are teenage girls who become pregnant before their growth is complete.

Adolescence has been shown to be a key period in acquiring adult dietary patterns, as pointed out in Chapter 2. One study showed that a somewhat consistent (year-to-year) dietary pattern is followed during the preschool and preadolescent periods, and that a major change that tends to persist into adulthood may occur during adolescence.

In general, teenagers are hungry, and they like to eat (Exhibit 16.5). Their favorite foods, according to surveys, include hamburgers, pizza, chicken, french fries, ice cream, spaghetti, and orange juice (Exhibit 16.6). The most unpopular food is liver, and all vegetables tend to be less popular than other foods.

Teenagers do not necessarily eat food as meals. Much of their diet may be in the form of snacks—from vending machines, school snack bars, fast-food outlets, or at home. A Gallup Poll, conducted in 1977 among teenagers, showed that one-third of them did not eat breakfast. Older teens, those between 16 and 19, and girls especially were the most likely to skip breakfast. For example, 45 percent of older teenage girls said they did not bother with breakfast.[5]

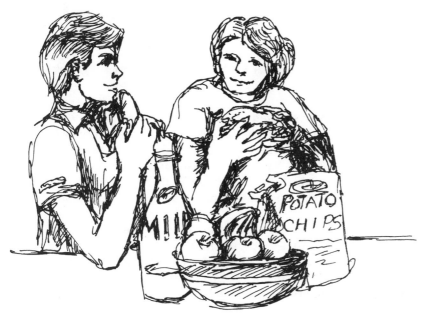

Exhibit 16.5. Most teenagers are hungry—and they like to eat!

[5]"Third of Teens Skip Breakfast, Poll Finds," Gallup Youth Survey. *Los Angeles Times*, December 1, 1977, part II, p. 10.

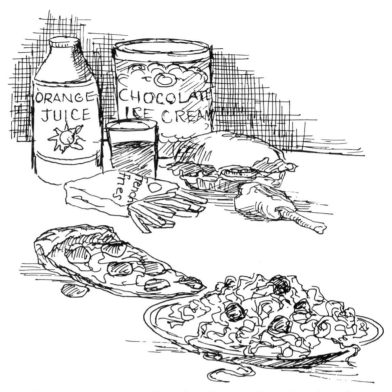

Exhibit 16.6.   Surveys show that these foods are favorites of teenagers. The most unpopular foods are liver and cooked vegetables.

The same survey showed that 95·percent of the 13 to 19 year-olds
ate fast foods as part of their diet. However, the teens interviewed said,
by a two-to-one margin, that they would rather eat at home—because
they thought fast foods had inferior taste and nutrition. Analysis of
some typical fast foods, however, shows that they do make important
nutrient contributions. They also tend to be high in fat, calories, and
salt.

Snacks chosen by teenagers frequently are the low-nutrient-density, high-sugar, high-fat foods, such as candy, soft drinks, and pastries, popular with other age groups. Yet studies show that when nutritious foods are readily available for snacks, at home or in school vending
machines, many hungry teenagers will choose these foods in preference
to those with low nutrient density. More information about snack foods
is included in Chapter 27.

To promote better nutrition among school children and better par-
ticipation in the school lunch program, the U.S. Department of Agriculture established a controversial requirement that schools receiving National School Lunch funding would have to limit "competitive sales"

from vending machines and snack bars to only the more nutritious snacks until after the last lunches were served.

An extensive study of teenage eating patterns conducted in California in the late 1960s showed that roughly one-third of the total group, and 90 percent of the black teenagers, had highly irregular eating patterns and that many youngsters were fending for themselves. Some were buying their own snacks, while others were helping themselves to whatever they could find at home.[6] With the ever-increasing number of working mothers, this situation has become even more common as later studies have confirmed. A study in the early 1970s showed that in families with employed mothers and teenage girls (13 to 18), the teenage girls frequently did the food shopping for the family. They also helped plan and prepare family meals.[7] Nutrition education is especially important for these teenagers who fend for themselves or who shop and prepare food for their families.

Another characteristic of many teenagers is that they lead very busy lives. They participate in sports and after-school activities and have part-time jobs and, as a result, are not home for family meals and have to eat on the run (Exhibit 16.7). Lack of time is a major reason why many of them skip breakfast. At school they don't want to take the time to stand in line to get a cafeteria lunch; so they eat snack foods instead. Often conscientious parents who would like to provide balanced meals for their teenagers find it difficult if not impossible to do so. The best they can do is to have nutritious, quick, easy snack foods readily available.

Teens are strongly influenced by peer pressures and may follow fad diets or eat foods they do not believe to be nutritious to be part of the group. Some may feel that rejection of parental eating practices is a way of expressing their independence. Parents who understand this need for independence, accent the positive, and try to build on and add to what teenagers already like and eat will probably be more effective than those who nag teenagers about bad habits.

APPEARANCE AND DIET

A notable characteristic of almost all adolescents is a shaky sense of self-esteem and an overconcern about their body size, sexual development, and personal appearance. This is easy to understand, consid-

[6]R. L. Huenemann, L. Shapiro, M. Hampton, B. Mitchell, "Food and Eating Practices of Teen-Agers." *Journal of the American Dietetic Association*, Vol. 53, No. 1, July, 1968, pp. 17-24.

[7]Study conducted by American Institute of Food Distributors and reported in *Fresh Produce Council Digest*, April, 1976, p. 7.

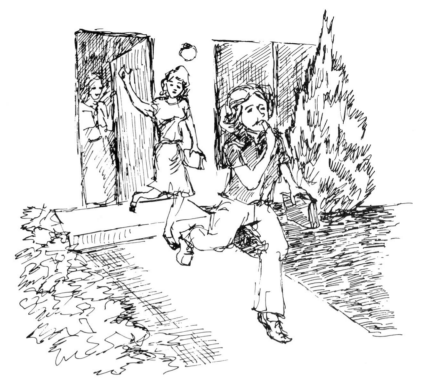

Exhibit 16.7. Lack of time is the reason many teenagers skip breakfast.

ering the physical and psychological changes that they are undergoing. Often their view of their body image is distorted or unrealistic.

Studies show, for example, that a large proportion of teenage girls think they are too fat or are afraid they might get too fat.[8] The cult of thinness in the American culture has led many a teenage girl to diet unwisely and unnecessarily to try to achieve an unattainable sylphlike silhouette (see Exhibit 16.8). A typical teenage girl who wants to be thinner will skip breakfast, eat an inadequate or no lunch, and then, driven by hunger, eat high-calorie, low-nutrient snack foods. She may also drink too little milk in an effort to reduce calories and as a result deplete calcium stores. Some teenage girls are prone to follow every new fad weight-control diet that comes along, and some may also try fasting (usually only briefly). A few may become so fanatic about dieting that they are diagnosed as having anorexia nervosa (see Chapter 5). Teenage girls who eat unwisely and then become pregnant are at high risk in terms of their own health and that of their baby.

[8]M. S. Read, F. P. Heald, "Adolescent Obesity--Summary of a Symposium." *Journal of the American Dietetic Association*, Vol. 47, No. 5, November, 1965, pp, 411-13.

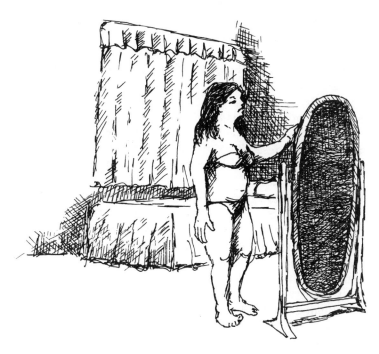

Exhibit 16.8. Many teenage girls think they are too fat, and this may cause them to diet unwisely.

Teenage boys, on the other hand, tend to think that they're too thin, and they want to gain weight, particularly to become more muscular.[9] Since their growth in height is so rapid, many boys go through a thin, scraggly stage before they start filling out. Their appetites are tremendous, and the drain on the family food budget can be disconcerting, but their intake of nutrients may be quite satisfactory because of the large amount of food they eat. Many boys this age need reassurance that in time they will stop growing up and will start growing out and become more symmetrical.

Another group of both boys and girls who are concerned about their appearance are the late maturers, who are behind their peers in growth and sexual development. They need to know that their time will come and that eventually they will catch up with their friends. All young people need help in learning to like and accept themselves as nature intended them to be. There is no point in building false hope during teen years that "eating the right foods" will change the genetic destiny of girls who have large frames and no hope of ever being thin and boys who are genetically small in stature and will never be tall.

[9]I. Valadian, "The Adolescent—His Growth and Development." Talk presented at the National Nutrition Education Conference, Washington, D.C., November 2-4, 1971.

Obesity During Adolescence

One group for which change in body size is possible, although difficult to achieve, is the obese. Often the period of maximum growth in height during the growth spurt and immediately thereafter is a good period to help the obese adolescent lose his fat since fat is not only growing at its minimum rate at this time, but actually shows a loss, especially in the male. Studies show that people who were obese during childhood and who remained obese after the growth spurt were most likely to continue to be .obese. Of these obese teens, 75 to 80 percent are likely to remain obese as adults.[10]

The idea that teenagers are obese because they eat so much is not necessarily accurate. Several studies have shown that obese teenagers did not eat more than their thin friends and, in fact, sometimes actually ate less.[11] The difference between thin and fat teenagers was in their level of activity. The obese teens studied were found to be far less active than normal-weight teens.

Obese teens tend to have very low self-esteem, may feel rejected and discriminated against by peers and adults, may withdraw and become socially isolated, and are less likely to participate in athletics. As a result, they may become even more obese. The vicious cycle is hard to disrupt (see Exhibit 16.9).

Because obese teenagers already have a low sense of self-esteem, parental nagging about their eating habits or moralizing and blaming their obesity on their lack of self-control or laziness makes them even more unhappy with themselves and more, rather than less, likely to continue in the cycle of obesity.

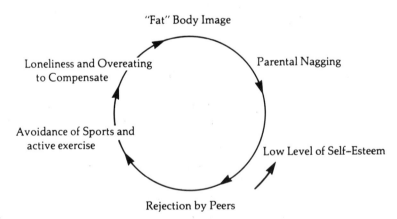

Exhibit 16.9.   The teenage obesity cycle can be difficult to interrupt.

[10]S. Abraham and M. Nordsieck, "Relationship of Excess Weight in Children and Adults." *Public Health Reports*, Vol. 75, 1960, pp. 263-73.

[11]J. Mayer, *Overweight—Causes, Cost, and Control.* Englewood Cliffs, NJ: Prentice-Hall, Inc. 1968, pp. 125-26.

What they need instead of lectures and diet books is supportive counseling, encouragement to participate in programs where they get regular exercise (often a special physical education activity for teens with weight problems is most helpful), and education and guidance about how they can choose foods that are nutritious but lower in calories (as discussed in Chapter 5). Keeping diet and activity records may be a helpful way for them to begin learning to be responsible for making their own decisions about their diets and exercise. But most important, they need to want to change their behavior and realize it's up to them and that no one can do it for them.

Complexion Problems

Acne and skin blemishes are worrisome, and appearance-conscious teens may make unhealthful changes in their diets, for example stop drinking milk, in an attempt to overcome their complexion problem. When parents tell a teenager that his bad complexion is caused by his poor diet, all they do is make him feel guilty. A good diet is necessary for optimal nutrition and healthy skin, but probably will have no immediate effect in improving a teenager's complexion.

Acne and pimples are not caused by eating foods such as chocolate, peanuts, soft drinks, whole milk, and french fries, according to research evidence. They are, instead, the result of the rapid and large increase in hormone production during adolescence. The *sebaceous* (oil-producing) glands of the skin are controlled by hormones and become very active during adolescence, resulting in oily skin, blackheads, pimples, and, in a small percentage of teenagers, an actual case of acne vulgaris.. Anxiety, tension, and emotional stress may be contributing factors also.

A well-controlled study of the relationship between chocolate in teenage diets and acne showed that eating high amounts of chocolate (1,200 calories) did not materially affect the course of acne or the output or composition of *sebum*, the oily substance produced by sebaceous glands.[12] In addition, the researchers inferred that a diet rich in vegetable fat probably does not alter sebaceous secretion, since the chocolate consumed in the study was also high in vegetable fat.

Even though acne is not considered to be caused by diet, treatment often includes food restrictions and diets that are not based on reliable evidence. In some cases, specific foods are found to aggravate the condition in certain individuals, perhaps because of an allergy, and eliminating these foods may help. But an excessively restricted diet may result in the teenager feeling more self-conscious about the problem and even more isolated and "different" from his peers, as well as deprive him of important nutrients.

---

[12]J. E. Fulton, *et. al*, "Effects of Chocolate on Acne Vulgaris." *Journal of the American Medical Association*, Vol. 210, 1969, pp. 2071-74.

Teenagers tend to tune out parents and teachers who talk to them about nutrition and eating wisely. But often they are easily influenced by athletic coaches and trainers whose diet advice sometimes is unreliable, inaccurate, or even potentially harmful.

Athletes and their coaches are prone to putting their faith in unproven dietary myths as they seek ways to improve strength and endurance to help them win contests. Over the years athletes have been told that protein foods, especially meat, will make them strong; vitamin C will prevent injuries; wheat germ oil will improve running performance; and vitamin E will give greater endurance. Controlled studies have disproven these beliefs and show that a well-balanced, normal diet with increased calories is what athletes need.[13]

Water Is Essential

During exercise, what an athlete needs, above all else, is water. Water is the only means the body has for getting rid of excess body heat through evaporation of sweat. During exercise body heat production is greatly speeded up, and an athlete sweats away large amounts of water. A distance runner, for example, may lose 8 to 13 pounds of water.

If this water is not replaced, the athlete becomes dehydrated, and his body temperature will increase above normal. This condition could lead to heat stroke. On a long-term basis, kidney stones may result from repeated formation of concentrated urine. Thus, the practice of restricting water intake during athletic events is detrimental to an athlete's health as well as his performance. Scientific evidence strongly supports the practice of replacing water lost during exercise by frequent, intermittent fluid intake.[14]

Thirst is not a reliable guide to an athlete's need for fluid replacement, and water breaks should be scheduled regularly during exercise. The amount of water needed varies with the temperature and strenuous level of the exercise.

Plain water is preferable to concentrated sugar solutions, which slow the rate of gastric emptying. The American College of Sports Medicine recommends use of fluids with less than 2.5 grams of glucose, sucrose, or other substances per 100 milliliters water.[15] Most popular liq-

[13] M. H. Williams, "Nutritional Faddism and Athletics." *Nutrition and the M.D.*, Vol. 4, No. 2, December, 1977, pp. 1-2.

[14] Food and Nutrition Board, "Water Deprivation and Performance of Athletes," A Statement of the Food and Nutrition Board, National Research Council. Washington, D.C.: National Academy of Sciences, 1974.

[15] "Nutrition and the Athlete." *Nutrition and the M.D.*, Vol. 3, No. 6, April, 1977, p. 3.

uids used by athletes exceed this ratio: orange and grapefruit juice, cola drinks, and ginger ale have 10 grams sugar per 100 milliliters and should be diluted with three parts water; tomato juice and electrolyte (sodium and potassium, plus glucose) "sports drinks" have 4 to 5 grams sugar per 100 milliliters and should be diluted with equal parts of water (see Exhibit 16.10). Since the loss of electrolytes is not usually the cause of fatigue, the electrolyte type drinks have not been shown to be more effective or useful to athletes than water or diluted sugar solutions, and some authorities recommend that they not be used.

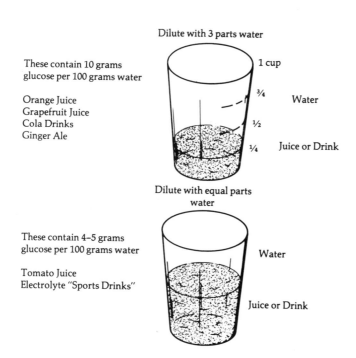

Exhibit 16.10. Most drinks used during active sports need to be diluted so they provide less than 2.5 grams of glucose per 100 grams of water.

Nutrient Needs of Athletes

Second to water, the athlete needs energy, and teenage athletes who are still growing need a great deal of energy. Energy requirements depend on the athlete's sex, age, and body size and on the type of sport and level of training (see Exhibit 16.11). For male athletes, energy needs can range anywhere from 3,000 to 4,000 calories to 5,000 or even 6,000 calories. Female athletes may need 3,000 to 4,000 calories.

A diet having 50 to 55 percent of calories from carbohydrates, 30 to 35 percent from fat, and 15 percent from protein is considered optimal (see Exhibit 16.12). During their growth spurt, teenage athletes may need a 20 percent protein diet. If an athlete's diet is adjusted in a balanced way to meet increased energy needs by adding more foods from all of the food groups, his additional requirements for nutrients will automatically be met. Vitamin supplements are not needed.

High-protein diets, which include large amounts of meat and/or protein supplements, have no advantage for the athlete. In fact, excess protein can be detrimental because it increases the athlete's water requirement for elimination of protein wastes and may add to the problem of dehydration during strenuous exercise. Loss of appetite and diarrhea also may result from excess protein use.

The athlete's balanced diet—even a balanced vegetarian diet— with the normal extra food intake for calories will supply sufficient protein for building muscle tissue and blood cells. Protein cannot make muscles strong; building strong muscles requires exercise, and exercise requires energy. Protein is not a primary fuel source for muscular exercise, and using protein for energy is costly and inefficient compared to using fats and carbohydrates.

Exhibit 16.11. Approximate Calories Expended Per Minute in Strenuous Sports

	CALORIES PER MINUTE OF ACTIVITY
Cycling	
5.5 mph	4.5
9.4 mph	7.0
13.1 mph	11.1
Football	8.9
Running	
Short distance	13.3–16.6
Cross-country	10.6
Tennis	7.1
Skating, fast	11.5
Skiing, moderate speed	10.8–15.9
Swimming	
Breast or backstroke	11.5
Crawl—55 yd/min	14.0
Wrestling	14.2

Exhibit 16.12.   Food Needs of Athletes

Plenty of water
More of all foods for extra calories
Iron-rich foods
Extra sodium and potassium
   Salt foods more liberally
   Some foods high in potassium

Iron-rich foods are important for teenage athletes, who already have a high iron requirement, because some iron is lost through sweating. Female athletes may become iron deficient during menstruation. Since training typically results in increases in hemoglobin, athletes also need more iron for building hemoglobin.

The electrolytic minerals sodium and potassium may be depleted during heavy exercise but usually can be replaced by more liberal salting of food and eating foods high in potassium, such as oranges and bananas. Use of salt tablets is not recommended by most authorities. The loss of sodium and potassium usually is not the cause of fatigue. However, cumulative potassium losses and excessive loss of body fluids may cause muscular weakness.

The Pregame Meal

In general, the pregame meal contributes little to the athlete's nutritional needs during the event, so foods eaten should be those well tolerated by the individual. The high-fat, high-protein meal—steak, for example—that once was thought to be needed before a game to add strength is now considered undesirable. Fat and protein are digested slowly and may interfere with respiration and place excessive stress on circulation if eaten within two hours of heavy exercise. Some protein foods form acids that may contribute to acidosis, which may, in turn, be a possible cause of fatigue.

Most authorities recommend that athletes eat a small, easily digested meal three or four hours before the event. A meal high in carbohydrates and low in protein and fat will be most easily digested and absorbed. A typical meal might include a sandwich, nonfat milk, banana, and cookies (see Exhibit 16.13).

Excited young athletes who are under emotional strain before a game may suffer from nausea, vomiting, or reduced gastrointestinal motility. The light, easily digested meal is desirable in this situation too. Some authorities have found that a pregame liquid meal having about 900 calories in 16 ounces of liquid is less likely to cause vomiting and gastrointestinal upset.[16]

Food and Fatigue

Different sports make different demands on the body's energy supply. Some sports of short duration, like sprinting, require a quick burst of energy; others require sustained, but not always continuous, energy for an hour or two; still others are prolonged, like marathon running or biking, and require endurance energy.

Fatigue or exhaustion correlates most closely with the athlete's inability to maintain normal blood sugar. During heavy exercise, the car-

[16]O. Mickelsen, "Nutrition and Athletics." *Food and Nutrition News,* Vol. 41, No. 7, April, 1970, pp. 1 and 4.

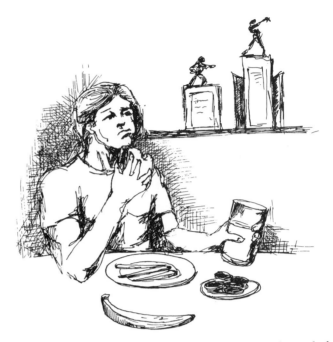

Exhibit 16.13.   A small, easily digested meal eaten 3-4 hours before an athletic event is recommended.

bohydrate (glycogen) stored in the liver and muscles is broken down to form glucose, or blood sugar. In endurance-type exercise, when the muscle glycogen is nearly depleted, the muscle fibers contract and an athlete is exhausted. In other sports, such as football, basketball, swimming, etc., muscle glycogen levels may be reduced over a time period during repeated days of heavy training. This happens when the athlete's energy requirements and rate of using muscle glycogen exceed his rate of carbohydrate intake. He becomes chronically fatigued, his performance level deteriorates, and he needs rest and a good diet in order to recuperate.

Using honey, sugar, glucose, or candy for "quick energy" before short- or moderate-term exercise appears to give little benefit and may actually have the opposite effect. Because these sugars stimulate insulin production, they can cause a reduction of blood sugar and reduce the time an athlete can exercise before becoming exhausted.[17]Also, the sugars tend to draw and hold water in the gastrointestinal tract and may cause cramps and discomfort.

During prolonged exercise, glucose replenishment during exercise can help keep the blood sugar level up and contribute to muscular energy. (Once the exercise has started, eating sugar does not increase insulin in the blood.) A fluid with no higher than 2.5 percent glucose or sugar is recommended.

[17]D. L. Costill, "Sports Nutrition: The Role of Carbohydrates." *Nutrition News*, Vol. 41, No. 1, February, 1978, pp. 1 and 4.

In recent years, a system for building glycogen stores in muscles with high-carbohydrate diets has become popular for athletes participating in endurance sports, especially marathon running. In this system, the athlete exercises the muscles one week in advance of the event to exhaust glycogen stores. Then he eats a modified diet of almost exclusively fat and protein for about three days to keep the glycogen content of exercising muscles low. A few days before the competition, fat and protein in the diet are reduced and replaced by large quantities of carbohydrates.

This dietary manipulation has been shown to double carbohydrate stores in muscles and improve endurance performance for some athletes.[18] But some risks are involved. Athletes may get diarrhea when they change from the low- to the high-carbohydrate diet. They also may get nausea and cramping. Water retention may cause sluggishness early in the event. More serious health risks involve disruption of heart function and the potential for muscle-fiber destruction. The effects over a competitor's lifetime are not known. Because of these risks, authorities advise caution in the use of this diet and recommend that it be used only for endurance events—the type of exercise where it is effective.[19] Use of this diet by teenagers is considered questionable by some authorities and they warn that it is not appropriate for very young athletes.

Weight Manipulation Diets for Athletes

In some sports, such as boxing, wrestling, and football, young athletes want to be placed in a particular weight class to have a competitive edge. As a result, they may manipulate their food and water intake unwisely and unhealthfully. Crash diets with drastic calorie reductions, induced vomiting, restriction of fluid intakes, and use of diuretics to qualify for a lower weight class can place serious stress on an athlete's cardiovascular system, result in dehydration, and cause kidney problems from reduced urine volume. Deaths of teenage athletes have been associated with dehydration abuses.[20]

On the other hand, weight-gaining abuses are also practiced in sports such as football. Use of high-fat diets to promote weight gains of 20 to 30 pounds can be harmful to the cardiovascular system and promote fat deposition rather than muscle building. Alternating crash dieting with gorging also is stressful to the body.

To sum up, athletes need the same nutrients and the same basic diets as other people, but they need more of all types of food in order to meet their increased energy needs and to supply the sodium, potassium, and iron lost in sweat. During exercise they need sufficient water to replace body fluids lost in sweat.

[18] P. Slovic, "What Helps the Long Distance Runner Run?" *Nutrition Today*, Vol. 10, No. 3, 1975, pp. 18-21.

[19] A. K. Kershnar, "Carbohydrate, Fat, and Protein Metabolism as Demanded by the Athlete." *Nutrition and the M.D.*, Vol. 2, No. 3, January, 1976, pp. 1-2.

[20] N. J. Smith, "Gaining and Losing Weight in Athletics." *Journal of the American Medical Association*, Vol. 236, July 12, 1976, p. 149.

There are no special foods or nutrients that have been scientifically proven to give athletes superior ability. However, the psychological aspect of foods should not be overlooked. In all athletic endeavors, a key factor in success is the athlete's mental set: his concentration and his confidence in his ability to win. When an athlete believes that a talisman, whether it is a certain nutrient, food, or something else, has the power to help him win, his performance may in truth improve when he uses it because of this faith. Thus, athletes and their coaches will probably continue to put their faith in the mystique of certain foods that give them "winning power" in spite of scientific evidence to the contrary.

Summary

Rapid growth and complex changes characterize adolescence. The age at which individuals enter and complete this stage varies widely, with girls generally about two years ahead of boys. Three phases have been identified: prepuberty, puberty, and postpuberty.

Requirements for all nutrients, particularly calcium and iron, increase during adolescence. Boys develop proportionately more lean tissue and have a particular need for protein and calories, reaching their maximum intake level at about age 16. The intake level for girls peaks around age 13.

Generalizations on the nutritional status of teenagers are hard to make because of variations in individual eating practices and scarcity of current research. Common problems include tooth decay, anemia, and obesity. Adolescent eating patterns often become adult practices. Teenagers commonly lead busy lives, skipping breakfast and depending on snacks—frequently those high in sugar and fat and low in other nutrients. They are subject to peer pressures and often are left to take charge of family meals or to fend for themselves if their mothers are employed.

Concern over appearance plays an important part in the life of the adolescent. Even though acne is not considered to be noticeably altered by diet, teenagers may restrict consumption of certain foods, hoping their skin will clear up. Teenage girls may go on fad diets or skip meals. Although obese teenagers usually do not eat excessive amounts, their level of activity is low, which often produces a vicious cycle. Boys are vulnerable to unreliable dietary advice regarding prowess in sports.

Nutrition for young athletes should be based upon a well-balanced diet, with additional calories to supply the extra energy needed for muscle development and sports activity. These calories should come primarily from extra servings of nutritious foods. Water is a critical requirement during exercise; if fruit juices or sweetened drinks are used, they should be diluted to prevent gastric problems. High-protein diets can be detrimental because of the water loss that results. Manipulating the diet for increased glycogen levels may improve endurance for some athletes, but risks are involved. Young athletes should avoid crash dieting to attain weight gain or loss for competitive purposes. The resulting body stress can be harmful or even fatal.

NUTRITION IN ADULTHOOD 17

Highlights

Nutritional needs during each phase of adult life

The aging process

Risks of energy imbalance, osteoporosis, and drug-induced malnutrition

Role of physical activity in aging

Aging is a normal part of the total life process. Adults age at different, individualized rates. So the phases of adulthood, like the phases of childhood, tend to blend together with no easy way to tell when one phase ends and another begins. Under one classification system, there are younger adults, ages 18 to 40 years; middle-aged adults, ages 40 to 60 years; and older adults, ages 60 to 80+ years.

Mature adults no longer need the extra nutrients for growth and development that they needed during childhood and adolescence. But good nutrition is vital to keep their bodies in good working order, supply energy, and enable them to resist disease and recuperate from illness.

NUTRITION OF YOUNG ADULTS

Young adults in their early twenties are much like postpuberty adolescents in their dietary habits and food needs. They may be involved in sports and recreation activities or be physically active in jobs and maintain relatively high calorie needs. Or they may settle into a more sedentary life-style as college students or clerical or other white collar workers and have much lower calorie needs. Some of their teenage eating habits, such as snacking and eating fast foods, may persist.

During this time a good diet is vitally important for young women of child-bearing age as preparation for pregnancy. But often young women are found to have a less than optimal diet. Many are likely to continue teenage habits such as meal-skipping and dieting to keep from gaining weight. If they use birth control pills, they may have increased needs for nutrients that are not being met through their diets. If they are young mothers, they may neglect their own diets while at the same time trying to see that their children eat well.

As a group, young adults often eat out and may encounter the same dietary pitfalls as teenagers (see Exhibit 17.1). According to a 1978 survey, persons who spend the most on meals away from home include young adults in the 25 to 34 age bracket and families without children. Families with more than one wage earner, a category into which many young couples fall, are also among those who eat out often.

Studies show that food intake begins to level off between the ages of 20 to 34 and that after reaching 35, both men and women eat less than they did before. Men drink only half as much milk as they did as teenagers. Women tend to eat less beef, pork, bread, and milk as they grow older.[1]

[1]"The Telltale Diet." *Farm Index*, Vol. 17, No. 9, September, 1978, pp. 8-9.

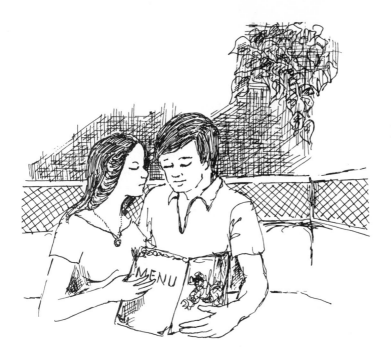

Exhibit 17.1.   Young adults tend to eat out more often and may frequently eat poorly balanced meals as a result.

NUTRITION OF MIDDLE-AGED ADULTS

Most middle-aged adults gradually slow down in their physical activity as their children grow up. Their jobs may become more sedentary, their housework less demanding, and their leisure time tends to be spent on activities such as reading, watching TV, handicrafts, and spectator sports rather than on vigorous physical activity.

Somewhere around their late fifties and early sixties, both men and women consume less than they did in their thirties and forties. One out of eight omits one meal or more a day, usually lunch. Because they tend to cook for fewer people after their children have left home, their diets are often poorer.

Nutrition-related ailments such as coronary heart disease, diabetes, and gallbladder and liver disorders may show up during these years, and some middle-aged adults may be at nutritional risk because of overuse of alcohol, drugs, and medication. Their interest in nutrition may be awakened through their concern for prevention or alleviation of health problems.

Older adults tend to worry about their health. They may be susceptible to the false hope offered by food faddists, pseudo-nutrition books, and people with products to sell who claim that a nutrient, food supplement, or "health food" will delay the degenerative effects of aging or prevent or cure illnesses such as cancer or arthritis.

While some older adults have a heightened concern about nutrition, others may lose interest in eating for a multitude of reasons. Surveys show that people over 65 as a group have poorer diets than younger people.[2] Their meals tend to be overloaded with carbohydrates—sugars and starches. Foods such as bread, crackers, doughnuts, breakfast cereals, sweet rolls, and cookies may make up the bulk of their diets because these foods are less expensive, require little preparation, keep without refrigeration, and are easy to chew. Diets of older adults often are found to be lacking in fruits and vegetables, milk and dairy products, and meats.

Why don't older people eat well? The causes may be social and psychological: singleness and loneliness, or apathy and lack of motivation (Exhibit 17.2). Older people often say: "It's no fun eating alone, . . . "It's too much bother to cook for just one" . . . "What difference does it make what I eat?" Older men who become widowers may eat poorly because they never learned to cook for themselves. Other older people may overeat as a way to alleviate their loneliness or boredom.

Lack of money is often a major reason why older people have poor diets. More than one-third of all Americans over 65 have incomes below the poverty level.[3] Many have fixed incomes that have not kept up with the rising cost of food, housing, and other necessities. An older adult may live in a room without cooking facilities and refrigeration and be forced to exist on foods that require no cooking. Many older people have no transportation to get to a food store or may be physically unable to walk to a store and carry groceries home.

Physical disabilities may affect an older person's ability to prepare food or to eat it, for example, the crippling effects of arthritis or a stroke, or lack of teeth or poorly fitting dentures, that make chewing slow and difficult. Also, older adults who get little exercise may not have very good appetites.

Lack of interest in eating and poor appetites often disappear when an older person can eat in a setting where good food is provided and

[2]P. O'Hanlon and M. B. Kohrs, "Dietary Studies of Older Americans." *American Journal of Clinical Nutrition*, Vol. 31, 1978, p. 1257.

[3]A. E. Gallo, L. E. Salathe, and W. T. Boehm, "Senior Citizens: Food Expenditure Patterns and Assistance." Agricultural Economic Report No. 426, U.S. Department of Agriculture. Washington D.C., 1979, pp. 1-3.

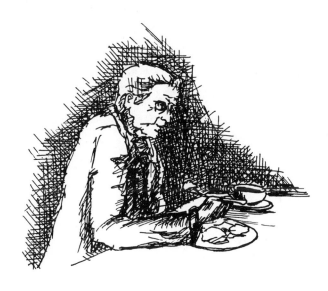

Exhibit 17.2. Some reasons older people don't eat well include poverty, loneliness, and physical disability.

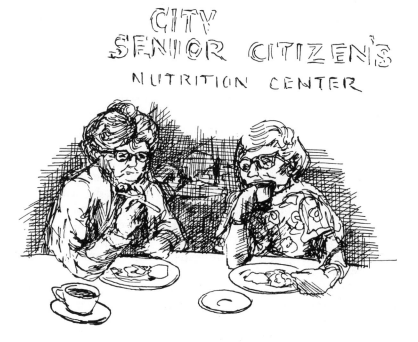

Exhibit 17.3. Older people get greater enjoyment from eating—and better nutrition—when they eat with others in a neighborhood nutrition center.

eating is a social experience, for example, in neighborhood nutrition centers funded under the Older American's Act (see Exhibit 17.3). For persons who are ill or handicapped and unable to cook for themselves, subsidized and volunteer "Meals on Wheels" programs in which hot meals are delivered are beneficial and would make a greater contribution toward improving the diet of older people if provided on a large scale nationwide. Unfortunately, to date these feeding programs do not begin to meet the nutritional needs of the nation's older people.

FOOD AND THE AGING PROCESS

The aging process adversely affects our ability to get nutrients from food, and, at the same time, the foods we eat affect how we age. Scientists do not completely understand the aging process—what causes it, exactly what changes take place, and the part that nutrients play.

Physiological Changes in Aging

Aging involves progressive changes in organs such as heart, lungs, kidney, and liver that lead to diminished effectiveness of their functioning as well as to the development of disease. These changes affect nutrition. They may interfere with nutrient intake; cause lessened ability to absorb, store, and use nutrients; or cause an increase in excretion and in the need for specific nutrients.

Food intake may be impaired as a result of crippling diseases such as arthritis or stroke, because of poorly functioning teeth, or because of reduced saliva flow and loss of sense of taste and smell, which may reduce appetite. Older people also may suffer from drug-induced malnutrition, as discussed in Chapter 20.

Digestion and absorption may be reduced in many ways. For example, starch digestion is impeded by reduced saliva production; iron absorption is decreased by a reduced production of hydrochloric acid in the stomach; impaired gallbladder functioning and reduced supplies of bile can diminish the body's ability to digest and absorb fat, protein, and fat-soluble vitamins; and many older people develop lactase deficiency and as a result suffer discomfort when they drink milk.

Aging is a complex biological process in which there is progressively less ability to repair body cells and in which more cells are destroyed than produced. Various theories have been advanced to explain this phenomenon. According to one theory, there are increased oxidation reactions in the body cells, especially if antioxidants are lacking. Under another theory, impairment of protein synthesis is thought to cause cells to die. And another theory holds that immunological processes progressively break down so that the elderly are more susceptible to infections.

The average adult has been found to lose active muscle tissue at the rate of about 3 percent every 10 years. If the individual maintains a constant weight, this means he is gradually getting fatter as fat tissue replaces muscle tissue. Inactivity is an important factor contributing to this loss of muscle tissue.

Inactivity also is a factor in an energy imbalance, where more calories are taken in than are used up, which leads to the commonly observed gain in weight as people get older. Another cause of the weight gain is the gradual slowing of the basal metabolic rate with age (see Chapter 4.).

Inactivity has other adverse effects on nutritional status. For example, it can promote depletion of calcium from bones and gradual bone loss. This, plus changes in the endocrine system and diets lacking in calcium, and possibly protein, are thought to be the causes of the high incidence of *osteoporosis*, a loss in bone density, in people over 65. This condition is six times more common in women than in men, and often leads to disabling bone fractures.

Nutritional Needs and Aging

Very little scientific evidence has been gathered about the specific nutritional needs of different ages of adults. Needs of older adults have been extrapolated from those of younger people. As you can see from Exihibit 17.4, Recommended Dietary Allowances for Adults, the nutrient recommendations do not change much during maturity.

Calorie requirements gradually decrease with age because of the decline in the basal metabolic rate and the lower level of activity. Since the need for B vitamins is in proportion to calorie needs, the requirement for these vitamins also is thought to decline with age, although some current evidence tends to contradict this belief.[4]

For older adults, the protein requirement has not been satisfactorily determined. Since the body protein mass is proportionately smaller in older persons, some authorities recommend a lower protein intake to reduce the need to excrete protein wastes and avoid overburdening the kidneys, which work less efficiently with age. Other authorities argue that the elderly need more protein in order to allow for a greater safety margin and to counteract the decreased absorption of protein and protein lossess due to illness.[5]

After menopause, a woman's need for iron is reduced and the recommendation for older women of 10 milligrams is the same as that for mature men. Iron deficiency anemia is often seen in the elderly and is believed to be the result of diets low in iron, poor absorption because of reduction of acid in the stomach, poor utilization of iron by the body,

[4]"Nutrition of the Elderly." *Dairy Council Digest*, Vol. 48, No. 1, January-February, 1977, p. 4.

[5]M. Winick, "Nutrition and Aging." *Contemporary Nutrition*, Vol. 2, No. 5, June, 1977.

Exhibit 17.4 Recommended Daily Dietary Allowances for Adults

NUTRIENT	UNIT	ALLOWANCE, MEN			ALLOWANCE, WOMEN		
		AGE			AGE		
		19–22	23–50	51+	19–22	23–50	51+
Food energy		2900	2700	2400[5]	2100	2000	1800[6]
Protein	g	56	56	56	44	44	44
Fat-soluble vitamins							
Vitamin A	μg RE[1]	1000	1000	1000	800	800	800
Vitamin E	mg & TE[2]	10	10	10	8	8	8
Vitamin D	μg[3]	7.5	5	5	7.5	5	5
Water-soluble vitamins							
Ascorbic acid	mg	60	60	60	60	60	60
Folacin		400	400	400	400	400	400
Niacin	mg equi NE[4]	19	18	16	14	13	13
Riboflavin	mg	1.7	1.6	1.4	1.3	1.2	1.2
Thiamin	mg	1.5	1.4	1.2	1.1	1.0	1.0
Vitamin B_6	mg	2.0	2.0	2.0	2.0	2.0	2.0
Vitamin B_{12}	μg	3.0	3.0	3.0	3.0	3.0	3.0
Minerals							
Calcium	mg	800	800	800	800	800	800
Phosphorus	mg	800	800	800	800	800	800
Iodine	μg	150	150	150	150	150	150
Iron	mg	10	10	10	18	18	10
Magnesium	mg	350	350	350	300	300	300
Zinc	mg	15	15	15	15	15	15

Source: *Recommended Dietary Allowances*, Ninth Edition (revised 1979). National Academy of Sciences, Washington, D.C.

[1] Retinol equivalents. 1 retinol equivalent = 1 μg retinol or 6 μg β-carotene.*

[2] α tocopherol equivalents. 1 mg d-α-tocopherol = 1 TE**

[3] As cholecalciferol. 10 μg cholecalciferol*** = 400 IU vitamin D.

[4] 1 NE (niacin equivalent) is equal to 1 μg of niacin or 60 μg of dietary tryptophan.

[5] 2050 for men 76+ years of age.

[6] 1600 for women 76+ years of age.

* = Beta carotene
** = Alpha-tocopherol
*** = Cholecalciferol

and chronic blood loss in some older people. Anemias caused by lack of folic acid or vitamin B_{12} (pernicious anemia) are also seen in older adults.

While the current RDA do not call for increased calcium for the elderly, some authorities believe that the requirement should go up due to decreased absorption with age.[6] Also, some authorities now believe

[6]"Nutrition of the Elderly." *Dairy Council Digest*, Vol. 48, No. 1, January-February, 1977, p. 3.

that a high-calcium diet may help to restore bone mass and prevent osteoporosis. Since older people often drink little milk (perhaps because of lactase deficiency), the main source of calcium, this nutrient is frequently found to be lacking in their diets.

In persons over age 65, 75 percent of the deaths are from coronary heart disease, often the result of slowly progressive *atherosclerosis*, the build up of fatty deposits in arteries (see Chapter 19). Because elderly people tend to have difficulty digesting and absorbing fat, the fat content of their diets should be reduced. Fatty foods such as gravies, pastries, cakes, cookies, and fried foods should be avoided both from the standpoint of their high fat content and the large number of calories they contain.

Vitamin deficiencies are seen in older people who do not eat enough fruits and vegetables and also in those who do not get enough fat or protein foods in their diets, who overuse laxatives, or who have impaired secretions of bile and impaired absorption. Thus an older person may lack vitamins A and C and at the same time have increased needs for these vitamins as well as for B vitamins, particularly folic acid, B_6, and B_{12} (see Exhibit 17.5).[7] Since more vitamin C is known to be needed in stressful situations, and aging can be considered stressful, the question of whether older people need extra vitamin C is being explored.

A low-fiber diet, attributable to consumption of insufficient amounts of fruits, vegetables, and whole grain cereals, can contribute to the constipation problem that plagues many older people who have reduced intestinal motility.

As the calorie needs and the amount of food consumed by an adult go down with age, the challenge of getting enough of the essential nutrients becomes greater. Thus, the older the person is, the less he can

Exhibit 17.5   Summary of Special Food Needs of Older Adults

May need more
  Protein
  Iron
  Calcium
  Vitamins: especially A and C and Folic Acid
  Fiber

May need less
  Fat
  Sugar
  Sodium
  Caloric intake

---

[7]M. Winick, "Nutrition and Aging." *Contemporary Nutrition*, Vol. 2, No. 6, June, 1977.

afford of the low-nutrient-density, high-calorie foods. A person with a small food budget can't afford them from standpoint of cost either. Thus, in order to adjust his diet to his decreasing need for energy, an older person needs to eat more of the foods that provide the maximum number of nutrients for the minimum number of calories.

Older people are at risk of developing drug-induced malnutrition, which is discussed in Chapter 20. When they receive continuing and extensive drug therapy, their nutritional status needs to be monitored to prevent this type of malnutrition.

Some older people may need food supplements. Studies show that many older people use self-prescribed supplements but that often they take nutrients they don't need, and don't get the ones they do need, such as folic acid, B_6, B_{12}, iron, and calcium. Or they may take excessively large doses in the belief that they may be able to prevent or cure some ailment. At best, overuse of supplements is a waste of money, at worst it is hazardous from the standpoint of overdosing or postponement of needed medical care.

Can Food Keep Us Young?

Man's search for the "fountain of youth" has included the hope of finding a diet or food that could prevent aging. This idea is not unreasonable since the food we eat provides the raw materials out of which our body cells are made. But so far, no such magic potion has been found. We know of no way to prevent aging through diet.

From time to time, in some remote area of the world, a group of people is found that has an unusually long life span. In the hope of finding the secret of their long life, scientists study their diets and their life-styles. Subsequently, a new dietary "discovery" for extending life, such as eating yogurt or vegetarianism, may be publicized. However, when these different groups of long-lived people are looked at as a whole, we find that they are not all alike in diet, but they are alike in being physically active. All work hard, trying to eke out a living from farming, and all are in very good physical condition. Rarely are they obese. Researchers believe that it is the physical activity and the absence of obesity that is probably the secret of their long life, and not any special food or diet.[8]

However, some characteristics of senility, thought to be due to old age, may instead be caused or intensified by nutritional failure. A good diet may be helpful in improving the mental outlook, if not the mental functioning, of an elderly person suffering from symptoms of senility.

[8]A. Leaf, "Observations of a Peripatetic Gerontologist." *Nutrition Today*, Vol. 1., No. 5, September-October, 1973, pp. 4-12.

Gerontologists, scientists who study the aging process, have evolved various theories about ways to prevent the development of senility. Those who believe that aging results from oxidative changes in the cells theorize that these changes could be modified through the use of vitamin E and other antioxidants.[9] Although this theory, developed in rat studies, has not been proven in humans, it led to the idea that vitamin E was the long-sought youth potion. But alas, taking vitamin E has not helped people prolong their youth.

Another theory holds that calorie restriction early in life, which results in delayed growth and a slower rate of maturity, can result in a longer age span. This idea also is based on animal studies and lacks adequate proof in humans.[10] But the belief that lifelong restriction of calories, so a person is never fat but always is on the slim side, will result in a longer and healthier life is supported by statistics that show a relationship between obesity and death due to heart disease, cancer, and other diseases.

From what scientists have learned so far, it seems that longevity has many causes: genetic, nutritional, exertional, environmental, and psychological, among others. The hope of finding the answer to long life, simply by changing our diet, does not appear to be realistic.

Summary

Young adults may retain eating patterns they developed as teenagers. They tend to eat out more often than other age groups, with consequent nutritional pitfalls. They also tend to reduce their consumption of certain foods such as milk. Middle-aged adults must deal with reduced energy needs and may be at nutritional risk due to overuse of alcohol, drugs, and medications. Older adults, understandably concerned about health, are vulnerable to claims by food faddists. Loneliness, economics, and physical disabilities may be key factors adversely affecting their nutritional status.

The aging process reduces one's ability to obtain nutrients from foods; at the same time, the foods eaten may affect aging. This process leads to a reduced ability to maintain body cells and gradual loss of active muscle tissue. Inactivity is a factor in tissue loss, energy imbalance, and bone loss, and there is a high incidence of *osteoporosis* among older adults, especially women.

Calorie requirements gradually decrease with age due to a decline in the basal metabolic rate and decreased physical activity. After meno-

[9] The Institute of Food Technologists Expert Panel on Food Safety and Nutrition and the Committee on Public Information, *Vitamin E.* Chicago, IL: Institute of Food Technologists, 1977.

[10] M. H. Ross in *Nutrition and Aging.* M. Winick (ed). New York: John Wiley & Sons, 1976, pp. 43-57.

pause, women's iron needs decrease. Calcium is the nutrient most frequently found to be lacking in diets of older adults. Due to the incidence of atherosclerosis and difficulty with fat digestion, the fat content in diets of older adults should be reduced. A low-fiber diet may cause reduced intestinal motility and the use of laxatives can lead to vitamin deficiencies. The older adult needs to choose foods that provide the maximum number of nutrients for the minimum number of calories. Although good nutrition is imperative to quality of life, it cannot prevent aging. Physical activity and prevention of obesity are other key factors in maintaining optimal health.

Part V

CONTEMPORARY ISSUES IN DIET AND HEALTH

DIETARY GOALS FOR THE UNITED STATES 18

Highlights

Background and development of current U.S.
dietary guidelines

Specific dietary recommendations

Suggested changes in food selection and preparation

Controversy over current U.S. dietary guidelines

Preventive nutrition—finding ways to eat to avoid or postpone killer diseases, particularly coronary heart disease, stroke, cancer, and diabetes—has become a challenge of growing interest to both health professionals and consumers during the last several decades.

DIETARY GOALS FOR THE UNITED STATES

The U.S. Congress also became involved in preventive nutrition as a result of hearings conducted by the Senate Select Committee on Nutrition and Human Needs. A report, *Dietary Goals for the United States,* was published by this committee in 1977 and revised in a second edition published in 1978.[1]

The committee members developed these goals, which were meant to serve as guidelines for people to use in making prudent, disease-preventing decisions about their diet, as a result of hearing volumes of testimony from a wide spectrum of the nation's food, nutrition, and health experts. The committee members concluded that changes in the American eating pattern of the past 75 years are of critical concern in terms of public health.

The goals include specific recommendations about changes that committee members thought Americans should make in their food consumption patterns.

Goal 1. To avoid overweight, consume only as much energy (calories) as is expended; if overweight, decrease energy intake and increase expenditure.

Goal 2. (a). Increase the consumption of complex carbohydrates and "naturally occurring" sugars (as opposed to added sugars) from about 28 percent to about 48 percent of energy intake; (b). Reduce the consumption of refined and processed sugars by about 45 percent to account for about 10 percent of total energy intake.

Goal 3. Reduce overall fat consumption from approximately 40 percent to about 30 percent of energy intake.

Goal 4. Reduce saturated fat consumption to account for about 10 percent of total energy intake, and balance that with polyunsaturated and monounsaturated fats, each of which should account for about 10 percent of energy intake.

Goal 5. Reduce cholesterol consumption to about 300 milligrams per day.

[1]Select Committee on Nutrition and Human Needs, United States Senate, 95th Congress, 1st Session: February, 1977, "Dietary Goals for the United States, Committee Report, 1977"; "Dietary Goals for the United States, second edition," Committee Report, 1978. Washington, D.C., 1977, 1978.

Goal 6. Limit intake of sodium by reducing the intake of table salt to about 5 grams per day.

The goals suggest the following changes in food selection and preparation:

1. Increase consumption of fruits and vegetables and whole grains.

2. Decrease consumption of refined and other processed sugars and foods high in such sugars.

3. Decrease consumption of foods high in total fat, and partially replace saturated fats, whether obtained from animals or vegetable sources, with polyunsaturated fats.

4. Decrease consumption of animal fat, and choose meats, poultry, and fish, which will reduce saturated fat intake.

5. Except for young children, substitute low-fat milk for whole milk and low-fat dairy products for high-fat dairy products.

6. Decrease consumption of butterfat, eggs, and other high cholesterol sources. Some consideration should be given to easing the cholesterol goal for premenopausal women, young children, and the elderly to obtain the nutritional benefits of eggs in the diet.

7. Decrease consumption of salt and foods high in salt content.

CONTROVERSY OVER DIETARY GOALS

After they were published, these goals became a highly controversial issue among the nation's health and nutrition professionals. Some of them believed the goals provided needed guidelines for the American public and would help to improve health and prevent disease. But other scientists disagreed, pointing to the inadequate scientific evidence showing that the dietary changes suggested could prevent diseases such as heart disease and cancer. Critics also stated that in many respects the goals were not based on contemporary scientific knowledge and if implemented by all Americans would not be in the public interest.[2]

A common criticism was that the goals were an attempt to provide guidelines for the prevention and cure of diseases considered to be public health hazards for certain groups of people, rather than recommendations for meeting the nutritional needs of all the population.[3] Other professionals, while not in disagreement with the intent of the goals,

[2]"U.S. Dietary Goals: For—Michael C. Latham, Lani S. Stephenson; Against—Alfred E. Harper." *Journal of Nutrition Education,* Vol. 9, No. 4, October-December, 1977, pp. 152-57.

[3]Council for Agricultural Science and Technology, "Dietary Goals for the United States: A Commentary," Report No. 71, November, 1977.

felt that they were unrealistic because they called for such drastic changes in the American diet. Exhibit 18.1 shows the differences in calorie sources between our current diet and that recommended by the guidelines.

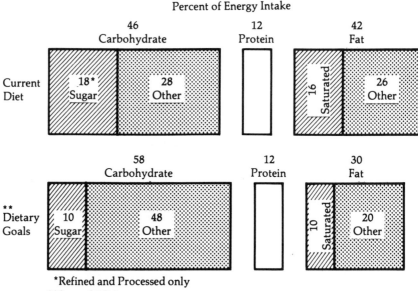

*Refined and Processed only
**Second Edition

Exhibit 18.1.   Distribution of energy from dietary substances in current diet and in the Dietary Goals, second edition. (*Source:* U.S. Department of Agriculture, *Family Economics Review.* Washington, D.C., Fall, 1978, p. 32.)

Summary

The report "Dietary Goals for the United States" was developed to provide guidelines for dietary decisions. Based upon testimony from food, nutrition, and health experts, it nevertheless has engendered criticism and controversy. Most health professionals agree that Americans are overweight; that their diets are too high in calories, sugar, fat, alcohol, and salt; and that dietary changes to reduce consumption of these products and increase consumption of fruits, vegetables, and whole-grain cereals would be healthful. But many do not agree that these changes will reduce the death rate resulting from major diseases.

DIET AND DISEASE 19

Highlights

Relationship between diet and heart disease

Significance of cholesterol, high- and low-density lipoproteins, and triglycerides in the blood

Research studies on cholesterol metabolism

Arguments for and against the Prudent Diet guidelines

Hypertension and its treatment

Diabetes—insulin deficient and insulin inefficient modes—and treatment

Hypoglycemia as a measure of low blood sugar

Food reactive and fasting reactive forms of hypoglycemia and diet alterations

Role of diet in cancer occurrence and treatment

Dietary quackery associated with rheumatic diseases

The relationship between diet and heart disease is the most widely debated diet-disease issue among professionals. It appears to be no closer to resolution today than it was 30 years ago, in spite of a great deal of research that has been done in the interim.

Coronary heart disease is the nation's number one cause of death and is an especially great health hazard to middle-aged men. Between the ages of 40 and 65, a man has a 25 percent chance of having some form of coronary heart disease. One-fourth of the people who have a heart attack die immediately, and of those who survive, one-third will die within a year.

Atherosclerosis

Atherosclerosis is a kind of hardening of the arteries in which fatty deposits, called plaques, build up in the arteries; it is believed to be a major factor in the development of coronary heart disease. These fatty deposits, which contain 70 percent cholesterol, clog the arteries and impede the flow of blood (see Exhibit 19.1). This causes the heart to work harder and may cause a rise in blood pressure. A blood clot, called a *thrombos*, then may get stuck in the clogged artery and close off the blood supply to the heart. This is called *coronary thrombosis* or a *coronary occlusion*. The heart muscle is damaged (called a *myocardial infarction*) when it doesn't get blood, and the person is said to have had a heart attack. Recent evidence has shown that many "heart attacks" may be due to spasm of the already clogged arteries rather than a clot as such.

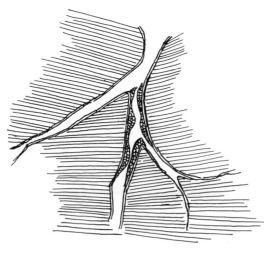

Exhibit 19.1.   In atherosclerosis, fatty deposits, called *plaques*, build up in the arteries and block or impede the flow of blood.

391
Coronary
Heart
Disease
and
Hypertension

If the heart muscle is so seriously damaged that the heart cannot function, the person will die. If the damage is less severe, a person may recover because the heart can keep functioning while the damaged muscle heals.

A key question, which researchers have tried to answer, is what causes the buildup of fatty deposits in arteries? Among a number of possible causes, the one that is now widely accepted as a prime cause is the amount of cholesterol and other fatty substances in the blood. When blood levels of cholesterol are high, the rate of atherosclerosis and heart disease also is high, as shown by the following observations:

1. Diseases associated with high blood cholesterol levels—the scientific term is *hypercholesterolemia,* i.e., hyper (high), cholesterol, emia (blood)—such as diabetes and hypothyroidism are also associated with atherosclerosis.

2. Persons with inborn errors of cholesterol metabolism develop extremely precocious atherosclerosis.

3. In countries where the population has high average blood cholesterol levels, the coronary heart disease rates also are high; and in countries where blood cholesterol levels are low, the death rate from coronary heart disease is low.[1]

4. In laboratory studies, when high levels of blood cholesterol or other fats are induced in mammals, especially primates, atherosclerotic deposits are produced. These deposits can be reduced by lowering blood cholesterol.[2]

5. A 20-year study of 5,000 people in Framingham, Massachusetts, showed that people with blood cholesterol levels of 260 (milligrams of cholesterol per 100 milliliters of blood) were three times more likely to have a coronary episode than those with cholesterol levels below 200. The higher the cholesterol level, the greater the risk of a coronary episode. But the high blood cholesterol level was a stronger predictor of coronary heart disease in younger people than in older people.[3]

All of these observations involve statistical correlations between blood cholesterol levels, atherosclerosis, and coronary heart disease, but they do not prove cause and effect. In other words, a high blood cholesterol level may be present but may not be the cause of the atherosclerosis. However, some recent discoveries on the metabolism of cholesterol promise to strengthen the causal relationship theory.[4]

[1]H.C. McGill, and G.E. Mott, "Diet and Coronary Heart Disease," in Nutrition Reviews' *Present Knowledge in Nutrition,* fourth edition. New York, Washington, D.C.: The Nutrition Foundation, Inc., 1976, pp. 376-91.

[2]*Ibid.*

[3]*Ibid.*

[4]*Ibid.*

Fatty Substances in the Blood

As we learned in Chapter 8, cholesterol is just one of several fatty substances that circulate in the blood. Others are triglycerides, phospholipids, and free fatty acids. Because they are not soluble in water, all fats are attached to proteins in large molecules called lipoproteins. The amount of these substances can be measured, and when their level is too high, the condition is called either *hyperlipoproteinemia*—hyper (high), lipo (fat), protein (protein), emia (blood)—or *hyperlipidemia.*

The differences between high density lipoproteins (HDL), low density lipoproteins (LDL), and very low density lipoproteins (VLDL) are described in Chapter 8. The ratio of HDL and LDL that a person has in his blood appears to have an effect on atherosclerosis and susceptibility to coronary heart disease. The cholesterol carried by HDL seems to be less harmful than the LDL cholesterol. HDL may even have a protective effect against coronary heart disease, while susceptibility to heart disease seems to be linked to high levels of LDL.[5]

For example, in the Framingham study, people with high levels of HDL were relatively free of heart disease, while those with high LDL were more likely to have heart disease.[6] Women, who have less atherosclerosis than men, also have a higher ratio of HDL to LDL than men. So do Greenland Eskimos and Swedish skiers. Diabetics and obese people have low ratios of HDL to LDL and more atherosclerosis. Rats, members of a species that is very resistant to the development of atherosclerosis, have higher ratios of HDL to LDL than humans.

Although it is still not clear whether high HDL levels prevent the onset of atherosclerosis in humans or animals, researchers are intensely interested in knowing why people with high levels of HDL are resistant to the disease and what alters the levels of lipoproteins in the blood. They also are trying to find out why the levels of HDL are high when the levels of LDL are low, and vice versa.

Diet and Blood Cholesterol and Triglycerides

The great unanswered question around which the diet-heart disease controversy revolves is, What part does diet play in the formation of cholesterol and triglycerides and in the ratio of HDL to LDL in the blood?

Researchers have found that people have at least five different types of hyperlipidemia.[7] The two most common forms both show in-

---

[5] J. Weininger, and G.M. Briggs, "Nutrition Update, 1977—Coronary Heart Disease." *Journal of Nutrition Education,* Vol. 9, No. 4, October-December, 1977, p. 173.

[6] M. Bureau, L. Finkler, L. Ryan, "Hyperlipoproteinemia and Heart Disease." *Notes on Nutrition,* Vol. 3, No. 5, May, 1978, p. 8.

[7] D.H. Blakenhorn, "Diagnosis and Dietary Management of Patients with Elevated Blood Lipids." *Nutrition and the M.D.,* Vol. 1, No. 1, November, 1974, p. 1.

creased levels of VLDL and LDL: one has elevated cholesterol levels and normal triglyceride levels, and the other has elevated triglycerides and normal cholesterol levels. The hyperlipidemia with elevated cholesterol levels can be found after excess intake of cholesterol and saturated fats and responds to a diet that is low in cholesterol and saturated fats and high in polyunsaturated fats. Thus it is theorized that polyunsaturated fats have the ability to reduce blood cholesterol levels in this type of hyperlipidemia, while saturated fats and cholesterol will raise them.

393
Coronary
Heart
Disease
and
Hypertension

In the person who has high blood-triglyceride levels, the situation is worsened by obesity, stress, alcohol, high-carbohydrate and high-calorie diets. What's needed here is a weight control diet with reduction of carbohydrate and calories, including fat calories, rather than the low-cholesterol, high polyunsaturated-fat diet.

In several other rare forms of hyperlipidemia, heredity may be involved, the person may not be at risk of developing coronary heart disease, and dietary changes may or may not be useful.

Thus, it is believed that recommendations for dietary changes for people with high levels of cholesterol and triglycerides should not be made without first testing their blood to determine which problem they have. The fact that there are large individual variations between normal people in levels of cholesterol in the blood also needs to be considered.

Some researchers believe that other dietary factors may be more important than cholesterol and saturated fats as causes of high blood fats and should be investigated more thoroughly. These include: not enough fiber; too high a ratio of sucrose to starch; lack of trace elements such as selenium, chromium, zinc, and copper; excess cadmium; improper ratio of zinc to copper; not enough vitamin C; and the use of soft water instead of hard water.[8] Some scientific evidence has developed to support each of these theories, but not enough to prove cause and effect.

Diets to Prevent Heart Disease

Even more controversial than the dietary recommendations for treatment of heart disease are the recommendations made for preventing it through dietary changes. Cholesterol control has been the focus of attention because of the correlation seen between high blood cholesterol levels and coronary heart disease and the fact that cholesterol is the principal component of artery-clogging plaques.

Dietary recommendations for cholesterol control include:

1. Adjust calories to achieve ideal weight.

2. Reduce total fat to 35 percent and increase polyunsaturated fat to 10 percent of total calories.

[8]H.A. Schroeder, "The Role of Trace Elements in Cardiovascular Diseases," in *The Nutrition Crisis*, T.P. Labuza, editor. St. Paul, MN: West Publishing Co., 1975, pp. 374-92.

3. Reduce cholesterol intake to 300 milligrams per day.

4. Avoid excess sugars.

5. Avoid excess salt.

These recommendations have been translated into a dietary pattern called the Prudent Diet and are the basis for many of the Dietary Goals set forth by the Senate Select Committee on Nutrition and Human Needs. In this diet, consumption of saturated fat-containing meats—beef, pork, lamb—is reduced to four, 4- to 6-ounce servings per week, and fish and chicken are recommended as substitutes since their ratio of polyunsaturated to saturated fats is higher. Butterfat, which is high in saturated fat and cholesterol, is drastically reduced through substitution of soft margarine for butter, cottage cheese for whole milk cheese, non-fat milk for whole milk, ice milk for ice cream (and only in small amounts). Consumption of cholesterol-containing foods such as egg yolks, organ meats (liver, heart), and certain shellfish is stringently limited, for example, to just three egg yolks per week, including eggs used in mixed dishes (see Exhibit 19.2). Polyunsaturated vegetable oils, such as safflower, soy, and corn and soft margarines made from them are recommended in place of hydrogenated vegetable shortenings and margarines.

The Prudent Diet originated in New York in 1957 as part of the Diet and Coronary Disease Study project conducted by the New York City Health Department, Bureau of Nutrition. It was attempted by a group of business and professional men, with no prior history of heart disease, who dubbed themselves the Anti-Coronary Club. The group was compared with controls of similar background who continued to eat their usual diet. At the end of seven years, those remaining in the study group had significantly reduced some risk factors of heart disease—blood cholesterol levels, obesity, and high blood pressure. However, this was not considered to be a well-controlled, scientific study.[9]

Exhibit 19.2   The Prudent Diet

Decrease Use Of	Increase Use Of
Red meats: beef, pork, lamb	Fish—except certain shellfish
Organ meats: liver, heart, etc.	Poultry
Eggs—especially yolks	Polyunsaturated margarine and oil
Shellfish: shrimp, lobster	Nonfat milk
Butter and hardened margarine	Cottage cheese
Whole milk	
Whole milk cheese	
Ice cream	

Evidence from the National Heart and Diet Study of 2,035 men between the ages of 45 and 54, who consumed a diet similar to the Prudent Diet, showed that a change in diet can reduce the risk factors of heart disease, especially by lowering blood cholesterol levels. Men who ate less cholesterol and total fat and used more polyunsaturated fat in place of saturated fat reduced their blood cholesterol levels by an average of 11 percent.[10]

395
Coronary
Heart
Disease
and
Hypertension

However, no studies to date have demonstrated that changes in diet that reduce risk factors, especially blood cholesterol levels, will significantly reduce the incidence of coronary heart disease. Proponents of dietary changes suggest that middle age may be too late to begin and that the changes may need to be made much earlier, in adolescence, childhood, or even in infancy, to be effective. This group recommends that young children at high risk of developing coronary heart disease because of heredity, high blood cholesterol, or high blood pressure should follow the Prudent Diet.

Studies do show that high blood cholesterol in adolescence can be reduced by diet.[11] But no studies have been conducted that show that this change will result in the reduction of heart disease in later life. Such studies would take a long time to complete, are costly, and are difficult to control.

The current stance of many health professionals is: any modification of diet that reduces blood cholesterol, body weight, or blood pressure probably will reduce the risk of coronary heart disease and is likely to do no harm. Furthermore, the earlier it is adopted, the more likely it is to be beneficial.

However, a core of nutrition and health scientists strongly disagrees with the mass prescription of the diet, most particularly the strict limitation on cholesterol-containing food and the change to large amounts of polyunsaturated fats. They argue that the majority of cholesterol in the body does not come from foods high in cholesterol, but instead from cholesterol made by the liver; that it has not been proven that cholesterol in the diet has a causal relationship with heart disease; and that limiting cholesterol will not necessarily reduce blood cholesterol levels and prevent heart disease.[12] Several studies, for example, have shown no rela-

[9]H.D. Hurt, "Heart Disease—Is Diet a Factor?" in *The Nutrition Crisis*, T.P. Labuza, editor. St. Paul, MN: West Publishing Co., 1975, p. 329.

[10]H.C. McGill and G.E. Mott, "Diet and Coronary Heart Disease," in Nutrition Reviews' *Present Knowledge in Nutrition*, fourth edition. New York, Washington, D.C.: The Nutrition Foundation, Inc., 1976, pp. 384-85.

[11]*Ibid.*, p. 387.

[12]D. Kritchevesky, "The Meaning of Serum Cholesterol." *Nutrition and the M.D.*, Vol. 2, No. 2, December, 1975, p. 1. And R. Reiser, "Normal vs. Pathological Variations in Serum Cholesterol Levels," same publication, p. 2.

tionship between egg consumption and blood cholesterol levels in men.[13]

The mechanism whereby polyunsaturated fats lower blood cholesterol and other fats has not been definitely established, nor is it clear what the relative importance of polyunsaturated fats is. Another unanswered question pertains to the safety of using large amounts of polyunsaturated fats. One study suggested they may contribute to the risk of cancer.

Those who oppose the dietary changes by the general population believe that not enough is known about the potential ill effects if they were adopted by everyone, including children. They recommend that dietary modifications be made on an individual basis only after serum-screening tests are made to determine what specific changes a person needs.[14]

During the past ten years, heart disease mortality has declined 20 percent in the United States. Both sides of the diet-heart disease controversy claim this as evidence bolstering their point of view. Those who believe that dietary changes can prevent heart disease point to changes in eating habits that also have taken place during this time: a decline in use of butter, fluid milk and cream, eggs, and animal fats; an increase in consumption of vegetable fats and oils.

Those on the other side note that the two sets of statistics do not prove a cause and effect relationship. They also point out that exercise has become more popular among men; that use of tobacco products has gone down; and that these and other broad changes that have taken place in the lives of Americans, including changes in economic and social status and in health care, may be the real reasons behind the drop in the coronary heart disease death rate.[15]

To Sum Up. Coronary heart disease seems to have no single cause, and instead appears to be the result of interaction between internal risk factors, such as genetic predisposition, obesity, levels of blood cholesterol and other fatty substances, high blood pressure, and diabetes, as well as external risk factors, such as diet, smoking, and lack of exercise (see Exhibit 19.3). Elimination or modification of as many of these risk factors as possible is thought to be the most effective way to reduce the chances of having a heart attack. Considerably more research is needed before scientists can say for sure what changes in diet are most effective in reducing the risk of developing heart disease.

---

[13]"Egg Consumption Has No Influence on Serum Cholesterol Levels." *Nutrition and the M.D.*, Vol. 3, No. 9., July, 1977, p. 4. And G. Slater, J. Mead, G. Dbopishwarkar, S. Robinson, R.B. Alfin-Slater, "Plasma Cholesterol and Triglycerides in Men with Added Eggs in the Diet." *Nutrition Reports International*, Vol. 14, 1976, pp. 249-60.

[14]R. Reiser, "Normal vs. Pathological Variations in Serum Cholesterol Levels." *Nutrition and the M.D.*, Vol. 2, No. 2, December, 1975, p. 2.

[15]S. Fogg, "Heart Disease Drops; Big Question is Why?" *Los Angeles Times*, November 24, 1978, Part XI, p. 11.

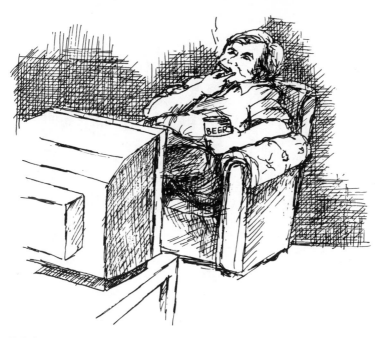

Exhibit 19.3. Diet is thought to be just one of a number of risk factors that may contribute to the development of heart disease. Some other factors include obesity, inactivity, cigarette smoking, overconsumption of alcoholic beverages, and heredity.

HYPERTENSION

Hypertension, or high blood pressure, is not a disease but rather a measurement of what may be an unhealthy physical condition. It is a symptom that accompanies many forms of heart and kidney disease.

Blood pressure is a combination of the muscle force exerted by blood on the walls of arteries as the heart contracts and relaxes and the resistance offered to this force by the other blood vessels in the body. There are two blood pressure readings: the *systolic*, which is taken when the heart muscle contracts and the pressure is at its highest point, and the *diastolic*, which is taken when the heart muscle relaxes and the pressure is at its lowest point (see Exhibit 19.4). Thus a reading of 120/80 means a systolic pressure of 120 millimeters of mercury and a diastolic pressure of 80 millimeters of mercury. The systolic pressure measures the muscle force and the diastolic pressure reflects the resistance of the many blood vessels throughout the body. A rise in the diastolic pressure is much more significant than increased systolic pressure.

Individuals vary in their blood pressure readings, but 120/80 is considered fairly normal for an adult between the ages of 18 and 45. Older adults tend to have somewhat higher readings. Blood pressure

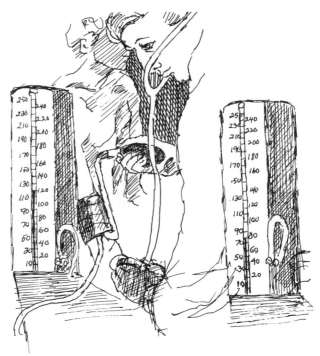

Exhibit 19.4.   The systolic blood pressure reading is taken when the heart muscle contracts and the pressure is at its highest point. The diastolic blood pressure reading is taken when the heart muscle relaxes and the pressure is at its lowest point.

changes constantly. It goes up when people exercise, are excited, or are emotionally upset and down when they are relaxed or sleeping.

Low blood pressure is a rare condition, but high blood pressure is common. Many people—an estimated 20 percent of adult Americans and 40 percent of older age groups—have blood pressure readings that are considered to be too high; that is, above 140/90 or 150/90. Some people are able to tolerate markedly high blood pressure for many years without apparent ill effect. But generally, consistently high blood pressure or a rapidly rising pressure is a cause for concern. It may be due to a heart that pumps too much blood or a normal heart output with narrowed blood vessels.

Blood vessels that are clogged with fatty deposits (atherosclerosis) can become resistant to the flow of blood (see Exhibit 19.5). The heart must then work harder to force the blood through the narrowed blood vessels, and the blood pressure goes up. This is one explanation of why high blood pressure is a risk factor or warning sign of coronary heart disease.

High blood pressure is also a risk factor in stroke, or *cerebrovascular disease*. In a stroke, an artery leading to or in the brain is blocked, usually by a hemorrhage or blood clot. Brain damage results if the blood supply

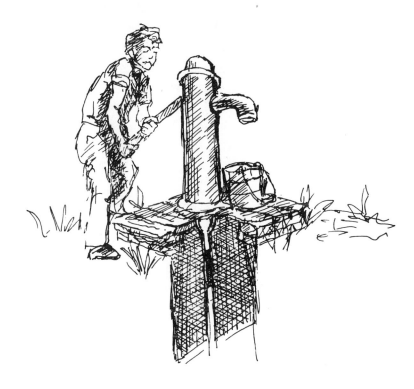

Exhibit 19.5. When pipes are clogged, it takes more pumping (pressure) to force water through them. In the same way, when arteries are clogged, the heart must pump harder; this causes blood pressure to go up.

is cut off for more than several minutes. The result may be full or partial paralysis due to loss of brain function, as well as many other neurological symptoms, including death in some cases.

Factors Contributing to High Blood Pressure

Obesity often is a contributing factor in high blood pressure. Every pound of extra weight turns into body tissue (usually fat tissue) and that tissue must have blood to nourish it. This blood is supplied through blood vessels. So when you gain weight you also add blood vessels. This means your heart must work harder to pump blood through the extra miles of blood vessels. An overweight person who has high blood pressure is likely to be able to bring his blood pressure down significantly by losing weight.

Sodium is also often a problem in high blood pressure. Some 15 to 20 percent of Americans are believed to have a genetic susceptibility to developing high blood pressure as a result of excess salt consumption. The effect of the condition appears to be on the kidney, altering its abil-

Exhibit 19.6.   Approximate Sodium Content of Common Foods

MEATS	AMOUNT	APPROXIMATE MILLIGRAMS
Beef, veal	3 ounces	75
Lamb, pork	3 ounces	75
Ham (cured)	3 ounces	675
Bacon	1 slice	75
Frankfurter	1	540
Bologna	1 slice	390
Chicken	3 ounces	75
Egg	1 whole	60
Fish (fresh) excpet shellfish	3 ounces	75
Dry beans, peas	½ cup	15
Peanuts, salted	¼ cup	275
unsalted	¼ cup	2

VEGETABLES AND FRUITS+		
Asparagus, corn, cucumber, green pepper, lima beans, okra, onions, peas, potatoes, pumpkin, rutabaga, green beans, sweet potato, squash, tomato, eggplant	1 cup	5
Broccoli, brussels sprouts, cabbage, cauliflower, lettuce, radishes, turnip greens	½ cup	5
Beets, carrots, celery, kale, spinach, turnips	½ cup	40
Fruits	1 medium serving or ½ cup	2

BREAD AND CEREALS		
Puffed wheat, puffed rice, shredded wheat	1 cup	1
Corn flakes	1 cup	165
Bran flakes	¾ cup	340
Whole wheat bread	1 slice	170
White bread (enriched)	1 slice	170
Macaroni	½ cup (cooked)	1
Rice	½ cup (cooked)	3

MILK, CHEESE, AND DAIRY PRODUCTS		
Low-fat milk	1 cup	120
Buttermilk	1 cup	225
Cheese—Cheddar, Muenster, Swiss, American	1 ounce	220
Cottage cheese, creamed	¼ cup	160
unsalted	¼ cup	30
Parmesan cheese	1 tablespoon	40
Low-fat cheese (sapsago, tilsiter, Port Salut)	1 ounce	200

Exhibit 19.6. Cont.

401
Hypertension

MEATS	AMOUNT	APPROXIMATE MILLIGRAMS
OTHER ITEMS		
Margarine, salted	1 tablespoon	110
unsalted	1 tablespoon	1
Salt	¼ teaspoon	575
Catsup	1 tablespoon	200
Worcestershire sauce	1 tablespoon	315
Peanut butter (regular)	1 tablespoon	18

Source: C. E. Bills, F. G. McDonald, W. Niedermeier, and M. C. Schwartz, "Sodium and Potassium in Foods and Water." *Journal of the American Dietetic Association,* Vol. 23, April, 1949, pp. 304-14.

+ Amounts listed are for fresh and canned or frozen foods without sodium or salt.

ity to handle sodium excretion. When a person has this condition, or has heart or kidney disease and cannot get rid of extra sodium, the sodium stays in body tissue and holds water. When the body holds water, the blood volume increases. This makes the heart work harder and raises blood pressure. The water also can cause swelling, or edema, and other problems. The inability of the body to utilize sodium properly may be the prime cause of hypertension today.

Thus a person with heart or kidney disease or high blood pressure is usually told to cut down on sodium in his diet, and this often helps to lower blood pressure (see Exhibit 19.6 for sodium content of popular foods.). The sodium restriction could be: very severe, an allowance of only 200 to 500 milligrams; moderate, 1,000 milligrams (1 gram); or more liberal, 2,000 to 3,000 milligrams (2 to 3 grams) per day. On the 2- to 3-gram sodium diet, a person would simply be required to add no extra salt to foods (a level teaspoon of salt contains 2.3 grams sodium) and avoid very salty foods (like pickles with 2 grams of sodium). On the very low sodium diet, the person would have to avoid or cut down on all foods with large amounts of sodium. (See Exhibit 19.7 showing foods considered high in sodium and Exhibit 19.8 for a comparison of the sodium content in common foods.) Label reading is important for the person on a low-sodium diet, to find foods that have added salt (plain salt or foods such as garlic salt and onion salt) or some other sodium-containing ingredient, such as mono*sodium* glutamate, *sodium* caseinate, or *sodium* benzoate.

Diuretics often are used to help a person with high blood pressure get rid of excess water in his tissues. Diuretics tend to deplete the body of potassium. To counteract this effect one method suggested is to use salt substitutes, in which potassium replaces sodium. This will reduce sodium intake and at the same time increase potassium intake.

One of the Dietary Goals for the United States is a limitation of salt intake to about 5 grams a day. This is well below the average American

Exhibit 19.7. Foods High in Sodium

MILK AND MILK PRODUCTS

Buttermilk (commercial)
Cheese foods
Cheese spreads
Cottage cheese
Natural cheese
Processed cheese
Canned puddings
Pudding mixes

BREADS AND CEREALS

Biscuit mix
Biscuits (commercial)
Bread crumbs, dry (commercial)
Bread sticks (commercial)
Cornbread (commercial)
Flour, self-rising
Muffins (commercial)
Ready-to-eat cereals
Saltines
Snack crackers
Rolls (commercial)
Stuffling mix (commercial)
Tortillas, flour (commercial)
Quick-cooking cereals
Instant hot cereal mixes
Pancake mixes
Waffles, frozen

MEAT AND MEAT SUBSTITUTES

Anchovies
Anchovy paste
Beef jerky
Bologna
Braunschweiger
Canadian bacon
Canned meat, fish and poultry
Caviar
Chipped beef
Corned beef
Dried fish
Frankfurters
Frozen breaded fish
Ham
Liverwurst
Luncheon meats
Meat spreads
Pastrami
Peanut butter
Pork and beans, canned
Salami
Salted nuts
Scallops
Smoked fish and meat

FRUITS AND VEGETABLES

Bean salad (commercial)
Coleslaw (commercial)
Canned soup
Canned vegetables
Canned vegetable juices
Dry soup mixes
Frozen international-style vegetables
Frozen vegetables in butter sauce
Instant mashed potatoes
Packaged potato mixes
Olives, black
Pickled beefs
Pickled cauliflower
Pickled onions
Pickles
Potato salad
Sauerkraut
Sauerkraut juice

CONVENIENCE FOODS

Canned barbecue beans
Canned beef stew
Canned chill con carne
Canned chicken chow mein
Canned corned beef hash
Frozen breakfast entrees
Instant breakfast drinks
Macaroni and cheese— canned, frozen and mixes
Pot pies, frozen
Ravioli, canned and frozen
Skillet dinner mixes
Shake 'n' bake mixes
Spaghetti sauce, canned and mixes
Spaghetti, canned
TV dinners

SEASONINGS AND CONDIMENTS

Salt
Butter-flavored salt
Celery salt
Garlic salt
Seasoned salt
MSG
Meat tenderizer
Baking powder
Baking soda
Barbecue sauce (commercial)
Capers
Catsup (commercial)
Chill sauce (commercial)
Chow-chow
Chutney
Gravy, canned or mix
Mustard, prepared (commercial)
Packaged sauce mixes
Soy sauce
Steak sauce
Worcestershire sauce

OTHERS

Bacon
Sausage
Imitation bacon bits
Salt pork
Chip dips
Bottled salad dressings
Salad dressing mixes

Source: C. E. Bills, F. G. McDonald, W. Niedermeier, and M. C. Schwartz, "Sodium and Potassium in Foods and Water." *Journal of the American Dietetic Association*, Vol. 23, April, 1949, pp. 304-14.

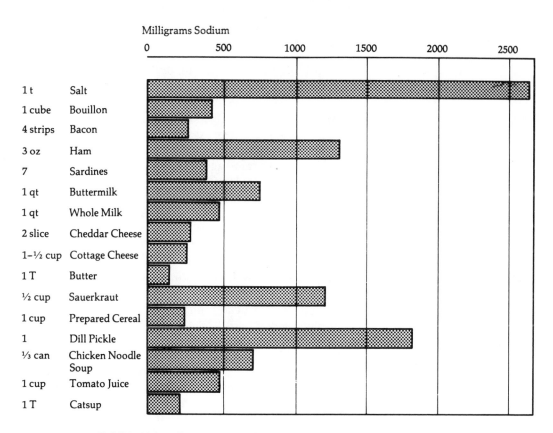

Milligrams Sodium

| | | 0 | 500 | 1000 | 1500 | 2000 | 2500 |

1 t	Salt
1 cube	Bouillon
4 strips	Bacon
3 oz	Ham
7	Sardines
1 qt	Buttermilk
1 qt	Whole Milk
2 slice	Cheddar Cheese
1-½ cup	Cottage Cheese
1 T	Butter
½ cup	Sauerkraut
1 cup	Prepared Cereal
1	Dill Pickle
⅓ can	Chicken Noodle Soup
1 cup	Tomato Juice
1 T	Catsup

Exhibit 19.8. Comparison of the sodium content in some common foods. (*Source:* U.S. Department of Agriculture, *Composition of Foods.* Agriculture Handbook No. 8, Washington, D.C., p. 7.)

intake of 10 to 20 grams per day and is believed by some authorities to be an unrealistic recommendation. The reason it was made was based on the theory, as yet not totally proven to everyone's satisfaction, that excess sodium may cause high blood pressure in genetically susceptible people. Recent evidence does seem to support this view. [16] Since American consumption of sodium is well above our needs, it was thought that a salt restriction would not be harmful and might be helpful to a certain percentage of Americans in preventing the development of high blood pressure.

[16]G.R. Meneely and H.D. Battarbee, "Sodium and Potassium," in Nutrition Reviews' *Present Knowledge in Nutrition,* fourth edition. New York, Washington, D.C.: The Nutrition Foundation, Inc., 1976, pp. 270-73.

Obesity, diabetes, high blood pressure, and coronary heart disease all appear to be interrelated. Diabetics are prone to develop atherosclerosis and high blood pressure. And the leading cause of death of diabetic adults is coronary heart disease. Conversely, a large proportion of people who suffer from coronary heart disease are diabetics. The death rate is almost 400 times greater for people who are both diabetic and obese than it is for people the same age who are not obese. Usually the death is from a cardiovascular cause.

Diabetes is a genetically caused disorder of carbohydrate metabolism associated with an elevation of blood sugar. The high blood sugar, *hyperglycemia,* results from deficient or inefficient insulin production. Insulin, which is produced by the pancreas, is the only hormone known to lower blood sugar. As people grow older (after age 40), their blood sugar level gradually increases so that "normal" levels at age 70 may be about 20 percent higher than what they were at age 40. Stress, such as heart attack, stroke, burns, or a head injury or other serious injury, also results in a rise in blood sugar.

Two basic forms of diabetes have been identified:

Insulin Deficient Diabetes. Called *growth onset* or *juvenile* diabetes because it most often begins in children during growth years, it also occurs in adults. The onset is usually acute. Carbohydrate metabolism is severely affected, and insulin is so minimal that symptoms can be controlled only through insulin treatment. The condition is irreversible and, with age, insulin production becomes less and less until finally there may be none. People having insulin deficient diabetes are usually thin.

Insulin Inefficient Diabetes. Often called *adult* or *maturity onset* diabetes, it usually occurs after age 30. The highest incidence of this type of diabetes is among adults in their fifties and sixties, with women being somewhat more susceptible than men. Most of the adults who develop this type of diabetes are obese. The incidence is 12 times as prevalent among those who are 50 percent over their ideal weight than it is among normal-weight adults (see Exhibit 19.9).

Obesity can lead to increased blood sugar levels because insulin does not work very well on the obese cells of a fat person. In order to compensate, an obese person may put out three times more insulin to get the same blood sugar level as a lean person. This additional stress may bring out a tendency a person has to be diabetic. In many cases, insulin injections are not required, and a weight control diet will lessen or even reverse the abnormal carbohydrate metabolism in this type of diabetes.

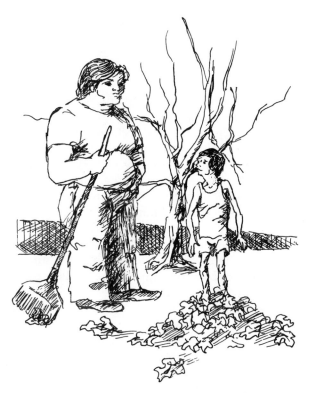

Exhibit 19.9. The incidence of insulin-inefficient diabetes (usually adult-onset) is 12 times more likely to occur in persons who are 50 percent or more over their ideal weight. On the other hand, insulin-deficient diabetics (usually juvenile-onset) are usually thin.

Treatment of Diabetes

A combination of diet and insulin is used to treat insulin deficient diabetes. Each day the person usually receives one and occasionally two injections, which contain a combination of long- and short-acting insulin. He then needs a diet to provide enough food to balance this insulin and to keep his blood sugar level relatively constant. Usually a diabetic needs to eat three regular meals a day plus mid-afternoon and bedtime snacks. Younger children sometimes need a mid-morning snack as well. For optimum control of blood sugar levels, total daily calories should be nearly constant.

Over the years, diet recommendations for diabetics have changed as new theories have replaced old ones. Current thinking gives emphasis to proper nutrition—to total adequacy of all nutrients needed to ensure good health and to maintaining proper weight in proportion to height. Diets that provide enough calories are important for a growing diabetic child, where underweight is more commonly seen than overweight. Since obese diabetics face greater risks from complications at every age, diets high in calories, especially from low-nutrient-density foods, should be avoided.

Some recent studies have shown that diets high in carbohydrates from starch and other polysaccharides have no detectable adverse effect on blood sugar levels of diabetics. In fact, in some cases high-starch diets actually seemed to bring about a lowering of blood sugar levels.[17] So the latest dietary recommendations for diabetic diets do not require strict restriction in carbohydrates as did earlier diets. However, because sugars are known to be rapidly absorbed and to result in a rapid rise in blood sugar, their use is generally limited in a diabetic diet.

Because sugar is prevalent in so many foods popular with children, providing a diabetic child with a diet that is both healthful and satisfying is a major challenge. The diabetic child, his parents, and the diabetic adult need to be taught about the importance of diet, particularly the timing of meals and quantities of food.

Because diabetic adults are at particular risk of developing atherosclerosis and cardiovascular disease, cholesterol control diets often are recommended. The suggested diet is similar to the Prudent Diet: lower in total fat (30 to 35 percent instead of 40 to 45 percent), lower in saturated fat and higher in polyunsaturated fat, and with restricted amounts of cholesterol-containing foods. Some practitioners are now recommending this diet for children with diabetes as well as for adults to help reduce the likelihood of their developing atherosclerosis in later years.

HYPOGLYCEMIA

Contrary to popular opinion, *hypoglycemia* is not a disease. It is a clinical measurement of low blood sugar. Many people are misdiagnosed as having low blood sugar based on complaints and not on adequate tests. The number with real problems is believed to be very small.

Low blood sugar is most commonly a complication of diabetes and results from an imbalance of insulin or oral drugs and food intake. An estimated 60 to 70 percent of the cases of hypoglycemia are found among diabetics. Too much insulin may be used; food intake may be delayed or too small; or the person may get more exercise than allowed for in his insulin dosage. (During exercise muscles metabolize glucose

---

[17]W.E. Connor and S.L. Connor, "Sucrose and Carbohydrate," in Nutrition Reviews' *Present Knowledge in Nutrition*, fourth edition. New York, Washington, D.C.: The Nutrition Foundation, Inc., 1976, pp. 38-39.

well without insulin, therefore a smaller dose may be needed.) A diabetic needs a constancy of calories, day by day and throughout the day, to maintain a relatively stable blood sugar level.

If the blood sugar level drops severely, the person may go into insulin shock, becoming uneasy, nervous, weak, hungry, trembly, dizzy, sweaty, faint, headachy, and emotionally unstable. The person needs an immediate form of sugar—candy, fruit juice or other sweetened liquid, or honey. Without sugar, the person may have convulsions, followed by coma and possibly death. Treatment of a person having insulin shock involves the administration of an intravenous glucose solution to immediately effect an increase in the blood sugar level.

In a nondiabetic person if blood sugar occurs *after fasting*, for example in the morning before breakfast, then it could be a symptom of a serious condition and needs further investigation. Potential causes include failure or insufficiency of the adrenal glands (a rare cause of *hypoglycemia*), drug abuse (of insulin or sulfonylurea oral medication used by diabetics), the use of alcohol in conjunction with fasting, liver disease, an enzyme or hormone deficiency, or tumors of the pancreas or other organs.

A second form of hypoglycemia is food reactive instead of fasting reactive. It takes place two to six hours *after eating*. Since many people who ingest sugar show a temporary lowering of blood sugar some hours afterwards without any symptoms, the occurrence of reactive hypoglycemia generally does not require treatment unless symptoms occur on a regular basis.

However, sometimes food-reactive hypoglycemia, when it occurs about four hours after a meal, is a sign of early diabetes. This may be treated with a diabetic diet and, when needed, a weight control diet. The result may be avoidance of a full-blown case of diabetes.

Nondiabetic, food-reactive hypoglycemia became a popular fad diagnosis during the 1970s. It was used to explain a lot of real or imagined symptoms, such as nervousness, perspiration, shakiness, headache, weakness, palpitations, hunger, changes in vision, and emotional exhaustion. However, low blood sugar is rarely the agent responsible for such symptoms and other reasons, such as simple anxiety, are far more common.

Many adults with these symptoms have been treated unnecessarily with drugs and diets that are expensive and potentially harmful. In a true case of food-reactive hypoglycemia, usually only minor alterations in diet are needed to avoid the symptoms. These include, first of all, not skipping meals and eating frequent, regular meals and snacks. Carbohydrate itself is not greatly restricted, but a reduction in sugar, including natural sugar-containing foods such as fruits—particularly dried fruits—is recommended. A restriction in alcohol consumption may also be recommended, particularly of drinks high in both sugar and alcohol such as sweet wines and liqueurs. Frequent snacks of protein-containing foods is the other essential ingredient to the management of this disorder.

The combination of a low-carbohydrate diet, which has been very popular with many dieters, plus alcohol has been found to bring on hypoglycemia attacks, including headache, nausea, nervousness, and apprehension. The physical effects of this combination on the body appear to be similar to those produced by higher blood alcohol levels than actually are present.

CANCER

The Role of Diet

Cancer is an umbrella term for a number of diseases involving the growth of malignant tumors or neoplasm. Grouped together, cancerous diseases are the second most common cause of death in the United States affecting all age groups. The risk of cancer goes up with age and the majority of cancer deaths occur among older people. The annual death rate from cancer is over ten times greater at age 50 and 100 times greater at age 65 than it is at age 25. Thus, as life expectancy rates go up, deaths caused by cancer can be expected to go up too. The most frequent death-causing cancers in the United States are lung cancer, cancers affecting the large bowel, and breast cancer, in that order.

For many years scientists have carried on an arduous research effort to find out what initiates malignant tumors and why tumors grow out of control, but the answers remain elusive. More and more, environmental factors, including nutrition and diet, are believed to be involved. Environmental factors are now thought to account for 80 percent of all cancers. By some estimates, over half of all cancers in women and 30 percent of cancers in men may be related to nutritional factors. Since different types of tumors behave differently, generalizations cannot be made about the effect of one agent on all tumors. Moreover, because clear evidence on the effect of nutrition on cancer is lacking at this time, specific dietary recommendations to minimize cancer risk, other than maintaining desirable body weight, cannot be made.

Diet is thought to play several roles in cancer development and control:

1. Certain nutrients, foods, food additives, or contaminants may have cancer-causing effects under certain circumstances by acting directly as *carcinogens* (cancer-causing agents) or by producing metabolic abnormalities that are carcinogenic.

2. A poor diet, or one lacking specific nutrients, may make a person more responsive to cancer-causing factors and more susceptible

to certain forms of cancer; conversely, a diet with a good balance of nutrients may aid in making a person more resistant to these factors.

3. Cancer and some forms of its treatment can have such detrimental effects on a person's desire or ability to eat or absorb nutrients that the person dies of malnutrition. This happens to about 10 percent of cancer patients. Nutrition therapy is a very important facet in the treatment of cancer patients.

Carcinogenic Effects of Diet

Two types of studies have been used to help identify cancer-causing agents in foods: epidemiologic, in which statistical comparisons are made between certain groups of people relating to their diets and cancer death rates; and laboratory studies or observations of animals or humans to test the effect of certain dietary factors. For obvious reasons, human studies are rare compared to animal studies.

Under the Delaney Amendment to the nation's pure food laws, the use in food of any substance that causes cancer in man or animal under any circumstances is forbidden (see Chapter 24).[18] As a result of this law, extensive animal tests have been conducted on many food additives to determine if they are carcinogenic. Long, drawn out controversies over the safety of substances such as saccharine and sodium nitrate (see Chapter 24) illustrate the difficulty scientists have in determining whether a given substance may cause cancer.

The same problem exists for other dietary factors that have been implicated as cancer-causing by comparison studies of populations. There are always many complexities and uncontrollable factors that make clear conclusions impossible. For example, statistics show that Mormons and Seventh Day Adventists have significantly lower death rates from cancer than the national average (their coronary heart disease rate also is lower).[19] Neither of these groups allow the drinking of coffee or alcohol, but we cannot conclude from this that coffee and alcohol cause cancer. There are many other variables to consider. For example, Mormons and Seventh Day Adventists do not smoke cigarettes; many Seventh Day Adventists are vegetarians; both groups emphasize the importance of a good diet; Mormons believe in having a strong family structure; and both groups are devout in following their religious beliefs. No one can say for sure exactly which aspects of their lives make them more resistant to cancer and coronary heart disease, but scientists are studying the matter and some day may have an answer.

Strong correlations have been found to exist between the following dietary factors in either epidemiological or laboratory studies or both.

[18]T.H. Jukes, "Carcinogens in Food and the Delaney Clause." *Journal of the American Medical Association*, Vol. 241, No. 6, February 9, 1979, pp. 617-19.

[19]G.B. Gori, "Diet and Cancer." *Journal of the American Dietetic Association*, Vol. 71, October, 1977, pp. 375-78.

However, in no case is the evidence strong enough for us to conclude that a cause and effect relationship has been proven.

Energy Imbalance. The strongest evidence gathered thus far in the quest for a diet–cancer link is in the relationship between an excess calorie intake and cancer. Obese people have higher cancer death rates, particularly for cancer of the endometrium, breast, and gallbladder. Obese men, but not obese women, show higher rates of colon cancer; overweight women may have cancer of the uterus more frequently.[20]

Animal studies, too, show the relationship between body weight and tumor risk. Heavy rats, for example, are more likely to develop tumors than lean rats. Animal studies also show that of all the types of diet modifications, calorie restriction throughout life is most likely to be effective in inhibiting the formation of many, but not all, types of tumors and in delaying their growth.[21]

High-fat diet. Statistical studies comparing different groups of people consistently link high-fat diets with high rates of colon and breast cancer.[22] Prostate cancer also may be related to high fat consumption. One theory explaining this relationship is that a high-fat (and possibly, high-cholesterol) diet from childhood may overstimulate our endocrine system, causing the glands to release increased amounts of hormones such as estrogen and prolactin.[23] (Women who are overweight also have higher estrogen levels than normal-weight women.) This may alter the body's biochemical balance, causing the breasts and other organs to be less immune to disease and more prone to the development of a cancerous tumor. Another theory suggests that the digestion of a high-fat diet may cause an increase in the formation of bile salts in the colon, which may be carcinogenic themselves or which may foster the growth of intestinal bacteria that produce cancer-causing substances.[24] Or it may be that the high fat is simply the major component of a cancer-causing, high-calorie diet.

One human study showed that a diet high in polyunsaturated fats resulted in a higher incidence of gallbladder disease and cancer deaths.[25] Other studies contradict as well as support this evidence. In a number of animal studies, incidence of malignant tumors was found to be

[20]"Nutrition, Diet, and Cancer." *Dairy Council Digest,* Vol. 46, No. 5, September-October, 1975, p. 26.

[21]*Ibid.*

[22]E.L. Wynder, "Dietary Habits in Cancer." *Nutrition Today,* Vol. 13, No. 5, September-October, 1978, p. 8.

[23]M.B. Lipsett, "Drugs and Hormones." *Nutrition Today,* Vol. 13, No. 5, September-October, 1978, p. 9.

[24]E.L. Wynder, "Dietary Habits in Cancer." *Nutrition Today,* Vol. 13, No. 5, September-October, 1978, p. 8.

[25]"Nutrition, Diet, and Cancer." *Dairy Council Digest,* Vol. 46, No. 5, September-October, 1975, p. 27.

greater when animals were fed polyunsaturated fats such as corn, saf-flower, soybean oil, or chicken fat, and smaller when they were fed sat-urated fats such as butter or coconut oil. One researcher theorized that the high polyunsaturated-fat intake could stimulate the formation of more bile salts. Another theorized that it might suppress the reaction of the immune system to cancer.[26]

As you can see, most of this evidence is tenuous and highly theo-retical. However, it does provide a basis for concern about the wisdom of changing our diets and greatly increasing our consumption of poly-unsaturated fats until more is known about how this might affect our risk of developing cancer.

Protein. Research to date does not show that protein plays an im-portant role in tumor formation and growth. However, one researcher has shown statistical relationships between colon cancer and popula-tions that consume large amounts of animal protein. He theorized that it is ammonia, one of the waste products of protein digestions, that is harmful. Other researchers disagree with the ammonia theory and be-lieve the explanation is that a high-meat diet is also high in fat.

Certain amino acid deficiencies have been shown to be tumor-sup-pressing in laboratory experiments. It has also been noted that severe protein deficiency can alter tumor incidence or site, perhaps by altering carcinogen metabolism.[27]

Vitamin A. Deficiency of vitamin A has been shown to be related to cancer of the stomach, salivary gland, nasopharynx, and lung. On the other hand, high levels of vitamin A appear to sometimes inhibit tumor growth and prevent epithelial cancer. *Retinoids,* vitamin A analogs, also appear to have anticancer abilities. It is theorized that vitamin A may inhibit enzymes that cause some substances to become carcinogenic and that it may stimulate the immune system to be more effective against tumor growth.

Vitamin C. This nutrient may have an inhibiting effect on the for-mation of nitrosamines when nitrites in food interact with amines in the stomach (see Chapter 24). This may help prevent stomach cancer. The increase in vitamin C in the American diet and the use of vitamin C supplements may help to explain why the incidence of stomach cancer has been going down in the United States. One human study showed that large doses of vitamin C (10 grams per day) extended the survival time of patients with various types of terminal cancer compared to con-trol subjects who did not receive vitamin C.[28]

---

[26]*Ibid.* pp. 26-27.

[27]*Ibid.*

[28]"How Dietary Factors Combat Cancer." *Science News,* Vol. 110, November 13, 1976, pp. 310-11.

Fiber. This dietary component has received wide publicity in recent years as a cancer preventative. The claims are based on comparative studies that showed very low rates of colon cancer among people, particularly Africans, who eat high-fiber diets. There is little laboratory research evidence to support this theory, and some health professionals believe other factors, especially little dietary fat or protein, may explain the low rates of colon cancer among some population groups. On the other hand, Finnish people who consume very high-fat diets have low colon-cancer rates, possibly because they also have high-fiber diets.[29]

While proof is lacking that fiber in the diet can prevent colon cancer, some current theories about how it might do so are:

1. Fiber increases the speed at which wastes move through the intestinal tract, thereby reducing the amount of time in which potentially harmful substances can be absorbed.

2. Fiber dilutes the intestinal contents, making them less irritating.

3. Certain fibers, such as lignin and pectin, may bind toxic substances, for example bile salts, chemically and prevent or impair their absorption.

4. Fiber may change the kind of bacteria growing in the intestine and prevent the growth of bacteria that might produce cancer-causing substances.

Raw Vegetables. One researcher found that people who eat uncooked vegetables appear to have less stomach cancer than the general population. Lettuce, tomatoes, carrots, cole slaw, and red cabbage in particular were found to be associated with low risk of stomach cancer. The researcher could not explain the reason for his finding.[30] Could it be due to the presence of a combination of factors such as fiber, vitamin A, and vitamin C?[31]

Milk. Some epidemiological studies have shown that this food may protect against stomach cancer also. In Japan, for example, the high rate of stomach cancer has declined, while the consumption of milk and milk products has increased considerably.[32] However, Japanese people also consume large amounts of salt, which could be a causative factor in stomach cancer.

While all of the studies to date provide clues to the mystery of cancer causation and prevention, they do not prove that any one dietary element is the answer. It seems that nutritional imbalances coupled with other environmental hazards may provide a long-term, low-level insult

[29]"Colon Cancer in Finland." *Science News*, Vol. 114, No. 3, July 15, 1978, p. 40.

[30]S. Graham, reported in *From Your Home Advisor*, April, 1973, p. 2.

[31]"Vitamin C Versus Cancer—Again." *Science News*, Vol. 114, No. 3, July 15, 1978, p. 40.

[32]G.B. Gori, "Diet and Cancer." *Journal of the American Dietetic Association*, Vol. 71, Oct. 1977, pp. 375-78.

that can weaken a susceptible individual's natural defenses against a cancer-causing agent.

Based on all of the current evidence, it appears that our best nutritional defense against cancer is to maintain optimum health by eating moderately, choosing a variety of foods from all the food groups, and restricting fats and calories to maintain our ideal weight.

RHEUMATIC DISEASES

Medical science has not solved the mystery of the cause and cure of rheumatic or arthritic diseases. Because of this, and because so many people suffer from these diseases, there is widespread dietary quackery in which nutrients, foods, or special diets are promoted as the latest "discovery" to cure arthritis. People who suffer from rheumatic disease are easily exploited because they are desperately seeking some way to alleviate their pain. And many times, people believe themselves to be cured when their condition suddenly disappears. They mistakenly attribute the remission of pain to the effectiveness of the treatment rather than to the well-known fact that in certain forms of rheumatism, the condition can disappear as suddenly as it can reappear—and for no apparent reason.

Fad dietary recommendations for treatment of arthritis, for which there is no scientific evidence (see Exhibit 19.10), include:

1. Cutting out milk or calcium. (In some forms of rheumatism, reduction of calcium can bring on severe complications.)

2. Taking large doses of vitamins, such as vitamins C, E, or D. Vitamin D in large doses is very toxic.

3. Taking cod liver oil, which is rich in vitamins D and A, and orange juice.

4. Drinking vinegar and honey.

5. Eating other special foods, such as cranberries, grape juice, cherries, or "natural foods."

Researchers have no evidence that any form of rheumatic disease is caused by inadequate nutrition; conversely, there is no specific dietary cure for any of them. Numerous diets have been tried: high- and low-protein, fat, or carbohydrate diets; modified-acid or alkaline-ash diets; reduced and increased calcium diets; diets with supplements of vitamins C and D. None has been effective.

However, a person who has good nutritional health is in a better position to fight the disease. The one most important diet-related health measure for arthritics, in addition to eating a balanced diet, is to maintain normal body weight. Obesity is often associated with osteoarthritis.

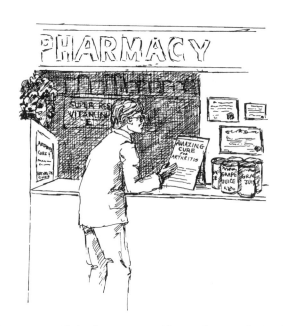

Exhibit 19.10.   While there is no evidence that any form of arthritis is caused or cured by special foods or nutrients, arthritis sufferers are easily exploited by such claims.

The excess weight puts additional strain on joints, accelerating the course of the disease, adding to the pain, and perhaps prolonging an attack. A weight control diet is usually suggested to an overweight arthritic. Rheumatoid and other forms of arthritis, on the other hand, may cause loss of appetite, weight loss, and result in a poor nutritional status. In this situation, treatment includes a high-calorie, high-nutrient diet, to build body tissue.

Gout, or gouty arthritis, is a hereditary disease seen most often in males over the age of 30 in which the person has a high uric acid blood level. Alcohol, obesity, high-fat and high-purine diets appear to be involved in the formation of the excess uric acid. This disease is generally treated with drugs. Diets limited in fats, calories, alcohol, and high-purine foods such as liver, kidney, brains, anchovies, sardines, meat extracts, and gravies may be recommended.

Summary

A heavily debated issue is the relationship between diet and *atherosclerosis*, the condition of clogged arteries leading to coronary heart disease. It is suspected that atherosclerosis is caused by the consumption of saturated fats and cholesterol-containing foods, which are thought to increase blood cholesterol and lead to arterial plaque buildup. The presence of high levels of triglycerides and low-density lipoproteins (LDL) in the blood are also considered key factors.

Dietary modifications called the *Prudent Diet* have been suggested for cholesterol control. These guidelines call for moderate calorie intake and reduced intake of fat, saturated fats, and cholesterol. Disagreement over these recommended changes centers around their potential adverse effects and lack of demonstrated proof of their effectiveness.

Hypertension, or high blood pressure, is a symptom, rather than a disease. While there is wide variation in blood pressure readings among individuals, 120/80 is considered fairly normal for adults. The first number (120) reflects *systolic* pressure, or muscular force; the second number (80) represents *diastolic* pressure, or blood vessel resistance. The level of diastolic pressure is considered the more significant of the two readings. Major contributors to high blood pressure are genetic predisposition, obesity, excess sodium, and diseases of the kidneys or other organs. Treatment often includes the use of diuretics, which may cause potassium depletion.

Diabetes is caused by disturbed carbohydrate metabolism with insufficient *insulin* production and an elevated level of sugar in the blood. There are two types of diabetes: *insulin deficient*, usually occurring in children and requiring both diet modification and insulin for treatment; and *insulin inefficient*, associated with obese adults over 30 and treated with weight control diet. Timing and quantities of food are essential in diabetes management.

Hypoglycemia is a measurement of low blood sugar, rather than a disease *per se*. Occurring when there is an imbalance of insulin with food intake, hypoglycemia may be either *food reactive* or *fasting reactive*. Treatment of food reactive hypoglycemia includes eating frequent regular meals, restricting intake of sugar and alcohol, and consuming protein snacks.

Over one-third of all cancers are estimated to be related to nutritional factors. Diet may have a direct carcinogenic effect, cause susceptibility, or interact with cancer or its treatment to cause malnutrition. The strongest relationship between diet and cancer is excess caloric intake. Also suspect are high levels of fat and protein, and deficiencies of vitamin A, vitamin C, and fiber.

Rheumatic diseases do not appear to be linked with diet. However, unproven dietary claims abound in this area. In *osteoarthritis*, obesity puts additional stress on joints, accelerating the onset of the disease. A well balanced diet of appropriate caloric content is the most effective nutritional approach to control of rheumatic diseases.

DIET
AND 20
DRUGS

Highlights

Types of drugs

Nutritional risks associated with drug use

Drug-food interactions

Nutritional consequences of alcohol use

Nutrition and hard drug addiction

Nutrient megadoses as drugs

Characteristics of well-designed and controlled research studies

Appropriate use of supplements

Amerca has become a nation of drug users and abusers. The drugs we use include over-the-counter and prescription medications, alcohol, and "hard" drugs. Even nutrients themselves, vitamins in particular, are sometimes used in large amounts as drugs instead of nutrients.

While drugs are used by all age groups, the health-conscious elderly are the most likely to be overusing over-the-counter drugs such as laxatives and vitamin supplements in addition to the prescription drugs they use to treat their many ailments (see Exhibit 20.1). Middle-aged women are the heaviest users of prescription drugs, including diet pills, sleeping pills, tranquilizers, barbituates, and antidepressants, while younger women are the most frequent users of oral contraceptives. Middle-aged men are most likely to be the alcohol abusers, although alcohol abuse has become a problem among middle-aged women, the elderly, and teenagers too. (Some 1.3 million 12- to 17-year-olds in the United States are estimated to have a drinking problem.) Teens and young adults are the age group that most frequently abuse hard drugs.

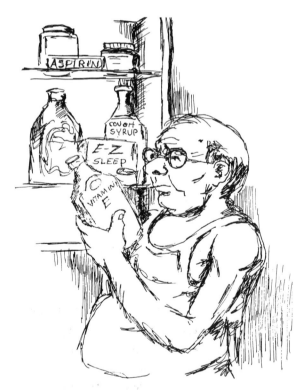

Exhibit 20.1.   The health-conscious elderly are among those Americans who are most likely to be overusing over-the-counter drugs, including vitamin supplements.

All drugs are toxic if used in excess and will almost always cause undesirable side effects, one of which may be nutritional deficiency. Persons most at nutritional risk from drug use are those who:

1. Lack reserve nutritional stores and are more vulnerable to nutritional assault. They are already undernourished, are chronically ill, or are in a period of rapid growth.

2. Use drugs over a long period of time. The longer a drug is used, the more likely it is to cause damage.

3. Use large amounts of one drug. Drug effects are exaggerated when excessive doses are taken.

4. Use several drugs at once. In that case, one drug may multiply the effects of another.

Drugs can cause nutritional deficiencies in several ways (see Exhibit 20.2). A very obvious effect is reduction of food intake because drugs either suppress the appetite, perhaps by interfering with taste, smell, or saliva production, or cause nausea, vomiting, and diarrhea. The most severe food-reduction response to drugs is seen in cancer patients undergoing chemotherapy. Amphetamines given to children as treatment for hyperactivity are a concern because they are appetite depressants and may cause growth retardation. Some drugs, such as digitalis and drugs used to reduce blood cholesterol, cause subtle, chronic anorexia (loss of appetite) that can result in a slow weight loss in those who use them. Other drugs increase appetite and may cause unwanted weight gains. Birth control pills sometimes have this effect. Tranquilizers may increase appetite in some people and may sedate others to the extent that their food intake is depressed.

Exhibit 20.2.   Detrimental Effects of Drugs on Nutritional Status

Stimulate appetite, causing increased food intake and weight
  gain
Suppress appetite, resulting in decreased food intake and
  weight loss
Cause nausea, vomiting, diarrhea, and nutrient loss
Reduce absorption in gastrointestinal tract
  Laxatives
  Antacids
  Diuretics
  Substances that bind nutrients
Interfere with metabolism of nutrients
  Cause damage to liver, pancreas, or other organs
  Act on specific nutrients
Interfere with synthesis of nutrients by bacteria in intestines

Drugs May Reduce Absorption of Nutrients. Laxatives, for example, speed up the emptying of the stomach and intestine so that nutrients have less time to be absorbed. Mineral oil combines with fat-soluble vitamins and keeps them from being absorbed because the mineral oil itself passes through the intestinal tract without being digested. Some drugs, such as antacids, change the acidity level in the gastrointestinal tract and affect the solubility of nutrients such as minerals. (Antacids may cause phosphate depletion, for example.) Some drugs, such as diuretics, increase the excretion of nutrients in urine by the kidneys. Sodium and potassium are depleted in this way. Cholestyramine, used to control cholesterol, may tie up folic acid and fat-soluble vitamins—A, D, K, and possibly E as well—and decrease their absorption.

Some Drugs Interfere With Metabolism of Nutrients. Drugs may damage the liver so it cannot metabolize vitamins, store nutrients, or synthesize protein; or they may damage the pancreas so it cannot make digestive enzymes. Sometimes drugs are used for the deliberate purpose of interfering with nutrient metabolism. For example, anticoagulants act by reducing vitamin K, the vitamin needed for blood clotting. Other drugs do this as an undesirable side effect. For example, L-dopa, used to treat Parkinson's disease, is an antagonist of vitamin B_6. If B_6 is used to prevent deficiency, it antagonizes or inactivates L-dopa. Anticonvulsant drugs used by epileptics may alter the metabolism of vitamins D, K, and folic acid, and they can also cause appetite loss. Pregnant women who use these drugs need to be alert to developing deficiencies of these nutrients. Aspirin interferes with vitamin C metabolism, and this is a concern to arthritic patients who use large amounts of aspirin over a long period of time.

Nutrient synthesis by bacteria in the intestine also may be adversely affected by certain drugs. Antibiotics in particular tend to kill "friendly" bacteria in the intestines at the same time that they are destroying disease-causing bacteria.

Oral Contraceptives are Hormones That Affect Numerous Metabolic Processes. They are known to reduce blood levels of thiamin, riboflavin, vitamins B_6, B_{12}, C, and folic acid and also to affect metabolism of protein, fat, and carbohydrates. Megaloblastic anemia, caused by folacin deficiency, has been found in some users of oral contraceptives. On the other hand, oral contraceptive users have been found to have higher blood levels of vitamin A and to need slightly less iron because they lose

Exhibit 20.3.   How Food Affects Drugs in the Body

Delays and/or reduces absorption
Improves absorption
Prevents nausea or vomiting
Causes toxic food-drug interaction

less blood during menstruation than non-pill users. A varied, balanced diet is considered to be the best method for counteracting the nutrient effects of using contraceptive pills; normally vitamin supplements are not necessary, except in cases of borderline deficiency.

HOW FOOD AFFECTS DRUG ABSORPTION AND ACTION

While drugs affect nutrition, food eaten during drug use can affect the drug action—sometimes decreasing it, sometimes increasing it, sometimes causing dangerous reactions (see Exhibit 20.3).

Often when a drug is taken at the same time as food, or shortly after eating, the food in the stomach will delay the absorption of the drug, and it also may reduce the amount absorbed. This is seen with the stimulant drug *methylphenidate* (Ritalin). Aspirin acts more slowly when taken with food. Some antibiotics, such as penicillin and tetracycline, will not be fully absorbed when taken with food. Certain foods may interfere with certain drugs: milk, for example, blocks the action of tetracyclines.

Some drugs are absorbed more readily when taken with food. Fat, for example, may promote absorption of certain compounds. Moreover, sometimes drugs are taken with food to prevent reactions such as nausea or vomiting. Some drugs are metabolized faster when the diet is high in protein and low in carbohydrate rather than the opposite. Certain foods, such as cabbage and brussel sprouts, contain substances that seem to speed up the metabolism of some drugs. And drastic changes in diet, for example, an increase in fiber, may affect the intestinal bacteria and change the rate or level of absorption of some drugs.

While dangerous drug-food reactions are uncommon, they have been observed. The most well known is the toxic reaction between drugs, most commonly tranquilizers, that block the activity of the enzyme *monoamine oxidase* (MAO) and foods containing a substance called *tyramine*. Tyramine can have a toxic effect in the body, causing rapid rise in blood pressure, headache, hemorrhage, and even death. We can eat foods containing tyramine, certain types of cheese and wine, without problems because the MAO enzyme counteracts its toxic action. But if someone takes a drug that keeps the MAO enzyme from doing its job, he can have a life-threatening reaction if he eats foods containing tyramine. Drugs that cause this reaction are *phenelzine* and *tranylcypromine* (tranquilizers), *paragyline* (an antihypertensive drug), *procarbazine* (an anticancer agent), *furazolidone* (an antibacterial agent), and some of the antidepressant drugs.

Obviously, it's very important that people be given explicit directions for each drug: when it should be taken—before, after, or during meals—and what foods, if any, need to be avoided when the drug is used (see Exhibit 20.4). When consumers buy prescription drugs, they

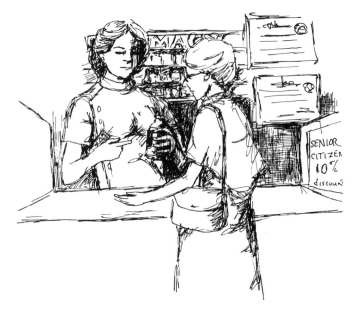

Exhibit 20.4.   Consumers should be given explicit directions for the use of foods with each drug from their physician and pharmacist—and they should follow those instructions.

should insist on receiving adequate directions from their physician and pharmacist and then be sure to follow them. When over-the-counter drugs are used, reading and following the directions that come with them is equally important. Federal food and drug regulations require that labels provide warnings about hazards involved in drug use.

NUTRITION AND ALCOHOLISM

Alcohol is both a food and a drug. It's considered a food because it does supply energy, 7 calories per gram, and some alcoholic beverages, such as beer and wine, also have other nutrients, including carbohydrates, protein, minerals, and vitamins (see Exhibit 20.5). However, these nutrients are present in minute quantities, and alcoholic beverages are high-calorie, low-nutrient-density foods.

Alcohol rates as the most commonly used drug in the United States. It is both toxic and addictive and it acts on our bodies as a depressant. About 1 in 10 people who drink become alcoholics, but there also are many people who consume too much alcohol on a regular basis. "Too much" for most people is when daily consumption amounts to 20 percent or more of calories (that's three or four drinks).

Alcoholism, or too much alcohol consumed regularly over an extended period of time, can lead to serious nutritional deficiencies as well as to physical ailments such as obesity, gout, alcoholic hepatitis, cirrho-

Exhibit 20.5. Nutrient Content of Some Alcoholic Beverages

	BEER 12 OZ	WHISKEY, GIN, RUM 1 JIGGER, 1½ FL OZ*	WINE, DRY 3½ OZ	WINE, SWEET 3½ OZ
Calories	150	97	87	141
Alcohol Calories	96	97	70	110
Protein (grams)	1.1	—	0.1	0.1
Fat (grams)	—	—	—	—
Carbohydrate (grams)	13.7	Trace	4.3	7.9
Vitamins				
Thiamin (milligrams)	0.01	—	Trace	0.01
Niacin (milligrams)	2.2	—	0.1	0.2
Riboflavin (milligrams)	0.11	—	0.01	0.02
Minerals				
Calcium (milligrams)	18	—	9	8
Iron (milligrams)	Trace	—	0.4	—
Potassium (milligrams)	90	—	94	77

Source: *Nutritive Value of American Foods in Common Units.* U.S. Department of Agriculture, Agriculture Handbook No. 456, Washington, D.C.
* 80 proof (33.4% alcohol by weight)

sis of the liver, and many neurological disorders, including a form of psychosis. Alcohol also appears to play a role in the development of coronary heart disease, cancer, and diabetes. Alcohol seems to work synergistically with cigarette smoking to enhance a person's chances of developing cancer of the oral cavity and pharynx, larynx, and esophagus. The effect of alcohol and tobacco combined is greater than the sum of the individual effects. Besides damaging the liver, alcohol may damage the stomach, pancreas, and intestinal tract. In addition, alcoholic intoxication is the leading cause of automobile accidents and is responsible for one in two automobile accident fatalities.

Nutritional disorders resulting from the overuse of alcohol come about in several ways (see Exhibit 20.6). First, alcohol acts as an appetite depressant and an alcoholic may eat very little, thereby getting too few

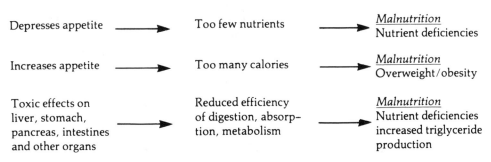

Exhibit 20.6. Effect of alcohol on nutritional status.

nutrients except calories. But alcohol requires nutrients for its metabolism, and the liver preferentially metabolizes alcohol. This depletes the nutrient supply needed for metabolism of other nutrients. The nonalcoholic overuser of alcohol, on the other hand, may have an improved appetite from a few drinks before meals, consume an excess of calories, and become overweight.

At one time it was thought that the liver disease resulting from alcoholism was totally due to the poor diet and state of malnutrition of the alcoholic. It is now known, however, that alcohol is *toxic* to the liver and other organs even in the presence of a good diet. Alcohol causes changes in the liver similar to those found in protein malnutrition.

Alcohol's toxic effect on the liver, stomach, pancreas, and intestines means they act less efficiently in digesting, metabolizing, and absorbing nutrients. Alcoholics are found to have symptoms of deficiency of B vitamins, especially thiamin, which may result in beriberi; anemia caused by lack of folic acid; night blindness from lack of vitamin A; loss of taste sensitivity and appetite from lack of zinc; tremors, known as DTs, from lack of magnesium; and shortages of protein, vitamin C, and potassium. There are also other nonspecific effects on the brain that can cause chronic disorders of the nervous system, including psychosis.

In the presence of alcohol, the liver increases its synthesis of triglycerides, and these fats are secreted in the blood, leading to hyperlipidemia and possibly atherosclerosis, high blood pressure, and coronary heart disease. The liver stores the fats too and becomes a *fatty liver*. A damaged liver is unable to store fat-soluble vitamins. Fat not absorbed may tie up calcium and result in kidney stone development. Impairment of glucose and glycogen stores in the liver lead to hypoglycemia, an increase of lactic acid level, and a rise in blood uric acid; this cycle can cause an alcoholic to be prone to gout.

Treatment of alcoholics includes nutritional rehabilitation, often with nutrient supplements, to rebuild the body's nutrient stores.

The person who drinks alcohol in excess without becoming a hardcore alcoholic also is at risk from the damaging effect of alcohol. As with all other aspects of nutrition and diet, moderation is the most healthful mode. Some recent research appears to show that moderate use of alcohol, up to three drinks a day depending on the person's size, may have a healthful effect on the body and help prevent heart attacks.

The beneficial effects of small amounts of alcohol may be related to its depressant or relaxing effect and its ability to lessen symptoms of exhaustion and tension. Pregnant women, however, need to be concerned about the toxic effect of even small amounts of alcohol on the developing fetus (discussed in Chapter 13).

In several studies in which case histories of hospitalized patients were reviewed, it was found that moderate users of alcohol were significantly less likely (30 percent in one study) to have had a heart attack than nondrinking patients.[1] It has also been found that alcohol in moderation does not seem to increase total cholesterol levels in the blood, although it increases triglycerides, but it does appear to be associated with a high level of high-density lipoproteins (HDL) and a low level of low-density lipoproteins (LDL).[2] As noted in Chapter 19, other studies have shown that higher levels of HDL are associated with heart disease resistance.

More research is needed on this subject, in view of some of the conflicting information. Scientists say it is still too early to endorse moderate use of alcohol as a heart attack preventative, especially because of its known medical risks.

NUTRITION AND "HARD" DRUG ADDICTION

Drug addiction among teenagers and young adults has become a serious problem in the United States since the 1960s. Over the years, the types of drugs used tend to change somewhat: some drugs, such as LSD, go out of favor and others take their place. Relatively little research has been done on the nutritional effects of the addictive drugs on the body, but it is known that young people who are seriously addicted and who become alienated from their families are likely to eat very poor diets and become malnourished as a result.

Health professionals who studied the diet habits of hard drug (heroin, cocaine, LSD) users in New York City found that the users had a craving for high-carbohydrate, low-nutrient-density snack foods such as cream or frosting-filled cakes, cookies, soft drinks, candy, potato chips, and pretzels. The addicts seemed to have the idea that these foods enhanced the drug effect. In addition, these foods are readily available "on the street," require no preparation, and are relatively low in cost. "Fast foods," such as hamburgers and hot dogs, were also eaten occasionally if an addict had enough money for both food and drugs. Milk, fruits, and vegetables were lacking in their diets.

Many of the addicts also were heavy users of alcohol and when tested clinically showed signs of liver malfunction and elevated levels of fats in their blood as well as nutrient deficiencies. The researchers concluded that the diet pattern of an addict carries a substantial risk of providing inadequate amounts of B vitamins, especially folic acid, and vitamins A and C. They recommended that rehabilitation programs for drug abusers include both a highly nutritious diet and the encourage-

[1]"Alcohol: A Heart Disease Preventive?" *Science News*, Vol. 112, August 13, 1977, pp. 102-3
[2]*Ibid.*

ment to eat a balanced diet, especially one that includes more fruits, vegetables, and milk.[3]

NUTRIENTS AS DRUGS

Sometimes nutrients, usually vitamins, are prescribed (or, more likely, self-prescribed) in large (or *mega*) doses for treatment or prevention of an ailment. When used in large amounts, nutrients go beyond functioning as nutrients and instead act as drugs. For example, when a vitamin is present in more than the small amount needed in the manufacture of coenzymes, its usual vitamin function, it cannot function as a vitamin and is either stored, excreted, or performs a nonvitamin chemical function.

Research to date has identified just a limited number of ways in which vitamins and other nutrients are known to function therapeutically in the body. But a visit to any health food store or reading the titles of books in the health or diet section of a bookstore could lead someone to believe that food supplements and vitamins can prevent or cure just about any disease, physical or mental, that a person might have. And there are many people who will testify to the "cure" or improved state of health they are in as a result of using large amounts of one or more vitamins or food supplements.

In this country it is not illegal for an individual to make false and unsubstantiated claims about the therapeutic value of a nutrient or food in person, in a book, or via the mass media (see Exhibit 20.7). The general public is often willing to believe such claims, especially when they are presented on an emotional level by show business personalities, doctors, or pseudo-professionals who claim unique "success" for their nutrient treatment method.

The only protection consumers have is the Food and Drug Administration (FDA) and Federal Trade Commission (FTC) regulations requiring labels and advertisements on food supplements to be truthful. The FDA does not allow false nutrition claims to be made on labels. The FTC theoretically does not allow false nutrition claims in advertisements. In actual practice, however, false claims often are made in advertisements until and unless the FTC rules that they are false and misleading and orders their discontinuation. By then the damage may be done.

The FDA truth-in-labeling requirement prohibits statements such as "cures colds" on a bottle of vitamin C tablets or "prevents heart disease" on a container of vitamin E because these claims have not been scientifically proven. In some cases, the FDA requires a disclaimer on

[3]R. Frankie and G. Christakis, "Some Nutritional Aspects of 'Hard' Drug Addiction." *Dietetic Currents*, Vol. 2, No. 3, July-August, 1975.

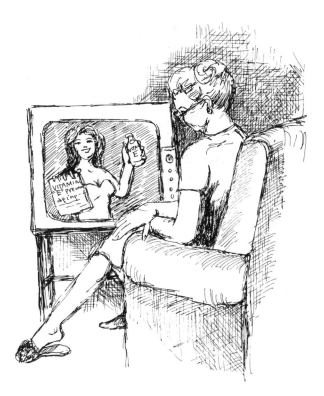

Exhibit 20.7. The general public is often willing to believe a show
business personality who gives nutrition advice.

the label. For example, on containers of lecithin the label must read,
"The need for lecithin in human nutrition has not been established."
The FDA requires this statement to counteract the many false claims
made about lecithin by its purveyors.

Labeling such as this does not appear to keep people from buying
substances that they believe to be healthful to them. Americans spend
over a billion dollars yearly on megadose food supplements. Those least
likely to be able to afford them, the elderly, often are the ones most
likely to buy them.

Ironically, the same groups who seem to be most concerned about
the potential harm of relatively small amounts of additives in foods are
most willing to use potentially toxic-size doses of nutrient supplements.
After the Food and Drug Administration prohibited over-the-counter
sale of megadose vitamin A and D supplements because of their known
toxicity, members of Congress were deluged by protests from purveyors
and consumers of these products. Subsequently, Congress passed a law
rescinding this regulation and prohibiting the FDA from requiring that
megadoses of nutrients be sold only as prescription drugs.

The promoters of megadoses of nutrients make two general claims, neither of which has factual evidence to support it, but both of which appear to be valid to some consumers. First, large doses may promote optimal health and prevent specific diseases. Second, there is wide individual variability in the need for nutrients, and some people may need much greater quantities than the averages represented in the Recommended Dietary Allowances (RDA).

The first claim is unsupported by the facts of human metabolism and is contradicted by the reality that large doses of nutrients are toxic. Ingestion of large amounts of any one foodstuff or nutrient, especially in concentrated form, is potentially harmful, not healthful. Optimal health is promoted by eating a balanced diet containing a variety of foods.

The second claim is based on a false allegation that the RDA do not take into account the wide variation in individual needs. All of the RDA, except for calories, are deliberately set high enough to accommodate a wide range of normal human variability. Only about 5 percent of people fall outside of these norms. The bulk of the evidence from worldwide dietary studies shows that individual variability in nutrient needs is not particularly great. In addition, there is also individual variability in toxic reactions to nutrients, which can increase the hazard to an individual who uses large doses.

Unsubstantiated claims about how megadoses of specific nutrients can prevent or cure disease tend to be based on:

1. Animal studies where data are misinterpreted or misunderstood, where unwarranted extrapolation to humans is made, or where results are overextended far beyond what they really demonstrated.

2. Human studies consisting of too small a sample to provide statistically significant results. In some cases claims have been based on one individual's personal experience.

3. Human studies that are uncontrolled or poorly controlled so that other variables may have influenced the results.

Well-designed, controlled studies have the following characteristics:

*At least two large groups are studied, one receives the nutrient, the other receives a *placebo*. A placebo is an inert substance made up to look exactly like the test substance. Placebos are often given by doctors in lieu of medication simply to make the patient think he is receiving some treatment. Often the thinking that he is being treated helps him get well. Many testimonials about how a nutrient has "cured" a person can be attributed to the placebo effect.

*The study is *double blind*. Neither the researchers nor the subjects know whether the pill is a nutrient or a placebo. The purpose of this is to eliminate the placebo effect.

*Measurable ways of determining change are used—not just subjective ratings such as subject "feels better" or "looks better."

*Data are analyzed by groups before the blind is broken. The purpose of this is to eliminate bias or preconceived ideas held by researchers.

Another way in which scientific research is tested so that it will be accepted as valid by the scientific community is for other researchers to repeat the study and get similar results. When the results of studies cannot be repeated with the same results, the conclusions are weakened by the possibility of an error or fluke in the research.

Thus, when reading about reports of research results in the newspaper or in popular magazines and books, be careful not to jump to unwarranted conclusions (see Exhibit 20.8). Check to find out whether these results are considered valid by other knowledgeable professionals.

Unsubstantiated Nutrient Megadose Claims

With few exceptions, the claims made for the ability of megadoses of nutrients to prevent or cure disease have not been supported by research that is acceptable to the majority of health professionals. In some cases, preliminary results of research have shown promise, but more research is needed before claims can be substantiated. Some examples of unsubstantiated megadose nutrient claims follow.

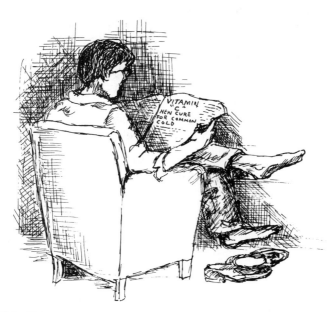

Exhibit 20.8. Newspaper headlines and articles in the popular press often present research information in a sensational way that may cause the reader to jump to unwarranted conclusions.

Vitamin C Prevents or Cures Colds. This has been a controversial subject among professionals for years, with some proponents believing that studies they or others have conducted do show that extremely large doses, 5 to 20 grams per day, of vitamin C can prevent colds.[4] However, a large proportion of health and nutrition professionals disagree, saying that no valid evidence exists to support these claims and that instead numerous studies show that vitamin C has no effect in keeping people from catching cold. They also point out the potential health hazards of using such extraordinarily large amounts of this nutrient.[5] There is some evidence that vitamin C acts as an antihistamine against cold symptoms, alleviating them to some degree. Opponents of use of vitamin C in treating colds point out that if this is the case, it would be cheaper, more effective, and probably safer to use one of the numerous antihistamines available for this purpose.[6]

Vitamin C Protects Against Heart Disease Resulting From Atherosclerosis. Some research has shown that vitamin C may have an effect on fat metabolism. In one study, vitamin C was found to help lower blood cholesterol levels in some groups, but not others; and in one case, it increased the cholesterol levels in patients who already had atherosclerosis.[7] Claims that vitamin C prevents atherosclerosis and heart disease are not warranted based on the limited evidence now available. More research is needed.

Vitamin E Prevents Male Impotence or Sterility and Abnormal Termination of Pregnancy. This idea developed as a result of animal studies that were incorrectly extrapolated to humans. On the basis of research results with humans over the past 35 years, leading scientific and medical opinion does not support this conclusion. Advocates of vitamin E supplementation in humans overlook the fact that an effect on reproduction in animals can be demonstrated only when the animals have been fed for long periods on *diets free of vitamin E.* The widespread presence of vitamin E in human diets prevents a deficiency such as seen in animals under experimental conditions from developing in man.

Vitamin E Prevents Heart Disease. In cattle and sheep severe heart muscle abnormalities that appear to be related to severe vitamin E deficiency have been observed. However, this effect has not been seen in

---

[4] L. Pauling, *Vitamin C and Common Cold and the Flu.* San Francisco, CA: W.H. Freeman and Co., 1976.

[5] R.E. Hodges, "Ascorbic Acid," in Nutrition Reviews' *Present Knowledge in Nutrition,* fourth edition. New York, Washington, D.C.: The Nutrition Foundation, Inc., 1976, pp. 119-30.

[8] T.W. Anderson, "New Horizons for Vitamin C." *Nutrition Today,* Vol. 12, No. 1, January-February, 1977, pp. 6-13.

[7] R.E. Hodges, "Ascorbic Acid," in Nutrition Reviews' *Present Knowledge in Nutrition,* fourth edition. New York, Washington, D.C.: The Nutrition Foundation, Inc., 1976, pp. 119-30.

animals more similar to humans such as monkeys. There is no scientific evidence that heart disease is a consequence of vitamin E deficiency, and to date extensive tests have failed to demonstrate that large amounts of vitamin E will prevent coronary heart disease.

Vitamin E Prevents or Slows Aging Process. This theory is based on the laboratory finding that vitamin E acts as an antioxidant, slowing the destruction of the fats in animal cells. This theory also holds that when diets are high in polyunsaturated fats more vitamin E is required. No animal or human studies show that animals live longer if they are given therapeutic doses of vitamin E, however. And while the idea that a diet high in polyunsaturated fats requires more vitamin E is thought to have some validity, nutritionists point out that a high polyunsaturated-fat diet is naturally higher in vitamin E since this nutrient is a natural component of vegetable oils, so supplements are not called for.

Megavitamins are Useful in Treating Psychiatric Ills. The first application of this theory was a treatment for schizophrenia using massive doses (3 grams per day) of niacin. Later, the treatment was expanded and termed *orthomolecular.* Large doses of niacin, pyridoxine, vitamin C, other water-soluble vitamins, and trace metals were used along with an antihypoglycemic diet, plus, when needed, electroconvulsive therapy and conventional psychiatric drugs. In such uncontrolled studies it was difficult to attribute any observed improvement to any one or any combinations of treatment. One investigator claimed to have observed significant benefit in a modest fraction of schizophrenics treated with megadoses of B vitamins, particularly niacin. But other investigators in numerous trials have failed to substantiate these findings.[8] The view held by all but a small proportion of health professionals is that presently there is no scientific basis for routine application of megavitamin therapy in psychiatric treatment.

Megadoses of Niacin Prolong Life of People With Coronary Heart Disease. In this treatment massive doses (3 grams per day) of niacin are used for the purpose of lowering blood cholesterol and lipoproteins. In a Coronary Drug Research project involving 1,119 subjects, a double blind test showed there was no evidence that niacin helped reduce total mortality.[9] While there was some evidence that niacin reduced the incidence of nonfatal myocardial infarction, balancing this were potential hazards: niacin-treated subjects showed increased incidence of atrial fibrillation and other arrhythmias; gastrointestinal problems; elevated serum enzymes, uric acid, and plasma glucose; and a greater risk of gouty arthri-

---

[8] D.B. McCormick, "B Vitamins and Schizophrenia." *Nutrition and the M.D.,* Vol. 3, No. 3, January, 1977, p. 1

[9] W.J. Darby, K.W. McNutt, E. N. Todhunter, "Niacin," in Nutrition Reviews' *Present Knowledge in Nutrition,* fourth edition. New York, Washington, D.C.: The Nutrition Foundation, Inc., 1976, pp. 168-70.

tis. Because the long-term effect of large doses of niacin is not known, current recommendations are that this treatment be used with great care and caution.

Hazards of Using Nutrients as Drugs

One of the major reasons why many health professionals object to the use of megadoses of nutrients is their potential toxic effect on the body. For some nutrients, such as the fat-soluble vitamins A and D, toxicity is well documented. For other nutrients, such as vitamin C and E, the belief has been that they are relatively harmless, even when used in large amounts. More recently, however, evidence is accumulating that suggests caution is needed when using even these apparently harmless nutrients in amounts well above the Recommended Dietary Allowances.

For example, it has been found that vitamin C in doses above 2 to 4 grams may induce kidney problems and the development of kidney stones, especially in susceptible males; may reverse the effect of anticoagulants that a person might be taking to prevent blood clots; may cause a false result in tests for diabetes and internal bleeding; and may increase the body's need for vitamin C and result in temporary *rebound scurvey*, a hazard to infants born to women who take large doses of vitamin C during pregnancy. One researcher found that continual massive doses of vitamin C appear to alter the vitamin C regulating system of the body, causing the buildup of an enzyme that speeds up the breakdown and excretion of the vitamin in the urine. As a result, the heavy vitamin C user may have a lower amount of vitamin C in his blood than someone who gets the normal RDA (60 milligrams), or the "saturation amount" (about 150 milligrams), a day. When the person stops taking the large amount of vitamin C, he can develop vitamin C deficiency within days or weeks. He may then be more susceptible to infection and develop temporary symptoms of deficiency—scurvy, bleeding gums, loose teeth, muscle pain, and rough skin.[10] Gradual withdrawal from large doses might help to prevent this condition.

Often the rationale used by people who take extra large doses of vitamins is that if a small amount is good for them, then a larger amount must be even better. However, when megadoses of nutrients are taken, which have a drug effect not a nutrient effect, then the elementary principle of pharmacology should be recognized: Increasing the dosage of a therapeutic compound leads to maximum effectiveness and a further increase leads to the production of toxic effects.

[10] V.D. Herbert, "Megavitamin Therapy." *Contemporary Nutrition*, Vol. 2, No. 10, October, 1977.

Americans are on a vitamin binge! We spend over $1.2 billion a year for vitamins and the amount is growing about 10 percent annually.[11] "Supernutrition" appears to be the goal of some vitamin fans; others use them because they are afraid their snack-food, fast-food, fabricated-food diets are deficient in these essential nutrients.

Because vitamins work in partnership with each other and with other nutrients in performing their functions in the body, the best way for us to get them in proper balance is to eat a wide variety of foods. Money spent on high-nutrient-density foods in the Four Food Groups can provide us with better nutrition than money spent on expensive vitamin supplements.

About a billion dollars worth of the vitamins sold directly to consumers are synthetic, that is, chemically formulated. The remainder are so-called "natural vitamins," extracted from foods, that often sell for double the price of synthetic vitamins.[12]

The Food and Drug Administration regulates the manufacture and labeling of vitamin and mineral supplements. All such products must meet the minimum standards set by law and must be accurately labeled with a list of nutrients by quantity and percentage of the RDA.

Every synthetic vitamin, by law, must have exactly the same chemical formula as its natural counterpart. And our bodies use either the natural or synthetic form equally well. In spite of this, many pill-takers insist that natural is better and are willing to pay the premium price for it. Often the product with a natural-sounding name (for example, "vitamin C with rose hips") consists mainly of synthetic vitamin with only a small amount of the more costly natural vitamin. Determination of ingredients may be made by reading the label.

Competition among the sellers of vitamins is intense, and many use major advertising campaigns to convince consumers that their products are superior and, therefore, worth a higher price. But are the differences real? It's unlikely, because 60 to 70 percent of all the vitamins sold in the United States are manufactured by one company.[13]

All together in the entire free world there are fewer than 30 producers of vitamins. No one company makes every vitamin, and each of the major vitamins is made by only a few companies.[14] Bulk vitamins

[11] H. Seneker, "Body Building at Hoffman-La Roche." *Forbes*, Vol. 123, No. 3, February 5, 1979, pp. 92-4.

[12] *Ibid.*

[13] *Ibid.*

[14] *Ibid.*

Exhibit 20.9.   Nutrient Supplements May be Needed by Certain People

Pregnant and lactating women
Children or teenagers who eat poorly balanced meals
Elderly persons with limited diets
People who eat out most of the time
People who are recovering from surgery, serious burns, or
    injuries
People with malfunctioning digestive systems or allergies

are purchased from manufacturers and packaged for consumer consumption under many labels.

What use is this information to consumers? It tells you that the only real difference between one brand of vitamin and another is the size of the dose and that you can save money by buying the least expensive vitamin sold in the dose you need.

Another way to save money is to buy vitamins only if you really need them, rather than using them as an insurance policy just in case your diet is inadequate. If your diet is inadequate, the nutrient supplements you use may not be the ones you need, so you may be buying a false sense of security if you buy vitamins.

On the other hand, vitamin and mineral deficiencies do exist, and some people may need to take supplements (see Exhibit 20.9). The groups most likely to need supplements are: children and teenagers who eat poorly balanced diets; elderly people who may have increased needs and inadequate diets; people who eat most of their meals in restaurants or institutions where foods are kept hot in steam tables and vitamins are likely to be lost through prolonged exposure to heat, light, and air; people who are recovering from surgery and other trauma such as serious burns; pregnant and lactating women; and people with allergies and malfunctioning digestive systems.

In cases where nutrient supplements do appear to be needed, products supplying moderate amounts, i.e, similar to the Recommended Dietary Allowances, are generally the safest choice. Larger megadoses should not be self-prescribed, but should be used only on the advice of a physician.

Some vitamins lose potency over time. Air (oxygen, that is), light, heat—all can destroy them. So supplements should be stored in a cool, dark place and should not be kept for a long period of time.

Protein Supplements

Another popular nutrient supplement is protein, marketed in tablet, powder, and liquid form. According to a 1979 report of the Federal Trade Commission (FTC), retail sales of protein supplements totaled an estimated $100 million in 1974 and have increased dramatically since then. The FTC attributed the increase in popularity of protein supplements to the growing interest in health foods and to the misleading advertising and labeling of these products, including claims that protein supplements will provide benefits such as weight reduction, good health, and improved athletic performance.[15]

From discussions in previous chapters we learned that: (1) very little protein is stored in the body and the excess is metabolized for energy or converted to body fat; (2) protein is not a nutrient that is likely to be lacking in the American diet; (3) exercise, not extra protein, builds strong muscles, so that athletes need more calories and proportionately more of all nutrients rather than protein supplements; (4) liquid protein diets have been found to be hazardous in weight control regimens. Thus, the evidence does not support the health claims made by the purveyors of protein supplements. An additional concern is that protein supplements may be hazardous to some, especially infants and persons suffering from severe liver or kidney problems.

For these reasons, the FTC staff report suggested that the Commission establish a trade regulation that would "ban deceptive and unfair claims about the need for and benefits from protein and require advertisers for these products to disclose appropriate health warnings." Their suggested warning was: "Do not use for infants under one year of age. Do not use without checking with your doctor if you have severe liver of kidney trouble." Their suggested disclosure was: "A fact you should know—very few Americans need extra protein. Almost all of us get all we need from the food we eat."[16]

The FTC report also suggested that labels disclose the percentage of protein in the product. If this information was on the label, consumers, with the help of a food composition table, could compare the amount and cost of the protein in the supplement with that available from a good and low-cost food source, such as nonfat dry milk. (Often the supplements are made from dry milk.) By making such a comparison, consumers would learn that protein supplements are a costly way to buy protein compared to buying it in food.

Summary

Americans use and overuse drugs of all types: prescription and over-the-counter medications, alcohol, "hard" drugs, and even nutrients—especially vitamins. Drugs can cause nutritional deficiencies, reduce absorption of nutrients, and even interfere with metabolism. Oral contraceptives, for instance, are hormones that affect numerous metabolic processes and may produce deficiencies of several B vitamins. Food itself can affect drug action, intensifying or decreasing it and sometimes causing dangerous reactions.

[15] Federal Trade Commission, "Protein Supplements May be Dangerous for Some, Unnecessary for Many More, Warns FTC Report." *FTC News Summary*. Washington, D.C.: Federal Trade Commission, July 24, 1979, pp. 1-2.

[16] *Ibid*.

Alcohol is the most commonly used drug. Its use may lead to serious nutritional deficiencies, be toxic to the liver, or increase the synthesis of triglycerides. Alcohol has been implicated in many physical ailments and accidents, and in combination with smoking, it can be quite damaging. Pregnant women should be wary about the toxic effects of alcohol on the developing fetus. In moderate amounts, alcohol may have some beneficial effects in the relief of stress.

Megadoses of vitamins may act as drugs. However, many false and unsubstantiated claims are made as to the extent of their therapeutic value. Labels on nutrient supplements are monitored by the Food and Drug Administration and must state accurate information. The Federal Trade Commission attempts to prevent false claims in advertising, but it can't always keep up with actual practice. There is little evidence to support the claims for the beneficial effects resulting from the consumption of large amounts of any one foodstuff or nutrient, and there are many reasons to be concerned about the potential harm or toxicity that may result.

Misinformation may result from misinterpreted or poorly controlled studies. Characteristics of a well-designed study are: at least two large groups are used; an experimental and a control dose are administered; the study is double blind; and data are measured and analyzed objectively. To be accepted as valid, other researchers should be able to repeat the study with similar results.

When vitamin and mineral supplements are needed, they should not be taken in amounts larger than the RDA except on the advice of a physician. Vitamins derived from food sources are as effective as those synthesized in the laboratory. Protein supplements are rarely needed and are a costly way to obtain protein.

Part VI

NUTRIENTS: ARE THEY THERE WHEN WE EAT THE FOOD?

VARIABLES AFFECTING NUTRIENTS IN FOOD 21

Highlights

Origin and accuracy of food composition tables and labeling data

Influence of genetics and growing conditions on nutrient content

Effect of depleted soil and organic fertilizer on nutrient content

Bioavailability of nutrients

Effects of harvesting, storage, and food processing methods on nutrient levels

"**N**o two alike." This phrase is often used to describe the infinite number of differences between people. It could also be applied to foods because so many variables affect the nutritional value of each food.

This makes our nutrition challenge much greater than simply selecting a variety of foods from the different food groups. We also need to be concerned with the way the food has been grown and handled, from the farm until we eat it. And, if we are trying to make some sort of estimate of our consumption of particular nutrients based on a record of the foods we eat, we also must be aware of the unreliability of food composition tables.

FACTORS THAT AFFECT NUTRIENT AVAILABILITY

Because of the many variables affecting the nutrient content of foods, food composition tables can only represent estimates, averages, or midpoints of ranges. So we need to use food composition statistics as guidelines, with a certain amount of skepticism, not as ultimate truth. Compiling all the data used in food composition tables is a vast undertaking. The first such tables were developed for U.S. foods in the late 1890s by W.O. Atwater, a pioneer nutrition scientist. The tables have been updated and reissued at intervals, primarily by the U.S. Department of Agriculture, in a publication known as *Agriculture Handbook No. 8—Composition of Foods: Raw, Processed, and Prepared.*[1] The food composition table in the Appendix is derived from the USDA data.

Continuing changes in varieties of foods grown, processing methods, and analysis methods, and in the development of new foods and new knowledge of nutrition, make it difficult to provide up-to-date data. Another problem is in producing reliable nationwide, year-round values.

Manufacturers who provide nutrition labels must use information based on a laboratory analysis of each food labeled. Therefore, label data are likely to be more current than, and may be different from, those found in published food composition tables. As noted in Chapter 3, values listed on labels allow a wide margin for variation among foods.

Genetics and Growing Conditions

The nutrient content of plant foods is greatly affected by the plant's genetic makeup, which is determined by its species and variety, as well as by the area of origin, stage of maturity when harvested and

---

[1] B.K. Watt and A.L. Merrill, *Composition of Foods: Raw, Processed, Prepared.* Agriculture Handbook No. 8, U.S. Department of Agriculture. Washington, D.C.: U.S. Government Printing Office, 1963.

Exhibit 21.1. Factors That Affect Nutrients in Food

	PLANTS	ANIMALS
Genetic makeup	Species Variety	Species Breed
Maturity	Ripeness	Age
Growing conditions	Soil Water Temperature Sunlight	Kind of feed
How food is handled	During harvesting, processing, shipping, storage	During processing

when eaten, and growing conditions. Factors such as temperature, amount of sunlight, amount of water, and type of soil and its fertility all can influence how well a plant grows and how nutritious it will be (see Exhibit 21.1).

Carrots, for example, have a range of vitamin A values of 2,200 to 47,000 International Units (IU) per 100 grams, depending on variety and stage of maturity. Potatoes can range in vitamin C content from 10 milligrams per 100 grams to 50 milligrams per 100 grams depending on variety and storage time. With oranges, the vitamin C value is related to area of origin, variety, and time of harvest. It decreases as the season progresses and the oranges become more mature. Through breeding, a variety of corn has been developed that is higher in the amino acid lysine, which is usually low in corn.

Nutrients in animal foods, while less variable than those in plants, are affected by the breed and age of the animal and the type of feed. In one experiment, for example, beef cattle were produced, using special feed, that had fat with higher levels of polyunsaturated fatty acids than ordinary beef. With milk, the protein and fat content varies with the breed and feed of the dairy cow. Vitamin A value in eggs changes with the hen's diet, and so forth.

For many years, " health food" proponents have claimed that our foods lack important nutrients because they have been grown on "depleted soils" or because they have been fertilized with "chemical" fertilizers instead of "organic" fertilizers such as manure. But agricultural research shows that there is little validity in this notion, and the only nutrients that may be affected by these factors are a few trace minerals.[2]

Studies show that plants grown on fertile soil produce more protein per acre—a higher yield—but the quality and quantity of protein

[2] Statement of the Food and Nutrition Board, National Research Council, "Soil Fertility and the Nutritive Value of Crops," *Journal of the American Dietetic Association*, Vol. 70, 1977, p. 469.

produced with any level of soil fertility is governed by plant genetics. Soil fertility has not been shown to be a determining factor in the level of vitamins in crops. Trace minerals in plants, however, may be affected by the presence of these minerals in the soil.

Most plants need only iron, copper, manganese, zinc, molybdenum, and boron for growth. When these minerals are lacking in the soil, the plant will not grow normally and a poor yield will result; but plants that are produced will not lack the normal complement of nutrients.

Plants can absorb trace elements they don't need from the soil, such as iodine, fluorine, cobalt, selenium, chromium, sodium, and chlorine, and later can serve as sources of these nutrients to humans who eat them. The level of these trace minerals can be influenced to some extent by their level in the soil. Thus, for example, foods grown in areas where the soil is lacking in iodine will be a poor source of iodine. However, foods lacking these trace elements could not be accurately described as nonnutritious.

Studies of the effects of organic and inorganic (chemical) fertilizers have failed to show any consistent difference in nutritive quality of the food. Results of a 10-year research program at the Michigan Experiment Station, a 25-year program at the U.S. Plant, Soil, and Nutrition Laboratory in Ithaca, N.Y., and a 34-year study on an experimental research farm in England showed that organically grown foods are identical in nutrition to those grown by conventional methods using inorganic chemicals.[3]

Plants require certain nutrients in the elemental form. These elements are absorbed by the plant as *inorganic* ions that move from soil water through plant roots into plant tissues. When plants are fertilized with organic fertilizers, such as manure, soil bacteria must first break the organic material down into the inorganic elements before the plant can absorb them. For this reason, chemical fertilizers fertilize plants more quickly and efficiently than organic fertilizers. And plants use the elements equally well regardless of whether they come from organic or inorganic fertilizers. Thus the idea that we will be better nourished if we eat organically fertilized foods has no scientific basis.

Bioavailability of Nutrients

Another variable that affects the nutritional value of a particular food is the *bioavailability* of its nutrients, that is, to what extent we can utilize the nutrients it contains. Because a laboratory analysis tells us

---

[3] Institute of Food Technologists' Expert Panel on Food Safety and Nutrition and the Committee on Public Information, *Organic Foods*, A Scientific Status Summary. Chicago, IL: Institute of Food Technologists, January, 1974.

that a food contains specific nutrients does not mean those nutrients are present in a form that is available to our bodies.

Many vitamins, for example, are present naturally in foods in "bound" forms, and scientists do not know for sure how effectively we can use each of these "bound" vitamins. Folic acid, as an example, is often found in food in complex compounds that must be reduced by intestinal enzymes to simpler forms before we can use the acid. It is thought that the degree to which intestinal enzymes can make folic acid available depends on the particular bound form that is present in a food.

Minerals, too, often are found in foods in forms that may adversely affect our ability to use them. In general, minerals from plant sources are less available than minerals from animal sources. For example, iron from meat (heme iron) is better absorbed than iron from nonmeat sources (nonheme iron), and in addition, the presence of heme iron significantly increases the absorption of nonheme iron in a mixed diet. Various plant compounds such as oxalic acid and phytic acid (see Chapter 23) in leafy vegetables, legumes, and cereals bind materials and inhibit their absorption.

Minerals and other nutrients also interact and affect each other's bioavailability. For example, when iron and vitamin C are present together, we absorb iron better, perhaps because vitamin C can reduce iron to a more available, ferrous form. When zinc intake is increased, our absorption of copper is decreased; on the other hand, increased calcium intake will reduce our intake of zinc, copper, and other trace minerals.

Very little is known about these nutrient interactions. But what is known points to our need to consume a mixed diet with *moderate amounts* of a *variety of foods* to obtain the best potential "mix" of nutrient interactions and to avoid potentially detrimental nutrient excesses.

How Food Is Handled

Everything that happens to a food from the time it is picked until the time it is eaten can have an effect on the nutrients it contains (see Exhibit 21.2). The most nutritious food would be one that we grew ourselves and ate within hours after picking. But few people can eat this way the year around. Often our food must be preserved, shipped, and stored for some time before it is purchased. We must rely on many people to do a good job of handling it.

The moment a plant is harvested, it begins to change nutritionally. For example, the sugar in freshly picked sweet corn will begin to turn to starch immediately, and the warmer the temperature, the faster the change occurs. Thus, harvest methods are important for some foods. Those foods that are moved quickly from a hot field into a cold environment or a processing plant will retain more nutritional value and quality.

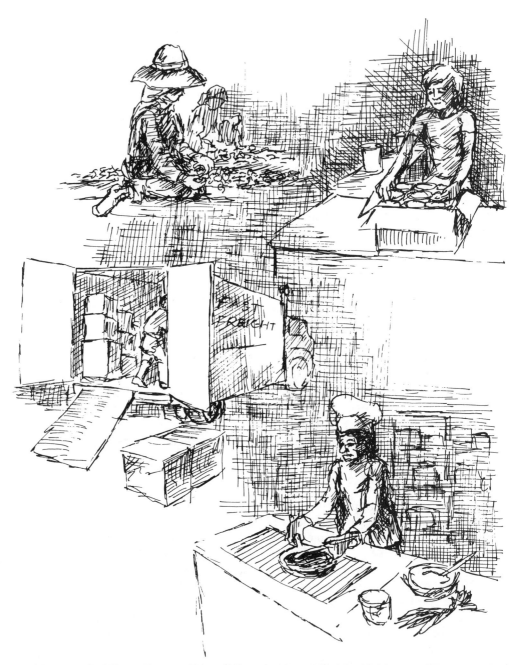

Exhibit 21.2. The way a food is handled from field to consumer affects its nutritional value.

The best tasting sweet corn, for example, results when farmers chill it, right in the field, after it has been picked.

Processing methods affect nutrients too. When conditions are well controlled, the resulting food will be high in nutrients; poor handling can have the opposite effect. Some preservation methods, such as sun drying, result in greater loss of nutrients than other methods. The kind of packaging used also can affect nutrients; for example, milk stored in an opaque carton will retain more riboflavin than that stored in glass because riboflavin is destroyed by the light that passes through glass. For some foods, keeping moisture out can be a factor in nutrient retention.

Once the food is prepared for fresh market or processed and packaged, it must be shipped and stored. There are then new opportunities for nutrient loss.

As an example, a major problem to the frozen food industry has been incorrect handling of products in transit, in warehouses, and in supermarkets. A frozen food, high in quality and nutrients as it leaves the processing plant, may have lost quality and nutrients by the time it reaches consumers if it is not held at all times at temperatures of zero degrees or colder. Somewhere en route the food may be allowed to stand on a warm shipping dock, be shipped in a truck or railroad car with insufficient refrigeration, or be held in a warehouse or supermarket freezer with inadequate temperature control.

Another variable is what happens to the food after it is bought. If groceries are kept in a hot car for an hour or two, quality and nutrients can be lost before the food even arrives home. And then, what about home storage? Are canned goods stored in a cool place? Does the freezer hold foods at zero degrees? And do we use foods, both fresh and processed, before they get old and have lost nutrients?

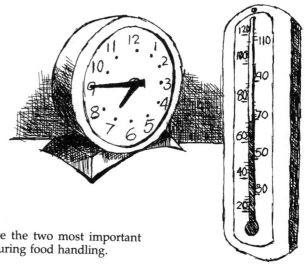

Exhibit 21.3. Time and temperature are the two most important variables that affect nutrients in foods during food handling.

Throughout the entire food shipping and storage cycle, the most important factors affecting nutrients are time and temperature (see Exhibit 21.3). The warmer the storage conditions, the faster and greater the loss of nutrients. The longer it takes for a food, fresh or processed, to reach the mouth of the consumer, the greater the likelihood of nutrient loss.

Summary

Food composition tables are based upon the analysis of foods, but they only represent estimates, since actual nutrient content can be influenced by an array of factors from plant varieties to food handling and preparation.

The nutrient content of plant foods is affected by genetic makeup, maturity, and growing conditions. Nutrients in animal foods tend to be less variable; they are influenced by breed, age of animal, and type of feed. Soil fertility does not significantly affect vitamin level in crops, although content of trace minerals may be modified. Studies show that organically grown foods are nutritionally identical to inorganically fertilized foods.

The bioavailability of nutrients in a particular food refers to the extent to which the nutrients can be readily used by our body, and it depends on the form in which the nutrients are present in that particular food. Minerals and other nutrients may interact and affect each other's bioavailability. It is recommended we consume a mixed diet with moderate amounts of a variety of foods in order to obtain maximum bioavailability and avoid potentially detrimental nutrient concentrations.

Harvesting, storage, and processing methods also affect nutrients. Time and temperature are key factors here. Cool conditions and short storage time generally lead to better nutrient retention.

LOSS AND RETENTION OF NUTRIENTS IN FOOD 22

Highlights

Mechanical separation and leaching losses, and effect of enzymatic action

Oxidation and nutrient destruction by light and heat

Influence of acids, alkalies, and other chemicals on nutrients

Drying methods

Factors affecting availability of each of the nutrients

Guidelines for retaining nutrients in foods during home preparation

Supermarket Nutrition: Fresh vs. Processed Foods

The pitfalls in making the assumption that we actually *know* the nutritional values of the foods we eat are obvious from the brief review in Chapter 21 of how nutrients are affected by genetics, growing conditions, and handling. Now let us look more closely at some of the ways nutrients are lost from food (see Exhibit 22.1).

Mechanical Separation and Leaching

Mechanical separation and leaching of nutrients from food is commonly seen in both commercial processing and home food preparation. Severe processing, where any part of the food is discarded, will cause a loss of protein, fat, carbohydrate, vitamins, and minerals and is particularly detrimental to trace minerals.

The milling of grain where the nutrient-rich bran and germ are separated from the nutrient-poor endosperm (white portion) results in a loss of protein, fiber, vitamins, fat, and minerals, especially trace minerals (see Chapter 7). When whey is separated from milk solids in cheesemaking, sugar, soluble proteins, minerals, and water-soluble vitamins are lost.

In home food preparation, trimming the more nutritious green leafy tops from root vegetables, such as beets, results in a major loss of nutrients. Peeling vegetables and fruits, for example removing skins from potatoes, is another way nutrients are lost mechanically. Chopping, shredding, and grating of salad vegetables causes a substantial loss of vitamin C because nutrient destructive enzymes are released from the tissues. Food tables do not reflect this loss. Juicing of vegeta-

Exhibit 22.1.   Summary of the Ways Nutrients are Lost From Foods

Mechanical
    Separation—Milling of grain
                  Removing whey or fat from milk solids
                  Trimming and peeling of fruits and vegetables
                  Juicing fruits or vegetables
    Leaching—Washing
             Soaking
             Cooking in water
Enzymatic Action
Oxidation—Increased by light and heat
Heat
Action of acids and alkalis
Action of other chemicals—Trace metals
                              Oxalates, phytates
                              Enzyme inhibitors
Removal of moisture

bles can cause the loss of vitamins C and A and calcium and phosphorus.

Water-soluble vitamins and minerals are lost in large quantities when vegetables are washed, soaked, and cooked in water and the cooking water is poured off. Starch may also be leached from vegetables such as potatoes when they are peeled and cut up for cooking. In canned vegetables and fruits, about one-third of the water-soluble vitamins and minerals will be dissolved in the liquid in the can and lost if this liquid is not consumed.

When meats are cooked, minerals and vitamins are lost as meat juices drain out, and fat and fat-soluble vitamins are lost as fat melts and drips out. The longer the cooking process, the greater the leaching of nutrients in drippings. If drippings are used, for example, in gravy, some of the nutrients will be recovered.

Enzymatic Action

Fresh fruits and vegetables are still alive, continue to respire after harvest, and their natural aging process continues. As they age, chemical reactions take place that change their nutritional composition. For example, fresh produce tends to become soft, and vitamin C and other nutrients are depleted. The warmer the temperature, the more rapid the changes.

Enzymes, which are organic catalysts produced inside living cells, are responsible for many of the changes that take place during aging. Enzymes enable cells to carry out life processes by accelerating chemical changes while not being changed themselves. They act in very small quantities and sometimes require the presence of other enzymes, called *coenzymes*. They are inactivated by heat, which breaks down their protein; but warm, not hot, temperatures increase their activity. Thus, there may be a temporary rapid increase in enzyme activity while a food is being heated to the temperature where enzymes are inactivated.

Low temperatures slow down but do not deactivate enzymes. So frozen vegetables slowly develop symptoms of aging, and nutrients such as vitamin C are oxidized unless enzymes are destroyed by blanching before the food is frozen. (Blanching is a brief heat treatment in hot water or steam.) When fruits are frozen, added sugar helps prevent enzyme action, so sugared fruits may be higher in nutrients than those frozen without sugar. The heat used in processing canned fruits and vegetables destroys enzymes.

Oxidation

The principal chemical change that takes place in many foods as they age is oxidation. In fresh fruits and vegetables, enzymes are the catalysts for this chemical reaction, which causes a loss of vitamins such as A, C, B_{12}, thiamin, and folic acid. When oxygen is removed from the air, oxidative changes are prevented or greatly reduced. Thus, fresh produce is sometimes stored in a *controlled atmosphere,* where inert gases such as carbon dioxide or nitrogen are introduced to take the place of oxygen. Canning and vacuum packaging prevent oxidation because air is removed.

In fats and oils, including meat fat, oxidation of unsaturated fats causes the development of rancidity and the production of toxic substances that destroy fat-soluble vitamins such as A, E, and D. To prevent this oxidation, foods such as nuts and peanut butter may be vacuum packed, and shortening and oil or oil-containing foods may have antioxidants such as BHA or BHT added (see Chapter 24). The more saturated a fat is, the more stable it is; so products high in saturated fat, coconut oil, for example, will not turn rancid readily.

Oxidation of fats also takes place when foods are frozen. The rancid odor and flavor that develops in frozen meats, poultry, and fish are a signal that the fats have oxidized. Pork and fish fat are particularly prone to oxidation, so freezer storage time of 3 to 6 months only is recommended for them, while beef and poultry can be stored 8 to 12 months before fats oxidize.

Light

Light catalyzes or accelerates the oxidation process, which leads to the breakdown of polyunsaturated fats and some vitamins. The light-sensitive vitamins are riboflavin, B_{12}, B_6, A, C, K, and D. Riboflavin and vitamin C are particularly sensitive to light. For example, if milk is allowed to stand out in the light, 50 to 70 percent of the riboflavin can be lost in just two hours.[1] As mentioned earlier, packaging materials that keep out light, such as opaque cartons for milk and brown or opaque bottles for oils and vitamin supplements, help protect light-sensitive nutrients from oxidation.

Heat

Temperature and oxidation are closely related, since heat speeds up the rate of oxidation and cold slows it down. In addition, heat degrades nutrients, causing substances such as fats and proteins to decompose. Many vitamins are destroyed by heat. The most heat-sensitive vitamins are C and thiamin, followed by vitamin A. Other vitamins that can be destroyed by heat are A, D, E, B_6, riboflavin, and folic acid. Minerals are not notably affected by heat.

The higher the temperature, the greater the nutrient destruction. For example, thiamin loss in pork roasted at 300°F is 36 percent, com-

[1]L.J. Bogert, G.M. Briggs, and D.H. Calloway, *Nutrition and Physical Fitness.* Philadelphia, PA: W.B. Saunders Company, 1966, p. 248.

pared to a 46 percent loss when the roasting temperature is 450°F.[2] The high heat used in toasting cereals and canning and drying milk causes changes in protein. During heating, amino acids and carbohydrate react, making a portion of the amino acids, lysine especially, unavailable for their essential functions. High heat in frying can cause fats to decompose and fat-soluble vitamins to be destroyed. Smoking is a sign that this decomposition is taking place.

The time that a food is exposed to heat also affects nutrient loss. The longer the food is exposed, the greater the nutrient loss. Thus, a quick-cooking method such as frying results in an 11 percent thiamin loss in meat, compared to a 60 percent loss in a long, slow-cooking process such as braising.[3] However, in this case, 20 percent of the thiamin loss remains in the drippings, which also increase with a long-cooking process.

When foods are canned, a heat treatment is always required with the temperature and time used dependent on the food being canned. Acid foods such as fruit can be processed at boiling water temperatures, while nonacid foods require pressure canning at temperatures well above boiling. Nutrients are destroyed during the heat processing of canned foods. For example, 50 percent of the vitamin C may be lost in a canned vegetable. Home-canned foods suffer more loss of nutrients than commercially canned because the recommendations for processing times are longer to allow a wide margin for safety.

However, once foods are canned, changes in nutrients take place slowly—unless the canned food is stored in a warm place. Thus, canned green beans stored at room temperature (70°F) will lose 10 percent of their vitamin C in 8 to 9 months, but if they are stored at 100°F, they will lose the same amount of vitamin C in only 2 to 5 months.[4]

Heating can improve the digestibility of some nutrients, however. For example, cooking improves the digestibility of the starch in potatoes, legumes, and cereals, and it destroys the antidigestive factor in legumes (see Chapter 23).

While heat speeds up loss of nutrients, cold temperatures help protect against that loss by slowing down chemical reactions. Thus, as pointed out in Chapter 12, fresh fruits and vegetables maintain higher nutrient content for a longer time when stored in cold temperatures. Frozen foods will have the highest overall nutritional quality of any processed food if they are consumed within the shelf-life period. The lower the freezer temperature, the longer the storage time and the higher the nutrient retention.

However, the loss of vitamin C can be faster in frozen foods than in canned foods, even at a zero-degree storage temperature, because

[2]R.M. Griswold, *The Experimental Study of Food.* Boston, MA: Houghton Mifflin Company, 1962, p. 137.

[3]*Ibid.*, p. 138.

[4]T.P. Labuza, *Food and Your Well-Being.* St. Paul, MN: West Publishing Co., 1977, pp. 328-29.

oxygen is present in frozen foods, while it is not present in canned foods. Thus, during the 6 to 9 month shelf life of frozen green beans, 30 to 45 percent of the vitamin C will be oxidized.[5]

Acidity-Aklalinity

The acidity or alkalinity of a food can have an effect on nutrients. Some nutrients, such as vitamins A, D, and folacin, are destroyed in acid solutions; others, such as vitamins C, D, riboflavin, and thiamin, are sensitive to alkalies; and others, such as vitamin C and thiamin, are also vulnerable in neutral foods and are protected by acids. Food preservation methods that rely on acids, such as fermentation of milk and pickling, help preserve some of the nutrients but lead to the destruction of others.

The use of alkaline materials such as lye for peeling fruit (for example, peaches and tomatoes) can have a detrimental effect on vitamin C and thiamin. The practice of adding a pinch of baking soda to water when cooking vegetables to retain the green color can result in loss of the alkaline-sensitive nutrients, vitamin C, thiamin, and riboflavin. On the other hand, the use of a bit of acid, such as lemon juice or cream of tartar, when cooking cauliflower to help keep it white, can have a beneficial effect on these nutrients.

When acid and heat are used in combination, for example, in making gelatin from animal by-products, the amino acid tryptophan is completely degraded and other amino acids also may be damaged. On the other hand, the acid cooking of meat can add calcium since the acid dissolves some of the calcium from the bones.

Acid foods such as tomatoes or spaghetti sauce, when cooked for a long time in iron utensils, will dissolve some of the iron from the utensil and be higher in this nutrient as a result.

Chemicals

Other compounds present in foods can cause the loss of nutrients in various ways. The effect of natural toxicants such as oxalates, phytates, enzyme inhibitors, and antivitamins on nutrients is discussed in Chapter 23. In polyunsaturated oils, trace metals will act as catalysts to speed up the oxidation process. To prevent this, chelating additives are used to tie up these metals and inactivate them. On the other hand, some compounds present in food can help protect nutrients. For example, sulfur dioxide produced when fruits are "sulfured" to keep the color from darkening when they are dried protects vitamins A and C from loss through oxidation.

[5]*Ibid.*, p. 330.

Drying

The removal of moisture from food for the purpose of preservation can destroy many of the nutrients, particularly vitamin C, thiamin, and vitamin A. Protein is not greatly affected by drying unless sugar is present. The amount of nutrient loss depends on the process, with the greatest loss resulting when food is dried in the presence of sunlight and oxygen and at high temperatures.

The largest loss of nutrients takes place when food is sun dried because it takes such a long time, and because sunlight catalyzes oxidation. Half or more of the vitamin C may be lost from fruits during sun drying, for example. The smallest loss of nutrients occurs during freeze drying because of the low temperature of the food. In this process, food is first frozen (very quickly using liquid nitrogen), then dehydrated. As little as 1 percent of the vitamin C in fruit or 5 percent of the thiamin in pork may be lost in freeze drying. The product retains, in addition to nutrients, its original size and shape and more of its natural flavor and color when freeze dried. However, the process is very costly compared to other drying methods.

Spray drying is another method that results in nutrient retention. In this process, which is used only for liquids such as milk, the food is dried to a very fine spray at a high temperature in just a few seconds.

In tray and tunnel drying, water is evaporated from food in 6 to 18 hours using hot air. The nutrient loss, 10 to 20 percent, is less than that in sun drying, but higher than that in spray drying and freeze drying.

Nutrient loss continues in dried foods during storage, and is affected by the water content of the food and the storage temperature. The greater the water content, the faster the nutrient loss. For example a powdered orange juice with 1 percent moisture might lose only 5 percent of its vitamin C in 9 months, compared to a 50 percent vitamin C loss in a week if its moisture content is 4 percent.[6] Therefore, a moisture-proof package or storage container for dried food is important to retain nutrients as well as to preserve the food.

The higher the storage temperature of dried foods, the faster the nutrient loss. For example, dried mashed potatoes will lose 25 percent of their vitamin C in 3 months if stored at 60°F, in less than 2 months at 70°F, and in zero months at 80° F.[7] This means dried foods should be stored in a cool as well as a dry place.

Dried vegetables lose carotene (pro-vitamin A) very rapidly during storage unless they are stored at a very cold temperature or are packaged in an airtight container filled with an inert gas such as carbon dioxide.

[6]*Ibid.*
[7]*Ibid.*

Exhibit 22.2.   Factors That Affect Nutrient Availability

NUTRIENT	RELATIVE STABILITY	FACTORS THAT AFFECT AVAILABILITY
Carbohydrate	Stable	Little change in ordinary cooking. Fermentation causes partial breakdown, but energy value is still available.
Protein	Stable	Little change in ordinary cooking. With high, dry heat, nonenzymatic browning may make amino acid lysine unavailable.
Fat Saturated	Stable	Little change in ordinary cooking. High heat can cause breakdown.
Polyunsaturated	Mod. Stable	Oxygen and light cause oxidation and rancidity. High heat causes breakdown.
Minerals	Stable	All are lost in milling; they are leached out in cooking water or drippings or whey. Not affected by oxidation, heat, light.
Calcium	Stable	Made insoluble by oxalic acid.
Iron	Stable	Made unavailable by phytic acid.
Magnesium	Stable	Made unavailable by phytic acid.
Potassium	Stable	Highly soluble, easily lost in cooking water, whey.
Vitamins Niacin	Stable	The most stable vitamin. Little loss in ordinary cooking. Lost in milling. Water soluble. Lost in leaching.
Biotin	Stable	Water soluble. Lost in leaching. Tied up by avidin in raw egg white; cooking destroys avidin.
Vitamin K	Stable	Fat soluble. Cooking destroys little. Light destroys.
Vitamin B$_6$	Mod. Stable	Water soluble. Lost in leaching. Light and heat destroy.
Vitamin E	Mod. Stable	Fat soluble. Lost in milling. Oxygen, heat destroy.
Pantothenic Acid	Mod. Stable	Water soluble. Lost in leaching. Lost in milling. Heat destroys.
Vitamin B$_{12}$	Mod. Unstable	Water soluble. Lost in leaching. Oxygen, light, and heat destroy. Not very stable in heat used in processing.
Vitamin D	Mod. Unstable	Fat soluble. Oxygen, light, heat, acids, and alkalies destroy.
Riboflavin	Mod. Unstable	Water soluble. Lost in leaching and milling. Light, heat, and alkalies destroy. Some foods show increase after cooking.
Folic Acid	Mod. Unstable	Water soluble. Lost in leaching and milling. Oxygen, heat, and acids destroy.
Vitamin A	Mod. Unstable	Fat soluble. Well retained in cooked vegetables. Oxygen, light, heat, and acids destroy.
Thiamin	Unstable	Water soluble. Lost in leaching and milling. Oxygen, light, heat, alkalies and neutral solutions destory. Acid protects.
Vitamin C	Very Unstable	Water soluble. Lost in leaching. Oxygen, light, heat, alkalies, and neutral solutions destroy. Acid protects.

SUMMARY OF CHANGES IN NUTRIENT AVAILABILITY

Exhibit 22.2 summarizes the effects of all these factors on the availability of specific nutrients. Carbohydrates, proteins, and saturated fats undergo little change in ordinary cooking processes. Minerals are stable to heat and oxidation but are prone to loss from mechanical separation and leaching and sometimes are made unavailable to the body through chemical reactions with compounds such as oxalates and phytates (oxalic and phytic acid). Vitamins are the most unstable of all the nutrients, with vitamin C and thiamin being the most easily lost (see also Exhibit 22.3).

Exhibit 22.3. Stability of Nutrients

NUTRIENT	EFFECT OF PH			AIR OR OXYGEN	LIGHT	HEAT	COOKING LOSSES, RANGE
	NEUTRAL PH 7	ACID <PH 7	ALKALINE >PH 7				
Vitamins							%
Vitamin A	S	U	S	U	U	U	0–40
Ascorbic acid (C)	U	S	U	U	U	U	0–100
Biotin	S	S	S	S	S	U	0–60
Carotenes (pro-A)	S	U	S	U	U	U	0–30
Choline	S	S	S	U	S	S	0–5
Cobalamin (B$_{12}$)	S	S	S	U	U	S	0–10
Vitamin D	S			U	U	U	0–40
Essential fatty acids	S	S	U	U	U	S	0–10
Folic acid	U	U	S	U	U	U	0–100
Inositol	S	S	S	S	S	U	0–95
Vitamin K	S	U	U	S	U	S	0–5
Niacin (PP)	S	S	S	S	S	S	0–75
Panthothenic acid	S	U	U	S	S	U	0–50
p-Amino benzoic acid	S	S	S	U	S	S	0–5
Pyridoxine (B$_6$)	S	S	S	S	U	U	0–40
Riboflavin (B$_2$)	S	S	U	S	U	U	0–75
Thiamin (B$_1$)	U	S	U	U	S	U	0–80
Tocopherols (E)	S	S	S	U	U	U	0–55
Essential amino acids							
Isoleucine	S	S	S	S	S	S	0–10
Leucine	S	S	S	S	S	S	0–10
Lysine	S	S	S	S	S	U	0–40
Methionine	S	S	S	S	S	S	0–10
Phenylalanine	S	S	S	S	S	S	0–5
Threonine	S	U	U	S	S	U	0–20
Tryptophan	S	U	S	S	U	S	0–15
Valine	S	S	S	S	S	S	0–10
Mineral salts	S	S	S	S	S	S	0–3

Source: A Hungry World. The Challenge to Agriculture. General Report by University of California Food Task Force, Berkeley, CA: 1974, p. 43.

S = stable (no important destruction).

U = unstable (significant destruction).

Understanding the ways nutrients are lost from foods can give some guidelines for handling foods to obtain the maximum nutritional benefit from them (see Exhibit 22.4). Home storage and preparation methods can be vitally important to our nutrition. Moreover, money as well as nutrients can be saved by following these guidelines.

Exhibit 22.4.   Guidelines for Retaining Nutrients in Food at Home

Store food in cool or cold place out of direct light.

Keep storage time short. Use rotation system so oldest foods are used first.

Avoid trimming or washing nutrients away.

Cook in ways that do not destroy nutrients.

Home Storage

We have seen that heat, light, oxygen (air), and the presence or absence of acids, alkalies, and moisture all have potentially adverse effects on some nutrients. Of these, storage temperature and length of time of storage are the most crucial for all forms of foods—fresh, fresh-cooked, canned, frozen, and dried.

Almost all fresh foods—fruits and vegetables, milk, cheese, meat, fish, poultry, eggs—and fresh-cooked foods need to be stored in a cold place. A refrigerator temperature of 32°–40° F is recommended to (a) retard growth of microorganisms that cause spoilage or food poisoning and (b) retain nutrients. Most fresh vegetables also need moist storage to help retain freshness and nutrients. Potatoes and dried onions need a cool—but not cold—dry, dark storage area.

Canned and dried foods need to be stored in a cool, dry, dark place. Frozen foods need a storage temperature of 0° F, or colder, and need to be wrapped in moisture- and vapor-proof materials.

All stored foods should be used within their optimum keeping time. The longer they are kept, the lower their nutrient level. This also applies to refrigerated leftovers, especially cooked vegetables. So an important practice to follow is to buy and cook food according to need so that foods don't have to be stored so long that they lose a large portion of their nutrients. Thus, buying the "large economy size" may not be wise if we end up with too many leftovers.

Shopping trips should be planned so groceries can be brought home immediately and stored in the refrigerator, freezer, or pantry before they have time to warm up to temperatures where nutrients are lost. When foods are stored, a rotation system should be used so the oldest foods are used up first.

Food Preparation

457
Guidelines
for
Retaining
Nutrients
in Foods

The major ways nutrients are lost in food preparation are through mechanical separation, leaching in liquid, oxidation when exposed to air and light, and use of too much heat—preparing food at too high a temperature or for too long a time, or both. Consider the following ideas when preparing foods to attain maximum nutrient retention:

1. Proceed gingerly in trimming and paring and throw away as little as possible. Leave skins on potatoes when they are boiled or fried, for example, and then eat the skins. Potatoes cooked with skins on retain more nutrients than peeled ones.

2. Chop, slice, grate, shred, puree, and juice fresh vegetables and fruits as close to eating time as possible. Keep foods that are prepared ahead of time closely covered and cold.

3. Avoid soaking foods in water or other liquids that will not be consumed. Do not wash foods that do not need washing, such as packaged rice. Cook rice in just the amount of water it will absorb so there is no nutrient-rich cooking water to pour off.

4. Use a small to moderate amount of water for boiling vegetables (one-half to one cup water per four servings) rather than cooking them in either large or tiny amounts of water ("waterless cooking").[8] If the amount of water is too small, the temperature of the vegetable increases more slowly than if a larger amount is used, and this allows more time for enzyme destruction of vitamin C. Also, vegetables are more palatable and more likely to be enjoyed and eaten if cooked in half their weight of water. Some leafy vegetables actually show greater vitamin C retention with more cooking water.

5. Cook fresh and frozen vegetables as quickly and as little as possible. Do not defrost frozen vegetables. Start cooking vegetables in boiling water; in fact, allow the water to boil for one minute or longer to drive off the dissolved oxygen. Use a lid on the pan to speed up the cooking; this can improve vitamin C retention by 10 to 20 percent. Cook vegetables only until they are crispy and tender. Overcooked vegetables have a mushy texture and a less appealing color, as well as fewer nutrients.

6. Consider nutrient loss in cooking water when cutting foods into pieces for cooking. Here two opposing forces are at work. When food is cut into pieces, more surface area is exposed, and this allows greater leaching of nutrients in cooking water. On the other hand, the food cooks so much faster when pieces are small that enzyme action stops more quickly and there is less nutrient loss from heat. These two

[8] R.M. Griswold, *The Experimental Study of Foods.* Boston, MA: Houghton Mifflin Company, 1962, pp. 183-4.

factors tend to balance each other out, except in the case of thinly cut vegetables, French-cut green beans, for example, where nutrient loss is notably greater.

7. Steam or stir-fry vegetables instead of boiling them to reduce leaching, especially when they are cut in small, thin pieces.

8. Use a moderate oven temperature, 325° F, when roasting meats and poultry, rather than higher temperatures where more nutrients are lost. When meats are cooked in liquid or by methods that produce a large amount of drippings (braising, for example) , use the liquid or drippings when possible (in gravy or soup, for example). However, you may want to remove the fat first to reduce calorie and saturated fat content.

9. Avoid holding cooked foods, especially vegetables, at "keep warm" temperatures for long periods of time. Instead, chill them, then reheat quickly when it is time to serve them.

10. Avoid overheating fats when frying. If fats smoke, it means they are breaking down and are too hot. Also, limit reuse of cooking oils. With high temperatures and repeated reuse, potentially toxic products are formed from the breakdown of polyunsaturated fats, and nutritive value is reduced.

11. If preserving fresh fruits and vegetables at home, try to do it the day they are picked when nutrient levels are highest. Work quickly with small batches so peeled, chopped, sliced, and pureed foods are heated promptly to destroy enzymes and prevent oxidation of nutrients. Do not skip the blanching step, brief boiling or steaming, when freezing vegetables, as it is needed to destroy enzymes that cause nutrient loss in frozen food. In canning, the hot-pack method is preferred because foods are heated more quickly to the point where enzyme action is stopped. And finally, use home preserved foods before the next crop is ready to be harvested.

SUPERMARKET NUTRITION: FRESH VERSUS PROCESSED FOODS

One of the statements we often hear, especially from those who consider themselves "health food" experts or who are critical of "big business," is that processed foods are greatly lacking in nutrients and that to be well nourished we need to eat fresh, rather than processed, foods.

From the information presented in the preceding sections, you can correctly conclude that this contention is not accurate for all foods. While it is true that nutrients are lost when food is processed, it is not true that processed foods are totally devoid of nutrients (see Exhibit 22.5).

Exhibit 22.5.   Effect of Processing on Vitamin C in Foods That are Good Sources of Vitamin C

	MILLIGRAMS VITAMIN C
4 oz Orange Juice (½ cup)	
Fresh	62
Frozen, reconstituted	60
Canned (unsweetened)	50
Dehydrated, reconstituted	55
4 oz Broccoli	
Raw	128
Boiled	102
Frozen, boiled	82
4 oz Potato	
Raw, peeled	23
Baked or boiled in skin	17
French fried, fresh	24
French fried, frozen	18
Chips	20
Dehydrated, flakes, prepared	6
Dehydrated, granules, prepared	4
4 oz Strawberries	
Fresh	67
Frozen, whole	62
Frozen, sliced	60
Canned	23
4 oz Spinach	
Raw	58
Boiled	32
Frozen, boiled	22
Canned	16

Source: *Nutritive Value of American Foods in Common Units.* U.S. Dept. of Agriculture, Agricultural Handbook No. 456, Washington, D.C., 1975.

In some cases, particularly that of refined cereals, only some of the nutrients lost in processing are replaced by enrichment, and the less-processed product is, in truth, considerably more nutritious. In the case of fabricated foods—those put together in factories from parts of food and laboratory-produced ingredients (for example, synthetic "orange juice")—many of the trace nutrients found in the food imitated are not present. But sometimes synthesized foods have additional nutrients at higher levels than those found in the natural food.

In the case of fresh versus processed fruits and vegetables, it is risky to assume that the fresh products always have a higher level of nutrients than the frozen or canned. As we learned earlier, nutrient loss from processed fruits and vegetables depends on the method of preservation as well as on the shipping and handling that the foods receive.

But nutrients also are lost from fresh fruits and vegetables that must be packed, shipped, and stored—sometimes for many days—before they are purchased. Nutrients are lost from fresh fruits and vegetables after they're bought, or even if they're grown in home gardens, if they are stored for some time, and especially if they're not stored in a cold place.

Another factor at the consumer end is loss of nutrients when fruits and vegetables are prepared for the table. For example, a canned vegetable might be quickly heated and eaten, while a fresh vegetable might be cooked in such a way that more nutrients are destroyed than were lost when the vegetable was canned. Thus, it is possible that some fresh fruits and vegetables have fewer nutrients when eaten than their processed counterparts.

In animal foods, which are normally cooked before eating, there is little nutritional difference between the fresh and processed products.

In the case of milk, there are those who claim that raw milk and products such as yogurt made from nonpasteurized milk are more healthful because pasteurization destroys nutrients such as vitamin C and thiamin as well as hormones and enzymes. But pasteurization does not destroy the nutrients milk is important for: calcium, protein, and riboflavin. The nutrients that pasteurization does decrease, thiamin and vitamin C, are found in milk in such small amounts that their loss is not worth worrying about. Also, vitamin C is not stable in raw milk either, and much is lost during storage. The claim that pasteurization destroys hormones and enzymes in milk is irrelevant because they have not been shown to play any role, other than as digested proteins, in our body processes.

Pasteurization does destroy *pathogens*, disease-causing bacteria, including the common food poisoning bacteria, salmonella. While these bacteria are usually few in number in fresh raw milk, they can multiply rapidly in milk that has not been properly refrigerated. They are of particular concern if raw milk is fed to infants, where the lukewarm milk may be allowed to stand long enough for bacteria to multiply, because infants are more vulnerable to attack by these pathogens.

Since there is no known nutritional advantage of raw milk—and in fact, raw milk lacks vitamin D, which is often added to pasteurized milk—and there are known health hazards, the conclusion could logically be drawn that the risk of using it outweighs the benefits. In many states raw milk is not allowed to be sold for this reason.

And so, the answer to the question—Which is more nutritious, fresh or processed food?—depends upon the food and the nutrients involved. The best plan is to follow the advice given elsewhere in this book: eat a wide variety of foods, including some fresh and some processed ones, and consider what nutrients might be missing or in short supply, when highly processed and fabricated foods are eaten.

Nutrients can be lost from foods in a number of ways. *Mechanical separation and leaching* procedures such as milling of grain, cheesemaking, peeling and chopping of vegetables, and soaking and canning of foods cause nutrient destruction or loss. *Enzymatic action* is responsible for chemical reactions even after food is harvested and processed. Heat processing deactivates enzymes, but may cause direct destruction of nutrients itself.

Oxidation is the principal chemical change taking place in many foods while they are stored or processed. Oxidation of fats and oils causes rancidity and destruction of fat-soluble vitamins, especially in polyunsaturated oils. *Light* accelerates the oxidative process and particularly affects riboflavin and vitamin C. *Heat* destroys many vitamins and also speeds the rate of oxidation. Thiamin and vitamin C are sensitive to canning and other heat processing methods. However, once foods are canned, their nutrients are relatively stable. Heating can improve the digestibility of some nutrients. Frozen foods generally have the highest overall nutritional quality of any processed food if not stored for long periods of time.

The *acidity or alkalinity* of foods has varying effects. Food preparation methods incorporating acids help preserve some nutrients, but may destroy others. *Chemical interactions* in foods can produce nutrient loss. *Drying,* especially sun drying, can be very destructive of nutrients; commercial processes such as freeze drying and spray drying minimize these losses.

Guidelines for retaining nutrients in foods include storing foods only for short periods of time in an appropriately cool environment, peeling and cutting foods as little as possible, avoiding soaking, using small to moderate amounts of water in preparation, consuming cooking liquids, and avoiding overcooking.

Part VII

WHAT'S IN FOODS BESIDES NUTRIENTS?

NATURAL TOXICANTS 23

Highlights

Chemicals, toxicity levels, and food hazards
Common naturally-occurring toxic materials in foods
Reasons for low potential hazard of natural toxicants in foods

There is no better way to scare people about food safety than to convince them that foods contain "chemicals" or, better yet, that the chemicals are poisons. This ploy is used often by those who have a book or product to sell. As a result, people are led to believe that anything chemical is harmful, and that only "natural" foods are safe.

Yet life is chemical; foods are chemicals; and nutrients are chemicals. Chemical reactions occur naturally in foods and in our bodies all the time, and without chemicals and chemical reactions life itself would be impossible. Not all chemicals and chemical reactions are harmful, but some are, and these are the ones we need to avoid.

When we eat food, we get many other substances besides nutrients. Foods naturally contain myriads of complex chemical compounds; a potato, for example, is known to have over 150 different chemicals (see Exhibit 23.1). In addition, foods contain other substances that are purposely added (additives—see Chapter 24) or that may get into them by accident (contaminants—see Chapter 25) somewhere along the line between production, marketing, and consumption.

Often people who extol the virtues of "natural foods" and worry about the dangers of chemicals added to our foods don't seem to realize that many of the natural chemicals in foods are more toxic than chemicals that are added (see Exhibit 23.2).

Consider the strawberry, for example. A ripe strawberry, just as it is picked, contains, among many other things: acetone, acetaldehyde, methyl butrate, ethyl caproate, hexyl acetate, methanol, acrolein, and crotonaldehyde. Every one of these natural substances is poisonous!

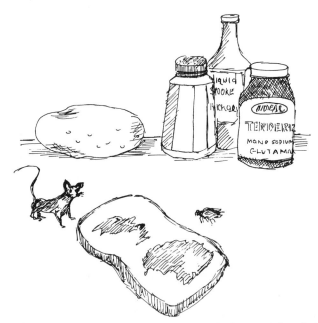

Exhibit 23.1. "Chemicals" in foods include natural substances, additives, and contaminants.

467
Not All
Toxic
Substances
Are
Hazardous

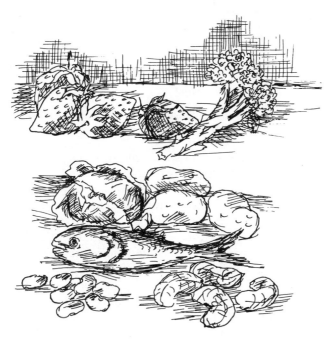

Exhibit 23.2. Poisonous chemicals are found naturally in all of these foods, and in many others; yet these foods are not hazardous when eaten in normal quantities.

Methanol, for example, is wood alcohol, and is deadly if too much is consumed. Crotonaldehyde is the chemical used in "Mickey Finns," and too large a dose will kill.

Chemical reactions are taking place in fresh foods right before our eyes, too, yet we cannot see these reactions. For example, in strawberries, right on the table, acetaldehyde is being oxidized into acetic acid and methanol to formaldehyde.

NOT ALL TOXIC SUBSTANCES ARE HAZARDOUS

In spite of the poisonous substances they contain and the chemical reactions taking place in them, strawberries don't poison us. Why? Because the amount of poisonous substances naturally found in them is too small to be harmful. Only if we ate enormous amounts of strawberries every day, perhaps to the exclusion of everything else, would these ingredients poison us.

The key point to remember is that a substance may be *toxic,* that is, inherently capable of producing injury when tested by itself, without being a *hazard,* that is, likely to produce injury under the normal circumstances of exposure, as in the diet (see Exhibit 23.3). The amount of the substance consumed, as well as its toxicity, determines its potential risk.

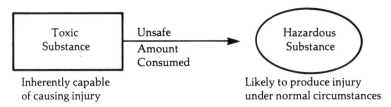

Inherently capable
of causing injury

Likely to produce injury
under normal circumstances

Exhibit 23.3.   A toxic substance is not necessarily hazardous unless
too much is consumed.

Substances that are safe in small amounts may not be safe in large
amounts. And we can eat too much of anything, as was demonstrated
most vividly in the case of a mentally ill woman whose compulsion for
drinking water caused her death. Investigation showed that she drank
as much as four gallons of water a day (supposedly to cleanse her body
of suspected cancer). She destroyed her body's chemical balance and,
as a result, her tissues swelled, particularly her lungs. This was followed
by a heart rhythm disturbance, and she died a slow, painful death from
water intoxication.[1] Yes, even something as necessary and benign as
water can be harmful if we consume too much of it.

Many of our favorite foods contain toxic compounds, and some are
highly toxic, but the foods are not hazardous.

COMMON NATURAL TOXICANTS IN FOODS

Goitrogens. Substances that cause antithyroid activity are found in
vegetables such as broccoli, cabbage, spinach, legumes, nuts, and milk.
A high incidence of goiter due to the high intake of cabbage has been
reported in New Zealand and India. Fortunately, goitrogenic activity in
foods is largely destroyed by cooking.

Estrogens. Small amounts of estrogens [but far greater concentrations than the amount of the controversial estrogen *diethylstibestrol*
(DES) in beef liver] have been detected in a wide variety of common
foods, including wheat, oats, barley, rice, soybeans, potatoes, apples,
plums, and cherries, as well as in a number of vegetable oils, such as
corn, olive, peanut, and cottonseed, and in liver and egg yolk. As far as
is known, such estrogenic activity in foods has not caused adverse effects in humans. High levels in animal forage have caused breeding difficulties in sheep, however.

Cyanogenetic Glycosides. When taken into the stomach, these liberate *hydrocyanic acid,* which is the basis of cyanide poisoning. Examples
of these poisons are *amygdalin* in the pits of fruits such as apricots,
peaches, plums, prunes, and bitter almonds; *phaseolutin* in lima beans;

[1] "4-Gallon-A-Day Water Binge Kills Woman." *Santa Ana* (California) *Register,*
February 25, 1977, Section A, pp. 1-2.

and *dhurrin* in millet and sorghum. (Amygdalin is the main component of *laetrile,* the controversial substance used in cancer treatment.) Cooking largely destroys these toxic chemicals.

Oxalates. Oxalates combine with calcium and prevent its absorption. They are present in significant amounts in spinach, rhubarb (the leaves are highly poisonous), chard, beet tops, parsley, cocoa, tea, almonds, cashew nuts, and other foods. Foods containing oxalates are not considered significant dietary hazards to man since collectively they do not ordinarily constitute a significant part of the diet. (More on these in Chapter 12.)

Enzyme Inhibitors. Various types of enzyme inhibitors are present in different foods. *Trypsin* inhibitors are found in legumes, such as soybeans, kidney, and lima beans. The uncooked meal of these legumes, at high dietary levels, inhibits growth of young animals. *Anticholinesterase* activity occurs naturally in a number of common fruits and vegetables, including broccoli, eggplant, sugar beets, asparagus, several varieties of potatoes, apples, and oranges.

Antivitamins. By inhibiting vitamins from being used by our bodies, antivitamins can produce vitamin deficiencies. For example, *avidin* in raw egg white combines with *biotin* and prevents its absorption. Orange peel contains *citral,* which antagonizes vitamin A. Soybeans contain a *lipoxidase,* which inactivates carotene. *Thiaminase,* found in clams and raw fish, can cause thiamin deficiency. Usually these factors are destroyed by cooking, or the amount eaten in the average diet is too small to cause a vitamin deficiency. For example, only if one ate quantities of raw eggs daily would the avidin in the whites cause biotin deficiency; eating an occasional raw egg would not cause a problem.

Essential Nutrients. These also can be toxic with long-term excess consumption. Known to be toxic are vitamins A and D, and the minerals iron, copper, zinc, fluoride, chromium, cadmium, and cobalt.

Other Natural Poisons. Some other natural poisons in some common foods include:

Nitrates in vegetables, especially greens such as spinach.
Phytates in cereals, which may interfere with the assimilation of calcium, magnesium, zinc, and iron.
Saponins and *hemagglutinins* in various legumes, especially soybeans.
Caffeine, theophylline, and *theobromine,* stimulants in coffee, tea, and cocoa.
Serotonin in banana, pineapple, tomato, pumpkin, squash, and cucumber.
Solanine, a bitter-tasting glycoalkaloid, found in all potatoes in small amounts and especially in the green portion that forms when potatoes are stored in the light.
Lycopene in tomato juice.

Hydroxphylisatin derivates in prunes, which have potent laxative properties.

Glycosides, which cause honey poisoning, may be present if bees collect nectar from the mountain laurel, rhododendron, azalea, and oleander.

As far as scientists know, there appears to be no real hazard from the many toxic substances naturally present in foods involved in the normal diet as consumed by healthy individuals because:

1. Concentrations of most toxic substances in commonly eaten foods are so low that a grossly exaggerated consumption of a food would be required to supply an unsafe amount.

2. Because many antagonistic interactions occur between chemical compounds in the diet, the toxicity of one element may be offset by an adequate amount of another. For example, the toxicity of cadmium in the diet is reduced by an adequate amount of zinc, and selenium counteracts the toxicity of methyl mercury in tuna.

3. The human body can tolerate small amounts of an unlimited number of chemical substances taken simultaneously, but it can tolerate only a limited amount of any one of them.

Our body defenses against these compounds are believed to be enzymes located in the skin, blood, lungs, liver, and kidney. These enzymes break down foreign compounds so they can be excreted and not build up to toxic levels. A diet adequate in proteins, unsaturated fats, vitamins, and minerals appears to be the best way for us to keep our enzymes in prime condition to detoxify toxic compounds.

Natural components of food can create a health hazard in the case of abnormal health or the physiologic makeup of an individual, for example, in the case of allergies or inborn errors of metabolism. More likely causes of hazard, however, are unbalanced or fad diets, leading to the toxicity of certain components through the overconsumption of a particular food. For example, the excess consumption of the nuts from apricot pits has led to cyanide poisoning. We can avoid these problems by eating a wide variety of foods and eating all foods in moderation.

Summary

Our world is composed of intricate combinations of basic building blocks termed chemicals. The chemicals in food are responsible for flavor, aroma, texture, and nutrient level. Many foods naturally contain small amounts of materials that are poisonous. However, a substance may be toxic without being a hazard. The potential risk of a substance is determined by the amount consumed as well as its toxicity. Even benign substances (water) can be harmful if consumed in excessive quantities.

Common natural toxicants include goitrogens, estrogens, glycosides, oxalates, enzyme inhibitors, antivitamins, essential nutrients, nitrates, phytates, and other natural poisons. The hazard from these appears to be negligible because of low concentrations, offsetting reactions between substances, the body's tolerance for them, and detoxifying enzymes.

INTENTIONAL ADDITIVES 24

Highlights

Additives and why they are used

Controversies regarding safety of additives, including the
  Delaney Clause

Risk–benefit dilemma illustrated with two additives, sodium
  nitrite and saccharin

Summary of kinds of additives and their functions in foods

When people express concern about dangerous chemicals in foods, they are usually referring to additives. An additive is a substance or combination of substances that is present in food as a result of processing, production, or packaging and that is not a contaminant. An additive is no more or no less of a chemical than nutrients and other substances in foods. Nearly 4,000 chemicals are added to foods for some specific effect, yet they make up only about 1 percent of the weight of our total diet. In other words, most additives are used in relatively small amounts.

Many additives are natural food substances, such as salt or sugar, or substances extracted from food; for example, carotene (the precursor of vitamin A), which is used as a yellow food coloring; and lecithin, which is used as an emulsifier. Other additives are synthesized by manufacturers to be chemically identical to natural substances; for example, ascorbic acid (vitamin C), which is used as an antioxidant; and calcium propionate, which is produced naturally when swiss cheese is made and is used as a mold inhibitor in bread. A third category of additives is made up of nonfood substances either found in nature or synthesized; for example, calcium carbonate, used to control acidity and alkalinity; and sulfur dioxide, which is used to retain the color in fruit.

Why are additives used? For many reasons—all related to improving the product (see Exhibit 24.1). Additives are used to improve flavor, color, and texture—in other words, to improve the organoleptic qualities. They are also used to improve nutritional value, prevent spoilage, and to extend shelf life. Without additives our foods would be less attractive, less flavorful, less nutritious, more likely to spoil, more difficult to prepare, and more expensive. Most convenience foods would not be possible without additives.

SAFETY OF ADDITIVES

There has been much public concern about additives because of recurring, widely publicized incidents relating to the safety of certain substances such as cyclamates, saccharine, red dyes, and sodium nitrite. Additives as a group have been condemned for their association with a few suspected substances. In fact, additives and pesticide residues are at the top of consumers' lists of food safety hazards, according to opin-

Exhibit 24.1.   Reasons for Using Additives in Foods

Improve flavor, color, texture
Improve nutritional value
Prevent spoilage and extend shelf life
Improve performance and/or ease of preparation

ion surveys,[1] and they receive the most attention in the media. Yet food technologists, the knowledgeable people in this field, say pesticide residues and food additives are the least likely to be real health threats.

Food technologists rank actual food safety hazards in order of their importance as follows:[2]

1. Microbiological (food poisoning)
2. Nutritional (poor food choices)
3. Environmental contaminants
4. Natural toxicants
5. Pesticide residues
6. Food additives

Food technologists point out that food additives as a group have been more thoroughly tested and are safer than the ingredients nature adds. However, new scientific findings make it essential to continually update the control of the use of specific additives.

Use of additives in food is regulated by the Food and Drug Administration (FDA) under the Food, Drug, and Cosmetic Act of 1938 and its subsequent amendments, the 1958 Food Additives Amendment and the 1960 Color Additives Amendment. The 1958 amendment made the FDA responsible for giving prior approval for the use of food additives according to specific and stringent regulations. To obtain approval for the use of any additive, manufacturers must petition the FDA with documented evidence that the additive is both needed and safe. Often, manufacturers spend many dollars and years of research before a food additive is FDA approved or rejected.

To prove the safety of an additive, three kinds of toxicity studies must be carried out:

1. An acute toxicity test to show the effects of a single large dose of the compound given to a sample of at least two species of laboratory animals (often rats and dogs)

2. Short-term toxicity studies (90 days) to show the effects of feeding diets with different concentrations of the chemical to at least two species of laboratory animals

3. Long-term toxicity studies (two years or more) to show effects of lifetime consumption of the chemical. An analysis of the effects on

[1]M.E. Simon and P.G. Kuehl, "FDA Survey of Consumer Opinion about the Safety of Foods," *FDA Consumer*, Vol. 7, No. 5, 1973, p. 15. And "1978 Consumer Food Labeling Survey, Summary Report," Consumer Research Staff, Division of Consumer Studies, Bureau of Foods, Food and Drug Administration. Washington, D.C., 1979, pp. 3-4.

[2]R.L. Hall, "Safe at the Plate." *Nutrition Today*, Vol. 12, No. 6, November-December, 1977, pp. 6-31.

fertility, reproduction, and lactation may also be required, as well as a study of how the compound is metabolized by the animal.

The FDA also regulates the amount of an additive that may be used. The quantity allowed may not exceed the smallest amount needed to accomplish its intended function. The additive must also be of an appropriate food grade and be handled as a food ingredient.

"Generally Recognized as Safe"

Over 700 additives, already in use in 1958 when the amendment went into effect, did not have to go through this rigid screening process. They were listed in a group referred to as GRAS (Generally Recognized as Safe) because they had been in use for many years without any known problems. Since that time however, some additives on the GRAS list were found to be potentially hazardous. As a result, a 1969 presidential decree directed the FDA to conduct a safety review of the GRAS substances.

This review, conducted by the Select Committee on GRAS Substances of the Federation of American Societies for Experimental Biology, assigned the GRAS substances to one of four categories:

1. Affirmed as generally regarded as safe and maintained on the GRAS list

2. Placed on a new GRAS list but with various restrictions

3. Converted to a regulated food additive status with strict controls over its use

4. Judged unsafe and banned from use in food.

In 1976, the Food and Drug Administration developed a new program to provide for the periodic review of all food additives to make certain they are safe by modern standards. Under this program, all food additives will undergo a scientific evaluation. If the results of tests are negative, the FDA will request a reevaluation by manufacturers. If new tests show that an additive needs to be restricted or removed from the market, the FDA will take that action.

The Delany Clause Controversy

Part of the 1958 Food Additives Amendment, the Delaney Clause, has brought about much of the current controversy regarding food additives. This clause forbids the use of any substance, in any amount, that causes cancer in man or animal under any circumstances.

There are those who argue that the Delaney Clause is too inflexible, especially its principle of zero tolerance. It was enacted at a time when the methods used to detect minute amounts of substances were far less sensitive than those now available. Today's technology makes it possible to detect parts per trillion, compared to parts per million in 1958.

If the Delaney Clause principle of zero tolerance was applied to natural foods, few would pass, its opponents argue, because many natural chemicals are toxic, and some are carcinogenic. Others argue that the evidence resulting from using large doses of a substance on laboratory animals is not always a reasonable test of carcinogenicity in humans.

Since it is impossible to avoid all risk, scientists suggest that a more reasonable approach to replace the zero tolerance principle of the Delaney Clause would be the application of the risk-benefit ratio: the degree of risk in proportion to the level of benefit.[3] Thus, if a high level of benefit is received from a food or additive, we may be willing to accept a greater degree of risk from eating it. Conversely, a product that provides little benefit in proportion to its risk would be one we would want to eliminate.

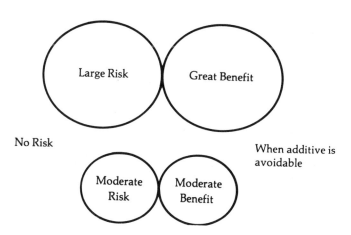

Exhibit 24.2. The level of risk we are willing to accept should be in proportion to its level of benefit, according to proponents of the risk–benefit ratio, rather than zero tolerance for additives.

Scientists propose this guideline for making risk–benefit decisions: great risk only for very great benefit; moderate risk for moderate benefit; and no risk at all if the additive is avoidable (Exhibit 24.2).

Problems relating to zero tolerance, especially as it pertains to carcinogens, and to decisions about food safety are not easily resolved by the Food and Drug Administration because:

[3]Institute of Food Technologists' Expert Panel on Food Safety and Nutrition, *The Risk-Benefit Concept Applied to Food*. Chicago, IL: Institute of Food Technologists, March, 1978.

1. The scientific data available are seldom adequate to make a positive decisive judgment on the safety of any food or additive.

2. Even when a substantial collection of safety data does exist, the scientists seldom agree on its meaning or significance.

3. Even assuming there are adequate scientific data and agreement on their meaning, there appears to be no consensus on the acceptable degree of risk with respect to the marketing of foods.

4. Whatever the latest safety issue may be, there is enormous and continuing public pressure for the FDA to resolve it promptly and decisively. Yet under the Food, Drug and Cosmetic Act, the FDA cannot take action—for example, ban a food additive—until scientific fact establishes that a product is unsafe.

5. Regardless of the decision, those who disagree with it will continue to vocally and emotionally pursue the matter through all available channels, while those who agree will remain silent.

THE RISK–BENEFIT DILEMMA—ILLUSTRATED BY TWO ADDITIVES

In the late 1970s, the federal government was enmeshed in major controversies over the use of two heavily used additives, sodium nitrite and saccharin, which illustrate the issues listed above. In both cases, government regulators and legislators have had to weigh health risks versus health benefits in order to establish regulations to protect the well-being of American consumers. As we go to press, neither of these issues has been resolved.

Sodium Nitrite

The use of this additive involves an unusual trade-off of health risks versus health benefits. The known, short-term *benefit* of using sodium nitrite in cured meats is the prevention of botulism food poisoning. The less certain, long-range *risk* is that sodium nitrite may be a cause of cancer. Some consumer groups and a few scientists have recommended that use of sodium nitrite in meats be banned by the federal government. A much larger number of scientists are recommending a more cautious approach: reducing sodium nitrite where possible, substituting other preservation methods where feasible, but continuing the use of sodium nitrite for the time being where botulism poisoning poses a serious health threat.

Those consumers who believe the danger of cancer is greater than the danger of botulism, and who therefore prefer to avoid nitrites, can buy a limited amount of nonnitrite-containing cured meats. (Fresh meats, such as those usually purchased in the meat section of the supermarket, do not contain nitrite.) Those who use these products should recognize the risk and observe these precautions to avoid botulism: (1) do not buy vacuum-packed, nonnitrite-cured meats—buy only those wrapped in materials that allow air to enter the package; (2) keep the meats cold, below 40° F; (3) use meat within a few days after purchase; and (4) cook the meat thoroughly before eating it.

Sodium nitrite is a reduced (deoxidized) form of *sodium nitrate*. Nitrates have been used as a meat-curing ingredient for a long time. The origin of this use is lost in history. Nitrates also occur naturally in some water supplies and in some leafy vegetables such as spinach, lettuce, collards, celery, radishes, beets, turnips, and eggplant. Nitrates in these foods are reduced to nitrites by bacteria in our own saliva, and they supply about 80 percent of the nitrites in our diets. The remainder come from cured meats.

In the late 1800s it was learned that nitrate was reduced to nitrite by bacterial action and that the pink color of cured meat was due to nitrite and not nitrate. This discovery led to the use of nitrite directly as a meat-curing ingredient in bacon, ham, sausage, frankfurters, corned beef, and the like (see Exhibit 24.3). In meat processing, nitrites are important as a color fixative, for flavor enhancement, and most important, as a preservative. In low-acid, low-oxygen (vacuum-packed), cured-meat products, nitrites are essential to prevent botulism. They also retard oxidation, which otherwise causes an undesirable flavor.

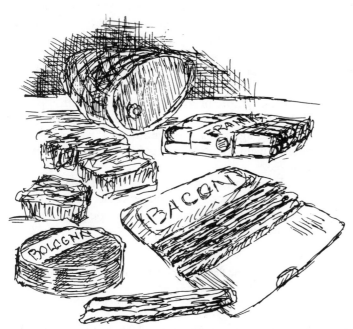

Exhibit 24.3.   Sodium nitrite is used as a curing agent in many popular meats to improve color, flavor, and keeping qualities, but its safety has been questioned.

Without nitrites, we could not have bacon, sausages, hams, and other meat products as we know them. No substitute for nitrites has been found by food researchers who have tested over 700 products. However, it has been learned that it is the quantity of nitrites used in processing the meat products and not the residual amount in the finished product that prevents botulism toxin from forming. Ascorbic acid or other similar compounds can appreciably reduce the amount of nitrites in the finished product. So ascorbic acid (vitamin C) is now being used in cured meats to help reduce nitrite levels.

The first research that raised the warning that nitrites could be a cause of cancer had to do with *nitrosamines.* Nitrosamines are formed when nitrites combine with amines (nitrogen-hydrogen groups) from protein breakdown. Several studies showed a relationship between nitrosamines and cancer in laboratory animals.[4] Nitrosamines appear to form in the body from ingested nitrites and secondary amines. Secondary amines could be formed in food during cooking.

Trace amounts of nitrosamines also have been found in a variety of foods, including cheese, fish meal, meat, sausage, flour, mushrooms, and alcoholic beverages. Nitrosamines also are formed in bacon when it is cooked. It seems that high heat plus the thin bacon strips are sufficient to produce the amines needed for nitrosamine formation. This can be prevented if bacon is cooked slowly, below 325°F. Most of the nitrosamines are found in the drippings.

Following the finding that nitrosamines might be cancer-causing, two lifetime rat-feeding studies of nitrite-cured meats were conducted, and they showed no carcinogenicity from either nitrite or nitrosamines.[5] But in 1978, results of a well-controlled study conducted at Massachusetts Institute of Technology provided the first direct link between nitrites and cancer. In this study, 13 percent of laboratory rats fed nitrites developed cancer of the lymphatic system compared with 8 percent on diets without nitrites. The difference is statistically significant. The researcher, while warning against a precipitous ban, recommended that the amount of nitrites used in cured meats be reduced and substitutes be used where feasible.[6]

The Food and Drug Administration, the U.S. Department of Agriculture, and the Congress, faced with this evidence plus the economic and safety implications of banning nitrites, are expected to move very slowly in resolving the issue.

[4]R.L. Shirley, "Nutritional and Physiological Effects of Nitrates, Nitrites, and Nitrosamines." *Bioscience,* Vol. 25, No. 12, December, 1975, pp. 789-94.

[5]Department of Public Relations, American Meat Institute, *Nitrite.* Washington, D.C.: American Meat Institute, January, 1978.

[6]Food and Drug Administration, "Statement on Nitrites" (press release). Washington, D.C.: Department of Health, Education and Welfare and U.S. Department of Agriculture, August 11, 1978.

One reason why the government is moving cautiously on nitrites is because of the enormous public outcry legislators encountered when the Food and Drug Administration took initial action to ban saccharin.

The health benefit of saccharin is much more nebulous than that of sodium nitrite. As a nonnutritive sweetener, it replaces all or part of the sugar in certain "diet" foods—canned fruits, desserts, and most especially soft drinks. Saccharin is used particularly by diabetics, who must avoid sugar but want to enjoy a sweet taste, and by people who are trying to control their calorie intake. However, there is no scientific evidence based on reliable, controlled studies that shows that saccharin is effective in the control of weight or blood sugar levels. However, in the public mind saccharin is useful and very important.

The health risk of saccharin is its potential carcinogenicity. In 1977, the FDA announced a proposal to prohibit the use of saccharin in foods and other ingestible products such as toothpaste, based on the results of a well-controlled study sponsored by the Canadian government. This study showed that saccharin, when fed to rats in high doses, caused malignant bladder tumors.[7] The FDA acted under the requirements of the Delaney Clause in issuing this proposal.

Public pressure, generated in part by the diet soft drink industry, caused Congress to act to delay the FDA ban for 18 months to allow time for further study. In the interim, Congress required that a warning sign be placed in all stores where saccharin-containing products are sold to the public and that new labels on these products describe the potential hazard of saccharin.

Subsequently, a panel of the National Academy of Sciences, appointed to review the saccharin issue at the request of Congress, reported that "saccharin must be viewed as a potential cause of cancer in humans" not only because it is a "low-potency" cancer-causing agent itself, but also because it may promote the cancer-causing action of other substances.[8] This panel is expected to make additional recommendations regarding the future use of saccharin in particular and government food safety policies in general before Congress takes final action. Congress has enacted a two-year extension of the time for saccharin's use.

[7]"Saccharin and Cancer: Confounding Data." *Science News,* Vol. 110, October 15, 1977, pp. 245-46.

[8]P.B. Hutt and E.A. Sloan, "NAS Issues Saccharin Report." (Report No. 1) *Nutrition Policy Issues,* No. 5, March, 1979. "National Academy of Sciences Issues Food Safety Report," (Report No. 2), *Nutrition Policy Issues,* No. 6, April, 1979.

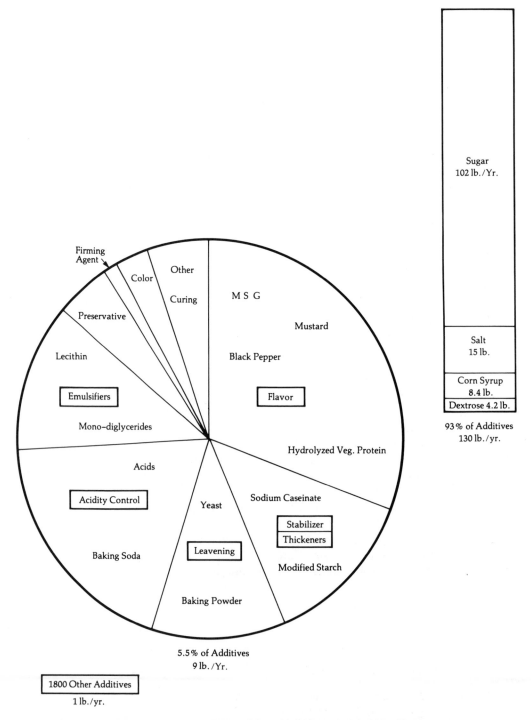

Firming Agent

Color

Other

Curing

M S G

Preservative

Mustard

Lecithin

Black Pepper

Emulsifiers

Flavor

Mono–diglycerides

Hydrolyzed Veg. Protein

Acids

Acidity Control

Sodium Caseinate

Yeast

Stabilizer

Thickeners

Leavening

Baking Soda

Modified Starch

Baking Powder

5.5% of Additives
9 lb./Yr.

Sugar
102 lb./Yr.

Salt
15 lb.

Corn Syrup
8.4 lb.

Dextrose 4.2 lb.

93% of Additives
130 lb./yr.

1800 Other Additives

1 lb./yr.

Exhibit 24.4. A small number of additives make up the largest quantity used in our foods.

We use a large quantity of a few additives and very minute quantities of a large number of them. As can be seen from Exhibit 24.4, the most commonly used additives are sugar, salt, and corn sweeteners (corn syrup, dextrose, and fructose). These compounds account for 93 percent by weight of all the food additives used in America. The next 5.5 percent is accounted for by 30 more additives, including monosodium glutamate, mustard, modified starch, yeasts, black pepper, citric and acetic acid, monoglycerides and diglycerides, sodium caseinate, sulfur dioxide, carbon dioxide, and lecithin. The other 1,900 direct additives make up the balance of 1.5 percent. [9]

All additives must serve a useful purpose to be accepted by the Food and Drug Administration. This purpose must be legitimate, that is, to enhance a food. Additives cannot be used to cover up a defect or to deceive the consumer in some way. Additives are classified according to their purpose. These purposes include: acting as preservatives and antioxidants; giving desired consistency to foods (emulsifying, stabilizing, thickening, controlling acidity); adding or restoring nutritive value; flavoring or coloring a food; and performing miscellaneous functions such as leavening, bleaching, or curing. Some additives perform more than one function. Sugar, for example, sweetens jelly and is also a preservative.

Preservatives. Because they help guard against microorganisms that cause spoilage or food poisoning, these are the most important additives. Sugar, salt, and vinegar have been used as preservatives for centuries. Sodium and calcium propionates are used in breads and other baked goods to inhibit mold growth. Sodium benzoate, benzoic acid, and sorbic acid inhibit bacterial or mold growth in margarine, certain fruit juices, syrup, pickles, and confections.

Antioxidants. A form of preservative, antioxidants are used to delay flavor and color changes resulting from oxidation. Sulfur dioxide is used to inhibit discoloration of dried fruits and vegetables and fruit juice. Ascorbic acid and citric acid often are used to prevent or delay enzymatic browning of fruits and vegetables. *Tocopherols,* such as vitamin E, *butylated hydroxyanisole* (BHA), and *butylated hydroxytoluene* (BHT) are used to prevent flavor changes resulting from the oxidation of fats and oils. They also make oils safer because when polyunsaturated oils are oxidized they can form a toxic product as well as a rancid flavor. BHA and BHT are used not only in fats and oils but also in foods containing fats and oils, such as cake mixes, peanut butter, breakfast cereals, potato chips, and whipped toppings.

---

[9] R.L. Hall, "Food Additives." *Nutrition Today,* Vol. 8, No. 4, July-August, 1973, pp. 20-28.

Emulsifiers, Thickeners, Leavening Agents, and Acids and Bases. All these agents are used to improve the texture of foods. Emulsifiers added to oil and vinegar mixtures—for example, to salad dressing—prevent separation; added to shortening, they permit even distribution of fat in a batter, giving improved volume and an even, fine grain; and added to pudding mixes, they help in the uniform dispersement of milk. Common emulsifiers are lecithin, polysorbates, diglycerides, and monoglycerides.

Stabilizers and thickeners are used to give a smooth, uniform texture to many foods, including salad dressings, yogurt and ice cream, puddings, chocolate milk, and sauce mixes. They include vegetable gums, starches, pectin, gelatin, algin, and carageean.

Leavening agents are well known for their ability to produce the carbon dioxide gas that causes cakes, breads, and similar foods to rise. They include yeast and baking powder ingredients (which also are acids and bases).

Acids and bases are buffers and neutralizing agents used to control the acidity or alkalinity in many processed foods. This can affect the texture, taste, and wholesomeness of the foods. This group of additives also gives or controls the acid or tart taste of soft drinks and instant fruit drinks. Some examples are citric acid, lactic acid, vinegar, sodium or ammonium bicarbonate, and calcium carbonate.

Additives for Nutritive Value. These replace or add to foods vitamins, minerals, or amino acids that are either partially lost through processing or that may be lacking in the diet. Examples are the B vitamins and iron, added to enrich white flour, bread, and other cereals; vitamin C, added to many fruit drinks; vitamin D, added to milk; vitamin A, added to nonfat milk and margarine to replace that found in butterfat; potassium iodide, added to salt; and vitamins, minerals, and amino acids, added to meat analogs made from soybeans and wheat gluten.

Flavors. Including all of the sweeteners and salt in this group, these substances are the most commonly used additives. There are some 1,400 natural and synthetic flavors available. They include herbs and spices, extracts (such as vanilla), essential oils (such as oil of lemon), hydrolized vegetable protein, and a myriad of synthesized substances that closely resemble food flavors, particularly fruit flavors. Flavor enhancers, such as monosodium glutamate, which do not add flavor themselves but bring out the natural flavor of the food, also are included in this group.

Food Colorings. Food colorings of both natural and synthetic origin are used extensively in processed foods such as jellies and jams, candy, soft drinks, fruit drinks, bakery goods, butter and margarine, cheese, ice cream, and gelatin desserts. Although more than 90 percent of food coloring is synthesized, some of the colors are identical to or made from substances found naturally in food. Much of the controversy about additives has stemmed from the use of synthetic colors whose purpose is merely cosmetic and whose safety is in doubt. Several widely used colors were banned by the Food and Drug Administration after tests showed they could be toxic. Publicity about the Feingold theory of the relationship between color additives and hyperkinesis (discussed in Chapter 15) also brought about an unfavorable consumer attitude towards food colors.

Maturing and Bleaching Agents. Such agents are important to the milling industry. Wheat flour in its natural freshly milled state has a pale yellowish tint. Upon storage for several months, flour slowly becomes white and undergoes an aging process that changes the gluten and improves the flour's baking qualities. Natural aging is slow and costly and results in a greater loss due to insect and rodent infestation. Compounds such as oxides of nitrogen, chlorine dioxide, nitrosyl chloride, and chlorine are used to accomplish the "whitening" and "aging" in almost a matter of seconds. They improve the flour without adversely affecting its nutritional value. Nevertheless, many consumers have been led to believe that unbleached flour is better because it's "natural."

Moisturizing Agents or Humectants. These prevent drying out of foods like coconut, marshmallows, and candy. Examples are glycerine and propylene glycol.

Anticaking Agents. These keep salts and powders free flowing. Calcium phosphates are used to do this job in instant breakfast drinks and lemonade and other soft drink mixes. Sodium silicoaluminate and dextrose may be used in salt to keep it from clumping in damp weather.

Clarifying Agents. These agents are used to remove small particles of minerals such as iron and copper that cause clouding in vinegar and other liquids.

Foaming Agents and Foam Inhibitors. Used to control the amount of air in products, these include the foaming agent sodium caseinate, which is used to help whipped topping to peak. Foam inhibitors remove the "head" from drinks such as orange and pineapple juice.

Sequestrants. These keep out traces of substances such as minerals that might promote unwanted oxidation.

Propellants, Aerating Agents, and Gases. Primarily, these are used to push products such as whipped cream out of aerosol cans. Gases such as carbon dioxide also may be used to exclude oxygen and prolong the shelf life of processed foods.

Nonnutritive Sweeteners. Saccharin and other nonnutritive sweeteners provide sweetening without calories for persons trying to reduce their intake of sugar.

Surface Finishing Agents. Waxes and more complex substances are used on fresh fruits and vegetables and eggs to protect the surface from bacterial invasion, reduce respiration, and prolong the keeping time.

From this brief summary it can be seen that additives perform many essential functions in our foods. Additives are a vital tool of the food-processing industry for providing us with a safe, wholesome, and varied food supply. The safety of additives is under continuing study. As someone discovers a new hazard, the testing is repeated. New hazards may have been discovered since this book was written. You will need to continually update your knowledge by reading current sources of nutritional information.

Summary

An additive is a substance or a combination of substances present in food as a result of processing, production, or packaging, and that is not a contaminant. Most of the nearly 4,000 additives are used in relatively small amounts. Many are extracted from food or synthesized in a form that is chemically identical to natural substances.

Additives are used to improve the flavor, color, texture, nutritional value, and storage qualities of foods. They are necessary in the production of most convenience foods.

The use and safety of food additives is regulated by the Food and Drug Administration under the nation's food safety laws. Toxicity studies are required to determine the safety of all new additives. The safety of additives that have been used for a long time and are "generally recognized as safe" (GRAS) is under scientific review.

The Delaney Clause of the food and drug laws forbids the use of any substance in any amount that causes cancer in man or animal under any circumstances. This rigid requirement for zero tolerance is the subject of controversy among scientists. Some recommend that a risk-benefit guideline be used instead: if a high level of benefit is derived from a food or additive, then we may be willing to accept a greater degree of risk from eating it.

Substances that present great risk should be used only if they provide a very great benefit. Sodium nitrite is an additive that provides a great benefit (protection from botulism), while its risk is still being evaluated; its use may be phased out if safe substitutes can be found. Saccharine's benefits are more questionable, and evidence of its risk is accumulating; but because of saccharine's popularity its use is being continued by Congressional action.

The most commonly used additives are sugar, salt, and corn sweeteners. These, plus 30 other common additives, make up 98.5 percent of all additives used. Additives are classified according to their function. The most important are preservatives; antioxidants; emulsifiers; thickeners; leavening agents; acids and bases; nutrients; flavors; colors; and bleaching, moisturizing, anticaking, and clarifying agents.

CONTAMINANTS 25

Highlights

Major types of contaminants in foods: pesticides, heavy metals, plastics, drugs, insects, and microorganisms

Origin of contaminants

Detrimental effects of contaminants on humans

Methods of avoiding contaminants or minimizing hazardous effects

Substances that are not purposely added to foods, known as incidental additives or contaminants, may get into food during growth, harvest, transportation, processing, packaging, or storage. Examples of contaminants include "filth" (soil, small stones, cigarette ashes, rodent hairs or feces, insect parts), pesticides, heavy metals such as mercury or lead, insects, microorganisms, and parasites (see Exhibit 25.1).

Some of the contaminants are harmful, most are esthetically undesirable, and government agencies are involved in their control. Guidelines established by the Food and Drug Administration provide standards for the maximum allowable amount of "filth," for example, and products found not meeting these standards during inspection are not allowed to be sold. Some have argued that the FDA standards for "filth" are too liberal; however a standard of zero contaminents would not be feasible to attain or enforce.

Exhibit 25.1.   Summary of the Common Contaminants in Food

Pesticides
Heavy Metals: mercury, lead, zinc
Plastics: phthalates, polychlorinated biphenyls (PCBs)
Drugs: antibiotics, hormones
Insects: weevils, pantry beetles
Parasites: trichinella, toxoplasma gondii, tapeworms
Microorganisms and toxins produced by microorganisms:
   "staph," salmonella, botulinum, perfringens,
Molds and Mycotoxins: alfatoxin

PESTICIDES

Pesticide contamination of food has received the most attention in the press, with the result that consumer concern is thought to be greatly out of proportion to the extent of the hazard.[1]

Pesticides are toxic chemicals and, like automobiles, can create environmental problems. But with pesticides, as with automobiles, in today's world it is difficult to get along without them. In spite of pest control programs, U.S. agriculture still loses possibly one-third of its potential crop production to various pests. Without modern pest control, including chemical pesticides, this annual loss probably would at least double.

Pesticides are used to produce not only more food, but also food

[1]R.L. Hall, "Safe at the Plate." *Nutrition Today*, Vol. 12, No. 6, November-December, 1977, pp. 6-31.

that is virtually free of insects or damage from insects and diseases. Often, especially in the United States, pesticides are used because of public demand, supported by government regulations, for uncontaminated and unblemished food. A consumer contribution to the problem would be the acceptance of the need for some inconvenience from annoying pests and, possibly, some visible evidence of insects or insect damage on food.

The Environmental Protection Agency (EPA) is responsible for administering two basic federal laws regulating the marketing and use of pesticides in the United States. The U.S. Department of Agriculture, the Food and Drug Administration, and state departments of agriculture and health also are involved in regulating and monitoring the use of pesticides and the amount of pesticide residue that is allowed to remain in or on plants, or in soil or water.

The most controversial question is, What amount of residue on food is "safe"? It probably never will be answered to everybody's satisfaction. The Environmental Protection Agency sets tolerance levels based on the toxicity of the product and restricts legal residues on food to no more than 1/100 of the largest amount that causes no effect on test animals. Most public health officials agree that this amount of residue, as a maximum, is harmless, and there have been no documented cases of consumer poisoning from pesticide residues on food.

Foods are inspected routinely for pesticide residues by state and federal inspectors as they are harvested, processed, and sold to consumers. In routine checks, the majority of food samples, according to the testing agencies, have been found to be completely free of pesticide residue or to have residues well below the tolerance level. Those foods that have pesticide residues in excess of the tolerance level are judged to be adulterated and are not allowed to be sold.

Another controversial question in regard to pesticides is how effective the regulatory system actually is in protecting the public from chemical hazards. For example, in 1978 the House of Representatives commerce subcommittee on oversight and investigations published a report that was highly critical of the way that the USDA, EPA, and FDA were monitoring toxic chemicals in food. The subcommittee reported that the EPA's system for establishing the safety of pesticides was out of date, that safety tests of many pesticides have never been conducted, and that many foods that contain illegal chemical residues are allowed to be marketed by the USDA.

Obviously, the question of the potential hazards from pesticides and other chemicals in foods will not be resolved quickly or easily. While scientists generally agree that there is little if any chance that chemical pesticides can be abandoned in the near future, they are directing their efforts to developing alternative ways to control pests—for example, biological control—that present less hazard to man and his environment.

Metallic substances such as mercury, lead, and aluminum are found in minute quantities in the environment—for example, in soil, water, and air—and are also found in all living matter, both animal and vegetable. Sometimes environmental conditions may cause abnormal amounts of these materials to be concentrated in food, with potentially hazardous results (see Exhibit 25.2).

Mercury

Mercury is absorbed by plants from the soil and air as they grow. Man and other animals get mercury from plants or animals when they eat them. This naturally occurring mercury does not appear to pose a toxic hazard. However, there have been cases of poisoning when large

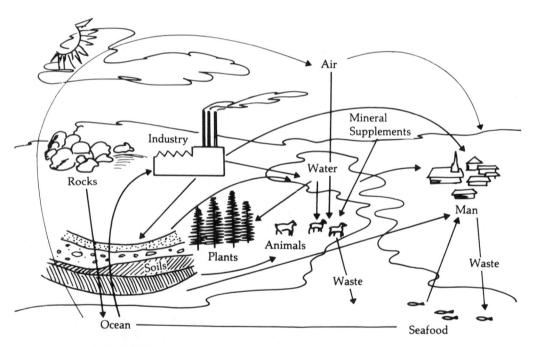

Exhibit 25.2. Trace elements move through countless cycles in the environment, and all of these cycles affect both the nutritional value and the safety of our food. (*Source: Toward the New: A Report on Better Foods and Nutrition from Agricultural Research*. U.S. Department of Agriculture, Agriculture Information Bulletin No. 341, Washington, D.C., 1970, p. 8.)

amounts of mercury compounds were dumped into the environment— for example, into fishing waters—or when seed grains treated with mercury compounds to prevent mold were accidently eaten by animals or people.

The Food and Drug Administration has a continuing program of analyzing foods for mercury content and has established a maximum safe limit of 5 parts per million. In the early 1970s a "mercury scare" concerning the safety of eating fish, particularly canned tuna and frozen swordfish, swept the country when they were found to have a mercury content exceeding 5 parts per million. Fish absorb mercury from water. Larger fish get mercury from the smaller fish that they eat. Swordfish and tuna have higher levels of mercury than other fish because as they grow larger they consume vast quantities of smaller fish. Although no harmful effects were observed in Americans who consumed tuna and swordfish, changes were made in fishing and selection practices of these species to eliminate those fish with higher levels of mercury.

Lead

Lead toxicity is a well-known syndrome in children who nibble on surfaces that have been painted with lead-containing paint. However, food can also be a source of toxic amounts of lead. For example, it has been found that plants can have high concentrations of lead when grown near highways where the soil also has been found to be high in lead. Leaded gasoline is thought to be the source of these concentrations. Lead was also found in evaporated milk and traced to lead used to seal the can. Another source of toxic amounts of lead are unglazed pottery and lead glazes of dishes that have been improperly fired. When an acid food, for example, orange juice, is stored in these products for a period of time, the acid may leach out toxic amounts of lead. The Food and Drug Administration has taken steps to try to eliminate these kinds of problems.

Aluminum

Utensils made of aluminum have often been accused of being unsafe because small amounts of aluminum are leached out, particularly when acid foods are cooked in them. However, there is an abundance of evidence that cooking in aluminum utensils is harmless. Aluminum is the third most abundant element in the earth's crust and it occurs naturally in many foods. In addition, aluminum compounds have a number of uses as direct food ingredients, for example, in baking powder. Many scientific studies have determined that the amount of aluminum ingested as a result of preparing foods in aluminum cookware is so small as to be of no significance in comparison with the amount of aluminum consumed from other sources.

Phthalates

A family of chemical compounds used in "plasticizers" in the manufacture of vinyl plastics, phthalates are an example of a man-made chemical that may find its way into our food.

Low levels of phthalates have been found in fish, probably as a result of the dumping of industrial wastes into water. Food wrappers and containers are sometimes made of vinyl plastics with the potential for the migration of the chemical into the food stored or wrapped in the material. As a result, containers made of these materials have been prohibited for use with certain foods, such as wine and soft drinks. The toxicity of phthalates has been tested extensively on laboratory animals, with the general finding that exposure does not produce significant toxic effects at high doses. Research on the safety of phythalates is continuing, however.

Polychlorinated Biphenyls (PCBs)

Another example of man-made chemicals that have found their way into the environment and from there into our food supply, PCBs are used as plasticizers and as electrical insulators and have a wide variety of other uses. They have been discovered in foodstuffs, rivers, wildfowl, and the human body. They are very stable chemically and persist in the environment for a long time. They are absorbed in body fat and will remain there for years.

Polychlorinated biphenyls have been found in milkfat and research evidence suggests they could be hazardous to infants. Studies with rhesus monkeys showed high mortality and disease, including that of the brain and nervous system, in offspring nursed by their mothers with milk that often contained 3.0 parts per million (ppm) PCBs. Because of these findings, the Food and Drug Administration has tentatively set a PCB level for whole cow's milk not to exceed 2.5 ppm.

Unfortunately, we cannot avoid chemicals such as this by eating only so-called natural foods. An Environmental Protection Agency survey of mother's milk in ten states along the Eastern seaboard showed undesirably high levels of PCBs in this natural milk in three states (2.3 to 2.6 ppm).[2] At this writing, however, there certainly has been no move to ban breast feeding because of this contamination.

While the one U.S. manufacturer of PCBs has sharply curtailed its sales since 1971, millions of pounds are imported. Congressional action was proposed to halt imports of PCBs in 1978.

[2]M. Jacobson, "Polluting Breast Milk: The PCB Story." *Nutrition Action*, Vol. 3, No. 12, December, 1976, p. 9.

Antibiotics, sulfonamides, and other antibacterial drugs are widely used to prevent infections and to increase the rate of weight gain in food-producing animals. If the drug is not properly used, it can be retained in the animal tissue and passed on to a person who eats the meat. This could create the potential for a harmful allergic reaction or contribute to a buildup of antibiotic-resistant bacteria in the intestinal tract of that person.

The Food and Drug Administration has been concerned with these possible adverse effects and has regulations regarding the use of these drugs. FDA approval is required for the use of specific drugs. Numerous drugs and combinations of drugs are not allowed to be used in animal production; for example, antibiotics most critically needed for treatment of disease in man are not permitted to be used in animals. Time periods for withdrawing approved drugs from medicated animal feeds are established to ensure against any residue in food, or to keep the residues at a safe level. Foods are considered adulterated and are removed from the marketplace if they contain unapproved residues of drugs.

More recent new concerns are that long-term feeding of low level antibacterials to food animals may cause the development of resistant intestinal organisms in the animal and that bacteria in foods could produce drug-resistant human diseases. These questions are now under investigation.

Growth Hormones

Hormones, for example, diethylstilbestrol (DES), are a type of drug used in raising animals to promote growth and reduce feed costs. DES, an estrogenic hormone, was suspected of being carcinogenic when it was discovered that the daughters of women who took DES during pregnancy to prevent miscarriage were prone to developing cancer of the vagina and cervix in adulthood. Because DES was considered potentially carcinogenic, strict regulations regarding its use were established by the Food and Drug Administration and the U.S. Department of Agriculture. Finally its use was banned in animal feeding in 1979.

Insects in stored foods are a common and annoying problem to consumers, but seldom (except in the case of cockroaches) a health hazard. The presence of insects can result in higher food costs or reduced nutrition, however, if contaminated foods must be thrown away.

Weevils and pantry beetles represent a large class of insects that invade foods such as cereals, pasta, dried fruit, nuts, seeds, crackers, and even spices. They generally get into these foods during storage, in warehouses and supermarkets, moving from container to container, eating, and laying their eggs. The eggs are tiny and not noticeable, so consumers may not discover the insects until they hatch and invade other foods in the home.

If insects are found in stored foods, immediate action is necessary, because generally there will be others hiding. *All* packages and containers of vulnerable foods should be checked, and those that are contaminated or suspect should be discarded or treated to kill bugs (either heated in a low (130° F) oven for two hours, with stirring to ensure thorough heat penetration, or frozen for two or more days). Heating and freezing will kill the insects in all stages of growth, from egg to adult. Foods should be stored in very tightly closed containers to prevent new contamination. The insects can be removed (for example sifted out) and the food safely eaten, as these pantry pests to not carry disease. While eating insects is not considered esthetically desirable in the United States, these insects are not nutritionally undesirable: they simply add a little extra protein! (In many cultures, insects are an accepted part of the diet.)

PARASITES

Parasites found occasionally in meat and fish are a much more serious health problem than insects. Because they are killed at temperatures above 140°/150°F, they are a problem to people only when raw or undercooked meat or fish are eaten.

Trichinella. Trichinosis can result from the consumption of raw pork or, uncommonly, raw beef and wild animals such as bears if the parasite trichinella is present. This parasite imbeds itself in the muscle and is not readily detected by visual inspection. The problem occurs rarely in the United States now that garbage fed to hogs must be pasteurized. However, an occasional case of trichinosis is reported by public health officials. For this reason, pork should never be eaten raw and should be cooked to a temperature higher than 150°F to ensure destruction of the parasite. Freezing pork for 10 to 20 days will also kill the trichinella.

Toxoplasma Gondii. Toxoplasmosis is a common parasite infection of humans and other animals caused by a protozoan, *toxoplasma gondii*. A major source of infection is raw meat. While the infection is generally mild in children and adults, it can cause birth defects in unborn babies. If a woman has the infection while pregnant, she can pass the infection along to her unborn baby where it can have devastating effects on the baby's nervous system, causing problems such as mental retardation, abnormal head growth, rashes, jaundice, eye problems, and convulsions. The infection can be avoided by always cooking meat to the well-done stage. Pregnant women should be particularly careful to avoid eating raw meat.

Tapeworms. Another parasite that humans can be infected with as a result of eating raw meat or fish, tapeworms are destroyed when the food is cooked.

Paralytic Shellfish Poisoning. This results from eating cooked or raw mussels and clams (bivalves) that have been feeding on the "red tide," an algae which blooms in the ocean during the summer months. When mussels and clams eat this algae, they produce alkaloid materials which can cause disturbances of vision, paralysis of chest muscles, and death in people who eat them. Gathering mussels and clams during the period of red tides is generally prohibited by state law.

MICROORGANISMS AND TOXINS PRODUCED BY MICROORGANISMS

Because foods are naturally loaded with microorganisms—yeasts, molds, and bacteria—it could be argued that microorganisms are a form of natural toxicant in food rather than contaminants. Some microorganisms are beneficial, and some are harmful. "Friendly" microorganisms play an important role in food preparation, processing, and preservation. They make bread rise and turn milk into yogurt or cheese, cabbage into saurkraut, cucumbers into pickles, and fruit juice into wine. Their growth in food supplies pleasing flavors and acid that preserves food. Friendly microorganisms are also used in the commercial production of vitamins, such as B_{12} and riboflavin, and amino acids. Some—certain yeasts and algae, for example—have even been used for food directly.

"Unfriendly" microorganisms cause food to spoil and can cause food to become harmful, resulting in illness and even death, either from the microorganisms themselves or from toxins they produce. Spoiled food results in waste and loss of the nutritional benefits of that food. But the illness and even death resulting from food poisoning caused by microorganisms are far more serious health hazards.

Some harmful microorganisms from food grow in the intestine and cause infections. Examples are salmonellosis, caused by salmonella bacteria, which are found in all animal foods; typhoid fever, caused by another species of salmonella bacteria; and hepatitis, caused by a virus that may be carried in food or water.

A second form of food-borne illness is intoxication, where the microorganisms grow in large numbers in food and produce a toxin that causes illness when the food is eaten. Examples are botulism, caused by *Clostridium botulinum*, perfringens poisoning caused by *Clostridium perfringens*, and staphylococcal food poisoning ("staph") caused by *Staphylococcus aureus*.

Exhibit 25.3.   Bacterial Foodborne Illness:

NAME OF ILLNESS	WHAT CAUSES IT	SYMPTOMS
Salmonellosis. Examples of foods involved: poultry, red meats, eggs, dried foods, dairy products.	*Salmonellae.* Bacteria widespread in nature, live and grow in intestinal tracts of human beings and animals.	Severe headache, followed by vomiting, diarrhea, abdominal cramps, and fever. Infants, elderly, and persons with low resistance are most susceptible. Severe infections cause high fever and may even cause death.
Perfringens poisoning. Examples of foods involved: stews, soups, or gravies made from poultry or red meat.	*Clostridium perfringens.* Spore-forming bacteria that grow in the absence of oxygen. Temperatures reached in thorough cooking of most foods are sufficient to destroy vegetative cells, but heat-resistant spores can survive.	Nausea without vomiting, diarrhea, acute inflammation of stomach and intestines.
Staphylococcal poisoning (frequently called staph). Examples of foods involved: custards, egg salad, potato salad, chicken salad, macaroni salad, ham, salami, cheese.	*Staphylococcus aureus.* Bacteria fairly resistant to heat. Bacteria growing in food produce a toxin that is extremely resistant to heat.	Vomiting, diarrhea, prostration, abdominal cramps. Generally mild and often attributed to other causes.
Botulism. Examples of foods involved: canned low-acid foods, smoked fish.	*Clostridium botulinum.* Spore-forming organisms that grow and produce toxin in the absence of oxygen, such as in a sealed container.	Double vision, inability to swallow, speech difficulty, progressive respiratory paralysis. Fatality rate is high in the United States (about 65 percent).

Causes, Symptoms, and Prevention

495

Microorganisms
and Toxins
Produced by
Microorganisms

CHARACTERISTICS OF ILLNESS	PREVENTIVE MEASURES
Transmitted by eating contaminated food, or by contact with infected persons or carriers of the infection. Also transmitted by insects, rodents, and pets. Onset: usually within 12 to 36 hours. Duration: 2 to 7 days.	Salmonellae in food are destroyed by heating the food to 140° F. and holding for 10 minutes or to higher temperatures for less time; for instance, 155° F. for a few seconds. Refrigeration at 40° F. inhibits the increase of Salmonellae, but they remain alive in foods in the refrigerator or freezer, and even in dried foods.
Transmitted by eating food contaminated with abnormally large numbers of the bacteria. Onset: usually within 8 to 20 hours. Duration: May persist for 24 hours.	To prevent growth of surviving bacteria in cooked meats, gravies, and meat casseroles that are to be eaten later, cool foods rapidly and refrigerate promptly at 40° F. or below, or hold them above 140° F.
Transmitted by food handlers who carry the bacteria and by eating food containing the toxin. Onset: usually within 3 to 8 hours. Duration: 1 to 2 days.	Growth of bacteria that produce toxin is inhibited by keeping hot foods above 140° F. and cold foods at or below 40° F. Toxin is destroyed by boiling for several hours or heating the food in a pressure cooker at 240° F. for 30 minutes.
Transmitted by eating food containing the toxin. Onset: usually within 12 to 36 hours or longer. Duration: 3 to 6 days.	Bacterial spores in food are destroyed by high temperatures obtained only in the pressure canner. More than 6 hours is needed to kill the spores at boiling temperature (212° F.). The toxin is destroyed by boiling for 10 to 20 minutes; time required depends on kind of food.

Source: Keeping Food Safe to Eat, U.S. Department of Agriculture, Home & Garden Bulletin No. 162, Washington, D.C., pp 8–9.

Exhibit 25.3 summarizes the causes, symptoms, and control methods for the four most common types of food poisoning. Of these, botulism is the only one likely to result from processed, rather than fresh foods.

For a food to become hazardous it must first be contaminated with microorganisms and then mishandled in a way that will allow the organisms to grow. Foods may become contaminated at any of the following stages:

1. During growth. Some organisms, such as botulinus bacteria, are soil organisms, and the spores move from the soil into plants; other organisms, such as salmonella, may be present in poultry houses or feed yards and may be ingested by animals.

2. During processing.

3. At the user level. Primarily from food handlers who may carry bacteria in the nose and throat, or intestines, on the skin, or in a cut or boil, and transfer them to food by sneezing or coughing, or with unwashed hands or clothing.

But just contamination is not enough to cause a problem. Conditions must be favorable so that bacteria grow and multiply in food. To grow, bacteria need food, water, a relatively neutral (not too acid or alkaline) condition, the right temperature, and enough time.

Food. Bacteria will grow readily in almost any food except one that is quite acidic, such as fruit or pickles. Moist proteins, meat, fish, eggs, poultry (especially when ground or chopped or sliced), milk, cream, and cream sauce are particularly vulnerable.

Moisture. Bacteria will not grow in dried foods, but may be present and begin to grow if moisture is added. They also do not grow in foods where moisture is unavailable, for example, when frozen or when tied up with sugar as in jelly or jam.

Temperature. A lukewarm or room temperature is ideal for bacterial growth. As you can see from Exhibit 25.4, the greatest danger zone is between 60° and 125°F. Below 40° and above 140°F, food-poisoning bacteria do not grow readily.

Time. Bacteria multiply very rapidly at ideal growth temperatures. In just 3 to 4 hours between the temperatures of 60°F and 120°F, a food could become unsafe.

Oxygen. Some bacteria, salmonella and staph, for example, are *aerobic* and need oxygen for growth; some, botulism and perfringens, grow in the absence of oxygen and are called *anaerobic*. This explains why botulism bacteria are most likely to grow in vacuum-packed and canned foods where oxygen has been eliminated.

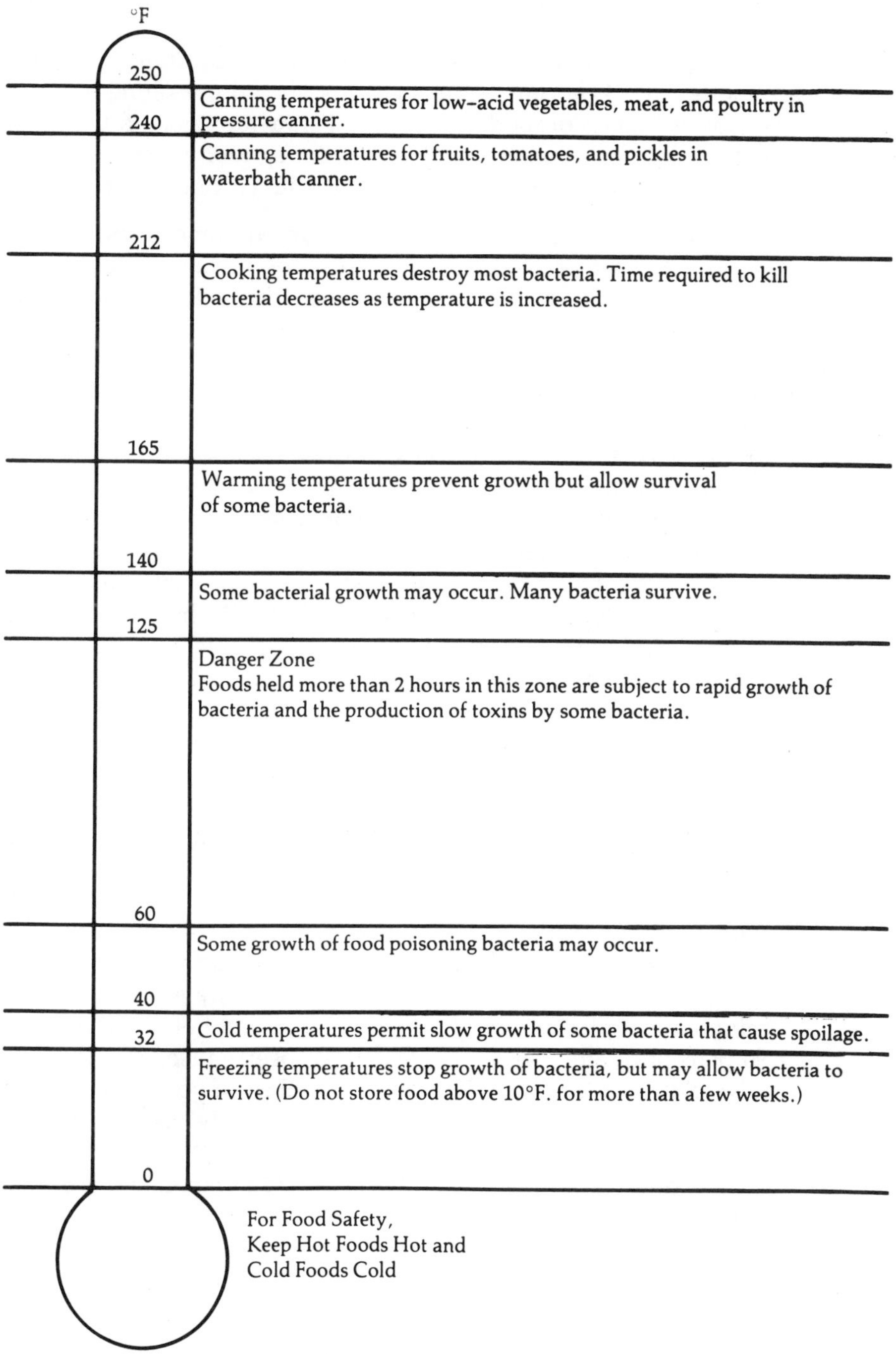

°F

250	
240	Canning temperatures for low–acid vegetables, meat, and poultry in pressure canner.
	Canning temperatures for fruits, tomatoes, and pickles in waterbath canner.
212	
	Cooking temperatures destroy most bacteria. Time required to kill bacteria decreases as temperature is increased.
165	
	Warming temperatures prevent growth but allow survival of some bacteria.
140	
125	Some bacterial growth may occur. Many bacteria survive.
	Danger Zone Foods held more than 2 hours in this zone are subject to rapid growth of bacteria and the production of toxins by some bacteria.
60	
	Some growth of food poisoning bacteria may occur.
40	
32	Cold temperatures permit slow growth of some bacteria that cause spoilage.
	Freezing temperatures stop growth of bacteria, but may allow bacteria to survive. (Do not store food above 10°F. for more than a few weeks.)
0	

For Food Safety,
Keep Hot Foods Hot and
Cold Foods Cold

Exhibit 25.4.   Temperature guide to food safety. (*Source: Keeping Food Safe to Eat*, Home and Garden Bulletin No. 162, U.S. Department of Agriculture, Washington, D.C., 1975, p. 5.)

497

Prevention of Food Poisoning

The Center for Disease Control of the U.S. Public Health Service reports that 94 percent of the incidents of food poisoning occur because people in homes or food service establishments do not follow good sanitation and health practices.[3] Yet preventing food poisoning is not difficult, once you understand what causes it. To prevent food poisoning:

1. Avoid contamination. Use clean equipment and clean hands; avoid sneezing or coughing into food; don't handle food when you have an open cut or sore on your hands; keep sick persons and pets out of the food preparation area; and keep out air and dust.

2. Handle food that you are preparing in such a way that bacteria will not multiply. This is accomplished by keeping vulnerable foods hot, above 0°F, or cold, below 40°F, and not allowing them to stand at room or lukewarm temperatures any longer than necessary—and never longer than one or two hours. Remember, there is no way to know for sure whether or not harmful bacteria are present in food; so always handle it as if they were present.

If you are suspicious that a food has been mishandled and is potentially unsafe, what should you do? Taste it? Smell it? Boil it? Unfortunately none of these methods is totally reliable. A food with enough bacteria or toxin to make you sick can look, smell, and taste perfectly normal. (Conversely, a putrid, foul-smelling food could be safe.) Also, boiling the food before eating it will not make it safe in every instance. Boiling does destroy bacteria that cause infections, such as salmonella, and it does destroy botulism toxin. But "staph" toxin is so highly heat resistant you would have to boil food for several hours to destroy this toxin.

Thus, the safest course to follow when there is a likelihood that food may cause food poisoning is to throw it out—without tasting it. If you use home-canned foods, particularly low-acid foods such as vegetables, meat, fish, or poultry, it is wise to always boil them 10 to 15 minutes as a precautionary measure to prevent botulism. An estimated 90 percent of all cases of botulism have been caused by home-canned, low-acid foods that were improperly handled. If you can foods at home, be sure to follow reliable, modern, scientifically tested directions and use the proper equipment. Keep in mind at all times that the botulism toxin is one of the most lethal poisons known to man: a tiny amount can kill you.

[3]T.P. Labusa, *Food and Your Well-Being*. St. Paul, MN: West Publishing Co., 1977, p. 253.

Molds are another form of microorganism that are both friendly and unfriendly. Friendly molds are used, for example, in cheesemaking to provide the desirable flavor of "blue" and roquefort cheese. Unfriendly molds cause spoilage of many foods that resist bacterial growth because they are too dry (like bread), their moisture is tied up by sugar (like jelly and jam), or they are too acidic (like fruit).

We have known about these molds for a long time. But in the last two decades, scientists have discovered some molds that produce mycotoxins, one of the most potent classes of toxins yet discovered. *Aflatoxins* are the best known of the mycotoxins, and they are known to be toxic to animals at extremely low levels—less than one part of toxin per million parts of food. Many farm animals, especially poultry, have died as a result of feed contaminated with aflatoxin, which caused liver tumors, lung edema, or disorders of the brain and other tissues.

More than 100 mold species that produce toxins have been found growing on food. The mycotoxins are found especially in foods not properly dried or stored. The molds that produce the mycotoxins thrive on moisture and on broken kernels of grains and legumes. Corn and peanuts are two most likely sources of food for these molds, but they also grow on other grains (wheat, rice, oats, barley), legumes (but not soybeans), nuts, and sweet potatoes. Because the toxin is so potent, contamination of just a small portion of the food can result in a whole batch becoming unsafe.

The Food and Drug Administration has in place a massive procedure for testing samples of local and imported foods and has set tolerance levels at 15 parts per billion for aflatoxin. Many major food companies have set up their own testing procedures also.

Not all forms of mold produce mycotoxins. For example, mold on jams, jellies, meat and fish, bacon, and fresh fruit is not mycotoxin-producing. Therefore, it is safe to remove the mold and eat the remaining food. Because molds on foods such as legumes, nut meats, grain, corn, and bread could be mycotoxin-producing, do not eat these foods if they are moldy. If mold is growing on a food preserved by acid, such as pickles, canned fruits, or tomatoes, throw the food out because mold growth could reduce the acidity of the food to the point where botulism bacteria could grow. If mold growth is extensive on jam and jellies, discard them too for the same reason.

To sum up, among the nonnutrient substances we find in foods, microorganisms present the greatest hazard to our health. The toxins produced by mold and bacteria are so powerful that a small amount can kill us or make us seriously ill. Bacterial infections are another health hazard caused by microorganisms. Safe food-handling practices at the consumer level are of prime importance in preventing the growth of microorganisms and protecting our health.

Summary
Contaminants are substances that are not purposely added to foods, but rather get into foods during growth, harvest, transportation, processing, packaging, or storage. Some are harmful.

Pesticides are important in protecting our food supply from destructive pests. Their use is closely regulated by the Environmental Protection Agency (EPA). Extensive safety tests are required, and tolerance levels for residues are set to provide a wide margin of safety. The question of the potential hazards from pesticides in foods is the subject of considerable debate that will not be resolved quickly or easily.

Heavy metals such as mercury, lead, and aluminum are found naturally in the environment and in both plant and animal foods. Excessive amounts, of lead, for example, do pose a toxic hazard. The Food and Drug Administration has established a program to monitor the food supply to determine the presence of mercury and lead, has set tolerance levels, and has taken steps to eliminate known sources.

The potential harmful effects of plastics such as phthalates and polychlorinated biphenyls (PCBs) and of antibiotics and growth hormones given to food animals are being studied, and regulations are being developed as a result of the research.

While seldom a health hazard to humans, insects in stored foods may destroy edible food, thereby reducing nutrients available and increasing food costs. Parasites such as trichinella and tapeworms are harmful, but are destroyed by cooking.

Of all the potentially harmful substances in foods, microorganisms are the most common and the most likely to cause harm. However, not all microorganisms are harmful; many are beneficial and are important in food production, processing, and preservation. The most likely source of bacteria-caused food poisoning is mishandling by the consumer. Bacteria need food, water, a relatively neutral environment, the proper temperature, and time for growth. Consumers can prevent the growth of food-poisoning bacteria by minimizing contamination and by handling and storing foods so that conditions are not favorable for their growth.

One of the most potent classes of toxins found in foods are produced by molds. Sources of these mycotoxins are grains, legumes, nuts, and foods made from these products when they are not properly dried or stored. The Food and Drug Administration and major food companies have established procedures for regular testing of vulnerable foods for the presence of mycotoxins.

WHO PROTECTS YOUR FOOD? 26

Highlights

Functions of government agencies involved in enforcing laws and
regulations protecting food safety

Supermarket Nutrition:

Natural, organic, and health foods

Why people use health foods

Relative cost and nutritional value of health foods

In Chapter 25, we referred to government agencies that are involved in enforcing laws relating to food safety. They include:

The Food and Drug Administration (FDA), which carries the prime responsibility for promulgating the regulations authorized by the food safety laws and seeing that they are enforced. However, the FDA does not have a large enough staff to continually inspect every food manufacturer and seller. Therefore, the agency uses the "spot check" method. Those firms that produce the most food and that have demonstrated the least effort in complying with regulations are the most likely to be inspected. Consumer complaints can also generate inspections. The FDA's jurisdiction is limited to foods shipped in interstate commerce, across state lines.

The United States Department of Agriculture (USDA) has jurisdiction over the safety of animal foods, meat, poultry, and eggs, with the exception of fish. The USDA develops regulations relating to the inspection and grading of these products and provides mandatory, continuous inspection of meat and poultry production plants to ensure the wholesomeness of these foods. Inspection is required for both fresh and processed meat and poultry products, and imported products must have USDA-approved inspection in the country of origin. The USDA's jurisdiction includes meat and poultry products produced and sold within states as well as those shipped across state lines. In addition, the USDA makes available, for a user fee, a voluntary continuous inspection of processed fruits and vegetables during processing.

The U.S. Department of Commerce's National Marine Fisheries Service is responsible for the safety of fish products. Unlike the USDA, this department does not require continuous inspection of fish processors. The inspection and grading service provided by this department is voluntary.

The Environmental Protection Agency (EPA) is responsible for establishing regulations for the use of substances that might be harmful to the environment, such as pesticides and other man-made chemicals; and monitoring their presence in air, water, soil, food, and so forth.

State departments of food, agriculture, and health are involved in protecting food that is grown, produced, and sold within the states. State laws vary considerably in the level of protection provided.

SUPERMARKET NUTRITION: "NATURAL," "ORGANIC," AND "HEALTH" FOODS

"Natural peanut butter," "organic applesauce," "natural cereal"—are these foods better for us than ordinary peanut butter, applesauce, and cereal? The manufacturers and promoters of these products would have us think so. They want us to believe that the foods so labeled are better tasting, more nutritious, or more healthful. But they cannot make such statements because they have no documented evidence to back them up—and labels must be truthful. Instead, they use terms like "natural," "organic," or "health food," which consumers associate with better nutrition. Since these terms have no legal definition they can be attached to just about any food, and often are, as a sales gimmick with no real meaning, except higher prices.

Specialty food producers are in general agreement with what these terms *should mean* (but often don't).

Organic foods means foods grown in soil fertilized only with manure or humus (organic fertilizers) and not treated with chemicals such as pesticides. "Organically grown" would be a more accurate term for these foods, since all foods fit the technical definition of "organic."

Natural foods means foods marketed without preservatives, emulsifiers, or other additives; or foods that are unprocessed or less processed, such as whole-grain cereals. A few foods could fit the definition of both natural and organically grown.

Health foods means foods for special diets such as vegetarian diets or foods having supposed special "health-giving" qualities (to prevent aging or to cure disease). These capabilities often are attributed, without scientific evidence, to foods such as dried ("dessicated") liver, brewer's yeast, bone meal, yogurt, blackstrap molasses, and the like. Foods in this group are often used as nutrient supplements. But again, the term is misleading, since all foods are health foods in the sense of supplying nutrients we need.

Because of abuses in the use of the terms natural, organic, and health foods on labels and in advertisements, the Federal Trade Commission has issued a report suggesting that these terms be defined more specifically and their use be controlled. To date, no decision has been made on this proposal.

Why Do People Buy Natural, Organic, and Health Foods?

An older person may not feel very well, but the doctor can find nothing wrong. At the health food store the friendly, sympathetic clerk is a good listener and offers personal attention. Thus, the older person believes that the health foods will make him feel better, and sometimes they do because of this belief. Then too, organic foods are more like the home-grown foods of the "olden days," which makes them seem better to an older person.

A young person may reject the life of the competitive, money-oriented establishment. He questions the big business profiteers, blames big chemical companies for pollution, and chooses natural foods as a way to reject big business and manipulative advertising. Friendly, personal stores emphasize "back to nature." For some young people, eating natural foods has been a substitute for self-destructive practices such as drug abuse.

A worried consumer may read about health dangers in food contaminants, pesticides, and additives and become excessively concerned and fearful about the safety or nutritional value of ordinary foods. Some devotees of health foods are looking for a cure-all to help overcome emotional difficulties.

Businessmen are quick to take advantage of any fad that helps sell products. Because "natural" and "organic" have been perceived as words with sales appeal, advertisements, and labels featuring these words (not only on foods but on cosmetics, detergents, and other products) were developed to expand sales to the average consumer. Then too, a food called "natural" or "organic" can be sold for a higher price than foods without these labels.

A U.S. Department of Agriculture survey, in which the costs of 29 commonly used foods—regular and those labeled "organic"—were compared at supermarkets, natural food stores, and health food stores, showed the price differences illustrated in Exhibit 26.1.

As an example, a quart of regular canned apple juice cost 29¢ at the supermarket; organic apple juice cost 65¢ at the supermarket, 51¢ at the natural food store, and 75¢ at the health food store.[4]

Exhibit 26.1. Comparison of Commonly Used Foods Purchased at Different Stores

TYPE OF FOOD AND PLACE OF PURCHASE	PRICE OF 1 BAG COMMONLY USED FOODS
Regular foods at supermarket	$11.00
Organic foods at supermarket	$20.30
Organic foods at natural food store	$17.80
Organic foods at health food store	$21.90

Are Natural or Organically Grown Foods More Nutritious?

The answer to this question can be found in information presented earlier in this chapter and in the preceding chapter. If the words natural or organic are used simply for descriptive purposes and sales appeal, it's obvious that there would be no nutritional differences between a food with these words and a food without these words on the label.

[4]Institute of Food Technologists' Expert Panel on Food Safety and Nutrition and the Committee on Public Information, *Organic Foods*, A Scientific Status Summary. Chicago, IL: Institute of Food Technology, January, 1974.

If the word natural is used to denote less processed, or less refined foods—for example, whole-grain cereals or natural orange juice, as opposed to synthesized sugar-water mixtures, and milk-based products instead of nondairy products—then the natural food probably is higher in nutrients. But if natural means no additives or chemicals, it could mean the food is actually less nutritious than a comparable food with additives if the additives are nutrients or are nutrient protective. (See Chapter 7 for an example of "natural" cereal.)

It is clear from the discussion of the effects of organic and inorganic fertilizers on nutrients in Chapter 21 that the claim that organically grown foods are more nutritious is not based on scientific evidence. The question of whether foods grown without pesticides are more healthful is yet to be resolved. However, several studies in which fresh produce marketed as "organic" was compared with ordinary produce showed that in some cases the "organic" produce had pesticide residue levels as high as, or higher than, those found on the ordinary produce. Researchers theorized that either the produce labeled "organic" had not been grown any differently than other produce and was falsely labeled, which is believed to be the case frequently, or that this produce was subject to "drift" of pesticides sprayed on crops grown in adjoining fields. In any event, the conclusion reached is that consumers who pay high prices for products labeled "organic" or "organically grown" are likely to be wasting their money on foods that may be poorer in quality or no different from ordinary foods.

As for quality and flavor differences claimed between "organically grown" and ordinary food, they may be more imagined than real. The key to high quality, good-tasting produce is planting flavorful varieties, harvesting them at the proper time, and eating them at their quality peak. This can easily be accomplished with home-grown fruits and vegetables, but not so easily with foods that are grown commercially and must be shipped and stored.

Thus the home gardener may attribute the flavor and quality differences in his fruits and vegetables to the fact that they were grown organically, when the differences are actually due to other factors. While it is practical for a home gardener to use manure and compost and pick off the bugs as they appear, this inefficient, costly growing method is not practical for feeding the hungry people of the world.

Summary

The federal agencies involved in enforcing laws relating to the safety of our food supply include the Food and Drug Administration (FDA), the U.S. Department of Agriculture (USDA), the U.S. Department of Commerce's National Marine Fisheries Service, and the Environmental Protection Agency (EPA). In addition, laws that vary from state to state are enforced by state departments of food, agriculture, or health.

The terms "natural," "organic," and "health foods" have no legal definition. They are used promiscuously to promote the sale of certain foods by implying that those foods are more nutritious than other foods.

Cost comparisons show that foods labeled "organic" sell for a higher price both at supermarkets and health food stores. But there is no scientific evidence that organically grown foods are more nutritious. Flavor differences claimed for organically grown foods may be imaginative rather than real, or they may be due to differences in variety, ripeness, or freshness (in the case of home-grown foods).

Part VIII

MEETING THE NUTRITION CHALLENGE

FOOD MANAGEMENT TO REACH NUTRITION GOALS 27

Highlights

Steps in providing balanced meals

Importance of breakfast and ways to improve breakfast habits

Nutritional value of away-from-home meals and how to improve it through wise food choices

Nutritional importance of snacks; nutritious snack foods to replace those low in nutrient density

Special nutritional problems faced by those who live alone; suggestions for overcoming them

510
Food
Management
to Reach
Nutrition
Goals

Knowing nutrient needs and the nutritional value of the foods we buy is just one aspect of eating a balanced diet. The other essential ingredient is management skill, accompanied by a daily effort to make balanced meals or snacks a reality for an individual or a family.

Managing meals involves the same sort of decision-making process used in managing money, time, or a business, and the same steps are followed: (1) setting goals; (2) planning how to reach them (choosing among alternatives); (3) carrying out the plan; and (4) evaluating progress towards goals (see Exhibit 27.1).

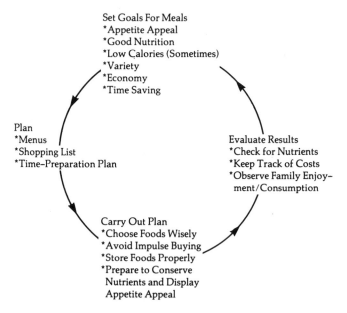

Set Goals For Meals
*Appetite Appeal
*Good Nutrition
*Low Calories (Sometimes)
*Variety
*Economy
*Time Saving

Plan
*Menus
*Shopping List
*Time–Preparation Plan

Evaluate Results
*Check for Nutrients
*Keep Track of Costs
*Observe Family Enjoy-
   ment/Consumption

Carry Out Plan
*Choose Foods Wisely
*Avoid Impulse Buying
*Store Foods Properly
*Prepare to Conserve
   Nutrients and Display
   Appetite Appeal

Exhibit 27.1.   Management steps to reach nutrition goals.

STEPS IN MANAGEMENT

Establishing Goals

When homemakers are asked, in surveys, what their goals are in providing food for their families, they answer: (1) balanced meals, which to them means good nutrition; (2) economy—staying within.a budget; (3) efficient use of time; (4) appetite appeal—foods that look good, taste good, and suit the family members' preferences; (5) variety; (6) low-calorie meals.[1]

[1]"Consumer Concerns Affect Food Purchases." *Farm Index*, Vol. 15, No. 11, November, 1976, pp. 4-9. And "Nutrition—The Redbook Nutrition Report," a National Study of Women Food Shoppers Conducted by the Gallup Organization, Inc. New York: The Redbook Publishing Co., 1976.

Two major surveys showed that balanced meals were the number one goal of 36 to 40 percent of the respondents. The two other most important considerations were family likes and staying within a budget. How do you rank the importance of these goals for your meals?

Planning

Having a plan is a key step in reaching all of these goals. Planning involves deciding ahead of time: what foods will be served during a day, week, or other time frame (a menu plan); what foods will be bought (a shopping list); when they will be prepared; and who will prepare them. In other words, it's a total management plan for meals. Without planning, a person is likely to waste time and money and may have a poor diet.

With planning a person can:

1. Be sure to include all of the foods needed for good health each day and have meals with more variety. The Four Food Groups (as outlined in Chapter 1) can serve as an easy guide for planning.

2. Take advantage of advertised specials if the plan is built around these foods. (One survey showed a 10 percent or larger saving was possible with this method.)

3. Get all the foods needed for a week or other time period in one trip to the store and with less backtracking down the aisles (if a shopping list is organized according to store layout). Frequent trips to the store not only waste time but also cost money because each trip exposes a person to the impulse-buying traps. A shopping list, followed with perseverence, can provide protection against buying high-cost, low-nutrient-value foods on impulse.

Intellectually, most people can agree that it makes sense to plan meals and make a list before going shopping. And, in fact, when homemakers are surveyed, they tend to describe themselves as careful shoppers, planning menus in advance, making shopping lists and sticking to them, buying advertised specials, comparing prices and nutritional content, and reading labels. But when their shopping behavior is actually examined, it turns out that the careful shoppers are in the minority.

In a 1976 USDA survey of 1,174 persons, only 18 percent fit the careful shopper image—the smallest group of shoppers. The largest group (39 percent) were pleasure motivated, buying favorite brands, even if they cost a little more, and experimenting with new and different products and recipes for their sensory appeal. The second largest group (32 percent) reported efficient use of time and money was their major consideration, with price being the strongest influence on their buying decisions.[2]

[2]"Consumer Concerns Affect Food Purchases." *Farm Index*, Vol. 15, No. 11, November, 1976, pp. 4-9.

512
Food
Management
to Reach
Nutrition
Goals

Planning does take some time and effort, but with practice it can be done quite speedily. Most people find it unrealistic to try to plan every meal and every snack for every day. A more realistic approach is to plan the main meal of the day and then buy enough "stock items" to put together for other meals and snacks. Another method is the "mix and match" approach, in which quantities of foods from the Four Food Groups are bought and put together into meals during the week. With this method a person is more likely to end up needing an extra shopping trip to pick up some missing foods or ingredients.

A planning method that frequently is used in food service establishments is the rotating-menu plan. Three or four weeks of menus and shopping lists to go with them are planned and then alternated during the year. Because this method lacks the flexibility of allowing for seasonal foods, advertised specials, unexpected leftovers, and the like, it is less desirable.

There are many different ways to plan and no one way is right. So choose the planning method that best suits your needs. Do try to make menu plans realistic, in terms of what you can afford and can do with the time you have available, and your menu plan and shopping list *flexible*—open to last minute changes if you come across better buys or cannot find something on your list.

Carrying Out the Plan

Armed with a shopping list as protection against impulse purchases, a consumer is ready to do battle with the supermarket. "Keep your eye on your list to avoid seeing the eye-level high-profit items," suggests one expert. Stoop to find the lower priced and more nutritious items on bottom shelves. Be careful of traps, such as out-of-place items (like doughnuts and sweet rolls nestled among the instant coffee) that give false "buy" signals. If possible, parents should leave children at home. They tend to distract shoppers from their serious decision-making task as well as nag parents into buying the foods they see advertised on TV.

As a further protection against impulse buying, eat before you shop. Hungry shoppers spend more and are likely to overbuy and succumb to impulse buying. The worst time to shop is right before dinner when a person is likely to be tired as well as hungry and less able to make careful choices.

Evaluating Progress

As you shop, use your nutrition knowledge and food labels to help you make decisions. At home, read nutrition labels on foods to help evaluate your purchases and improve planning and future decisions.

One method of evaluation is to keep track of spending in the different food categories to see how much you spend for food and how

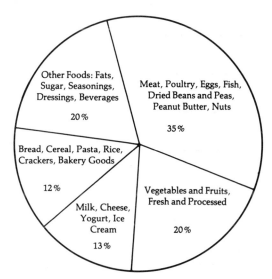

Exhibit 27.2. Families that get the best diets for their money divide their food dollars in this manner, according to U.S. Department of Agriculture studies.

you are dividing your food dollar. Exhibit 27.2 shows how families that get the best diets for their money divide their food dollars.

If your spending is far off from the averages in several categories (when one is high, something else must be lower), you might want to find out why. Most commonly, families overspend for meat and protein foods. Often spending for milk products and fruits and vegetables is too low. Overspending in the "other foods" category may mean you are buying too many soft drinks, snack foods, and high-calorie extras and getting too few other nutritious foods as a result.

In addition to evaluating the cost of food and how food dollars are divided, the food manager also will want to examine the meals served: for nutritional value, using the Four Food Groups as a guide and seeing that each is sufficiently represented; for appetite appeal (did meals look good, taste good, and did family members enjoy them?); and for the time and effort required to prepare and clean up afterwards. The checklist in Exhibit 27.3 provides an easy way to see if goals for meals were reached and also serves as a guide for meal planning.

BETTER BREAKFASTS = BETTER NUTRITION

In many homes, the meal that most needs the attention of the food manager is breakfast. Often, the organized family breakfast, with everyone sitting down together to eat, is a special occasion rather than an everyday event. As a result, both children and adults frequently start their day with either no breakfast or an inadequate one.

Appetite Appeal With Contrast In:

Colors ————————————

Textures ————————————

Shapes ————————————

Temperatures ————————————

Flavors ————————————

Nutritional Balance ————————————

Ease of Preparation
   (Time and Dishes) ————————————

Economy ————————————
                        ————————————

Total ———————————— Exhibit 27.3. How do your meals rate?

Yet breakfast is really our most important meal. Our stomachs are empty after a night without food. To properly equip us for the long hours and hard work ahead, breakfast should supply at least one-fourth of our day's food needs. When breakfast is skimpy, high-calorie, low-nutrient-density snacks are likely to be eaten in mid-morning, and the nutrients missed at breakfast are never made up.

Children and adults skip breakfast for many different reasons or combinations of reasons such as:

1. Lack of time. Everyone is too rushed to eat

2. Lack of appetite. Many people claim they're just not hungry early in the morning

3. Lack of appeal of foods served for breakfast. Many people are bored with typical breakfast foods

4. No one fixes breakfast for the family so some members don't eat

5. The mistaken notion that skipping breakfast is a good way to cut calories and lose weight.

After a period of time, eating no food in the early morning becomes a habit that many people adjust to. Yet a carefully documented study at Iowa State University showed that students who skipped breakfast were likely to have a poor attitude toward school work and decreased scholastic attainment. (School teachers often complain that by mid-morning their students are too hungry and restless to concerntrate on their studies.) Efficiency in physical performance and work output decreased when breakfast was omitted. But the omission of breakfast was of no value in weight control.[3]

Other studies showed that the type of foods served for breakfast did not affect physiological responses if protein was adequate. A protein intake of 20 to 25 grams (for an adult, proportionately less for children) was found to be needed to maintain blood sugar levels for 3 to 4 hours after the meal and to prevent the mid-morning slump. A typical school child's breakfast of sugared cereal may have less than half the recommended amount of protein.

A balanced breakfast is one which includes foods from each of the Four Food Groups, and it doesn't have to consist of typical breakfast foods at all! A food manager with imagination can plan breakfasts to include new and different foods that are little more work than the usual breakfast yet will stimulate family members' appetites and interest in eating breakfast. Some suggestions for "different" foods for breakfast are listed in Exhibit 27.4.

Exhibit 27.4. Nontraditional Foods Can Make Breakfast Nutritious and Varied

BREAKFAST MENU	FRUIT/ VEGETABLE GROUP	MILK* GROUP	PROTEIN GROUP	BREAD/ CEREAL GROUP
Cream of tomato soup	X	X		
Crackers and cheese		X		X
Cottage cheese and fruit	X	X		X
Toast or English muffin				
Peanut butter, French			X	X
toast			X	
Orange juice	X			
Milk		X		
Tomato juice				
Toasted cheese sandwich	X	X		X
Left over meat/pasta			X	X
casserole				
½ Grapefruit	X			
Milk		X		
Cream of potato soup	X	X		
Crackers				X
Canned tuna			X	
Tortilla with beans			X	X
Orange juice	X			
Milk		X		

* Milk group can be source of protein for meal.

[3]*Breakfast Source Book.* Chicago, IL: Cereal Institute, 1959.

516
Food
Management
to Reach
Nutrition
Goals

Studies show that children who eat breakfast with the whole family eat better breakfasts than those who don't, and also that children eat better breakfasts when mother or some other adult prepares and supervises the meal than when the child prepares his own breakfast.[4] So it behooves parents to see that children get a good breakfast by:

Making breakfast a family routine so everyone gets in the habit of eating it together

Having an adult or older teenager be in charge of making breakfast for everyone

Seeing that all family members get up early enough so that they have time to eat breakfast

Being organized—planning breakfasts in advance so they can be prepared quickly and easily, doing some jobs ahead of time, delegating some jobs to others

Setting a good example by eating breakfast themselves.

In some areas low-cost breakfasts are served at school as an extension of the School Lunch Program. They may be a good alternative in family situations where parents are unable to provide a nutritious breakfast for children.

EATING OUT: NUTRITIONALLY ADEQUATE OR NOT?

More and more, Americans are eating food not prepared in their own homes. A 1978 survey showed that consumers spend 27 percent of their household food dollar on meals away from home, compared to 20 percent 15 years ago.[5] People who eat a substantial portion of their meals away from home face a particular challenge in achieving a balanced diet (see Exhibit 27.5). In general, away-from-home meals tend to be less well balanced nutritionally.

Exhibit 27.5. Overview of Nutrients in Typical Restaurant Meals And Fast-Food Meals

MEALS ARE HIGH IN	MEALS ARE LOW IN
Protein	Fiber
Sodium	Vitamins A, C, E and
Fat	Folic Acid
Sugar	Calcium
Starch	Iron
(and calories)	Other trace minerals

Source: E. A. Young, E. H. Brennan, G. L. Irving, "Perspectives on Fast Foods," *Dietetic Currents*, Vol. 5, No. 5, Sept.–Oct. 1978.

[4]"Better Breakfasts Make Better Students." *Today's Homemaker*, January, 1970.

[5]"The High Cost of Eating." *Today's Homemaker*, November, 1978.

Vegetables often are not served at all, especially at fast-food restaurants, with the exception of potatoes, lettuce salad, and cabbage slaw; and when they are served, they may be overcooked or held too long on a steam table or refrigerator and as a result have reduced levels of unstable nutrients such as vitamin C.

Fruits, especially fresh ones, rarely appear except as main dish salads, calorie-laden pie, or a high-priced side dish at breakfast.

Soft drinks, coffee, tea, or alcoholic drinks are often chosen as beverages rather than milk or fruit juice. Nonfat or low-fat milk often are not available. High-calorie shakes are a favorite choice at fast-food outlets. One study showed that it was the choice of drink that determined whether a fast-food meal was excessively high in calories.[6]

Oversize portions, especially of pasta, meats, and other protein foods, are common. People either overeat or waste food.

High-calorie foods, rich in fats and sugar, are found in abundance—for example, french fried and hash browned potatoes, baked potatoes loaded with sour cream, hot breads and rolls with lots of butter, cream soups, rich salad dressing, fried fish or chicken with crispy, fat-laden coatings, malts and shakes, cakes, pies, and other rich desserts. And for breakfast there are bacon, pork sausage, fried eggs, sweet rolls or doughnuts, and pancakes or waffles with plenty of butter and syrup.

Foods high in saturated fats are popular. These include meats, especially fat-streaked steaks and fatty hamburger, butter, cheese, sour cream, and coffee creamers. *Cholesterol* is abundant in many of these foods, too, as well as in eggs and shellfish.

Salt and monosodium glutamate, both high in sodium, are used liberally in seasonings.

If you eat out only occasionally, you are not likely to suffer nutritionally from this imbalance of nutrients. But if you eat out frequently, then you should be concerned and should learn to evaluate restaurant meals on the basis of the Four Food Groups and add some of the needed foods or be sure other meals make up for the missing foods. If you have a weight problem, choose foods carefully and be sure that the other foods you eat are relatively low in calories.

You can choose nutritious meals away from home if you avoid establishments where the choices are limited to foods that are greasy, starchy, high protein, and high calorie. When possible, eat in cafeterias or restaurants that offer a wider choice of fruits, vegetables, and salads. Plan your food choices before you start through the serving line—and try to avoid looking at the tempting desserts!

Also, pay attention to the way food is prepared. If calories are a problem, choose baked or broiled meats instead of those that are batter-fried, or don't eat the coating. Select baked potatoes instead of fried, poached eggs instead of fried. Avoid foods with rich sauces and gravies.

[6]E.A. Young, E.H. Brennan, G.L. Irving, "Perspectives on Fast Foods." *Dietetic Currents*; Vol. 5, No. 5, September-October, 1978.

518
Food
Management
to Reach
Nutrition
Goals

Exhibit 27.6.   Calories in Snack Foods

SNACK FOOD CALORIES ADD UP FAST!	CALORIES	A BETTER CHOICE—	CALORIES
Mid-morning			
Donut and	150	2 Graham crackers	55
Coffee with creamer	20	Coffee, black	5
Mid-afternoon			
8-oz Carton of fruit-flavored yogurt	230	Banana	85
Before dinner			
Handful (2 oz) peanuts	332	20 stick pretzels	20
12-oz beer	170	8-oz tomato juice	45
Evening			
½ cup ice cream	135	1 cup popcorn (plain)	90
with 2 T chocolate sauce	125		
Day's Total	1162		300

Watch out for the so-called low-calorie specials. Often they are higher in calories than other menu choices—for example, when they include a broiled hamburger plus a large serving of cottage cheese. Another way to save calories is to request a vegetable, such as tomatoes, in place of the french fried potatoes.

The additions to food, which contribute sugar and fat, are another source of calories and include: dressing on salads; sugar and cream in coffee; gravy, butter, or sour cream on potatoes; butter, jelly, honey, on bread, toast, or biscuits; and whipped cream on desserts. Ask for salad dressing to be served separately, instead of mixed with the salad, so you can control the amount.

If you are concerned about calories, choose foods carefully. For example, for appetizers choose tomato juice, fruit cup, clear soup, shrimp or fish cocktail. For lunch, a good choice is fish or chicken salad with no dressing, fruit salad or tomato slices with cottage cheese, or a vegetable plate. For dinner, choose chicken, fish, or veal instead of steaks or roasts, and when you eat the latter, trim away all visible fat. Limit your starchy food intake to one starch—rice or potato, for example, and no bread, or vice versa; or eat half-size servings of each. Skip dessert, or choose a simple one such as baked apple, baked custard, angel food or sponge cake without frosting, or fruit gelatin without whipped cream.

Typical fast-food menus of cheeseburgers, hamburgers, tacos, pizza, fried chicken, or fried fish tend to be relatively high in calories. However, their nutritional value in most other respects has been found to be reasonably good. It is a mistake to consider these foods, which are so popular with teenagers and young adults, to be worthless or "junk foods." Nutrients likely to be lacking or low in fast-food meals are vitamins C, A, and folic acid. A typical meal of a cheeseburger, french fries, and chocolate shake will yield a whopping 1,200 calories, which may be well tolerated by a teenage boy, but be too high for his teenage girlfriend with a weight problem. Dieters who eat in fast-food outlets had best find ways to avoid some of the high-calorie extras, for example by substituting milk for the shake and a salad or cabbage slaw for the french fries, thereby saving about 500 calories.

SNACKING: FUN OR FOLLY?

Snacking, as we learned in Chapter 2, has become a way of life for many Americans, with snacks sometimes supplanting as well as supplementing regular meals. Snacking in itself is not necessarily bad for us, but it does have some nutritional hazards.

1. We may eat too much without realizing it. Snack foods often are high in calories. The small amounts we eat off and on throughout the day may not seem like much, but they may add up to an astounding total as illustrated in Exhibit 27.6. If the total number of calories consumed in a day is greater than our energy need, we will gain weight.

2. We may cheat ourselves of needed nutrients if our snack foods are of the high-fat, high-sugar, low-nutrient-density type that provide an excess of calories in proportion to the number of other nutrients they contain. (Some people call these "junk foods" or "empty calorie foods," but the more accurate term is "low-nutrient-density foods." You know them: soft drinks, fruit-flavored drinks, corn and potato chips, cookies, cream-filled cupcakes, candy, and so forth.)

3. We may contribute to a tooth decay problem by constantly munching sticky, gooey, high-sugar, high-starch foods. These foods are known to cling to the teeth and provide food for oral bacteria to grow on and produce acid that eats away tooth enamel (see Chapter 15). The amount of tooth decay in susceptible persons has been shown to be directly proportional to the number of different exposures to these kinds of foods.[7] The oftener you snack on them, the more likely you are to develop tooth decay problems.

The way to avoid losing out nutritionally, if snacking is a major part of your life-style, is to select snack foods from the Four Food Groups so that they will contribute important amounts of nutrients to your diet. Only after you have met the day's requirements for necessary foods should you add the low-nutrient-density foods. If weight control is a problem, you must be especially frugal when it comes to spending your calories on the high-sugar, high-fat snack foods.

[7]D. P. DePaola and M.C. Alfano, "Diet and Oral Health." *Nutrition Today,* Vol. 23, No. 3, May-June, 1977, pp. 6-32.

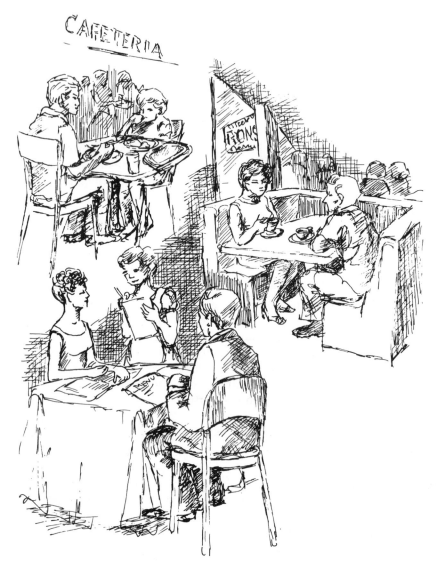

Exhibit 27.7. Meals away from home take many forms, from fast foods to gourmet foods in elegant restaurants.

Sometimes nutrition labels can help identify snack foods which give a good nutrient return for calories. But often snack foods do not have nutrition labels (remember the labels are voluntary) since manufacturers may make no special dietary claims about them.

As with other foods, if you don't buy the fattening type snack foods, you won't eat them. So it is important to control your impulse to

Exhibit 27.8.   Which Snack Foods Do You Choose?

	CALORIES	COST*
Fresh vegetable nibbles (carrots, or celery)	20	6¢
vs		
10 potato chips	100	25¢
8-oz tomato juice	40	10¢
vs		
12-oz soft drink	150	20–25¢
Fresh fruit—apple, orange, banana	75	10–15¢
vs		
Candy bar	150	20–25¢
1 oz raisins	80	20¢
vs		
Cream-filled snack cake	190	15–20¢

* Southern California prices, Summer, 1979.

buy the appetite-appealing snack foods when you're shopping and, instead, stock up on the nutritious kind of foods for snacks—foods that nevertheless are convenient, ready to eat, and fun (like cheese and fresh or dried fruit). An added bonus for buying nutritious snack foods is that they are a better buy; you get more food for your money. Some comparisons to illustrate this are shown in Exhibit 27.8.

Some people need snacks (see Exhibit 27.9). *Young children* often have a small capacity for food and small appetites. They simply cannot eat enough at a meal to hold them over until the next meal and to give them all the food they need for growth and activities. One study found that children who enjoyed snacks in the middle of the afternoon actually ate larger evening meals than usual. The snacks probably prevented fatigue, which tends to reduce the appetite.

Active teenagers, especially boys and those involved in athletics, who are growing rapidly need enormous quantities of food. Three meals a day just are not enough to satisfy their appetites.

Older people often feel more comfortable on five or six small meals instead of three bigger ones.

Ulcer patients and persons with other gastrointestinal disorders are usually advised to eat small meals frequently.

Dieters may find that frequent small meals help curb their appetites and keep them from gorging themselves on a calorie-laden dinner.

Underweight people sometimes have small appetites and need to eat oftener than three times a day.

The timing of between-meal eating is important. Food eaten 30 to 60 minutes before a meal tends to dull the appetite. Thin people and children who need to eat well at mealtime should avoid snacking within an hour before a meal. Overweight people who want to lose weight might have a snack before a meal so they eat less at the meal. This is the principle of the "two-slices-of-bread-before-a-meal diet."

522
Food
Management
to Reach
Nutrition
Goals

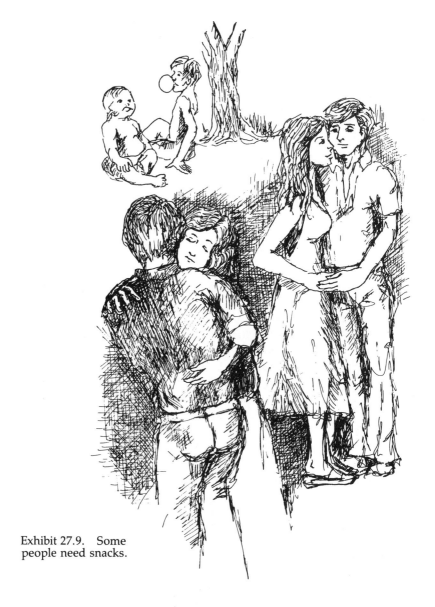

Exhibit 27.9.   Some
people need snacks.

EAT ALONE AND LIKE IT

According to recent census data, one out of five American households has just one person (Exhibit 27.10).[8] People who live alone may have problems with food preparation that larger family groups don't have, such as:

[8]P.C.Glick, "Some Recent Changes in American Families, *Current Population Reports.* Special Studies, Series P-23, No. 52, U.S. Department of Commerce, Bureau of the Census. Washington, D.C.: US. Government Printing Office, 1976.

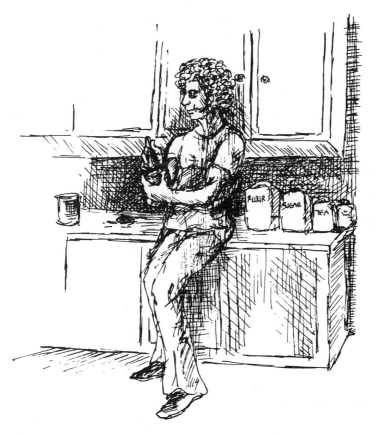

Exhibit 27.10.   Single adults often don't have the incentive or take
the time to cook for themselves.

No incentive to cook for themselves

Few or no cooking skills

Limited time for shopping and cooking

Minimum cooking equipment

Limited money to spend on food

Problems buying small quantities of food

Too many leftovers.

For one or more of these reasons the single adult may be eating a
poorly balanced or unappealing diet much of the time. This could be
having negative effects on both his physical and mental well-being. Eating well can brighten a person's mental outlook. Tasty meals give a
person something to look forward to. After all, eating is one of life's
greatest pleasures. And cooking can be a creative avocation. In sum, it's
worth the bother for a single person to fix good food for himself.

524
Food
Management
to Reach
Nutrition
Goals

To overcome special "single" problems, take the management approach and begin with planning, using the Four Food Groups. Avoid the common, nutritionally hazardous mistake made by many singles, of limiting food choices to just a few easy-to-fix favorite foods. Eating a variety of foods from the different groups is necessary to ensure a balanced diet.

People who have no incentive to cook for themselves need to begin by convincing themselves that eating well is really important and is something they value. They need to develop a routine that includes breakfast, lunch, and dinner and not let themselves slip into a catch-as-catch-can pattern, especially one that includes heavy dependence on the high-calorie, low-nutrient-density snack foods.

Often the meals eaten alone are drab. So taking the trouble to make food look appealing and taste good—having foods with color, flavor, and texture contrasts and at least one hot food in each meal, and adding a bit of garnish or especially-liked extras—will help make the meal more fun to eat.

People who don't know how to cook and don't want to take the trouble to learn can still eat nutritiously. One approach is to eat one good, balanced meal at a restaurant or cafeteria or senior citizen food serving center every day and then choose foods that don't require cooking skills for other meals. Some examples are: frozen dinners or main dishes; canned main dishes (soups, meat, tuna or other fish); dairy and delicatessen items such as cheese, cottage cheese, yogurt, lunch meats, hot dogs, salads, etc.; dried fruit, fresh fruits and vegetables; breads and cereals (crackers, frozen waffles, prepared breakfast cereals, breakfast in a package); dry milk; nuts (peanut butter and sunflower seeds). Even with a limited amount of cooking equipment, simple meals can be prepared from these foods.

A common complaint of singles is that they have problems buying small quantities of foods and as a result have too many leftovers and may end up wasting foods. Some suggestions for overcoming this problem are:

Buy foods with long keeping times, such as eggs, carrots, cabbage, celery, apples, oranges, grapefruit, dried fruit, dry milk, processed cheese and cheese spreads.

Buy foods that are easy to cook in small amounts, such as eggs, hot dogs, chicken parts, fish filets, chops, steaks, ground beef, potatoes, instant rice, loose-pack frozen vegetables, and small cans of fruits and vegetables.

Team up with a friend and share fresh foods with short keeping times, such as lettuce, cauliflower, broccoli, and meat.

Plan ahead so that several different meals are made with leftovers. This helps to save time and work as well as food. If freezer space is available, leftovers can be packaged in meal-size portions, for example on TV dinner trays, and frozen for future use.

From these suggestions you can see that the single person who is really concerned about achieving nutritious meals can do so in spite of having some unique problems. As with most activities, it is a matter of motivation. Some sample menus that would be easy for a single person to make are shown in Exhibit 27.11.

Exhibit 27.11.   Meals for Singles that Turn Leftovers Into "Planned Overs"

Meal 1	Baked chicken breasts or thighs Baked rice Canned peas Fresh fruit
Meal 2	Casserole made of leftover chicken, rice, peas mixed with ½ can of cream of chicken, celery or mushroom soup and seasoned with instant (dehydrated) minced onion Lettuce salad
Meal 3	Creamed tuna on toast (heat ½ can tuna with leftover soup, season with instant onion) Raw carrot sticks Fresh fruit
Meal 4	Tuna salad made from leftover ½ can of tuna mixed with pickle relish and salad dressing Cream of tomato soup Crackers

Summary

Management, a decision making process, involves setting goals, making a plan, carrying it out, and evaluating results. Applying these steps to food selection and meal preparation can help us achieve a nutritionally balanced and appealing diet within the confines of our time and money resources. Most important is planning: deciding in advance what foods to buy, making a list, and avoiding impulse purchases not included in our plan. The way we allocate our food dollars among the food groups can affect both our nutritional intake and how much we spend for food.

Breakfast is our most important meal, and it should supply about one-fourth of our day's nutrient needs with enough protein to prevent mid-morning fatigue. Having a family breakfast routine that includes enough time to sit down together, to eat with an adult in charge of preparation and with some nontraditional foods used, can help family members learn to enjoy eating breakfast.

Eating out is becoming more and more common among Americans. Foods eaten out tend to be high in fat, sodium, protein, starch, sugar, and calories and low in fiber, vitamins, and minerals. Serving sizes tend to be too large, and many high-calorie extras are added. Yet nutritious away-from-home meals can be achieved if the consumer chooses wisely, eating more salads, vegetables, and fruits and avoiding foods high in fats and sugar. Fast food meals can be improved with the

526
Food
Management
to Reach
Nutrition
Goals

addition of salad or cabbage slaw in place of french fries, and milk in place of a soft drink or milk shake.

Snacks are an important part of the daily food intake of many people, especially children and teen-agers, and they should provide nutrients other than calories. The best snack foods are those of high nutrient density from the Four Food Groups, such as fresh fruits and vegetables and fruit juices. These foods also give us more food value for our money than candy, soft drinks, and corn or potato chips. Sticky, sugary snack foods, besides being low in nutrient density, may be a cause of tooth decay in susceptible people.

One of five American households consists of just one person. The single adult may have a less nutritious diet because of various food preparation problems such as lack of incentive or lack of food preparation skills. These shortcomings can be overcome with motivation, planning, and development of a lifestyle that includes taking the time and making the effort to eat balanced meals.

NUTRITION CHALLENGES: YESTERDAY, TODAY AND TOMORROW 28

Highlights

Accomplishments of nutrition scientists to date, and questions still unanswered

Gap between nutrition knowledge and ordinary food consumer

Questions to help consumers separate fact from fiction

Need for moderate approach and attention to the total nutrition picture

During the last fifty years, nutrition science has undergone revolutionary change. Advancements in scientific methods for studying body tissue and body processes and for analyzing the composition of food have opened the door to an explosion in the development of new knowledge.

Nutrition researchers have discovered many essential nutrients, including over 20 vitamins and minerals. They have learned about some of the ways nutrients act in the body. They have determined how much of some of the nutrients we need and how to prevent nutritional-deficiency diseases. They have learned how to either synthesize or supply these nutrients independently from the foods in which they naturally occur.

Today, the major nutritional-deficiency diseases have been controlled and are no longer commonly seen in the United States. The knowledge, but not the wherewithal, exists to wipe out nutritional-deficiency diseases worldwide.

QUESTIONS STILL UNANSWERED

But even with these scientific advancements, our knowledge is incomplete and is based in part on theories rather than solid evidence. Scientists are still seeking the answers to questions such as:

1. How much of each nutrient is optimal for each stage of growth and development?

2. What is the requirement for those essential nutrients about which little is known?

3. How can the nutritional status of an individual be accurately measured?

4. What is the nutrition status of the general population of the United States and of various subgroups, such as preschool children or the elderly, and how can we monitor it on an ongoing basis?

5. What is the real nutritional value of the foods we eat?

6. What is the nutritional impact of the widespread consumption of processed, fabricated, and fortified foods?

7. What does constitute a fully adequate diet?

8. What is the role of diet in the prevention of chronic degenerative diseases and obesity?

9. How adequate are the diets consumed by Americans?

10. How or why do food preferences develop, and how can they be influenced?

Expanding the knowledge base in order to answer these questions is the challenge facing nutrition scientists of today and tomorrow. But an even greater challenge is bridging the gap between scientific knowledge and the nutrition knowledge of the ordinary food consumer. Only a small proportion of consumers have a real understanding of sound nutrition practices, and even those who have the knowledge often do not apply it!

Why? Because nonnutritional factors are predominantly responsible for our food decisions. We eat food because we like it, not because we think it is good for us. Yet most nutrition education is based on the idea that if we know more about the nutrient needs of the body we will apply that knowledge to improve our health.

Another roadblock to the adoption of sound nutrition practices by consumers is the large amount of nutrition misinformation conveyed to us by a dedicated vocal group of food faddists, "health food" enthusiasts, and entrepreneurs with products and publications to sell. Their propaganda methods, often based on emotional appeals, particularly fear, have been notably more effective than those of nutrition educators.

Food faddism is nothing new. Throughout history, magical properties and curative qualities have been attributed to foods. Every age and country has had food myths that have been proven worthless in time. And we, too, have our food myths, often conveyed to us by pseudo-scientists who take a little scientific information and build a story they know people want to hear. For example, they may tell us that we can cure arthritis or prevent cancer by eating certain foods.

Throughout this book, references have been made to many of the popular misconceptions about nutrients, foods, diets, and the relationship of diet and disease. They are listed for ready reference in Exhibit 28.1.

While many of these notions have been around for a long time, some are relatively new. Some are discarded and fade away, only to return again with a slightly different twist.

FACT OR FICTION?

One thing we can be sure of is that new misconceptions, new fad diets, new "miracle cures" are bound to appear every year along with news about true scientific discoveries in nutrition. How can you, as an informed nutrition consumer, separate fact from fiction?

Here are some questions to ask about this information:

1. What is the source? Is the person a recognized nutrition authority who is associated with an authentic scientific research establishment such as a university? (Be careful, many pseudo-nutritionists adopt titles that sound authentic, and claim to be members of associations that seem, from their titles, to be legitimate research organizations when they really are not.)

2. What is the claim? Does it seem reasonable? Does it agree with other facts about nutrition that you have learned?

Exhibit 28.1.   Misconceptions About Foods, Nutrients, and Diets

MISCONCEPTION	DISCUSSED ON PAGE:
Vitamins and Minerals	
Vitamin K	255
Pantothenic acid	267
Biotin	268
Vitamin C	430
Vitamin E	430
Megadoses of vitamins to treat psychiatric ills	431
Natural versus synthetic vitamins	433
Selenium supplements	236
Fluoride: safety	236
Macronutrients	
Low carbohydrate diets	121
High fiber diets	128
Lecithin as a health food supplement	157
Fat digestion	157
High-protein diets	104
Athlete's need for protein	366
Water for athletes	364
Diets	
Fad weight diets	104
Weight gain in pregnancy	391
Salt use in pregnancy	297
Nonfat milk for fat babies	323
Solid foods for babies	319
Diets/foods for arthritis sufferers	413
Foods	
Chocolate, fatty foods and acne	363
Glucose: electrolyte drinks for athletes	365
Special foods for athletic prowess	364
Special foods as "youth potions"	380
Yogurt and acidolphilus milk	240
Effect of chocolate on calcium in milk	241
Calories in imitation milk and ice cream	245
Raw versus pasteurized milk	460
Calories in dry roasted nuts	193
Nutritional value of brown versus white eggs	199
Calories in "diet bread"	137
Bleached vs. unbleached flour	483
Raw sugar and honey	148
Foods: Processing, Growing	
Depleted soils	441
Organic fertilizers	442
Sun drying compared to heat drying	453
Fresh versus processed foods	458
Sodium nitrite	476
Saccharin	479
BHA and BHT (additives)	481
Pesticide residues	486
Aluminum utensils	489
Natural and organic foods	504

3. What is the evidence to support the claim? Is it based on scientific research? Theory? Imagination? The popular press often reports new and different "therapeutic triumphs" that must be carefully evaluated and verified before they are accepted as fact. The public often is misled when the news media play up a medical report or scientific study that was specifically stated by the authors to be preliminary in nature and was limited to results observed in just a few people, or in animals, not people.

4. What do other authorities have to say about the information? New scientific information may be disputed by other scientists until it is verified by further research. Pseudo-scientific information is rejected by scientists.

5. Is there a profit motive? Is a sale of a product or publication involved? Writers for pseudo-scientific products and publications have a flair for words and can write volumes of nonsense and somehow make it sound reasonable to many who read it. The writing may be confusing, yet subtly convincing, with hidden meanings, hints of other inferred benefits, and claims that the product is a cure-all, a miracle, or a newly discovered "secret formula." A money-back guarantee or free trial also may be offered.

6. Are the readers/users encouraged to treat themselves based on the information? Be extremely wary when this approach is used. Self-treatment of a real ailment with unproved products or methods can be harmful and may delay much needed medical care. Self-treatment of an imagined ailment is a waste of money and it can be harmful, too, if the product used is toxic, for example, large doses of vitamin A or D.

FOCUS ON THE BIG PICTURE

While there are still many gaps in our nutrition knowledge, the evidence is quite clear that the moderate approach is the healthiest. We need to avoid extremes in both total quantity of food eaten and in the use of any one food or nutrient.

Choosing food for good nutrition is like working a jigsaw puzzle, with each of the 50-plus essential nutrients representing one piece of the puzzle. Some pieces are very large, some are very tiny, but the puzzle is not complete unless all the pieces are in their proper place (see Exhibit 28.2). Each piece of the puzzle has its specialized role to play in coordination with all of the other pieces to complete the whole, just as all the nutrients work together in the body to provide complete nutrition.

By focusing our attention on the total nutrition picture, the completed puzzle, and choosing a variety of foods every day from the different food groups, there's a good chance that we can meet our personal nutrition challenge and be well nourished in the midst of plenty.

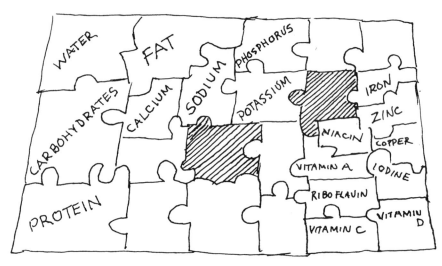

Exhibit 28.2. The nutrients work together in our bodies like pieces
in a jigsaw puzzle; the whole is not complete without all of the parts.

Summary   Nutrition knowledge is constantly expanding and evolving. Although many life-saving and life-enhancing discoveries have been made in the area of controlling nutritional deficiency diseases, for example, our knowledge is incomplete and often contradictory. Complex challenges in addition to that of advancing the knowledge base face nutrition scientists today. Chief among these are bridging the gap between scientific knowledge and application by the food consumer.

Since external factors are often responsible for food decisions, these must be addressed. With the abundance of nutritional misinformation, separating fact from fiction is a prime task of today's consumer. The consumer should carefully examine the source, evidence, scientific support, and motives involved with nutritional claims. In the final analysis, the keys to good nutrition continue to be variety and moderation.

NUTRITIVE VALUE OF FOODS

EXPLANATION OF THE TABLES

Foods listed.—Foods are grouped under the following main headings:

>Dairy products
>Eggs
>Fats and oils
>Fish, shellfish, meat, and poultry
>Fruits and fruit products
>Grain products
>Legumes (dry), nuts, and seeds
>Sugars and sweets
>Vegetables and vegetable products
>Miscellaneous items

Most of the foods listed are in ready-to-eat form. Some are basic products widely used in food preparation, such as flour, fat, and cornmeal.

The weight in grams for an approximate measure of each food is shown. A footnote indicates if inedible parts are included in the description and the weight. For example, item 246 is half a grapefruit with peel having a weight of 241 grams. A footnote to this item explains that the 241 grams include the weight of the peel.

The approximate measure shown for each food is in cups, ounces, pounds, some other well-known unit, or a piece of certain size. The cup measure refers to the standard measuring cup of 8 fluid ounces or one-half liquid pint. The ounce refers to one-sixteenth of a pound avoirdupois, unless fluid ounce is indicated. The weight of a fluid ounce varies according to the food measured. Some helpful volume and weight equivalents are shown in table 1.

Volume

Level measure	Equivalent
1 gallon (3.786 liters; 3,786 milliliters)	4 quarts
1 quart (0.946 liter; 946 milliliters)	4 cups
1 cup (237 milliliters)	8 fluid ounces ½ pint 16 tablespoons
2 tablespoons (30 milliliters)	1 fluid ounce
1 tablespoon (15 milliliters)	3 teaspoons
1 pound regular butter or margarine	4 sticks 2 cups
1 pound whipped butter or margarine	6 sticks 2 8-ounce containers 3 cups

Weight

Avoirdupois weight	Equivalent
1 pound (16 ounces)	453.6 grams
1 ounce	28.35 grams
3½ ounces	100 grams

533

Item No. (A)	Foods, approximate measures, units, and weight (edible part unless footnotes indicate otherwise) (B)		Water (C)	Food energy (D)	Pro-tein (E)	Fat (F)
			Grams	Per-cent	Cal-ories	Grams	Grams

DAIRY PRODUCTS (CHEESE, CREAM, IMITATION CREAM, MILK; RELATED PRODUCTS)

Item No.	Foods	measure	Grams	Percent	Calories	Protein	Fat
	Cheese:						
	Natural:						
1	Blue-----------------------	1 oz----------------------	28	42	100	6	8
	Cheddar:						
3	Cut pieces----------------	1 oz----------------------	28	37	115	7	9
4		1 cu in-------------------	17.2	37	70	4	6
5	Shredded------------------	1 cup---------------------	113	37	455	28	37
	Cottage (curd not pressed down):						
	Creamed (cottage cheese, 4% fat):						
6	Large curd--------------	1 cup---------------------	225	79	235	28	10
7	Small curd--------------	1 cup---------------------	210	79	220	26	9
8	Low fat (2%)-------------	1 cup---------------------	226	79	205	31	4
9	Low fat (1%)-------------	1 cup---------------------	226	82	165	28	2
10	Uncreamed (cottage cheese dry curd, less than 1/2% fat).	1 cup---------------------	145	80	125	25	1
11	Cream---------------------	1 oz----------------------	28	54	100	2	10
	Pasteurized process cheese:						
22	American------------------	1 oz----------------------	28	39	105	6	9
23	Swiss---------------------	1 oz----------------------	28	42	95	7	7
24	Pasteurized process cheese food, American.	1 oz----------------------	28	43	95	6	7
25	Pasteurized process cheese spread, American.	1 oz----------------------	28	48	82	5	6
	Cream, sweet:						
26	Half-and-half (cream and milk)-	1 cup---------------------	242	81	315	7	28
27		1 tbsp--------------------	15	81	20	Trace	2
	Whipping, unwhipped (volume about double when whipped):						
30	Light---------------------	1 cup---------------------	239	64	700	5	74
31		1 tbsp--------------------	15	64	45	Trace	5
32	Heavy---------------------	1 cup---------------------	238	58	820	5	88
33		1 tbsp--------------------	15	58	80	Trace	6
34	Whipped topping, (pressurized)-	1 cup---------------------	60	61	155	2	13
35		1 tbsp--------------------	3	61	10	Trace	1
36	Cream, sour---------------------	1 cup---------------------	230	71	495	7	48
37		1 tbsp--------------------	12	71	25	Trace	3
	Cream products, imitation (made with vegetable fat):						
	Sweet:						
	Creamers:						
38	Liquid (frozen)------------	1 cup---------------------	245	77	335	2	24
39		1 tbsp--------------------	15	77	20	Trace	1
40	Powdered-------------------	1 cup---------------------	94	2	515	5	33
41		1 tsp--------------------	2	2	10	Trace	1
	Whipped topping:						
42	Frozen--------------------	1 cup---------------------	75	50	240	1	19
43		1 tbsp--------------------	4	50	15	Trace	1
44	Powdered, made with whole milk.	1 cup---------------------	80	67	150	3	10
45		1 tbsp--------------------	4	67	10	Trace	Trace
46	Pressurized---------------	1 cup---------------------	70	60	185	1	16
47		1 tbsp--------------------	4	60	10	Trace	1
48	Sour dressing (imitation sour cream) made with nonfat dry milk.	1 cup---------------------	235	75	415	8	39

[1]Vitamin A value is largely from beta-carotene used for coloring. Riboflavin value for items 40-41 apply to products with added riboflavin.

534

Saturated (total) (G) Grams	Unsaturated Oleic (H) Grams	Unsaturated Linoleic (I) Grams	Carbohydrate (J) Grams	Calcium (K) Milligrams	Phosphorus (L) Milligrams	Iron (M) Milligrams	Potassium (N) Milligrams	Vitamin A value (O) International units	Thiamin (P) Milligrams	Riboflavin (Q) Milligrams	Niacin (R) Milligrams	Ascorbic acid (S) Milligrams
5.3	1.9	0.2	1	150	110	0.1	73	200	0.01	0.11	0.3	0
6.1	2.1	.2	Trace	204	145	.2	28	300	.01	.11	Trace	0
3.7	1.3	.1	Trace	124	88	.1	17	180	Trace	.06	Trace	0
24.2	8.5	.7	1	815	579	.8	111	1,200	.03	.42	.1	0
6.4	2.4	.2	6	135	297	.3	190	370	.05	.37	.3	Trace
6.0	2.2	.2	6	126	277	.3	177	340	.04	.34	.3	Trace
2.8	1.0	.1	8	155	340	.4	217	160	.05	.42	.3	Trace
1.5	.5	.1	6	138	302	.3	193	80	.05	.37	.3	Trace
.4	.1	Trace	3	46	151	.3	47	40	.04	.21	.2	0
6.2	2.4	.2	1	23	30	.3	34	400	Trace	.06	Trace	0
5.6	2.1	.2	Trace	174	211	.1	46	340	.01	.10	Trace	0
4.5	1.7	.1	1	219	216	.2	61	230	Trace	.08	Trace	0
4.4	1.7	.1	2	163	130	.2	79	260	.01	.13	Trace	0
3.8	1.5	.1	2	159	202	.1	69	220	.01	.12	Trace	0
17.3	7.0	.6	10	254	230	.2	314	260	.08	.36	.2	2
1.1	.4	Trace	1	16	14	Trace	19	20	.01	.02	Trace	Trace
46.2	18.3	1.5	7	166	146	0.1	231	2.690	0.06	0.30	0.1	1
2.9	1.1	.1	Trace	10	9	Trace	15	170	Trace	.02	Trace	Trace
54.8	22.2	2.0	7	154	149	.1	179	3,500	.05	.26	.1	1
3.5	1.4	.1	Trace	10	9	Trace	11	220	Trace	.02	Trace	Trace
8.3	3.4	.3	7	61	54	Trace	88	550	.02	.04	Trace	0
.4	.2	Trace	Trace	3	3	Trace	4	30	Trace	Trace	Trace	0
30.0	12.1	1.1	10	268	195	.1	331	1,820	.08	.34	.2	2
1.6	.6	.1	1	14	10	Trace	17	90	Trace	.02	Trace	Trace
22.8	.3	Trace	28	23	157	.1	467	[1]220	0	0	0	0
1.4	Trace	0	2	1	10	Trace	29	[1]10	0	0	0	0
30.6	.9	Trace	52	21	397	.1	763	[1]190	0	[1].16	0	0
.7	Trace	0	1	Trace	8	Trace	16	[1]Trace	0	[1]Trace	0	0
16.3	1.0	.2	17	5	6	.1	14	[1]650	0	0	0	0
.9	.1	Trace	1	Trace	Trace	Trace	1	[1]30	0	0	0	0
8.5	.6	.1	13	72	69	Trace	121	[1]290	.02	.09	Trace	1
.4	Trace	Trace	1	4	3	Trace	6	[1]10	Trace	Trace	Trace	Trace
13.2	1.4	.2	11	4	13	Trace	13	[1]330	0	0	0	0
.8	.1	Trace	1	Trace	1	Trace	1	[1]20	0	0	0	0
31.2	4.4	1.1	11	266	205	.1	380	[1]20	.09	.38	.2	2

Item No. (A)	Foods, approximate measures, units, and weight (edible part unless footnotes indicate otherwise) (B)		Water (C)	Food energy (D)	Protein (E)	Fat (F)
			Percent	Calories	Grams	Grams
	Milk:					
	Fluid:					
50	Whole (3.3% fat)------------	1 cup---------------------	244	88	150	8	8
	Lowfat (2%):					
51	No milk solids added-------	1 cup---------------------	244	89	120	8	5
	Milk solids added:					
52	Label claim less than 10 g of protein per cup.	1 cup---------------------	245	89	125	9	5
53	Label claim 10 or more grams of protein per cup (protein fortified).	1 cup---------------------	246	88	135	10	5
	Lowfat (1%):					
54	No milk solids added------	1 cup---------------------	244	90	100	8	3
	Milk solids added:					
55	Label claim less than 10 g of protein per cup.	1 cup---------------------	245	90	105	9	2
	Nonfat (skim):					
57	No milk solids added------	1 cup---------------------	245	91	85	8	Trace
	Milk solids added:					
58	Label claim less than 10 g of protein per cup.	1 cup---------------------	245	90	90	9	1
60	Buttermilk------------------	1 cup---------------------	245	90	100	8	2
	Canned:					
	Evaporated, unsweetened:					
61	Whole milk-----------------	1 cup---------------------	252	74	340	17	19
62	Skim milk------------------	1 cup---------------------	255	79	200	19	1
63	Sweetened, condensed---------	1 cup---------------------	306	27	980	24	27
	Milk beverages:					
	Chocolate milk (commercial):					
67	Regular---------------------	1 cup---------------------	250	82	210	8	8
68	Lowfat (2%)-----------------	1 cup---------------------	250	84	180	8	5
71	Chocolate-------------------	1 cup of milk plus 3/4 oz of powder.	265	81	235	9	9
	Shakes, thick:[8]					
73	Chocolate, container, net wt., 10.6 oz.	1 container---------------	300	72	355	9	8
74	Vanilla, container, net wt., 11 oz.	1 container---------------	313	74	350	12	9
	Milk desserts, frozen:					
	Ice cream:					
	Regular (about 11% fat):					
75	Hardened-------------------	1/2 gal-------------------	1,064	61	2,155	38	115
76		1 cup---------------------	133	61	270	5	14
77		3-fl oz container---------	50	61	100	2	5
78	Soft serve (frozen custard)	1 cup---------------------	173	60	375	7	23

[2]Applies to product without added vitamin A. With added vitamin A, value is 500 International Units (I.U.).
[3]Applies to product without vitamin A added.
[4]Applies to product with added vitamin A. Without added vitamin A, value is 20 International Units (I.U.).
[5]Yields 1 qt of fluid milk when reconstituted according to package directions.
[6]Applies to product with added vitamin A.
[7]Weight applies to product with label claim of 1 1/3 cups equal 3.2 oz.
[8]Applies to products made from thick shake mixes and that do not contain added ice cream.
 Products made from milk shake mixes are higher in fat and usually contain added ice cream.

Fatty Acids												
Satu-rated (total)	Unsaturated		Carbo-hydrate	Calcium	Phos-phorus	Iron	Potas-sium	Vitamin A value	Thiamin	Ribo-flavin	Niacin	Ascorbic acid
	Oleic	Lino-leic										
(G)	(H)	(I)	(J)	(K)	(L)	(M)	(N)	(O)	(P)	(Q)	(R)	(S)
Grams	Grams	Grams	Grams	Milli-grams	Milli-grams	Milli-grams	Milli-grams	Inter-national units	Milli-grams	Milli-grams	Milli-grams	Milli-grams
5.1	2.1	.2	11	291	228	.1	370	[2]310	.09	.40	.2	2
2.9	1.2	.1	12	297	232	.1	377	500	.10	.40	.2	2
2.9	1.2	.1	12	313	245	.1	397	500	.10	.42	.2	2
3.0	1.2	.1	14	352	276	.1	447	500	.11	.48	.2	3
1.6	.7	.1	12	300	235	.1	381	500	.10	.41	.2	2
1.5	.6	.1	12	313	245	.1	397	500	.10	.42	.2	2
.3	.1	Trace	12	302	247	.1	406	500	.09	.37	.2	2
0.4	0.1	Trace	12	316	255	0.1	418	500	0.10	0.43	0.2	2
1.3	.5	Trace	12	285	219	.1	371	[3]80	.08	.38	.1	2
11.6	5.3	0.4	25	657	510	.5	764	[3]610	.12	.80	.5	5
.3	.1	Trace	29	738	497	.7	845	[4]1,000	.11	.79	.4	3
16.8	6.7	.7	166	868	775	.6	1,136	[3]1,000	.28	1.27	.6	8
5.3	2.2	.2	26	280	251	.6	417	[3]300	.09	.41	.3	2
3.1	1.3	.1	26	284	254	.6	422	500	.10	.42	.3	2
5.5	—	—	29	304	265	.5	500	330	.14	.43	.7	2
5.0	2.0	.2	63	396	378	.9	672	260	.14	.67	.4	0
5.9	2.4	.2	56	457	361	.3	572	360	.09	.61	.5	0
71.3	28.8	2.6	254	1,406	1,075	1.0	2,052	4,340	.42	2.63	1.1	6
8.9	3.6	.3	32	176	134	.1	257	540	.05	.33	.1	1
3.4	1.4	.1	12	66	51	Trace	96	200	.02	.12	.1	Trace
13.5	5.9	.6	38	236	199	.4	338	790	.08	.45	.2	1

Item No.	Foods, approximate measures, units, and weight (edible part unless footnotes indicate otherwise)		Water	Food energy	Pro-tein	Fat
(A)	(B)		(C)	(D)	(E)	(F)
		Grams	Per-cent	Cal-ories	Grams	Grams
	Milk desserts, frozen:					
	Ice cream:					
79	Rich (about 16% fat), hardened.	1/2 gal -------------------- 1,188	59	2,805	33	190
80		1 cup --------------------- 148	59	350	4	24
	Ice milk:					
81	Hardened (about 4.3% fat)----	1/2 gal -------------------- 1,048	69	1,470	41	45
82		1 cup --------------------- 131	69	185	5	6
83	Soft serve (about 2.6% fat)	1 cup --------------------- 175	70	225	8	5
84	Sherbet (about 2% fat)-------	1/2 gal ------------------- 1,542	66	2,160	17	31
85		1 cup --------------------- 193	66	270	2	4
	Milk desserts, other:					
86	Custard, baked---------------	1 cup --------------------- 265	77	305	14	15
	Puddings:					
	From mix (chocolate) and milk:					
90	Regular (cooked)---------	1 cup --------------------- 260	70	320	9	8
91	Instant-----------------	1 cup --------------------- 260	69	325	8	7
	Yogurt:					
	With added milk solids:					
	Made with lowfat milk:					
92	Fruit-flavored[9]----------	1 container, net wt., 8 oz 227	75	230	10	3
93	Plain--------------------	1 container, net wt., 8 oz 227	85	145	12	4

EGGS

Item No.	Foods		Water	Food energy	Pro-tein	Fat
	Eggs, large (24 oz per dozen):					
	Raw:					
96	Whole, without shell-------	1 egg --------------------- 50	75	80	6	6
97	White---------------------	1 white ------------------- 33	88	15	3	Trace
98	Yolk----------------------	1 yolk -------------------- 17	49	65	3	6
	Cooked:					
99	Fried in butter-----------	1 egg --------------------- 46	72	85	5	6
100	Hard-cooked, shell removed_	1 egg --------------------- 50	75	80	6	6
101	Poached-------------------	1 egg --------------------- 50	74	80	6	6
102	Scrambled (milk added) in butter. Also omelet.	1 egg --------------------- 64	76	95	6	7

FATS, OILS; RELATED PRODUCTS

Item No.	Foods		Water	Food energy	Pro-tein	Fat
	Butter:					
	Regular (1 brick or 4 sticks per lb):					
103	Stick (1/2 cup)------------	1 stick ------------------- 113	16	815	1	92
104	Tablespoon (about 1/8 stick).	1 tbsp -------------------- 14	16	100	Trace	12
105	Pat (1 in square, 1/3 in high; 90 per lb).	1 pat --------------------- 5	16	35	Trace	4
	Whipped (6 sticks or two 8-oz containers per lb).					
106	Stick (1/2 cup)------------	1 stick ------------------- 76	16	540	1	61
107	Tablespoon (about 1/8 stick).	1 tbsp -------------------- 9	16	65	Trace	8
108	Pat (1 1/4 in square, 1/3 in high; 120 per lb).	1 pat --------------------- 4	16	25	Trace	3

[9]Content of fat, vitamin A, and carbohydrate varies. Consult the label when precise values are needed for special diets.
[10]Applies to product made with milk containing no added vitamin A.
[11]Based on year-round average.

Fatty Acids												
Saturated (total)	Unsaturated		Carbohydrate	Calcium	Phosphorus	Iron	Potassium	Vitamin A value	Thiamin	Riboflavin	Niacin	Ascorbic acid
	Oleic	Linoleic										
(G)	(H)	(I)	(J)	(K)	(L)	(M)	(N)	(O)	(P)	(Q)	(R)	(S)
Grams	Grams	Grams	Grams	Milligrams	Milligrams	Milligrams	Milligrams	International units	Milligrams	Milligrams	Milligrams	Milligrams
118.3	47.8	4.3	256	1,213	927	.8	1,771	7,200	.36	2.27	.9	5
14.7	6.0	.5	32	151	115	.1	221	900	.04	.28	.1	1
28.1	11.3	1.0	232	1,409	1,035	1.5	2,117	1,710	.61	2.78	.9	6
3.5	1.4	.1	29	176	129	.1	265	210	.08	.35	.1	1
2.9	1.2	0.1	38	274	202	0.3	412	180	0.12	0.54	0.2	1
19.0	7.7	.7	469	827	594	2.5	1,585	1,480	.26	.71	1.0	31
2.4	1.0	.1	59	103	74	.3	198	190	.03	.09	.1	4
6.8	5.4	.7	29	297	310	1.1	387	930	.11	.50	.3	1
4.3	2.6	.2	59	265	247	.8	354	340	.05	.39	.3	2
3.6	2.2	.3	63	374	237	1.3	335	340	.08	.39	.3	2
1.8	.6	.1	42	343	269	.2	439	[10]120	.08	.40	.2	1
2.3	.8	.1	16	415	326	.2	531	[10]150	.10	.49	.3	2
1.7	2.0	.6	1	28	90	1.0	65	260	.04	.15	Trace	0
0	0	0	Trace	4	4	Trace	45	0	Trace	.09	Trace	0
1.7	2.1	.6	Trace	26	86	.9	15	310	.04	.07	Trace	0
2.4	2.2	.6	1	26	80	.9	58	290	.03	.13	Trace	0
1.7	2.0	.6	1	28	90	1.0	65	260	.04	.14	Trace	0
1.7	2.0	.6	1	28	90	1.0	65	260	.04	.13	Trace	0
2.8	2.3	.6	1	47	97	.9	85	310	.04	.16	Trace	0
57.3	23.1	2.1	Trace	27	26	.2	29	[11]3,470	.01	.04	Trace	0
7.2	2.9	.3	Trace	3	3	Trace	4	[11]430	Trace	Trace	Trace	0
2.5	1.0	.1	Trace	1	1	Trace	1	[11]150	Trace	Trace	Trace	0
38.2	15.4	1.4	Trace	18	17	.1	20	[11]2,310	Trace	.03	Trace	0
4.7	1.9	.2	Trace	2	2	Trace	2	[11]290	Trace	Trace	Trace	0
1.9	.8	.1	Trace	1	1	Trace	1	[11]120	0	Trace	Trace	0

Item No. (A)	Foods, approximate measures, units, and weight (edible part unless footnotes indicate otherwise) (B)		Water (C)	Food energy (D)	Pro- tein (E)	Fat (F)
		Grams	Per- cent	Cal- ories	Grams	Grams
109	Fats, cooking (vegetable shortenings).	1 cup-------------------- 200	0	1,770	0	200
110		1 tbsp------------------- 13	0	110	0	13
111	Lard-------------------------	1 cup-------------------- 205	0	1,850	0	205
112		1 tbsp------------------- 13	0	115	0	13
	Margarine: Regular (1 brick or 4 sticks per lb):					
113	Stick (1/2 cup)-------------	1 stick------------------ 113	16	815	1	92
114	Tablespoon (about 1/8 stick)-	1 tbsp------------------- 14	16	100	Trace	12
115	Pat (1 in square, 1/3 in high; 90 per lb).	1 pat-------------------- 5	16	35	Trace	4
116	Soft, two 8-oz containers per lb.	1 container-------------- 227	16	1,635	1	184
117		1 tbsp------------------- 14	16	100	Trace	12
	Oils, salad or cooking:					
120	Corn-------------------------	1 cup-------------------- 218	0	1,925	0	218
126	Safflower---------------------	1 cup-------------------- 218	0	1,925	0	218
127		1 tbsp------------------- 14	0	120	0	14
128	Soybean oil, hydrogenated (partially hardened).	1 cup-------------------- 218	0	1,925	0	218

	Salad dressings:
	  Commercial:
	    Blue cheese:					

132	Regular--------------------	1 tbsp------------------- 15	32	75	1	8
133	Low calorie (5 Cal per tsp)	1 tbsp------------------- 16	84	10	Trace	1
	French:					
134	Regular--------------------	1 tbsp------------------- 16	39	65	Trace	6
135	Low calorie (5 Cal per tsp)	1 tbsp------------------- 16	77	15	Trace	1
	Italian:					
136	Regular--------------------	1 tbsp------------------- 15	28	85	Trace	9
137	Low calorie (2 Cal per tsp)	1 tbsp------------------- 15	90	10	Trace	1
138	Mayonnaise-------------------	1 tbsp------------------- 14	15	100	Trace	11
	Mayonnaise type:					
139	Regular--------------------	1 tbsp------------------- 15	41	65	Trace	6
140	Low calorie (8 Cal per tsp)	1 tbsp------------------- 16	81	20	Trace	2
141	Tartar sauce, regular--------	1 tbsp------------------- 14	34	75	Trace	8
	Thousand Island:					
142	Regular--------------------	1 tbsp------------------- 16	32	80	Trace	8
143	Low calorie (10 Cal per tsp)	1 tbsp------------------- 15	68	25	Trace	2

FISH, SHELLFISH, MEAT, POULTRY; RELATED PRODUCTS

	Fish and shellfish: Clams:					
146	Raw, meat only---------------	3 oz--------------------- 85	82	65	11	1
147	Canned, solids and liquid-----	3 oz--------------------- 85	86	45	7	1
148	Crabmeat (white or king), canned, not pressed down.	1 cup-------------------- 135	77	135	24	3
149	Fish sticks, breaded, cooked, frozen (stick, 4 by 1 by 1/2 in).	1 fish stick or 1 oz------- 28	66	50	5	3
150	Haddock, breaded, fried[14]-------	3 oz--------------------- 85	66	140	17	5
151	Ocean perch, breaded, fried[14]---	1 fillet------------------ 85	59	195	16	11

[12] Based on average vitamin A content of fortified margarine. Federal specifications for fortified margarine require a minimum of 15,000 International Units (I.U.) of vitamin A per pound.

[13] Fatty acid values apply to product made with regular-type margarine.

[14] Dipped in egg, milk or water, and breadcrumbs; fried in vegetable shortening.

540

Fatty Acids												
Satu-rated (total)	Unsaturated		Carbo-hydrate	Calcium	Phos-phorus	Iron	Potas-sium	Vitamin A value	Thiamin	Ribo-flavin	Niacin	Ascorbic acid
	Oleic	Lino-leic										
(G)	(H)	(I)	(J)	(K)	(L)	(M)	(N)	(O)	(P)	(Q)	(R)	(S)
Grams	Grams	Grams	Grams	Milli-grams	Milli-grams	Milli-grams	Milli-grams	Inter-national units	Milli-grams	Milli-grams	Milli-grams	Milli-grams
48.8	88.2	48.4	0	0	0	0	0	—	0	0	0	0
3.2	5.7	3.1	0	0	0	0	0	—	0	0	0	0
81.0	83.8	20.5	0	0	0	0	0	0	0	0	0	0
5.1	5.3	1.3	0	0	0	0	0	0	0	0	0	0
16.7	42.9	24.9	Trace	27	26	.2	29	[12]3,750	.01	.04	Trace	0
2.1	5.3	3.1	Trace	3	3	Trace	4	[12]470	Trace	Trace	Trace	0
.7	1.9	1.1	Trace	1	1	Trace	1	[12]170	Trace	Trace	Trace	0
32.5	71.5	65.4	Trace	53	52	.4	59	[12]7,500	.01	.08	.1	0
2.0	4.5	4.1	Trace	3	3	Trace	4	[12]470	Trace	Trace	Trace	0
27.7	53.6	125.1	0	0	0	0	0	—	0	0	0	0
20.5	25.9	159.8	0	0	0	0	0	—	0	0	0	0
1.3	1.6	10.0	0	0	0	0	0	—	0	0	0	0
31.8	93.1	75.6	0	0	0	0	0	—	0	0	0	0
1.6	1.7	3.8	1	12	11	Trace	6	30	Trace	.02	Trace	Trace
.5	.3	Trace	1	10	8	Trace	5	30	Trace	.01	Trace	Trace
1.1	1.3	3.2	3	2	2	.1	13	—	—	—	—	—
.1	.1	.4	2	2	2	.1	13	—	—	—	—	—
1.6	1.9	4.7	1	2	1	Trace	2	Trace	Trace	Trace	Trace	—
.1	.1	.4	Trace	Trace	1	Trace	2	Trace	Trace	Trace	Trace	—
2.0	2.4	5.6	Trace	3	4	.1	5	40	Trace	.01	Trace	—
1.1	1.4	3.2	2	2	4	Trace	1	30	Trace	Trace	Trace	—
.4	.4	1.0	2	3	4	Trace	1	40	Trace	Trace	Trace	—
1.5	1.8	4.1	1	3	4	.1	11	30	Trace	Trace	Trace	Trace
1.4	1.7	4.0	2	2	3	.1	18	50	Trace	Trace	Trace	Trace
.4	.4	1.0	2	2	3	.1	17	50	Trace	Trace	Trace	Trace
—	—	—	2	59	138	5.2	154	90	.08	.15	1.1	8
0.2	Trace	Trace	2	47	116	3.5	119	—	.01	.09	.9	—
.6	0.4	0.1	1	61	246	1.1	149	—	.11	.11	2.6	—
—	—	—	2	3	47	.1	—	0	.01	.02	.5	—
1.4	2.2	1.2	5	34	210	1.0	296	—	.03	.06	2.7	2
2.7	4.4	2.3	6	28	192	1.1	242	—	.10	.10	1.6	—

Item No.	Foods, approximate measures, units, and weight (edible part unless footnotes indicate otherwise)			Water	Food energy	Protein	Fat
(A)	(B)			(C)	(D)	(E)	(F)
			Grams	Percent	Calories	Grams	Grams
152	Oysters, raw, meat only (13-19 medium Selects).	1 cup	240	85	160	20	4
153	Salmon, pink, canned, solids and liquid.	3 oz	85	71	120	17	5
154	Sardines, Atlantic, canned in oil, drained solids.	3 oz	85	62	175	20	9
155	Scallops, frozen, breaded, fried, reheated.	6 scallops	90	60	175	16	8
	Shrimp:						
157	Canned meat	3 oz	85	70	100	21	1
158	French fried[16]	3 oz	85	57	190	17	9
159	Tuna, canned in oil, drained solids.	3 oz	85	61	170	24	7
160	Tuna salad[17]	1 cup	205	70	350	30	22
	Meat and meat products:						
161	Bacon, (20 slices per lb, raw), broiled or fried, crisp.	2 slices	15	8	85	4	8
	Beef,[18] cooked:						
	Cuts braised, simmered or pot roasted:						
162	Lean and fat (piece, 2 1/2 by 2 1/2 by 3/4 in).	3 oz	85	53	245	23	16
163	Lean only from item 162	2.5 oz	72	62	140	22	5
	Ground beef, broiled:						
164	Lean with 10% fat	3 oz or patty 3 by 5/8 in	85	60	185	23	10
165	Lean with 21% fat	2.9 oz or patty 3 by 5/8 in	82	54	235	20	17
	Roast, oven cooked, no liquid added:						
	Relatively fat, such as rib:						
166	Lean and fat (2 pieces, 4 1/8 by 2 1/4 by 1/4 in).	3 oz	85	40	375	17	33
167	Lean only from item 166	1.8 oz	51	57	125	14	7
	Relatively lean, such as heel of round:						
168	Lean and fat (2 pieces, 4 1/8 by 2 1/4 by 1/4 in).	3 oz	85	62	165	25	7
	Steak:						
	Relatively fat—sirloin, broiled:						
170	Lean and fat (piece, 2 1/2 by 2 1/2 by 3/4 in).	3 oz	85	44	330	20	27
171	Lean only from item 170	2.0 oz	56	59	115	18	4
179	Chili con carne with beans, canned.	1 cup	255	72	340	19	16
180	Chop suey with beef and pork (home recipe).	1 cup	250	75	300	26	17
181	Heart, beef, lean, braised	3 oz	85	61	160	27	5
	Lamb, cooked:						
	Leg, roasted:						
184	Lean and fat (2 pieces, 4 1/8 by 2 1/4 by 1/4 in).	3 oz	85	54	235	22	16
185	Lean only from item 184	2.5 oz	71	62	130	20	5

[15] If bones are discarded, value for calcium will be greatly reduced.
[16] Dipped in egg, breadcrumbs, and flour or batter.
[17] Prepared with tuna, celery, salad dressing (mayonnaise type), pickle, onion, and egg.
[18] Outer layer of fat on the cut was removed to within approximately 1/2 in of the lean. Deposits of fat within the cut were not removed.

542

Fatty Acids												
Satu-rated (total)	Unsaturated Oleic	Lino-leic	Carbo-hydrate	Calcium	Phos-phorus	Iron	Potas-sium	Vitamin A value	Thiamin	Ribo-flavin	Niacin	Ascorbic acid
(G)	(H)	(I)	(J)	(K)	(L)	(M)	(N)	(O)	(P)	(Q)	(R)	(S)
Grams	Grams	Grams	Grams	Milli-grams	Milli-grams	Milli-grams	Milli-grams	Inter-national units	Milli-grams	Milli-grams	Milli-grams	Milli-grams
1.3	.2	.1	8	226	343	13.2	290	740	.34	.43	6.0	——
.9	.8	.1	0	^{15}167	243	.7	307	60	.03	.16	6.8	——
3.0	2.5	.5	0	372	424	2.5	502	190	.02	.17	4.6	——
——	——	——	9	——	——	——	——	——	——	——	——	——
.1	.1	Trace	1	98	224	2.6	104	50	.01	.03	1.5	——
2.3	3.7	2.0	9	61	162	1.7	195	——	.03	.07	2.3	——
1.7	1.7	.7	0	7	199	1.6	——	70	.04	.10	10.1	——
4.3	6.3	6.7	7	41	291	2.7	——	590	.08	.23	10.3	2
2.5	3.7	.7	Trace	2	34	.5	35	0	.08	.05	.8	——
6.8	6.5	.4	0	10	114	2.9	184	30	.04	.18	3.6	——
2.1	1.8	.2	0	10	108	2.7	176	10	.04	.17	3.3	——
4.0	3.9	.3	0	10	196	3.0	261	20	.08	.20	5.1	——
7.0	6.7	.4	0	9	159	2.6	221	30	.07	.17	4.4	——
14.0	13.6	.8	0	8	158	2.2	189	70	.05	.13	3.1	——
3.0	2.5	.3	0	6	131	1.8	161	10	.04	.11	2.6	——
2.8	2.7	.2	0	11	208	3.2	279	10	.06	.19	4.5	——
11.3	11.1	.6	0	9	162	2.5	220	50	.05	.15	4.0	——
1.8	1.6	.2	0	7	146	2.2	202	10	.05	.14	3.6	——
7.5	6.8	.3	31	82	321	4.3	594	150	.08	.18	3.3	——
8.5	6.2	.7	13	60	248	4.8	425	600	.28	.38	5.0	33
1.5	1.1	.6	1	5	154	5.0	197	20	.21	1.04	6.5	1
7.3	6.0	.6	0	9	177	1.4	241	——	.13	.23	4.7	——
2.1	1.8	.2	0	9	169	1.4	227	——	.12	.21	4.4	——

Item No.	Foods, approximate measures, units, and weight (edible part unless footnotes indicate otherwise)		Water	Food energy	Protein	Fat
(A)	(B)		(C)	(D)	(E)	(F)
		Grams	Percent	Calories	Grams	Grams
188	Liver, beef, fried[20] (slice, 6 1/2 by 2 3/8 by 3/8 in).	3 oz	85	56	195	22	9
	Pork, cured, cooked:						
189	Ham, light cure, lean and fat, roasted (2 pieces, 4 1/8 by 2 1/4 by 1/4 in).[22]	3 oz	85	54	245	18	19
	Luncheon meat:						
190	Boiled ham, slice (8 per 8-oz pkg.).	1 oz	28	59	65	5	5
	Pork, fresh,[18] cooked:						
	Chop, loin (cut 3 per lb with bone), broiled:						
192	Lean and fat	2.7 oz	78	42	305	19	25
193	Lean only from item 192	2 oz	56	53	150	17	9
	Roast, oven cooked, no liquid added:						
194	Lean and fat (piece, 2 1/2 by 2 1/2 by 3/4 in).	3 oz	85	46	310	21	24
195	Lean only from item 194	2.4 oz	68	55	175	20	10
	Sausages (see also Luncheon meat (items 190-191)):						
198	Bologna, slice (8 per 8-oz pkg.).	1 slice	28	56	85	3	8
199	Braunschweiger, slice (6 per 6-oz pkg.).	1 slice	28	53	90	4	8
202	Frankfurter (8 per 1-lb pkg.), cooked (reheated).	1 frankfurter	56	57	170	7	15
204	Pork link (16 per 1-lb pkg.), cooked.	1 link	13	35	60	2	6
	Salami:						
205	Dry type, slice (12 per 4-oz pkg.).	1 slice	10	30	45	2	4
	Veal, medium fat, cooked, bone removed:						
208	Cutlet (4 1/8 by 2 1/4 by 1/2 in), braised or broiled.	3 oz	85	60	185	23	9
	Poultry and poultry products:						
	Chicken, cooked:						
210	Breast, fried,[23] bones removed, 1/2 breast (3.3 oz with bones).	2.8 oz	79	58	160	26	5
211	Drumstick, fried,[23] bones removed (2 oz with bones).	1.3 oz	38	55	90	12	4
212	Half broiler, broiled, bones removed (10.4 oz with bones).	6.2 oz	176	71	240	42	7
213	Chicken, canned, boneless	3 oz	85	65	170	18	10
214	Chicken a la king, cooked (home recipe).	1 cup	245	68	470	27	34
218	Chicken potpie (home recipe), baked,[19] piece (1/3 or 9-in diam. pie).	1 piece	232	57	545	23	31
	Turkey, roasted, flesh without skin:						
219	Dark meat, piece, 2 1/2 by 1 5/8 by 1/4 in.	4 pieces	85	61	175	26	7
220	Light meat, piece, 4 by 2 by 1/4 in.	2 pieces	85	62	150	28	3

[19]Crust made with vegetable shortening and enriched flour.
[20]Regular-type margarine used.
[21]Value varies widely.
[22]About one-fourth of the outer layer of fat on the cut was removed. Deposits of fat within the cut were not removed.
[23]Vegetable shortening used.

	Fatty Acids											
Satu-rated (total)	Unsaturated Oleic	Unsaturated Lino-leic	Carbo-hydrate	Calcium	Phos-phorus	Iron	Potas-sium	Vitamin A value	Thiamin	Ribo-flavin	Niacin	Ascorbic acid
(G)	(H)	(I)	(J)	(K)	(L)	(M)	(N)	(O)	(P)	(Q)	(R)	(S)
Grams	Grams	Grams	Grams	Milli-grams	Milli-grams	Milli-grams	Milli-grams	Inter-national units	Milli-grams	Milli-grams	Milli-grams	Milli-grams
2.5	3.5	.9	5	9	405	7.5	323	[24]45,390	.22	3.56	14.0	23
6.8	7.9	1.7	0	8	146	2.2	199	0	.40	.15	3.1	——
1.7	2.0	.4	0	3	47	.8	——	0	.12	.04	.7	——
8.9	10.4	2.2	0	9	209	2.7	216	0	0.75	0.22	4.5	——
3.1	3.6	.8	0	7	181	2.2	192	0	.63	.18	3.8	——
8.7	10.2	2.2	0	9	218	2.7	233	0	.78	.22	4.8	——
3.5	4.1	.8	0	9	211	2.6	224	0	.73	.21	4.4	——
3.0	3.4	.5	Trace	2	36	.5	65	——	.05	.06	.7	——
2.6	3.4	.8	1	3	69	1.7	——	1,850	.05	.41	2.3	——
5.6	6.5	1.2	1	3	57	.8	——	——	.08	.11	1.4	——
2.1	2.4	.5	Trace	1	21	.3	35	0	.10	.04	.5	——
1.6	1.6	.1	Trace	1	28	.4	——	——	.04	.03	.5	——
4.0	3.4	.4	0	9	196	2.7	258	——	.06	.21	4.6	——
1.4	1.8	1.1	1	9	218	1.3	——	70	.04	.17	11.6	——
1.1	1.3	.9	Trace	6	89	.9	——	50	.03	.15	2.7	——
2.2	2.5	1.3	0	16	355	3.0	483	160	.09	.34	15.5	——
3.2	3.8	2.0	0	18	210	1.3	117	200	.03	.11	3.7	3
12.7	14.3	3.3	12	127	358	2.5	404	1,130	.10	.42	5.4	12
11.3	10.9	5.6	42	70	232	3.0	343	3,090	.34	.31	5.5	5
2.1	1.5	1.5	0	——	——	2.0	338	——	.03	.20	3.6	——
.9	.6	.7	0	——	——	1.0	349	——	.04	.12	9.4	——

Item No.	Foods, approximate measures, units, and weight (edible part unless footnotes indicate otherwise)		Water	Food energy	Protein	Fat
(A)	(B)		(C)	(D)	(E)	(F)
		Grams	Percent	Calories	Grams	Grams

FRUITS AND FRUIT PRODUCTS

Item No.	Foods, approximate measures, units, and weight		Grams	Percent	Calories	Grams	Grams
	Apples, raw, unpeeled, without cores:						
223	2 3/4-in diam. (about 3 per lb with cores).	1 apple-----------------	138	84	80	Trace	1
225	Applejuice, bottled or canned[24]---	1 cup------------------	248	88	120	Trace	Trace
	Applesauce, canned:						
226	Sweetened-------------------	1 cup------------------	255	76	230	1	Trace
227	Unsweetened-----------------	1 cup------------------	244	89	100	Trace	Trace
	Apricots:						
228	Raw, without pits (about 12 per lb with pits).	3 apricots--------------	107	85	55	1	Trace
229	Canned in heavy sirup (halves and sirup).	1 cup------------------	258	77	220	2	Trace
	Dried:						
230	Uncooked (28 large or 37 medium halves per cup).	1 cup------------------	130	25	340	7	1
231	Cooked, unsweetened, fruit and liquid.	1 cup------------------	250	76	215	4	1
232	Apricot nectar, canned-----------	1 cup------------------	251	85	145	1	Trace
	Avocados, raw, whole, without skins and seeds:						
233	California, mid- and late-winter (with skin and seed, 3 1/8-in diam.; wt., 10 oz).	1 avocado-----------------	216	74	370	5	37
235	Banana without peel (about 2.6 per lb with peel).	1 banana---------------	119	76	100	1	Trace
237	Blackberries, raw----------------	1 cup------------------	144	85	85	2	1
238	Blueberries, raw-----------------	1 cup------------------	145	83	90	1	1
	Cantaloup. See Muskmelons (item 271).						
	Cherries:						
239	Sour (tart), red, pitted, canned, water pack.	1 cup------------------	244	88	105	2	Trace
240	Sweet, raw, without pits and stems.	10 cherries----------------	68	80	45	1	Trace
241	Cranberry juice cocktail, bottled, sweetened.	1 cup------------------	253	83	165	Trace	Trace
242	Cranberry sauce, sweetened, canned, strained.	1 cup------------------	277	62	405	Trace	1
	Dates:						
243	Whole, without pits-------------	10 dates-----------------	80	23	220	2	Trace
244	Chopped-----------------------	1 cup------------------	178	23	490	4	1
245	Fruit cocktail, canned, in heavy sirup.	1 cup------------------	255	80	195	1	Trace
	Grapefruit:						
	Raw, medium, 3 3/4-in diam. (about 1 lb 1 oz):						
246	Pink or red-------------------	1/2 grapefruit with peel[28]	241	89	50	1	Trace
247	White-------------------------	1/2 grapefruit with peel[28]	241	89	45	1	Trace
248	Canned, sections with sirup-----	1 cup------------------	254	81	180	2	Trace
	Grapefruit juice:						
249	Raw, pink, red, or white--------	1 cup------------------	246	90	95	1	Trace

[24]Also applies to pasteurized apple cider.
[25]Applies to product without added ascorbic acid. For value of product with added ascorbic acid, refer to 1
[26]Based on product with label claim of 45% of U.S. RDA in 6 fl oz.
[27]Based on product with label claim of 100% of U.S. RDA in 6 fl oz.
[28]Weight includes peel and membranes between sections. Without these parts, the weight of the edible portio is 123 g for item 246 and 118 g for item 247.
[29]For white-fleshed varieties, value is about 20 International Units (I.U.) per cup; for red-fleshed varieties, 1,080 I.U.

	Fatty Acids											
Satu-rated (total)	Unsaturated		Carbo-hydrate	Calcium	Phos-phorus	Iron	Potas-sium	Vitamin A value	Thiamin	Ribo-flavin	Niacin	Ascorbic acid
	Oleic	Lino-leic										
(G)	(H)	(I)	(J)	(K)	(L)	(M)	(N)	(O)	(P)	(Q)	(R)	(S)
Grams	Grams	Grams	Grams	Milli-grams	Milli-grams	Milli-grams	Milli-grams	Inter-national units	Milli-grams	Milli-grams	Milli-grams	Milli-grams
—	—	—	20	10	14	.4	152	120	.04	.03	.1	6
—	—	—	30	15	22	1.5	250	—	.02	.05	.2	[25]2
—	—	—	61	10	13	1.3	166	100	.05	.03	.1	[25]3
—	—	—	26	10	12	1.2	190	100	.05	.02	.1	[25]2
—	—	—	14	18	25	.5	301	2,890	.03	.04	.6	11
—	—	—	57	28	39	.8	604	4,490	.05	.05	1.0	10
—	—	—	86	87	140	7.2	1,273	14,170	.01	.21	4.3	16
—	—	—	54	55	88	4.5	795	7,500	.01	.13	2.5	8
—	—	—	37	23	30	.5	379	2,380	.03	.03	.5	[26]36
5.5	22.0	3.7	13	22	91	1.3	1,303	630	.24	.43	3.5	30
—	—	—	26	10	31	.8	440	230	.06	.07	.8	12
—	—	—	19	46	27	1.3	245	290	0.04	0.06	0.6	30
—	—	—	22	22	19	1.5	117	150	.04	.09	.7	20
—	—	—	26	37	32	.7	317	1,660	.07	.05	.5	12
—	—	—	12	15	13	.3	129	70	.03	.04	.3	7
—	—	—	42	13	8	.8	25	Trace	.03	.03	.1	[27]81
—	—	—	104	17	11	.6	83	60	.03	.03	.1	6
—	—	—	58	47	50	2.4	518	40	.07	.08	1.8	0
—	—	—	130	105	112	5.3	1,153	90	.16	.18	3.9	0
—	—	—	50	23	31	1.0	411	360	.05	.03	1.0	5
—	—	—	13	20	20	.5	166	540	.05	.02	.2	44
—	—	—	12	19	19	.5	159	10	.05	.02	.2	44
—	—	—	45	33	36	.8	343	30	.08	.05	.5	76
—	—	—	23	22	37	.5	399	([29])	.10	.05	.5	93

Item No. (A)	Foods, approximate measures, units, and weight (edible part unless footnotes indicate otherwise) (B)		Water (C)	Food energy (D)	Protein (E)	Fat (F)
		Grams	Percent	Calories	Grams	Grams
	Grapes, European type (adherent skin), raw:					
255	Thompson Seedless---------------	10 grapes------------------ 50	81	35	Trace	Trace
256	Tokay and Emperor, seeded types-	10 grapes[30]---------------- 60	81	40	Trace	Trace
	Grapejuice:					
257	Canned or bottled--------------	1 cup---------------------- 253	83	165	1	Trace
	Frozen concentrate, sweetened:					
258	Undiluted, 6-fl oz can--------	1 can---------------------- 216	53	395	1	Trace
259	Diluted with 3 parts water by volume.	1 cup---------------------- 250	86	135	1	Trace
260	Grape drink, canned--------------	1 cup---------------------- 250	86	135	Trace	Trace
	Lemon juice:					
262	Raw-----------------------------	1 cup---------------------- 244	91	60	1	Trace
263	Canned, or bottled, unsweetened-	1 cup---------------------- 244	92	55	1	Trace
264	Frozen, single strength, unsweetened, 6-fl oz can.	1 can---------------------- 183	92	40	1	Trace
	Lemonade concentrate, frozen:					
265	Undiluted, 6-fl oz can----------	1 can---------------------- 219	49	425	Trace	Trace
266	Diluted with 4 1/3 parts water by volume.	1 cup---------------------- 248	89	105	Trace	Trace
	Limejuice:					
269	Raw-----------------------------	1 cup---------------------- 246	90	65	1	Trace
271	Cantaloup, orange-fleshed (with rind and seed cavity, 5-in diam., 2 1/3 lb).	1/2 melon with rind[33]----- 477	91	80	2	Trace
272	Honeydew (with rind and seed cavity, 6 1/2-in diam., 5 1/4 lb).	1/10 melon with rind[33]---- 226	91	50	1	Trace
	Oranges, all commercial varieties, raw:					
273	Whole, 2 5/8-in diam., without peel and seeds (about 2 1/2 per lb with peel and seeds).	1 orange------------------ 131	86	65	1	Trace
274	Sections without membranes------	1 cup---------------------- 180	86	90	2	Trace
	Orange juice:					
275	Raw, all varieties--------------	1 cup---------------------- 248	88	110	2	Trace
276	Canned, unsweetened-------------	1 cup---------------------- 249	87	120	2	Trace
	Frozen concentrate:					
277	Undiluted, 6-fl oz can--------	1 can---------------------- 213	55	360	5	Trace
278	Diluted with 3 parts water by volume.	1 cup---------------------- 249	87	120	2	Trace
282	Papayas, raw, 1/2-in cubes--------	1 cup---------------------- 140	89	55	1	Trace
	Peaches:					
	Raw:					
283	Whole, 2 1/2-in diam., peeled, pitted (about 4 per lb with peels and pits).	1 peach------------------- 100	89	40	1	Trace

[30]Weight includes seeds. Without seeds, weight of the edible portion is 57 g.

[31]Applies to product without added ascorbic acid. With added ascorbic acid, based on claim that 6 fl oz of reconstituted juice contain 45% or 50% of the U.S. RDA, value in milligrams is 108 or 120 for a 6-fl oz can (item 258), 36 or 40 for 1 cup of diluted juice (item 259).

[32]For products with added thiamin and riboflavin but without added ascorbic acid, values in milligrams would be 0.60 for thiamin, 0.80 for riboflavin, and trace for ascorbic acid. For products with only ascorbic acid added, value varies with the brand. Consult the label.

[33]Weight includes rind. Without rind, the weight of the edible portion is 272 g for item 271 and 149 g for item 272.

[34]Represents yellow-fleshed varieties. For white-fleshed varieties, value is 50 International Units (I.U.) for 1 peach, 90 I.U. for 1 cup of slices.

Fatty Acids												
Satu-rated (total)	Unsaturated		Carbo-hydrate	Calcium	Phos-phorus	Iron	Potas-sium	Vitamin A value	Thiamin	Ribo-flavin	Niacin	Ascorbic acid
	Oleic	Lino-leic										
(G)	(H)	(I)	(J)	(K)	(L)	(M)	(N)	(O)	(P)	(Q)	(R)	(S)
Grams	Grams	Grams	Grams	Milli-grams	Milli-grams	Milli-grams	Milli-grams	Inter-national units	Milli-grams	Milli-grams	Milli-grams	Milli-grams
—	—	—	9	6	10	.2	87	50	.03	.02	.2	2
—	—	—	10	7	11	.2	99	60	.03	.02	.2	2
—	—	—	42	28	30	.8	293	—	.10	.05	.5	[25]Trace
—	—	—	100	22	32	.9	255	40	.13	.22	1.5	[31]32
—	—	—	33	8	10	.3	85	10	.05	.08	.5	[31]10
—	—	—	35	8	10	.3	88	—	[32].03	[32].03	.3	([32])
—	—	—	20	17	24	.5	344	50	.07	.02	.2	112
—	—	—	19	17	24	.5	344	50	.07	.02	.2	102
—	—	—	13	13	16	.5	258	40	.05	.02	.2	81
—	—	—	112	9	13	.4	153	40	.05	.06	.7	66
—	—	—	28	2	3	.1	40	10	.01	.02	.2	17
—	—	—	22	22	27	.5	256	20	.05	.02	.2	79
—	—	—	20	38	44	1.1	682	9,240	.11	.08	1.6	90
—	—	—	11	21	24	.6	374	60	.06	.04	.9	34
—	—	—	16	54	26	.5	263	260	.13	.05	.5	66
—	—	—	22	74	36	.7	360	360	.18	.07	.7	90
—	—	—	26	27	42	.5	496	500	.22	.07	1.0	124
—	—	—	28	25	45	1.0	496	500	.17	.05	.7	100
—	—	—	87	75	126	.9	1,500	1,620	.68	.11	2.8	360
—	—	—	29	25	42	.2	503	540	.23	.03	.9	120
—	—	—	14	28	22	.4	328	2,450	.06	.06	.4	78
—	—	—	10	9	19	.5	202	[34]1,330	.02	.05	1.0	7

Item No. (A)	Foods, approximate measures, units, and weight (edible part unless footnotes indicate otherwise) (B)			Water (C)	Food energy (D)	Protein (E)	Fat (F)
			Grams	Percent	Calories	Grams	Grams
	Peaches:						
	Raw:						
284	Sliced	1 cup	170	89	65	1	Trace
	Canned, yellow-fleshed, solids and liquid (halves or slices):						
285	Sirup pack	1 cup	256	79	200	1	Trace
	Frozen, sliced, sweetened:						
289	10-oz container	1 container	284	77	250	1	Trace
290	Cup	1 cup	250	77	220	1	Trace
	Pears:						
	Raw, with skin, cored:						
291	Bartlett, 2 1/2-in diam. (about 2 1/2 per lb with cores and stems).	1 pear	164	83	100	1	1
294	Canned, solids and liquid, sirup pack, heavy (halves or slices).	1 cup	255	80	195	1	1
	Pineapple:						
295	Raw, diced	1 cup	155	85	80	1	Trace
	Canned, heavy sirup pack, solids and liquid:						
296	Crushed, chunks, tidbits	1 cup	255	80	190	1	Trace
	Slices and liquid:						
297	Large	1 slice; 2 1/4 tbsp liquid.	105	80	80	Trace	Trace
298	Medium	1 slice; 1 1/4 tbsp liquid.	58	80	45	Trace	Trace
299	Pineapple juice, unsweetened, canned.	1 cup	250	86	140	1	Trace
	Plums:						
	Raw, without pits:						
300	Japanese and hybrid (2 1/8-in diam., about 6 1/2 per lb with pits).	1 plum	66	87	30	Trace	Trace
	Canned, heavy sirup pack (Italian prunes), with pits and liquid:						
302	Cup	1 cup[36]	272	77	215	1	Trace
303	Portion	3 plums; 2 3/4 tbsp liquid.[36]	140	77	110	1	Trace
	Prunes, dried, "softenized," with pits:						
304	Uncooked	4 extra large or 5 large prunes.[36]	49	28	110	1	Trace
305	Cooked, unsweetened, all sizes, fruit and liquid.	1 cup[36]	250	66	255	2	1
306	Prune juice, canned or bottled	1 cup	256	80	195	1	Trace
	Raisins, seedless:						
307	Cup, not pressed down	1 cup	145	18	420	4	Trace
308	Packet, 1/2 oz (1 1/2 tbsp)	1 packet	14	18	40	Trace	Trace
	Raspberries, red:						
309	Raw, capped, whole	1 cup	123	84	70	1	1
310	Frozen, sweetened, 10-oz container	1 container	284	74	280	2	1
	Rhubarb, cooked, added sugar:						
311	From raw	1 cup	270	63	380	1	Trace

[27]Based on product with label claim of 100% of U.S. RDA in 6 fl oz.

[35]Value represents products with added ascorbic acid. For products without added ascorbic acid, value in milligrams is 116 for a 10-oz container, 103 for 1 cup.

[36]Weight includes pits. After removal of the pits, the weight of the edible portion is 258 g for item 302, 133 g for item 303, 43 g for item 304, and 213 g for item 305.

Fatty Acids												
Saturated (total)	Unsaturated		Carbo-hydrate	Calcium	Phos-phorus	Iron	Potas-sium	Vitamin A value	Thiamin	Ribo-flavin	Niacin	Ascorbic acid
	Oleic	Lino-leic										
(G)	(H)	(I)	(J)	(K)	(L)	(M)	(N)	(O)	(P)	(Q)	(R)	(S)
Grams	Grams	Grams	Grams	Milli-grams	Milli-grams	Milli-grams	Milli-grams	Inter-national units	Milli-grams	Milli-grams	Milli-grams	Milli-grams
—	—	—	16	15	32	.9	343	[34]2,260	.03	.09	1.7	12
—	—	—	51	10	31	.8	333	1,100	.03	.05	1.5	8
—	—	—	64	11	37	1.4	352	1,850	0.03	0.11	2.0	[35]116
—	—	—	57	10	33	1.3	310	1,630	.03	.10	1.8	[35]103
—	—	—	25	13	18	.5	213	30	.03	.07	.2	7
—	—	—	50	13	18	.5	214	10	.03	.05	.3	3
—	—	—	21	26	12	.8	226	110	.14	.05	.3	26
—	—	—	49	28	13	.8	245	130	.20	.05	.5	18
—	—	—	20	12	5	.3	101	50	.08	.02	.2	7
—	—	—	11	6	3	.2	56	30	.05	.01	.1	4
—	—	—	34	38	23	.8	373	130	.13	.05	.5	[27]80
—	—	—	8	8	12	.3	112	160	.02	.02	.3	4
—	—	—	56	23	26	2.3	367	3,130	.05	.05	1.0	5
—	—	—	29	12	13	1.2	189	1,610	.03	.03	.5	3
—	—	—	29	22	34	1.7	298	690	.04	.07	.7	1
—	—	—	67	51	79	3.8	695	1,590	.07	.15	1.5	2
—	—	—	49	36	51	1.8	602	——	.03	.03	1.0	5
—	—	—	112	90	146	5.1	1,106	30	.16	.12	.7	1
—	—	—	11	9	14	.5	107	Trace	.02	.01	.1	Trace
—	—	—	17	27	27	1.1	207	160	.04	.11	1.1	31
—	—	—	70	37	48	1.7	284	200	.06	.17	1.7	60
—	—	—	97	211	41	1.6	548	220	.05	.14	.8	16

Item No. (A)	Foods, approximate measures, units, and weight (edible part unless footnotes indicate otherwise) (B)		Water (C) Per-cent	Food energy (D) Cal-ories	Pro-tein (E) Grams	Fat (F) Grams
		Grams				
	Strawberries:					
313	Raw, whole berries, capped-----	1 cup----------------------	149	90	55	1	1
	Frozen, sweetened:					
314	Sliced, 10-oz container------	1 container---------------	284	71	310	1	1
315	Whole, 1-lb container (about 1 3/4 cups).	1 container---------------	454	76	415	2	1
316	Tangerine, raw, 2 3/8-in diam., size 176, without peel (about 4 per lb with peels and seeds).	1 tangerine---------------	86	87	40	1	Trace
317	Tangerine juice, canned, sweet-ened.	1 cup----------------------	249	87	125	1	Trace
318	Watermelon, raw, 4 by 8 in wedge with rind and seeds (1/16 of 32 2/3-lb melon, 10 by 16 in).	1 wedge with rind and seeds[37]	926	93	110	2	1

GRAIN PRODUCTS

Item No. (A)	Foods, approximate measures, units, and weight (edible part unless footnotes indicate otherwise) (B)		Water (C) Per-cent	Food energy (D) Cal-ories	Pro-tein (E) Grams	Fat (F) Grams
	Bagel, 3-in diam.:					
319	Egg-----------------------------	1 bagel--------------------	55	32	165	6	2
	Biscuits, baking powder, 2-in diam. (enriched flour, vege-table shortening):					
322	From home recipe---------------	1 biscuit------------------	28	27	105	2	5
323	From mix----------------------	1 biscuit------------------	28	29	90	2	3
	Breads:					
325	Boston brown bread, canned, slice, 3 1/4 by 1/2 in.[38]	1 slice--------------------	45	45	95	2	1
	Cracked-wheat bread (3/4 en-riched wheat flour, 1/4 cracked wheat):[38]					
326	Loaf, 1 lb-------------------	1 loaf---------------------	454	35	1,195	39	10
327	Slice (18 per loaf)----------	1 slice--------------------	25	35	65	2	1
	French or vienna bread, en-riched:[38]					
328	Loaf, 1 lb-------------------	1 loaf---------------------	454	31	1,315	41	14
	Slice:					
329	French (5 by 2 1/2 by 1 in)	1 slice--------------------	35	31	100	3	1
	Raisin bread, enriched:[38]					
333	Loaf, 1 lb-------------------	1 loaf---------------------	454	35	1,190	30	13
334	Slice (18 per loaf)----------	1 slice--------------------	25	35	65	2	1
	Rye Bread:					
	American, light (2/3 enriched wheat flour, 1/3 rye flour):					
335	Loaf, 1 lb-------------------	1 loaf---------------------	454	36	1,100	41	5
336	Slice (4 3/4 by 3 3/4 by 7/16 in).	1 slice--------------------	25	36	60	2	Trace
	White bread, enriched:[38]					
	Soft-crumb type:					
339	Loaf, 1 lb-------------------	1 loaf---------------------	454	36	1,225	39	15
340	Slice (18 per lb) -------	1 slice--------------------	25	36	70	2	1
341	Slice, toasted----------	1 slice--------------------	22	25	70	2	1
342	Slice (22 per lb) -------	1 slice--------------------	20	36	55	2	1
	Whole-wheat bread:					
	Soft-crumb type:[38]					
357	Loaf, 1 lb-------------------	1 loaf---------------------	454	36	1,095	41	12
358	Slice (16 per loaf)-------	1 slice--------------------	28	36	65	3	1

[37]Weight includes rind and seeds. Without rind and seeds, weight of the edible portion is 426 g.
[38]Made with vegetable shortening.
[39]Applies to product made with white cornmeal. With yellow cornmeal, value is 30 International Units (I.U.).

Fatty Acids												
Satu-rated (total)	Unsaturated		Carbo-hydrate	Calcium	Phos-phorus	Iron	Potas-sium	Vitamin A value	Thiamin	Ribo-flavin	Niacin	Ascorbic acid
	Oleic	Lino-leic										
(G)	(H)	(I)	(J)	(K)	(L)	(M)	(N)	(O)	(P)	(Q)	(R)	(S)
Grams	Grams	Grams	Grams	Milli-grams	Milli-grams	Milli-grams	Milli-grams	Inter-national units	Milli-grams	Milli-grams	Milli-grams	Milli-grams
—	—	—	13	31	31	1.5	244	90	0.04	0.10	0.9	88
—	—	—	79	40	48	2.0	318	90	.06	.17	1.4	151
—	—	—	107	59	73	2.7	472	140	.09	.27	2.3	249
—	—	—	10	34	15	.3	108	360	.05	.02	.1	27
—	—	—	30	44	35	.5	440	1,040	.15	.05	.2	54
—	—	—	27	30	43	2.1	426	2,510	.13	.13	.9	30
0.5	0.9	0.8	28	9	43	1.2	41	30	.14	.10	1.2	0
1.2	2.0	1.2	13	34	49	.4	33	Trace	.08	.08	.7	Trace
.6	1.1	.7	15	19	65	.6	32	Trace	.09	.08	.8	Trace
.1	.2	.2	21	41	72	.9	131	[39]0	.06	.04	.7	0
2.2	3.0	3.9	236	399	581	9.5	608	Trace	1.52	1.13	14.4	Trace
.1	.2	.2	13	22	32	.5	34	Trace	.08	.06	.8	Trace
3.2	4.7	4.6	251	195	386	10.0	408	Trace	1.80	1.10	15.0	Trace
.2	.4	.4	19	15	30	.8	32	Trace	.14	.08	1.2	Trace
3.0	4.7	3.9	243	322	395	10.0	1,057	Trace	1.70	1.07	10.7	Trace
.2	.3	.2	13	18	22	.6	58	Trace	.09	.06	.6	Trace
0.7	0.5	2.2	236	340	667	9.1	658	0	1.35	0.98	12.9	0
Trace	Trace	.1	13	19	37	.5	36	0	.07	.05	.7	0
3.4	5.3	4.6	229	381	440	11.3	476	Trace	1.80	1.10	15.0	Trace
.2	.3	.3	13	21	24	.6	26	Trace	.10	.06	.8	Trace
.2	.3	.3	13	21	24	.6	26	Trace	.08	.06	.8	Trace
.2	.2	.2	10	17	19	.5	21	Trace	.08	.05	.7	Trace
2.2	2.9	4.2	224	381	1,152	13.6	1,161	Trace	1.37	.45	12.7	Trace
.1	.2	.2	14	24	71	.8	72	Trace	.09	.03	.8	Trace

Item No.	Foods, approximate measures, units, and weight (edible part unless footnotes indicate otherwise)		Water	Food energy	Pro-tein	Fat
(A)	(B)		(C)	(D)	(E)	(F)
			Grams	Per-cent	Cal-ories	Grams	Grams

			Grams	Percent	Calories	Grams	Grams
	Breakfast cereals:						
	Hot type, cooked:						
	Corn (hominy) grits, degermed:						
363	Enriched----------------	1 cup-----------------	245	87	125	3	Trace
364	Unenriched--------------	1 cup-----------------	245	87	125	3	Trace
365	Farina, quick-cooking, en-riched.	1 cup-----------------	245	89	105	3	Trace
366	Oatmeal or rolled oats--------	1 cup-----------------	240	87	130	5	2
367	Wheat, rolled-------------	1 cup-----------------	240	80	180	5	1
368	Wheat, whole-meal------------	1 cup-----------------	245	88	110	4	1
	Ready-to-eat:						
369	Bran flakes (40% bran), added sugar, salt, iron, vitamins.	1 cup-----------------	35	3	105	4	1
370	Bran flakes with raisins, add-ed sugar, salt, iron, vita-mins.	1 cup-----------------	50	7	145	4	1
	Corn flakes:						
371	Plain, added sugar, salt, iron, vitamins.	1 cup-----------------	25	4	95	2	Trace
372	Sugar-coated, added salt, iron, vitamins. mins.	1 cup-----------------	40	2	155	2	Trace
374	Corn, shredded, added sugar, salt, iron, thiamin, niacin.	1 cup-----------------	25	3	95	2	Trace
375	Oats, puffed, added sugar, salt, minerals, vitamins.	1 cup-----------------	25	3	100	3	1
	Rice, puffed:						
376	Plain, added iron, thiamin, niacin.	1 cup-----------------	15	4	60	1	Trace
377	Presweetened, added salt, iron, vitamins.	1 cup-----------------	28	3	115	1	0
378	Wheat flakes, added sugar, salt, iron, vitamins.	1 cup-----------------	30	4	105	3	Trace
	Wheat, puffed:						
379	Plain, added iron, thiamin, niacin.	1 cup-----------------	15	3	55	2	Trace
380	Presweetened, added salt, iron, vitamins.	1 cup-----------------	38	3	140	3	Trace
381	Wheat, shredded, plain-------	1 oblong biscuit or 1/2 cup spoon-size biscuits.	25	7	90	2	1
382	Wheat germ, without salt and sugar, toasted.	1 tbsp--------------------	6	4	25	2	1
	Cakes made from cake mixes with enriched flour:[46]						
	Angelfood:						
385	Whole cake (9 3/4-in diam. tube cake).	1 cake----------------	635	34	1,645	36	1
386	Piece, 1/12 of cake----------	1 piece------------------	53	34	135	3	Trace
	Cupcakes, made with egg, milk, 2 1/2-in diam.						
389	Without icing---------------	1 cupcake----------------	25	26	90	1	3
390	With chocolate icing--------	1 cupcake----------------	36	22	130	2	5

[40]Applies to white varieties. For yellow varieties, value is 150 International Units (I.U.).
[41]Applies to products that do not contain di-sodium phosphate. If di-sodium phosphate is an ingredient, value is 162 mg.
[42]Value may range from less than 1 mg to about 8 mg depending on the brand. Consult the label.
[43]Value varies with the brand. Consult the label.
[44]Value varies with the brand. Consult the label.
[45]Applies to product with added ascorbic acid. Without added ascorbic acid, value is trace.
[46]Excepting angelfood cake, cakes were made from mixes containing vegetable shortening; icings, with butter.

Satu-rated (total) (G)	Unsaturated Oleic (H)	Lino-leic (I)	Carbo-hydrate (J)	Calcium (K)	Phos-phorus (L)	Iron (M)	Potas-sium (N)	Vitamin A value (O)	Thiamin (P)	Ribo-flavin (Q)	Niacin (R)	Ascorbic acid (S)
Grams	Grams	Grams	Grams	Milli-grams	Milli-grams	Milli-grams	Milli-grams	Inter-national units	Milli-grams	Milli-grams	Milli-grams	Milli-grams
Trace	Trace	.1	27	2	25	.7	27	[40]Trace	.10	.07	1.0	0
Trace	Trace	.1	27	2	25	.2	27	[40]Trace	.05	.02	.5	0
Trace	Trace	.1	22	147	[41]113	([42])	25	0	.12	.07	1.0	0
.4	.8	.9	23	22	137	1.4	146	0	.19	.05	.2	0
—	—	—	41	19	182	1.7	202	0	.17	.07	2.2	0
—	—	—	23	17	127	1.2	118	0	.15	.05	1.5	0
—	—	—	28	19	125	12.4	137	1,650	.41	.49	4.1	12
—	—	—	40	28	146	17.7	154	2,350	.58	.71	5.8	18
—	—	—	21	([43])	9	0.6	30	1,180	0.29	0.35	2.9	9
—	—	—	37	1	10	1.0	27	1,880	.46	.56	4.6	14
—	—	—	22	1	10	.6	—	0	.11	.05	.5	0
—	—	—	19	44	102	2.9	—	1,180	.29	.35	2.9	9
—	—	—	13	3	14	.3	15	0	.07	.01	.7	0
—	—	—	26	3	14	[44]1.1	43	1,250	.38	.43	5.0	[45]15
—	—	—	24	12	83	([43])	81	1,410	.35	.42	3.5	11
—	—	—	12	4	48	.6	51	0	.08	.03	1.2	0
—	—	—	33	7	52	[44]1.6	63	1,680	.50	.57	6.7	[45]20
—	—	—	20	11	97	.9	87	0	.06	.03	1.1	0
—	—	—	3	3	70	.5	57	10	.11	.05	.3	1
—	—	—	377	603	756	2.5	381	0	.37	.95	3.6	0
—	—	—	32	50	63	.2	32	0	.03	.08	.3	0
.8	1.2	.7	14	40	59	.3	21	40	.05	.05	.4	Trace
2.0	1.6	.6	21	47	71	.4	42	60	.05	.06	.4	Trace

Item No.	Foods, approximate measures, units, and weight (edible part unless footnotes indicate otherwise)		Water	Food energy	Pro-tein	Fat
(A)	(B)		(C)	(D)	(E)	(F)
		Grams	Per-cent	Cal-ories	Grams	Grams
	Devil's food with chocolate icing:					
391	Whole, 2 layer cake (8- or 9-in diam.).	1 cake------------------- 1,107	24	3,755	49	136
392	Piece, 1/16 of cake----------	1 piece------------------ 69	24	235	3	8
	Gingerbread:					
394	Whole cake (8-in square)-------	1 cake------------------ 570	37	1,575	18	39
395	Piece, 1/9 of cake-------------	1 piece----------------- 63	37	175	2	4
	Cookies made with enriched flour:[50] [51]					
	Brownies with nuts:					
	Home-prepared, 1 3/4 by 1 3/4 by 7/8 in:					
412	From home recipe------------	1 brownie---------------- 20	10	95	1	6
413	From commercial recipe-------	1 brownie---------------- 20	11	85	1	4
414	Frozen, with chocolate icing,[52] 1 1/2 by 1 3/4 by 7/8 in.	1 brownie---------------- 25	13	105	1	5
	Chocolate chip:					
415	Commercial, 2 1/4-in diam., 3/8 in thick.	4 cookies---------------- 42	3	200	2	9
416	From home recipe, 2 1/3-in diam.	4 cookies---------------- 40	3	205	2	12
420	Oatmeal with raisins, 2 5/8-in diam., 1/4 in thick.	4 cookies---------------- 52	3	235	3	8
422	Sandwich type (chocolate or vanilla), 1 3/4-in diam., 3/8 in thick.	4 cookies---------------- 40	2	200	2	9
	Cornmeal:					
	Degermed, enriched:					
426	Dry form----------------------	1 cup---------------------- 138	12	500	11	2
427	Cooked-----------------------	1 cup---------------------- 240	88	120	3	Trace
	Crackers:[38]					
430	Graham, plain, 2 1/2-in square--	2 crackers---------------- 14	6	55	1	1
431	Rye wafers, whole-grain, 1 7/8 by 3 1/2 in.	2 wafers------------------ 13	6	45	2	Trace
432	Saltines, made with enriched flour.	4 crackers or 1 packet---- 11	4	50	1	1
	Danish pastry (enriched flour), plain without fruit or nuts:[54]					
433	Packaged ring, 12 oz------------	1 ring-------------------- 340	22	1,435	25	80
434	Round piece, about 4 1/4-in diam. by 1 in.	1 pastry------------------ 65	22	275	5	15
435	Ounce-------------------------	1 oz---------------------- 28	22	120	2	7
	Doughnuts, made with enriched flour:[38]					
436	Cake type, plain, 2 1/2-in diam., 1 in high.	1 doughnut---------------- 25	24	100	1	5
437	Yeast-leavened, glazed, 3 3/4-in diam., 1 1/4 in high.	1 doughnut---------------- 50	26	205	3	11
	Macaroni, enriched, cooked (cut lengths, elbows, shells):					
440	Hot macaroni------------------	1 cup---------------------- 140	73	155	5	1

[38]Made with vegetable shortening.
[50]Products are commercial unless otherwise specified.
[51]Made with enriched flour and vegetable shortening except for macaroons which do not contain flour or shortening.
[52]Icing made with butter.
[53]Applies to yellow varieties; white varieties contain only a trace.
[54]Contains vegetable shortening and butter.

Saturated (total) (G) Grams	Unsaturated		Carbohydrate (J) Grams	Calcium (K) Milligrams	Phosphorus (L) Milligrams	Iron (M) Milligrams	Potassium (N) Milligrams	Vitamin A value (O) International units	Thiamin (P) Milligrams	Riboflavin (Q) Milligrams	Niacin (R) Milligrams	Ascorbic acid (S) Milligrams
	Oleic (H) Grams	Linoleic (I) Grams										
50.0	44.9	17.0	645	653	1,162	16.6	1,439	1,660	1.06	1.65	10.1	1
3.1	2.8	1.1	40	41	72	1.0	90	100	.07	.10	.6	Trace
9.7	16.6	10.0	291	513	570	8.6	1,562	Trace	0.84	1.00	7.4	Trace
1.1	1.8	1.1	32	57	63	.9	173	Trace	.09	.11	.8	Trace
1.5	3.0	1.2	10	8	30	.4	38	40	.04	.03	.2	Trace
.9	1.4	1.3	13	9	27	.4	34	20	.03	.02	.2	Trace
2.0	2.2	.7	15	10	31	.4	44	50	.03	.03	.2	Trace
2.8	2.9	2.2	29	16	48	1.0	56	50	.10	.17	.9	Trace
3.5	4.5	2.9	24	14	40	.8	47	40	.06	.06	.5	Trace
2.0	3.3	2.0	38	11	53	1.4	192	30	.15	.10	1.0	Trace
2.2	3.9	2.2	28	10	96	.7	15	0	.06	.10	.7	0
.2	.4	.9	108	8	137	4.0	166	[53]610	.61	.36	4.8	0
Trace	.1	.2	26	2	34	1.0	38	[53]140	.14	.10	1.2	0
.3	.5	.3	10	6	21	.5	55	0	.02	.08	.5	0
—	—	—	10	7	50	.5	78	0	.04	.03	.2	0
.3	.5	.4	8	2	10	.5	13	0	.05	.05	.4	0
24.3	31.7	16.5	155	170	371	6.1	381	1,050	.97	1.01	8.6	Trace
4.7	6.1	3.2	30	33	71	1.2	73	200	.18	.19	1.7	Trace
2.0	2.7	1.4	13	14	31	.5	32	90	.08	.08	.7	Trace
1.2	2.0	1.1	13	10	48	.4	23	20	.05	.05	.4	Trace
3.3	5.8	3.3	22	16	33	.6	34	25	.10	.10	.8	0
—	—	—	32	11	70	1.3	85	0	.20	.11	1.5	0

Item No.	Foods, approximate measures, units, and weight (edible part unless footnotes indicate otherwise)		Water	Food energy	Pro-tein	Fat
(A)	(B)		(C)	(D)	(E)	(F)
			Grams	Per-cent	Cal-ories	Grams	Grams

	Macaroni (enriched) and cheese:						
441	Canned[55]	1 cup	240	80	230	9	10
442	From home recipe (served hot)[56]	1 cup	200	58	430	17	22
	Muffins made with enriched flour:[38]						
	From recipe:						
444	Bran	1 muffin	40	35	105	3	4
445	Corn (enriched degermed corn-meal and flour), 2 3/8-in diam., 1 1/2 in high.	1 muffin	40	33	125	3	4
446	Plain, 3-in diam., 1 1/2 in high.	1 muffin	40	38	120	3	4
448	Noodles (egg noodles), enriched, cooked.	1 cup	160	71	200	7	2
449	Noodles, chow mein, canned	1 cup	45	1	220	6	11
	Pancakes, (4-in diam.):[38]						
452	Made from mix with enriched flour, egg and milk added.	1 cake	27	51	60	2	2
	Pies, piecrust made with enriched flour, vegetable shortening (9-in diam.):						
	Apple:						
453	Whole	1 pie	945	48	2,420	21	105
454	Sector, 1/7 of pie	1 sector	135	48	345	3	15
	Cherry:						
459	Whole	1 pie	945	47	2,465	25	107
460	Sector, 1/7 of pie	1 sector	135	47	350	4	15
	Lemon meringue:						
463	Whole	1 pie	840	47	2,140	31	86
464	Sector, 1/7 of pie	1 sector	120	47	305	4	12
	Pumpkin:						
471	Whole	1 pie	910	59	1,920	36	102
472	Sector, 1/7 of pie	1 sector	130	59	275	5	15
475	Pizza (cheese) baked, 4 3/4-in sector; 1/8 of 12-in diam. pie.[19]	1 sector	60	45	145	6	4
	Popcorn, popped:						
476	Plain, large kernel	1 cup	6	4	25	1	Trace
478	Sugar coated	1 cup	35	4	135	2	1
	Pretzels, made with enriched flour:						
480	Thin, twisted, 3 1/4 by 2 1/4 by 1/4 in.	10 pretzels	60	5	235	6	3
481	Stick, 2 1/4 in long	10 pretzels	3	5	10	Trace	Trace
	Rice, white, enriched:						
482	Instant, ready-to-serve, hot	1 cup	165	73	180	4	Trace
	Long grain:						
483	Raw	1 cup	185	12	670	12	1
484	Cooked, served hot	1 cup	205	73	225	4	Trace
	Parboiled:						
485	Raw	1 cup	185	10	685	14	1
486	Cooked, served hot	1 cup	175	73	185	4	Trace
	Rolls, enriched:[38]						
	Commercial:						
487	Brown-and-serve (12 per 12-oz pkg.), browned.	1 roll	26	27	85	2	2
489	Frankfurter and hamburger (8 per 11 1/2-oz pkg.).	1 roll	40	31	120	3	2

[19]Crust made with vegetable shortening and enriched flour.
[38]Made with vegetable shortening.
[55]Made with corn oil.
[56]Made with regular margarine.
[59]Product may or may not be enriched with riboflavin. Consult the label.

	Fatty Acids		Carbo-hydrate	Calcium	Phos-phorus	Iron	Potas-sium	Vitamin A value	Thiamin	Ribo-flavin	Niacin	Ascorbic acid
Satu-rated (total)	Unsaturated											
	Oleic	Lino-leic										
(G)	(H)	(I)	(J)	(K)	(L)	(M)	(N)	(O)	(P)	(Q)	(R)	(S)
Grams	Grams	Grams	Grams	Milli-grams	Milli-grams	Milli-grams	Milli-grams	Inter-national units	Milli-grams	Milli-grams	Milli-grams	Milli-grams
4.2	3.1	1.4	26	199	182	1.0	139	260	.12	.24	1.0	Trace
8.9	8.8	2.9	40	362	322	1.8	240	860	.20	.40	1.8	Trace
1.2	1.4	.8	17	57	162	1.5	172	90	.07	.10	1.7	Trace
1.2	1.6	.9	19	42	68	.7	54	[57]120	.10	.10	.7	Trace
1.0	1.7	1.0	17	42	60	0.6	50	40	0.09	0.12	0.9	Trace
—	—	—	37	16	94	1.4	70	110	.22	.13	1.9	0
—	—	—	26	—	—	—	—	—	—	—	—	—
.7	.7	.3	9	58	70	.3	42	70	.04	.06	.2	Trace
27.0	44.5	25.2	360	76	208	6.6	756	280	1.06	.79	9.3	9
3.9	6.4	3.6	51	11	30	.9	108	40	.15	.11	1.3	2
28.2	45.0	25.3	363	132	236	6.6	992	4,160	1.09	.84	9.8	Trace
4.0	6.4	3.6	52	19	34	.9	142	590	.16	.12	1.4	Trace
26.1	33.8	16.4	317	118	412	6.7	420	1,430	.61	.84	5.2	25
3.7	4.8	2.3	45	17	59	1.0	60	200	.09	.12	.7	4
37.4	37.5	16.6	223	464	628	7.3	1,456	22,480	.78	1.27	7.0	Trace
5.4	5.4	2.4	32	66	90	1.0	208	3,210	.11	.18	1.0	Trace
1.7	1.5	0.6	22	86	89	1.1	67	230	0.16	0.18	1.6	4
Trace	.1	.2	5	1	17	.2	—	—	—	.01	.1	0
.5	.2	.4	30	2	47	.5	—	—	—	.02	.4	0
—	—	—	46	13	79	.9	78	0	.20	.15	2.5	0
—	—	—	2	1	4	Trace	4	0	.01	.01	.1	0
Trace	Trace	Trace	40	5	31	1.3	—	0	.21	([59])	1.7	0
.2	.2	.2	149	44	174	5.4	170	0	.81	.06	6.5	0
.1	.1	.1	50	21	57	1.8	57	0	.23	.02	2.1	0
.2	.1	.2	150	111	370	5.4	278	0	.81	.07	6.5	0
.1	.1	.1	41	33	100	1.4	75	0	.19	.02	2.1	0
.4	.7	.5	14	20	23	.5	25	Trace	.10	.06	.9	Trace
.5	.8	.6	21	30	34	.8	38	Trace	.16	.10	1.3	Trace

Item No. (A)	Foods, approximate measures, units, and weight (edible part unless footnotes indicate otherwise) (B)		Grams	Water (C) Per-cent	Food energy (D) Cal-ories	Pro-tein (E) Grams	Fat (F) Grams
	Spaghetti, enriched, cooked:						
493	Firm stage, "al dente," served hot.	1 cup--------------------	130	64	190	7	1
494	Tender stage, served hot-------	1 cup--------------------	140	73	155	5	1
	Spaghetti (enriched) in tomato sauce with cheese:						
495	From home recipe--------------	1 cup--------------------	250	77	260	9	9
496	Canned-----------------------	1 cup--------------------	250	80	190	6	2
	Spaghetti (enriched) with meat balls and tomato sauce:						
497	From home recipe--------------	1 cup--------------------	248	70	330	19	12
498	Canned-----------------------	1 cup--------------------	250	78	260	12	10
499	Toaster pastries-------------	1 pastry----------------	50	12	200	3	6
	Waffles, made with enriched flour, 7-in diam.:[38]						
500	From home recipe--------------	1 waffle----------------	75	41	210	7	7
501	From mix, egg and milk added---	1 waffle----------------	75	42	205	7	8
	Wheat flours:						
	All-purpose or family flour, enriched:						
502	Sifted, spooned--------------	1 cup--------------------	115	12	420	12	1
503	Unsifted, spooned------------	1 cup--------------------	125	12	455	13	1
506	Whole-wheat, from hard wheats, stirred.	1 cup--------------------	120	12	400	16	2

LEGUMES (DRY), NUTS, SEEDS; RELATED PRODUCTS

Item No. (A)	(B)		Grams	(C)	(D)	(E)	(F)
	Almonds, shelled:						
507	Chopped (about 130 almonds)-----	1 cup--------------------	130	5	775	24	70
508	Slivered, not pressed down (about 115 almonds).	1 cup--------------------	115	5	690	21	62
	Beans, dry:						
	Common varieties as Great North-ern, navy, and others:						
	Cooked, drained:						
509	Great Northern--------------	1 cup--------------------	180	69	210	14	1
510	Pea (navy)------------------	1 cup--------------------	190	69	225	15	1
	Canned, solids and liquid:						
	White with—						
511	Frankfurters (sliced)-----	1 cup--------------------	255	71	365	19	18
512	Pork and tomato sauce-----	1 cup--------------------	255	71	310	16	7
513	Pork and sweet sauce------	1 cup--------------------	255	66	385	16	12
514	Red kidney----------------	1 cup--------------------	255	76	230	15	1
515	Lima, cooked, drained----------	1 cup--------------------	190	64	260	16	1
518	Cashew nuts, roasted in oil-------	1 cup--------------------	140	5	785	24	64
	Coconut meat, fresh:						
519	Piece, about 2 by 2 by 1/2 in---	1 piece-----------------	45	51	155	2	16
520	Shredded or grated, not pressed down.	1 cup--------------------	80	51	275	3	28
523	Peanuts, roasted in oil, salted (whole, halves, chopped).	1 cup--------------------	144	2	840	37	72
524	Peanut butter--------------------	1 tbsp------------------	16	2	95	4	8
525	Peas, split, dry, cooked----------	1 cup--------------------	200	70	230	16	1
528	Sunflower seeds, dry, hulled------	1 cup--------------------	145	5	810	35	69
	Walnuts:						
531	Persian or English, chopped (about 60 halves).	1 cup--------------------	120	4	780	18	77

[60]Value varies with the brand. Consult the label.

Fatty Acids												
Saturated (total)	Unsaturated Oleic	Unsaturated Linoleic	Carbohydrate	Calcium	Phosphorus	Iron	Potassium	Vitamin A value	Thiamin	Riboflavin	Niacin	Ascorbic acid
(G)	(H)	(I)	(J)	(K)	(L)	(M)	(N)	(O)	(P)	(Q)	(R)	(S)
Grams	Grams	Grams	Grams	Milligrams	Milligrams	Milligrams	Milligrams	International units	Milligrams	Milligrams	Milligrams	Milligrams
—	—	—	39	14	85	1.4	103	0	.23	.13	1.8	0
—	—	—	32	11	70	1.3	85	0	.20	.11	1.5	0
2.0	5.4	.7	37	80	135	2.3	408	1,080	.25	.18	2.3	13
.5	.3	.4	39	40	88	2.8	303	930	.35	.28	4.5	10
3.3	6.3	.9	39	124	236	3.7	665	1,590	.25	.30	4.0	22
2.2	3.3	3.9	29	53	113	3.3	245	1,000	.15	.18	2.3	5
—	—	—	36	[60]54	[60]67	1.9	[60]74	500	.16	.17	2.1	([60])
2.3	2.8	1.4	28	85	130	1.3	109	250	.17	.23	1.4	Trace
2.8	2.9	1.2	27	179	257	1.0	146	170	.14	.22	.9	Trace
0.2	0.1	0.5	88	18	100	3.3	109	0	0.74	0.46	6.1	0
.2	.1	.5	95	20	109	3.6	119	0	.80	.50	6.6	0
.4	.2	1.0	85	49	446	4.0	444	0	.66	.14	5.2	0
5.6	47.7	12.8	25	304	655	6.1	1,005	0	.31	1.20	4.6	Trace
5.0	42.2	11.3	22	269	580	5.4	889	0	.28	1.06	4.0	Trace
—	—	—	38	90	266	4.9	749	0	.25	.13	1.3	0
—	—	—	40	95	281	5.1	790	0	.27	.13	1.3	0
—	—	—	32	94	303	4.8	668	330	.18	.15	3.3	Trace
2.4	2.8	.6	48	138	235	4.6	536	330	.20	.08	1.5	5
4.3	5.0	1.1	54	161	291	5.9	—	—	.15	.10	1.3	—
—	—	—	42	74	278	4.6	673	10	.13	.10	1.5	—
—	—	—	49	55	293	5.9	1,163	—	.25	.11	1.3	—
12.9	36.8	10.2	41	53	522	5.3	650	140	.60	.35	2.5	—
14.0	.9	.3	4	6	43	.8	115	0	.02	.01	.2	1
24.8	1.6	.5	8	10	76	1.4	205	0	.04	.02	.4	2
13.7	33.0	20.7	27	107	577	3.0	971	—	.46	.19	24.8	0
1.5	3.7	2.3	3	9	61	.3	100	—	.02	.02	2.4	0
—	—	—	42	22	178	3.4	592	80	.30	.18	1.8	—
8.2	13.7	43.2	29	174	1,214	10.3	1,334	70	2.84	.33	7.8	—
8.4	11.8	42.2	19	119	456	3.7	540	40	.40	.16	1.1	2

Item No.	Foods, approximate measures, units, and weight (edible part unless footnotes indicate otherwise)			Water	Food energy	Pro- tein	Fat
(A)	(B)			(C)	(D)	(E)	(F)
			Grams	Per- cent	Cal- ories	Grams	Grams

SUGARS AND SWEETS

Item No.	Foods	measure		Grams	Percent	Calories	Protein	Fat
	Candy:							
537	Caramels, plain or chocolate	1 oz		28	8	115	1	3
	Chocolate:							
538	Milk, plain	1 oz		28	1	145	2	9
542	Fudge, chocolate, plain	1 oz		28	8	115	1	3
543	Gum drops	1 oz		28	12	100	Trace	Trace
544	Hard	1 oz		28	1	110	0	Trace
545	Marshmallows	1 oz		28	17	90	1	Trace
	Chocolate-flavored beverage powders (about 4 heaping tsp per oz):							
546	With nonfat dry milk	1 oz		28	2	100	5	1
547	Without milk	1 oz		28	1	100	1	1
548	Honey, strained or extracted	1 tbsp		21	17	65	Trace	0
549	Jams and preserves	1 tbsp		20	29	55	Trace	Trace
551	Jellies	1 tbsp		18	29	50	Trace	Trace
552		1 packet		14	29	40	Trace	Trace
	Sirups:							
	Chocolate-flavored sirup or topping:							
553	Thin type	1 fl oz or 2 tbsp		38	32	90	1	1
	Molasses, cane:							
555	Light (first extraction)	1 tbsp		20	24	50	—	—
556	Blackstrap (third extraction)	1 tbsp		20	24	45	—	—
557	Sorghum	1 tbsp		21	23	55	—	—
558	Table blends, chiefly corn, light and dark.	1 tbsp		21	24	60	0	0
	Sugars:							
559	Brown, pressed down	1 cup		220	2	820	0	0
	White:							
560	Granulated	1 cup		200	1	770	0	0
561		1 tbsp		12	1	45	0	0
562		1 packet		6	1	23	0	0
563	Powdered, sifted, spooned into cup.	1 cup		100	1	385	0	0

VEGETABLE AND VEGETABLE PRODUCTS

Item No.	Foods	measure		Grams	Percent	Calories	Protein	Fat
	Asparagus, green:							
	Cooked, drained:							
	Spears, 1/2-in diam. at base:							
566	From raw	4 spears		60	94	10	1	Trace
567	From frozen	4 spears		60	92	15	2	Trace
568	Canned, spears, 1/2-in diam. at base.	4 spears		80	93	15	2	Trace
	Beans:							
	Snap:							
	Green:							
	Cooked, drained:							
571	From raw (cuts and French style).	1 cup		125	92	30	2	Trace
	From frozen:							
572	Cuts	1 cup		135	92	35	2	Trace
573	French style	1 cup		130	92	35	2	Trace
574	Canned, drained solids (cuts).	1 cup		135	92	30	2	Trace
	Bean sprouts (mung):							
578	Raw	1 cup		105	89	35	4	Trace
579	Cooked, drained	1 cup		125	91	35	4	Trace
	Beets:							
	Canned, drained solids:							
582	Whole beets, small	1 cup		160	89	60	2	Trace
583	Diced or sliced	1 cup		170	89	65	2	Trace

562

Saturated (total)	Unsaturated		Carbohydrate	Calcium	Phosphorus	Iron	Potassium	Vitamin A value	Thiamin	Riboflavin	Niacin	Ascorbic acid
	Oleic	Linoleic										
(G)	(H)	(I)	(J)	(K)	(L)	(M)	(N)	(O)	(P)	(Q)	(R)	(S)
Grams	Grams	Grams	Grams	Milligrams	Milligrams	Milligrams	Milligrams	International units	Milligrams	Milligrams	Milligrams	Milligrams
1.6	1.1	.1	22	42	35	.4	54	Trace	.01	.05	.1	Trace
5.5	3.0	.3	16	65	65	.3	109	80	.02	.10	.1	Trace
1.3	1.4	.6	21	22	24	.3	42	Trace	.01	.03	.1	Trace
—	—	—	25	2	Trace	.1	1	0	0	Trace	Trace	0
—	—	—	28	6	2	.5	1	0	0	0	0	0
—	—	—	23	5	2	.5	2	0	0	Trace	Trace	0
.5	.3	Trace	20	167	155	.5	227	10	.04	.21	.2	1
.4	.2	Trace	25	9	48	.6	142	—	.01	.03	.1	0
0	0	0	17	1	1	.1	11	0	Trace	.01	.1	Trace
—	—	—	14	4	2	.2	18	Trace	Trace	.01	Trace	Trace
—	—	—	13	4	1	.3	14	Trace	Trace	.01	Trace	1
—	—	—	10	3	1	.2	11	Trace	Trace	Trace	Trace	1
.5	.3	Trace	24	6	35	.6	106	Trace	.01	.03	.2	0
—	—	—	13	33	9	.9	183	—	.01	.01	Trace	—
—	—	—	11	137	17	3.2	585	—	.02	.04	.4	—
—	—	—	14	35	5	2.6	—	—	—	.02	Trace	—
0	0	0	15	9	3	.8	1	0	0	0	0	0
0	0	0	212	187	42	7.5	757	0	.02	.07	.4	0
0	0	0	199	0	0	.2	6	0	0	0	0	0
0	0	0	12	0	0	Trace	Trace	0	0	0	0	0
0	0	0	6	0	0	Trace	Trace	0	0	0	0	0
0	0	0	100	0	0	.1	3	0	0	0	0	0
—	—	—	2	13	30	.4	110	540	.10	.11	.8	16
—	—	—	2	13	40	.7	143	470	.10	.08	.7	16
—	—	—	3	15	42	1.5	133	640	.05	.08	.6	12
—	—	—	7	63	46	.8	189	680	.09	.11	.6	15
—	—	—	8	54	43	.9	205	780	.09	.12	.5	7
—	—	—	8	49	39	1.2	177	690	.08	.10	.4	9
—	—	—	7	61	34	2.0	128	630	.04	.07	.4	5
—	—	—	7	20	67	1.4	234	20	.14	.14	.8	20
—	—	—	7	21	60	1.1	195	30	.11	.13	.9	8
—	—	—	14	30	29	1.1	267	30	.02	.05	.2	5
—	—	—	15	32	31	1.2	284	30	.02	.05	.2	5

Item No.	Foods, approximate measures, units, and weight (edible part unless footnotes indicate otherwise)		Water	Food energy	Protein	Fat
(A)	(B)		(C)	(D)	(E)	(F)
		Grams	Percent	Calories	Grams	Grams
	Broccoli, cooked, drained:					
	From raw:					
587	Stalk, medium size------------ 1 stalk-------------------	180	91	45	6	1
588	Stalks cut into 1/2-in pieces- 1 cup--------------------	155	91	40	5	Trace
	From frozen:					
589	Stalk, 4 1/2 to 5 in long----- 1 stalk------------------	30	91	10	1	Trace
590	Chopped---------------------- 1 cup-------------------	185	92	50	5	1
	Cabbage:					
	Common varieties:					
	Raw:					
593	Coarsely shredded or sliced- 1 cup--------------------	70	92	15	1	Trace
594	Finely shredded or chopped-- 1 cup--------------------	90	92	20	1	Trace
595	Cooked, drained-------------- 1 cup--------------------	145	94	30	2	Trace
	Carrots:					
	Raw, without crowns and tips, scraped:					
600	Whole, 7 1/2 by 1 1/8 in, or 1 carrot or 18 strips---- strips, 2 1/2 to 3 in long.	72	88	30	1	Trace
601	Grated----------------------- 1 cup--------------------	110	88	45	1	Trace
602	Cooked (crosswise cuts), drained 1 cup--------------------	155	91	50	1	Trace
	Canned:					
603	Sliced, drained solids-------- 1 cup--------------------	155	91	45	1	Trace
604	Strained or junior (baby food) 1 oz (1 3/4 to 2 tbsp)---	28	92	10	Trace	Trace
	Cauliflower:					
605	Raw, chopped-------------------- 1 cup--------------------	115	91	31	3	Trace
	Cooked, drained:					
606	From raw (flower buds)-------- 1 cup--------------------	125	93	30	3	Trace
607	From frozen (flowerets)------- 1 cup--------------------	180	94	30	3	Trace
	Celery, Pascal type, raw:					
608	Stalk, large outer, 8 by 1 1/2 1 stalk------------------ in, at root end.	40	94	5	Trace	Trace
609	Pieces, diced------------------ 1 cup--------------------	120	94	20	1	Trace
	Collards, cooked, drained:					
610	From raw (leaves without stems)- 1 cup--------------------	190	90	65	7	1
611	From frozen (chopped)---------- 1 cup--------------------	170	90	50	5	1
	Corn, sweet:					
	Cooked, drained:					
612	From raw, ear 5 by 1 3/4 in--- 1 ear[61]-------------------	140	74	70	2	1
	From frozen:					
613	Ear, 5 in long-------------- 1 ear[61]-------------------	229	73	120	4	1
614	Kernels--------------------- 1 cup--------------------	165	77	130	5	1
	Canned:					
615	Cream style------------------- 1 cup--------------------	256	76	210	5	2
	Whole kernel:					
616	Vacuum pack----------------- 1 cup--------------------	210	76	175	5	1
	Cucumber slices, 1/8 in thick (large, 2 1/8-in diam.; small, 1 3/4-in diam.):					
619	Without peel------------------- 6 1/2 large or 9 small pieces.	28	96	5	Trace	Trace
	Lettuce, raw:					
	Butterhead, as Boston types:					
624	Head, 5-in diam--------------- 1 head[63]----------------	220	95	25	2	Trace
625	Leaves----------------------- 1 outer or 2 inner or 3 heart leaves.	15	95	Trace	Trace	Trace

[61]Weight includes cob. Without cob, weight is 77 g for item 612, 126 g for item 613.
[62]Based on yellow varieties. For white varieties, value is trace.
[63]Weight includes refuse of outer leaves and core. Without these parts, weight is 163 g.

Fatty Acids												
Satu-rated *(total)*	Unsaturated		Carbo-hydrate	Calcium	Phos-phorus	Iron	Potas-sium	Vitamin A value	Thiamin	Ribo-flavin	Niacin	Ascorbic acid
	Oleic	Lino-leic										
(G)	(H)	(I)	(J)	(K)	(L)	(M)	(N)	(O)	(P)	(Q)	(R)	(S)
Grams	Grams	Grams	Grams	Milli-grams	Milli-grams	Milli-grams	Milli-grams	Inter-national units	Milli-grams	Milli-grams	Milli-grams	Milli-grams
—	—	—	8	158	112	1.4	481	4,500	.16	.36	1.4	162
—	—	—	7	136	96	1.2	414	3,880	.14	.31	1.2	140
—	—	—	1	12	17	.2	66	570	.02	.03	.2	22
—	—	—	9	100	104	1.3	392	4,810	.11	.22	.9	105
—	—	—	4	34	20	0.3	163	90	0.04	0.04	0.02	33
—	—	—	5	44	26	.4	210	120	.05	.05	.3	42
—	—	—	6	64	29	.4	236	190	.06	.06	.4	48
—	—	—	7	27	26	.5	246	7,930	.04	.04	.4	6
—	—	—	11	41	40	.8	375	12,100	.07	.06	.7	9
—	—	—	11	51	48	.9	344	16,280	.08	.08	.8	9
—	—	—	10	47	34	1.1	186	23,250	.03	.05	.6	3
—	—	—	2	7	6	.1	51	3,690	.01	.01	.1	1
—	—	—	6	29	64	1.3	339	70	.13	.12	.8	90
—	—	—	5	26	53	.9	258	80	.11	.10	.8	69
—	—	—	6	31	68	.9	373	50	.07	.09	.7	74
—	—	—	2	16	11	.1	136	110	.01	.01	.1	4
—	—	—	5	47	34	.4	409	320	.04	.04	.4	11
—	—	—	10	357	99	1.5	498	14,820	.21	.38	2.3	144
—	—	—	10	299	87	1.7	401	11,560	.10	.24	1.0	56
—	—	—	16	2	69	.5	151	[62]310	.09	.08	1.1	7
—	—	—	27	4	121	1.0	291	[62]440	.18	.10	2.1	9
—	—	—	31	5	120	1.3	304	[62]580	.15	.10	2.5	8
—	—	—	51	8	143	1.5	248	[62]840	.08	.13	2.6	13
—	—	—	43	6	153	1.1	204	[62]740	.06	.13	2.3	11
—	—	—	1	5	5	0.1	45	Trace	0.01	0.01	0.1	3
—	—	—	4	57	42	3.3	430	1,580	.10	.10	.5	13
—	—	—	Trace	5	4	.3	40	150	.01	.01	Trace	1

Item No.	Foods, approximate measures, units, and weight (edible part unless footnotes indicate otherwise)		Water	Food energy	Pro-tein	Fat
(A)	(B)		(C)	(D)	(E)	(F)
		Grams	Per-cent	Cal-ories	Grams	Grams
	Crisphead, as Iceberg:					
626	Head, 6-in diam--------------- 1 head[64]----------------	567	96	70	5	1
627	Wedge, 1/4 of head------------ 1 wedge-----------------	135	96	20	1	Trace
628	Pieces, chopped or shredded--- 1 cup-------------------	55	96	5	Trace	Trace
629	Looseleaf (bunching varieties including romaine or cos), chopped or shredded pieces. 1 cup-------------------	55	94	10	1	Trace
630	Mushrooms, raw, sliced or chopped- 1 cup------------------- Onions: Mature: Raw:	70	90	20	2	Trace
633	Chopped--------------------- 1 cup-------------------	170	89	65	3	Trace
637	Parsley, raw, chopped------------- 1 tbsp------------------	4	85	Trace	Trace	Trace
638	Parsnips, cooked (diced or 2-in lengths). 1 cup------------------- Peas, green: Canned:	155	82	100	2	1
639	Whole, drained solids--------- 1 cup-------------------	170	77	150	8	1
640	Strained (baby food)---------- 1 oz (1 3/4 to 2 tbsp)--	28	86	15	1	Trace
641	Frozen, cooked, drained------- 1 cup------------------- Peppers, sweet (about 5 per lb, whole), stem and seeds removed:	160	82	110	8	Trace
643	Raw-------------------------- 1 pod-------------------	74	93	15	1	Trace
644	Cooked, boiled, drained------- 1 pod------------------- Potatoes, cooked:	73	95	15	1	Trace
545	Baked, peeled after baking (about 1 potato---------------- 2 per lb, raw). Boiled (about 3 per lb, raw):	156	75	145	4	Trace
646	Peeled after boiling---------- 1 potato----------------	137	80	105	3	Trace
647	Peeled before boiling--------- 1 potato---------------- French-fried, strip, 2 to 3 1/2 in long:	135	83	90	3	Trace
648	Prepared from raw------------- 10 strips---------------	50	45	135	2	7
649	Frozen, oven heated----------- 10 strips---------------	50	53	110	2	4
650	Hashed brown, prepared from frozen. 1 cup------------------- Mashed, prepared from— Raw:	155	56	345	3	18
651	Milk added------------------ 1 cup-------------------	210	83	135	4	2
652	Milk and butter added------- 1 cup-------------------	210	80	195	4	9
653	Dehydrated flakes (without milk), water, milk, butter, and salt added. 1 cup-------------------	210	79	195	4	7
654	Potato chips, 1 3/4 by 2 1/2 in oval cross section. 10 chips----------------	20	2	115	1	8
657	Radishes, raw (prepackaged) stem ends, rootlets cut off. 4 radishes--------------	18	95	5	Trace	Trace
658	Sauerkraut, canned, solids and liquid. 1 cup------------------- Southern peas. See Blackeye peas (items 585-586). Spinach:	235	93	40	2	Trace
659	Raw, chopped-------------------- 1 cup------------------- Cooked, drained:	55	91	15	2	Trace
660	From raw--------------------- 1 cup------------------- From frozen:	180	92	40	5	1
661	Chopped--------------------- 1 cup-------------------	205	92	45	6	1

[64]Weight includes core. Without core, weight is 539 g.
[65]Value based on white-fleshed varieties. For yellow-fleshed varieties, value in International Units (I.U.) is 70 for item 633, 50 for item 634, and 80 for item 635.

Fatty Acids												
Satu-rated (total)	Unsaturated		Carbo-hydrate	Calcium	Phos-phorus	Iron	Potas-sium	Vitamin A value	Thiamin	Ribo-flavin	Niacin	Ascorbic acid
	Oleic	Lino-leic										
(G)	(H)	(I)	(J)	(K)	(L)	(M)	(N)	(O)	(P)	(Q)	(R)	(S)
Grams	Grams	Grams	Grams	Milli-grams	Milli-grams	Milli-grams	Milli-grams	Inter-national units	Milli-grams	Milli-grams	Milli-grams	Milli-grams
—	—	—	16	108	118	2.7	943	1,780	.32	.32	1.6	32
—	—	—	4	27	30	.7	236	450	.08	.08	.4	8
— —	—	—	2	11	12	.3	96	180	.03	.03	.2	3
—	—	—	2	37	14	.8	145	1.050	.03	.04	.2	10
—	—	—	3	4	81	.6	290	Trace	.07	.32	2.9	2
—	—	—	15	46	61	.9	267	[65]Trace	.05	.07	.3	17
—	—	—	Trace	7	2	.2	25	300	Trace	.01	Trace	6
—	—	—	23	70	96	.9	587	50	.11	.12	.2	16
—	—	—	29	44	129	3.2	163	1,170	.15	.10	1.4	14
—	—	—	3	3	18	.3	28	140	.02	.03	.3	3
—	—	—	19	30	138	3.0	216	960	.43	.14	2.7	21
—	—	—	4	7	16	.5	157	310	.06	.06	.4	94
—	—	—	3	7	12	.4	109	310	.05	.05	.4	70
—	—	—	33	14	101	1.1	782	Trace	.15	.07	2.7	31
—	—	—	23	10	72	.8	556	Trace	.12	.05	2.0	22
—	—	—	20	8	57	.7	385	Trace	.12	.05	1.6	22
1.7	1.2	3.3	18	8	56	.7	427	Trace	.07	.04	1.6	11
1.1	.8	2.1	17	5	43	.9	326	Trace	.07	.01	1.3	11
4.6	3.2	9.0	45	28	78	1.9	439	Trace	.11	.03	1.6	12
.7	.4	Trace	27	50	103	.8	548	40	.17	.11	2.1	21
5.6	2.3	0.2	26	50	101	0.8	525	360	0.17	0.11	2.1	19
3.6	2.1	.2	30	65	99	.6	601	270	.08	.08	1.9	11
2.1	1.4	4.0	10	8	28	.4	226	Trace	.04	.01	1.0	3
—	—	—	1	5	6	.2	58	Trace	.01	.01	.1	5
—	—	—	9	85	42	1.2	329	120	.07	.09	.5	33
—	—	—	2	51	28	1.7	259	4,460	.06	.11	.3	28
—	—	—	6	167	68	4.0	583	14,580	.13	.25	.9	50
—	—	—	8	232	90	4.3	683	16,200	.14	.31	.8	39

Item No.	Foods, approximate measures, units, and weight (edible part unless footnotes indicate otherwise)			Water	Food energy	Protein	Fat
(A)	(B)			(C)	(D)	(E)	(F)
			Grams	Percent	Calories	Grams	Grams
	Squash, cooked:						
664	Summer (all varieties), diced, drained.	1 cup--------------------	210	96	30	2	Trace
665	Winter (all varieties), baked, mashed.	1 cup--------------------	205	81	130	4	1
	Sweetpotatoes:						
	Cooked (raw, 5 by 2 in; about 2 1/2 per lb):						
666	Baked in skin, peeled---------	1 potato----------------	114	64	160	2	1
	Canned:						
669	Solid pack (mashed)-----------	1 cup--------------------	255	72	275	5	1
670	Vacuum pack, piece 2 3/4 by 1 in.	1 piece-----------------	40	72	45	1	Trace
	Tomatoes:						
671	Raw, 2 3/5-in diam. (3 per 12 oz pkg.).	1 tomato[66]------------	135	94	25	1	Trace
672	Canned, solids and liquid------	1 cup--------------------	241	94	50	2	Trace
673	Tomato catsup--------------------	1 cup--------------------	273	69	290	5	1
674		1 tbsp------------------	15	69	15	Trace	Trace
	Tomato juice, canned:						
675	Cup----------------------------	1 cup--------------------	243	94	45	2	Trace
676	Glass (6 fl oz)---------------	1 glass-----------------	182	94	35	2	Trace
677	Turnips, cooked, diced-----------	1 cup--------------------	155	94	35	1	Trace
680	Vegetables, mixed, frozen, cooked-	1 cup--------------------	182	83	115	6	1

MISCELLANEOUS ITEMS

Item No.	Foods			Water	Food energy	Protein	Fat
699	Gelatin dessert prepared with gelatin dessert powder and water.	1 cup---------------------	240	84	140	4	0
	Olives, pickled, canned:						
701	Green--------------------------	4 medium or 3 extra large or 2 giant.[69]	16	78	15	Trace	2
702	Ripe, Mission------------------	3 small or 2 large[69]-------	10	73	15	Trace	2
	Pickles, cucumber:						
703	Dill, medium, whole, 3 3/4 in long, 1 1/4-in diam.	1 pickle------------------	65	93	5	Trace	Trace
704	Fresh-pack, slices 1 1/2-in diam., 1/4 in thick.	2 slices------------------	15	79	10	Trace	Trace
705	Sweet, gherkin, small, whole, about 2 1/2 in long, 3/4-in diam.	1 pickle------------------	15	61	20	Trace	Trace
	Soups:						
	Canned, condensed:						
	Prepared with equal volume of milk:						
708	Cream of chicken-------------	1 cup---------------------	245	85	180	7	10
709	Cream of mushroom-----------	1 cup---------------------	245	83	215	7	14
710	Tomato----------------------	1 cup---------------------	250	84	175	7	7
	Prepared with equal volume of water:						
711	Bean with pork---------------	1 cup---------------------	250	84	170	8	6
712	Beef broth, bouillon, consomme.	1 cup---------------------	240	96	30	5	0
713	Beef noodle-------------------	1 cup---------------------	240	93	65	4	3
714	Clam chowder, Manhattan type (with tomatoes, without milk).	1 cup---------------------	245	92	80	2	3

[66]Weight includes cores and stem ends. Without these parts, weight is 123 g.
[67]Based on year-round average. For tomatoes marketed from November through May, value is about 12 mg; from June through October, 32 mg.
[68]Applies to product without calcium salts added. Value for products with calcium salts added may be as much as 63 mg for whole tomatoes, 241 mg for cut forms.
[69]Weight includes pits. Without pits, weight is 13 g for item 701, 9 g for item 702.

Fatty Acids												
Satu-rated (total)	Unsaturated Oleic	Unsaturated Lino-leic	Carbo-hydrate	Calcium	Phos-phorus	Iron	Potas-sium	Vitamin A value	Thiamin	Ribo-flavin	Niacin	Ascorbic acid
(G)	(H)	(I)	(J)	(K)	(L)	(M)	(N)	(O)	(P)	(Q)	(R)	(S)
Grams	Grams	Grams	Grams	Milli-grams	Milli-grams	Milli-grams	Milli-grams	Inter-national units	Milli-grams	Milli-grams	Milli-grams	Milli-grams
—	—	—	7	53	53	.8	296	820	.11	.17	1.7	21
—	—	—	32	57	98	1.6	945	8,610	.10	.27	1.4	27
—	—	—	37	46	66	1.0	342	9,230	.10	.08	.8	25
—	—	—	63	64	105	2.0	510	19,890	.13	.10	1.5	36
—	—	—	10	10	16	.3	80	3,120	.02	.02	.2	6
—	—	—	6	16	33	.6	300	1,110	.07	.05	.9	[6][7]28
—	—	—	10	[6][8]14	46	1.2	523	2,170	.12	.07	1.7	41
—	—	—	69	60	137	2.2	991	3,820	.25	.19	4.4	41
—	—	—	4	3	8	.1	54	210	.01	.01	.2	2
—	—	—	10	17	44	2.2	552	1,940	.12	.07	1.9	39
—	—	—	8	13	33	1.6	413	1,460	.09	.05	1.5	29
—	—	—	8	54	37	.6	291	Trace	.06	.08	.5	34
—	—	—	24	46	115	2.4	348	9,010	.22	.13	2.0	15
0	0	0	34	—	—	—	—	—	—	—	—	—
.2	1.2	.1	Trace	8	2	.2	7	40	—	—	—	—
.2	1.2	.1	Trace	9	1	.1	2	10	Trace	Trace	—	—
—	—	—	1	17	14	.7	130	70	Trace	.01	Trace	4
—	—	—	3	5	4	.3	—	20	Trace	Trace	Trace	1
—	—	—	5	2	2	.2	—	10	Trace	Trace	Trace	1
4.2	3.6	1.3	15	172	152	0.5	260	610	0.05	0.27	0,7	2
5.4	2.9	4.6	16	191	169	.5	279	250	.05	.34	,7	1
3.4	1.7	1.0	23	168	155	.8	418	1,200	.10	.25	1,3	15
1.2	1.8	2.4	22	63	128	2.3	395	650	.13	.08	1.0	3
0	0	0	3	Trace	31	.5	130	Trace	Trace	.02	1.2	—
.6	.7	.8	7	7	48	1.0	77	50	.05	.07	1.0	Trace
.5	.4	1.3	12	34	47	1.0	184	880	.02	.02	1.0	—

Item No.	Foods, approximate measures, units, and weight (edible part unless footnotes indicate otherwise)		Water	Food energy	Pro-tein	Fat
(A)	(B)		(C)	(D)	(E)	(F)
		Grams	Per-cent	Cal-ories	Grams	Grams
	Soups:					
	Canned, condensed:					
	Prepared with equal volume of water:					
718	Split pea-------------------- 1 cup--------------------	245	85	145	9	3
719	Tomato----------------------- 1 cup--------------------	245	91	90	2	3
720	Vegetable beef--------------- 1 cup--------------------	245	92	80	5	2
721	Vegetarian------------------- 1 cup--------------------	245	92	80	2	2
	Dehydrated:					
	Prepared with water:					
724	Chicken noodle------------ 1 cup--------------------	240	95	55	2	1
725	Onion--------------------- 1 cup--------------------	240	96	35	1	1
726	Tomato vegetable with noodles. 1 cup--------------------	240	93	65	1	1

[70]Value may vary from 6 to 60 mg.

Fatty Acids												
Satu-rated (total)	Unsaturated		Carbo-hydrate	Calcium	Phos-phorus	Iron	Potas-sium	Vitamin A value	Thiamin	Ribo-flavin	Niacin	Ascorbic acid
	Oleic	Lino-leic										
(G)	(H)	(I)	(J)	(K)	(L)	(M)	(N)	(O)	(P)	(Q)	(R)	(S)
Grams	Grams	Grams	Grams	Milli-grams	Milli-grams	Milli-grams	Milli-grams	Inter-national units	Milli-grams	Milli-grams	Milli-grams	Milli-grams
1.1	1.2	.4	21	29	149	1.5	270	440	.25	.15	1.5	1
.5	.5	1.0	16	15	34	.7	230	1,000	.05	.05	1.2	12
—	—	—	10	12	49	.7	162	2,700	.05	.05	1.0	—
—	—	—	13	20	39	1.0	172	2,940	.05	.05	1.0	—
—	—	—	8	7	19	.2	19	50	.07	.05	.5	Trace
—	—	—	6	10	12	.2	58	Trace	Trace	Trace	Trace	2
—	—	—	12	7	19	.2	29	480	.05	.02	.5	5

Food and Nutrition Board, National Academy of Sciences-National Research Council Recommended Daily Dietary Allowances[a] Revised 1979

	AGE (YEARS)	WEIGHT (KG)	WEIGHT (LBS)	HEIGHT (CM)	HEIGHT (IN)	PROTEIN (G)	FAT-SOLUBLE VITAMINS VITAMIN A (µG R.E.)[b]	VITAMIN D (µG)[c]	VITAMIN E (MG α T.E.)[d]	VITAMIN C (MG)	WATER-SOLUBLE VITAMINS THIAMIN (MG)	RIBOFLAVIN (MG)	NIACIN (MG N.E.)[e]	VITAMIN B$_6$ (MG)	FOLACIN[f] (µG)	VITAMIN B$_{12}$ (µG)
Infants	0.0-0.5	6	13	60	24	kg×2.2	420	10	3	35	0.3	0.4	6	0.3	30	0.5[g]
	0.5-1.0	9	20	71	28	kg×2.0	400	10	4	35	0.5	0.6	8	0.6	45	1.5
Children	1-3	13	29	90	35	23	400	10	5	45	0.7	0.8	9	0.9	100	2.0
	4-6	20	44	112	44	30	500	10	6	45	0.9	1.0	11	1.3	200	2.5
	7-10	28	62	132	52	34	700	10	7	45	1.2	1.4	16	1.6	300	3.0
Males	11-14	45	99	157	62	45	1000	10	8	50	1.4	1.6	18	1.8	400	3.0
	15-18	66	145	176	69	56	1000	10	10	60	1.4	1.7	18	2.0	400	3.0
	19-22	70	154	177	70	56	1000	7.5	10	60	1.5	1.7	19	2.2	400	3.0
	23-50	70	154	178	70	56	1000	5	10	60	1.4	1.6	18	2.2	400	3.0
	51+	70	154	178	70	56	1000	5	10	60	1.2	1.4	16	2.2	400	3.0
Females	11-14	46	101	157	62	46	800	10	8	50	1.1	1.3	15	1.8	400	3.0
	15-18	55	120	163	64	46	800	10	8	60	1.1	1.3	14	2.0	400	3.0
	19-22	55	120	163	64	44	800	7.5	8	60	1.1	1.3	14	2.0	400	3.0
	23-50	55	120	163	64	44	800	5	8	60	1.0	1.2	13	2.0	400	3.0
	51+	55	120	163	64	44	800	5	8	60	1.0	1.2	13	2.0	400	3.0
Pregnant						+30	+200	+5	+2	+20	+0.4	+0.3	+2	+0.6	+400	+1.0
Lactating						+20	+400	+5	+3	+40	+0.5	+0.5	+5	+0.5	+100	+1.0

MINERALS

CALCIUM (MG)	PHOS-PHORUS (MG)	MAG-NESIUM (MG)	IRON (MG)	ZINC (MG)	IODINE (μG)
360	240	50	10	3	40
540	360	70	15	5	50
800	800	150	15	10	70
800	800	200	10	10	90
800	800	250	10	10	120
1200	1200	350	18	15	150
1200	1200	400	18	15	150
800	800	350	10	15	150
800	800	350	10	15	150
800	800	350	10	15	150
1200	1200	300	18	15	150
1200	1200	300	18	15	150
800	800	300	18	15	150
800	800	300	18	15	150
800	800	300	10	15	150
+400	+400	+150	h	+5	+25
+400	+400	+150	h	+10	+50

Source: Recommended Dietary Allowances, Ninth Edition (revised 1979). National Academy of Sciences, Washington, D.C.

a The allowances are intended to provide for individual variations among most normal persons as they live in the United States under usual environmental stresses. Diets should be based on a variety of common foods in order to provide other nutrients for which human requirements have been less well defined.

b Retinal equivalents. 1 Retinol equivalent = 1 μg retinol or 6 μg carotene.

c As cholecalciferol. 10 μg cholecalcifoerol = 400 I.U. vitamin D.

d α tocopherol equivalents.

e 1 NE (niacin equivalent) is equal to 1 μg of niacin or 60 μg of dietary tryptophan.

f The folacin allowances refer to dietary sources as determined by *lactobacillus casei* assay after treatment with enzymes ("conjugases") to make polyglutamyl forms of the vitamin available to the test organism.

g The RDA for vitamin B_{12} in infants is based on average concentration of the vitamin in human milk. The allowances after weaning are based on energy intake (as recommended by the American Academy of Pediatrics) and consideration of other factors such as intestinal absorption; see text.

h The increased requirement during pregnancy cannot be met by the iron stores of many women; therefore the use of 30–60 mg of supplemental iron is recommended. Iron needs during lactation are not substantially different from those of nonpregnant women, but continued supplementation of the mother for 2–3 months after parturition is advisable in order to replenish stores depleted by pregnancy.

Estimated Safe and Adequate Daily Dietary Intakes of Additional Selected Vitamins and Minerals[a]

| | | VITAMINS | | | | |
	AGE (YEARS)	VITAMIN K (μG)	BLOTIN (μG)	PANTO-THENIC ACID (MG)	COPPER (MG)	MANGANESE (MG)
Infants	0–0.5	12	35	2	0.5–0.7	0.5–0.7
	0.5–1	10–20	50	3	0.7–1.0	0.7–1.0
Children	1–3	15–30	65	3	1.0–1.5	1.0–1.5
and	4–6	20–40	85	3–4	1.5–2.0	1.5–2.0
Adolescents	7–10	30–60	120	4–5	2.0–2.5	2.0–3.0
	11+	50–100	100–200	4–7	2.0–3.0	2.5–5.0
Adults		70–140	100–200	4–7	2.0–3.0	2.5–5.0

Source: Recommended Dietary Allowances, Ninth edition (revised 1979). National Academy of Sciences, Washington, D.C.

Because there is less information on which to base allowances, these figures are not given in the main table of the RDA and are provided here in the form of ranges of recommended intakes.

Since the toxic levels for many trace elements may be only several times usual intakes, the upper levels for the trace elements given in this table should not be habitually exceeded.

TRACE ELEMENTS[b]				ELECTROLYTES		
FLUORIDE (MG)	CHROMIUM (MG)	SELENIUM (MG)	MOLYBDENUM (MG)	SODIUM (MG)	POTASSIUM (MG)	CHLORIDE (MG)
0.1–0.5	0.01–0.04	0.01–0.04	0.03–0.06	115–350	350–925	275–700
0.2–1.0	0.02–0.06	0.02–0.06	0.04–0.08	250–750	425–1275	400–1200
0.5–1.5	0.02–0.08	0.02–0.08	0.05–0.1	325–975	550–1650	500–1500
1.0–2.5	0.03–0.12	0.03–0.12	0.06–0.15	450–1350	775–2325	700–2100
1.5–2.5	0.05–0.2	0.05–0.2	0.1 –0.3	600–1800	1000–3000	925–2775
1.5–2.5	0.05–0.2	0.05–0.2	0.15–0.5	900–2700	1525–4575	1400–4200
1.5–4.0	0.05–0.2	0.05–0.2	0.15–0.5	1100–3300	1875–5625	1700–5100

575

Mean Heights and Weights and Recommended Energy Intake

Category	Age (years)	Weight (kg)	Weight (lb)	Height (cm)	Height (in)	Energy Needs (with range) (kcal)	Energy Needs (with range) (MJ)
Infants	0.0–0.5	6	13	60	24	kg × 115 (95–145)	kg × .48
	0.5–1.0	9	20	71	28	kg × 105 (80–135)	kg × .44
Children	1–3	13	29	90	35	1300 (900 –1800)	5.5
	4–6	20	44	112	44	1700 (1300–2300)	7.1
	7–10	28	62	132	52	2400 (1650–3300)	10.1
Males	11–14	45	99	157	62	2700 (2000–3700)	11.3
	15–18	66	145	176	69	2800 (2100–3900)	11.8
	19–22	70	154	177	70	2900 (2500–3300)	12.2
	23–50	70	154	178	70	2700 (2300–3100)	11.3
	51–75	70	154	178	70	2400 (2000–2800)	10.1
	76+	70	154	178	70	2050 (1650–2450)	8.6
Females	11–14	46	101	157	62	2200 (1500–3000)	9.2
	15–18	55	120	163	64	2100 (1200–3000)	8.8
	19–22	55	120	163	64	2100 (1700–2500)	8.8
	23–50	55	120	163	64	2000 (1600–2400)	8.4
	51–75	55	120	163	64	1800 (1400–2200)	7.6
	76+	55	120	163	64	1600 (1200–2000)	6.7
Pregnancy						+300	
Lactation						+500	

Source: Recommended Dietary Allowances, Ninth edition (revised 1979). National Academy of Sciences, Washington, D.C.

The data in this table have been assembled from the observed median heights and weights of children shown in Table 1, together with desirable weights for adults given in Table 2 for the mean heights of men (70 inches) and women (64 inches) between the ages of 18 and 34 years as surveyed in the U.S. population (HEW/ NCHS data).

The energy allowances for the young adults are for men and women doing light work. The allowances for the two older age groups represent mean energy needs over these age spans, allowing for a 2% decrease in basal (resting) metabolic rate per decade and a reduction in activity of 200 kcal/day for men and women between 51 and 75 years, 500 kcal for men over 75 years and 400 kcal for women over 75 (see text). The customary range of daily energy output is shown for adults in parentheses, and is based on a variation in energy needs of ± 400 kcal at any one age (see text and Garrow, 1978), emphasizing the wide range of energy intakes appropriate for any group of people.

Energy allowances for children through age 18 are based on median energy intakes of children these ages followed in longitudinal growth studies. The values in parentheses are 10th and 90th percentiles of energy intake, to indicate the range of energy consumption among children of these ages (see text).

RELIABLE NUTRITION INFORMATION SOURCES

Nutrition is a very popular topic. You will find many nutrition books on the shelves in bookstores, health food stores, and even supermarkets. You will also see articles in magazines and newspapers. Some of these materials present reliable information; some, while seeming to be very believable, may contain inaccurate or misleading information. One of your goals in studying nutrition should be to equip yourself with a basic understanding of nutrition principles to enable you to evaluate the nutrition information that you read and hear. Some questions you might ask about the author or source of the information can be found in the last chapter of this book.

The following books are suggested for additional reading on general nutrition topics. Suggestions for supplementary reading on specific subjects can be found under headings for each section of this book.

Bogert, L. H., George Briggs and Doris Calloway, *Nutrition and Physical Fitness*, tenth edition, Philadelphia, PA: W.B. Saunders Co., 1978.

Clydesdale, F.J. and F. J. Francis, *Food, Nutrition and You*, Englewood Cliffs, NJ: Prentice-Hall, Inc., 1977.

Deutsch, Ronald M., *Realities of Nutrition*, Palo Alto, CA: Ball Publishing Co., 1976.

Guthrie, Helen A., *Introductory Nutrition*, fourth edition, St. Louis, MO: The C.V. Mosby Co., 1978.

Guthrie, Helen A., *Programmed Nutrition*, second edition, St. Louis, MO: The C.V. Mosby Co., 1978.

Labuza, T.P. and H. Elizabeth Sloan, *Food for Thought*, Westport, CT: AVI Publishing Co., 1977.

Labuza, T.P., *Food and Your Well-Being*, St. Paul, MN: West Publishing Co., 1977.

Martin, Ethel A., *Nutrition in Action*, fourth edition, New York: Holt, Rinehardt and Winston, 1978.

Mayer, Jean, *A Diet for Living*, New York: David McKay Co., Inc., 1975.

McNutt, Kristen W. and David R. NcNutt, *Nutrition and Food Choices*, Chicago, IL: Science Research Associates, 1978.

Nutrition Reviews' *Present Knowledge in Nutrition*, fourth edition, New York and Washington, D.C.: The Nutrition Foundation, Inc., 1976.

Robinson, C.H., *Fundamentals of Normal Nutrition*, third edition, New York: Macmillan Publishing Co., 1978.

Robinson, C.H. and M. Lawler, *Normal and Therapeutic Nutrition*, 15th edition, New York: Macmillan Publishing Co., 1977.

Stare, Frederick J. and Margaret McWilliams, *Living Nutrition*, second edition, New York: John Wiley and Sons, 1977.

Stare, Frederick J. and Elizabeth M. Whelan, *Eat OK-Feel OK*, North Quincy, MA: The Christopher Publishing Co., 1978.

Whitney, E.N. and E.M.N. Hamilton, *Understanding Nutrition*, St. Paul, MN: West Publishing Co., 1977.

Williams, S.R., *Nutrition and Diet Therapy*, third edition, St. Louis, MO: The C.V. Mosby Co., 1977.

The following references contain charts and tables for information on Recommended Dietary Allowances and nutritive value of foods.

Adams, Catherine F., *Nutritive Value of American Foods in Common Units*, Agriculture Handbook No. 456, Washington, D.C.: U.S. Department of Agriculture, Superintendent of Documents, U.S. Government Printing Office, 1975.

Agricultural Research Service, *Nutritive Value of Foods*, Home and Garden Bulletin No. 72, Washington, D.C.: U.S. Department of Agriculture, Superintendent of Documents, U.S. Government Printing Office, 1977. (Much of this is reproduced as Appendix B.)

Church, C.F. and H.N. Church, *Food Values of Portions Commonly Used*, Philadelphia, PA: J. B. Lippincott Co., 1970.

Food and Nutrition Board, National Research Council, *Recommended Dietary Allowances*, ninth edition, National Academy of Sciences, Washington, D.C.: 1979.

Watt, Bernice K. and Annabel L. Merrill, *Composition of Foods-Raw, Processed, Prepared*, Agriculture Handbook No. 8, Washington, D.C.: U.S. Department of Agriculture, Superintendent of Documents, U.S. Government Printing Office, 1963. (Revision underway.)

The following periodicals provide reliable articles that will update your nutrition knowledge.

American Journal of Clinical Nutrition, Bethesda, MD: American Society for Clinical Nutrition, Inc.

FDA Consumer, Washington, D.C.: Food and Drug Administration, U.S. Government Printing Office.

Journal of the American Dietetic Association, Chicago, IL: American Dietetic Association.

Journal of the American Home Economics Association, Washington, D.C.: American Home Economics Association.

Journal of Nutrition, Bethdsda, MD: American Institute of Nutrition.

Journal of Nutrition Education, Berkeley, CA: Society for Nutrition Education.

Nutrition Reviews, New York, NY: The Nutrition Foundation, Inc.

Nutrition Today, Annapolis, MD: Nutrition Today Society.

Some medical journals which include nutrition information include the *Journal of the American Dental Association, Journal of the American Medical Association, Journal of Pediatrics, Lancet, New England Journal of Medicine,* and *Pediatrics.*

SECTION I   FOODS, NUTRITION, AND CONSUMER CHOICES

Consumer Food Choices

Gift, H.H., M.B. Washbon, G.G. Harrison, *Nutrition, Behavior, and Change,* Englewood Cliffs, N.J.: Prentice-Hall, Inc., 1976.

Hochbaum, Godfrey, "Human Behavior and Nutrition Education," *Nutrition News*, Vol. 40, No. 1, February, 1977.

Kare, M.R. and O. Maller (eds.), *The Chemical Senses and Nutrition,* New York: Academic Press, 1977.

Lowenberg, M.E., E.N. Todhunter, E.D. Wilson, J.R. Savage, J.L. Lubawski, *Food and Man,,* second edition, New York: John Wiley & Sons, Inc., 1974.

Redman, B.J., *Consumer Behavior: Theory and Applications,* Westport, CT: AVI Publishing Co., 1979.

Food and Population

Borgstrom, G., *The Food and People Dilemma*, Belmont, CA: Dixburg Press, Division of Wadsworth Publishing Co., Inc., 1973.

National Research Council, *World Food and Nutrition Study, the Potential Contributions of Research*, Washington, D.C.: National Academy of Sciences, 1977.

University of California Food Task Force, *A Hungry World: The Challenge to Agriculture*, Berkeley, CA: Division of Agricultural Sciences, University of California, July, 1974.

Nutrients and Labeling

Food and Drug Administration, *Nutrition Labeling—Terms You Should Know*, FDA Consumer Memo, DHEW Publication No. (FDA)74-2010, Washington, D.C.: U.S. Government Printing Office, March, 1974.

Hansen, R.G., B. W. Wyse, A. W. Sorenson, *Nutritional Quality Index of Foods*, Westport, CT: AVI Publishing Co., 1979.

Harper, A.E., "Uses and Misuses of Recommended Dietary Allowances," *Contemporary Nutrition*, Vol. 3 No. 7, July, 1978.

National Nutrition Consortium/with Ronald M. Deutsch, *Nutrition Labeling: How It Can Work for You*, Bethesda, MD: National Nutrition Consortium, Inc., 1975.

Pennington, J.A., *Dietary Nutrient Guide*, Westport, CT: AVI Publishing Co., 1976.

Peterkin, B., "The RDA or U.S. RDA?" *Journal of Nutrition Education*, Vol. 9, January-March, 1977, p. 10.

Peterkin, B., J. Nicholas, and C. Cromwell, *Nutrition Labeling: Tools for Its Use*, Agricultural Information Bulletin No. 382, U.S. Department of Agriculture, Washington, D.C.: U.S. Government Printing Office, April, 1975.

SECTION II   ENERGY AND BODY WEIGHT

Bruch, Hilde, "Anorexia Nervosa," *Nutrition Today,*, Vol. 13, No. 5, September-October, 1978.

Bruch, Hilde, *Eating Disorders: Obesity and Anorexia Nervosa,* New York: Basic Books, Inc., 1973.

"Current Concepts of Obesity," *Dairy Council Digest*, Vol 46, No. 4, July-August, 1975.

Deutsch, R. M., *The Fat Counter Guide*, Palo Alto, CA: Bull Publishing Co., 1978.

Ferguson, J. M., *Habit, Not Diets*, Palo Alto, CA: Bull Publishing Co., 1976.

Ferguson, J. M., *Learning to Eat*, Palo Alto, CA: Bull Publishing Co., 1975.

Katch, F.I. and W. D. McArdle, *Nutrition, Weight Control and Exercise*, Boston, MA: Houghton Mifflin Co., 1977.

Konishi, F., *Exercise Equivalents of Foods: A Practical Guide for the Overweight*, Carbondale, IL: Southern Illinois University Press, 1975.

Lucas, Alexander R., "Anorexia Nervosa," *Contemporary Nutrition*, Vol. 3 No. 8, August, 1978.

The Medicine Show, Mount Vernon, NY: Consumers Union, September, 1976.

"Nutrition, Weight Control, and You!" (pamphlet), Manhasset, NY: Weight Watchers International, Inc. 1975.

Osman, J.D. *Thin from Within*, New York: Hart Publishing Co., Inc., 1976.

Spannhake, E. G., *Eye It Before You Diet (A Nutritional Analysis of Nine Popular Diets)*, Washington, D.C.: The Sugar Association, Inc., 1977.

Stuart, R. B., *Act Thin, Stay Thin*, New York: W. W. Norton & Co., Inc., 1978.

Stuart, R.B. and B. Davis, *Slim Chance in a Fat World: Behavioral Control of Obesity*, Champaign, IL: Research Press, 1972.

"What's New in Weight Control?" *Dairy Council Digest*, Vol. 49, No. 2, March-April, 1978.

SECTION III   THE NUTRIENTS AND THE FOODS THAT SUPPLY THEM

The Nutrients

See books suggested for reading on general nutrition topics at the beginning of this section.

Harland, B. and A. Hecht, "Grandma Called It Roughage," *FDA Consumer*, HEW Publication No. (FDA) 78-2087, Washington, D.C.: U.S. Government Printing Office, July-August, 1977.

Institute of Food Technologists, *Dietary Fiber*, A Scientific Status Summary by the Institute of Food Technologists' Expert Panel on Food Safety and Nutrition and the Committee on Public Information, Chicago, IL: January, 1979.

McNutt, Kristen, "Perspective-Fiber," *Journal of Nutrition Education*, Vol. 8, No. 4, October-December, 1976, pp. 3-8.

Southgate D., B. Bailey, E. Collinson, et all, "A Guide to Calculating Intakes of Dietary Fiber," *Journal of Human Nutrition*, Vol 30, 1976, p. 303.

Spiller, G.A., R.J. Amen (eds.), *Fiber in Human Nutrition*, New York: Plenum Press, 1976.

Fiber

Cook, James D., "Food Iron Availability," *Food & Nutrition News*, Vol. 49, No. 3, February, 1978.

Hambridge, K. M., "Trace Elements in Pediatric Nutrition," *Advances in Pediatrics*, Vol. 24, Yearbook, Chicago, IL: Medical Publishers, Inc., 1977.

International Nutritional Anemia Consultive Group, *Guidelines for the Eradication of Iron Deficiency Anemia*, New York and Washington, D.C.: Nutrition Foundation, December, 1977.

Krehl, W.A., "Sodium: A Most Extraordinary Dietary Essential," *Nutrition Today*, Vol 1, December 1966, pp. 16-18.

Linkswiler, H. and M. Zemel, "Calcium to Phosphorus Ratios," *Contemporary Nutrition*, Vol. 4, No. 5, May, 1979.

Mertz, Walter, "Trace Elements," *Contemporary Nutrition*, Vol. 3, No. 2, February, 1978.

Murphy, E. W., B.W. Willis, and B.K. Watt, "Provisional Tables on Zinc Content of Foods," *Journal of the American Dietetic Association*, Vol. 66, 1975, pp. 345-55.

Minerals

Vitamins

Agricultural Research Service, *Pantothenic Acid, Vitamin B₆ and Vitamin B₁₂ in Foods*, Home Economics Research Report No. 36, U.S. Department of Agriculture, Washington, D.C.: U. S. Government Printing Office, 1969.

Food and Nutrition Board, National Research Council, *Folic Acid*, Washington, D.C.: National Academy of Sciences, 1977.

"Functions and Interrelationships of Vitamins," *Dairy Council Digest*, Vol. 43, No. 5, September-October, 1972.

Institute of Food Technologists, *Vitamin E*, A Scientific Status Summary by the Institute of Food Technolosists' Expert Panel on Food Safety and Nutrition and the Committee on Public Information, Chicago, IL: January, 1977.

Perloff, B.P. and R.R. Butrum, "Folacin in Selected Foods," *Journal of the American Dietetic Association*, Vol. 70, February, 1977, p. 161.

"Recent Developments in Vitamin D," *Dairy Council Digest*, Vol. 47, No. 3, May-June, 1976.

Robinson, J.R., "Water, the Indispensable Nutrient," *Nutrition Today*, 5(1970): 16.

"Vitamin E: What's Behind All Those Claims for It?" *Consumer Reports*, Vol. 38, No. 1, January, 1973, pp. 60-66.

Vegetarianism

American Academy of Pediatrics, Committee on Nutrition, "Nutritional Aspects of Vegetarianism, Health Foods, and Fad Diets," *Pediatrics*, Vol. 59, No. 3, March, 1977, pp. 460-64.

Lappe, F.M., *Diet for A Small Planet*, Westminster, MD: Ballantine Books, 1975.

Peng, A., "Plant Proteins and Their Utilization," Columbus, OH: The Ohio State University, Cooperative Extension Service, Bulletin No. 524, 1970.

Register, U.D., and L.M. Sonnenberg, "The Vegetarian Diet," *Journal of the American Dietetic Association*, Vol. 62, No. 3, March, 1973, and reprinted in *The Nutrition Crisis* (T.P. Labusa, Ed.), pp. 257-273.

Smith, E., "A Guide to Good Eating the Vegetarian Way," *Journal of Nutrition Education*, Vol. 7, No. 3, July-September, 1975, pp. 109-11.

Food Choices

"Coffee Creamers," *Consumer Reports*, Vol. 40, No. 3 March, 1975, pp. 196-98.

Graham, D. M. and A. A. Hertzler, "Why Enrich or Fortify Foods?" *Journal of Nutrition Education*, Vol 9, No. 4, October-December, 1977.

Lessons on Meat, Chicago, IL: National Livestock and Meat Board, 1973.

Peterkin, B., "Bargain Hunting: Meat and Meat Alternates," *Family Economics Review*, Fall, 1978, pp. 26-30.

Stillings, B. and M. H. Thompson, *Seafoods for Health*, National Marine Fisheries Service, U.S. Department of Commerce, Washington, D.C.: U.S. Government Printing Office, GPO No. 823-118.

"Which Cereals Are Most Nutritious?" *Consumer Reports*, Vol. 40, No. 2, February, 1975, pp. 76-82.

U.S. Department of Agriculture, Washington, D.C.: U.S. Government Printing Office:

Home and Garden Bulletins—

"Beef and Veal in Family Meals," No. 118, 1967

"Breads, Cakes, and Pies in Family Meals," No. 186, 1971

"Cheese in Family Meals," No. 112, 1977

"Eggs in Family Meals," No. 103, 1967

"Family Fare—A Guide to Good Nutrition," No. 1, 1970

"Food for the Family—A Cost Saving Plan," No. 209, 1976

"Fruits in Family Meals," No. 125, 1968

"Milk in Family Meals," No. 127, 1967

"Pork in Family Meals," No. 160, 1969

"Poultry in Family Meals," No. 110, 1967

"Soybeans in Family Meals," No. 208, 1974

"Vegetables in Family Meals," No. 105, 1968

Yearbooks of Agriculture—

Food for Us All, 1969

Shopper's Guide, 1974

SECTION IV   NUTRITION THROUGHOUT THE LIFE CYCLE

Pregnancy

Committee on Maternal Nutrition, Food and Nutrition Board, National Research Council, *Maternal Nutrition and the Course of Pregnancy*, Washington, D.C.: National Academy of Sciences, 1970.

Jacobson, H. N. "Current Concepts in Nutrition—Diet in Pregnancy," *The New England Journal of Medicine*, Vol. 297, No. 19, November 10, 1977, pp. 1051-53.

Maternal and Child Health Unit, California Department of Health, *Nutrition during Pregnancy and Lactation*, Sacramento, CA: California Department of Health, 1975.

Pitkin, R. M., "Nutrition in Pregnancy," *Dietetic Currents*, Vol. 4, No. 1, January-February, 1977.

Shank, R. E. "A Chink in Our Armor," *Nutrition Today*, Vol. 5, No. 2., Summer, 1970, pp. 2-11.

Winick, M. (Editor), *Nutrition and Fetal Development*, New York: John Wiley & Sons, 1974.

Worthington, B. S., J. Vermeersch and S.R. Williams, *Nutrition in Pregnancy and Lactation*, St. Louis, MO: The C.V. Mosby Co., 1977.

Zackler, J. and W. Brandstadt, (Editors), *The Teenage Pregnant Girl*, Springfield, IL: Charles C. Thomas, 1975.

Infants and Children

Filer, L.J. Jr. (Editor), *Infant Nutrition-A Foundation for Lasting Health,* Part I-"The First Year of Life," and Part II-"Health Consequences," Bloomfield, N.J.: Health Learning Systems, Inc., 1977.

Foman, S. J., *Infant Nutrition,* second edition, Philadelphia, PA: W.B. Saunders Co., 1974.

"Is Breast Feeding Best for Babies?" *Consumer Reports,* Vol. 2, No. 3, March, 1977, pp. 152-57.

McWilliams, M., *Nutrition for the Growing Years,* second edition, New York: John Wiley and Sons, Inc., 1975.

National Center for Health Statistics: *Height and Weight of Children, United States,* Vital and Health Statistics, United States Department of Health, Education, and Welfare Publication No. 1000, Series 11, No. 104.

National Center for Health Statistics, *Growth Charts, 1976,* U.S. Department of Health, Education, and Welfare Monthy Vital Statistics Report (HRA) 76-1120, Vol. 25, No. 3, June 22, 1976

Own, G. and G. Lippmann, "Nutritional Status of Infants and Young Children, USA," *Pediatric Clinics of North America,* Vol. 24, No. 1, February, 1977, pp. 211-27.

Peterkin, B. and S. Walker, "Food for the Baby-Cost and Nutritive Value Considerations," *Family Economics Review,* Fall, 1976, pp. 3-8.

Pipes, P. L. *Nutrition in Infancy and Childhood,* St. Louis, MO: The C.V. Mosby Co., 1977.

Sunderlin, S. (Editor), *Nutrition and Intellectual Growth in Children,* Washington, D.C.: Association for Childhood Education International, 1969.

Wing. J. P., "Human Versus Cow's Milk in Infant Nutrition and Health: Update 1977," *Current Problems in Pediatrics,* Vol. 8, No. 1, November, 1977.

Dental Disease in Children

De Paola, D. P. and M.C. Alfano, "Diet and Oral Health," *Nutrition Today,* Vol. 12, No. 3, May-June, 1977, pp. 6-32.

"Diet and Dental Health," Chicago, IL: American Dental Association, 1975.

Nizel, A., "Preventing Dental Caries—Nutrition Factors," in *The Pediatric Clinics of North America,* Vol. 24, No. 1, Symposium in Nutrition in Pediatrics, February, 1977, Philadelphia, PA: W. B. Saunders Co., 1977.

"Nutrition and Oral Health," *Dairy Council Digest,* Vol. 49, No. 3, May-June, 1978.

Hyperactivity in Children

Feingold, B. F., *Why Your Child is Hyperactive,* New York: Random House, 1975.

Hartley, J. P. and C.G. Mathews, "The Feingold Hypothesis: Current Studies," *Contemporary Nutrition,* Vol. 3, No. 4, April, 1978.

Institute of Food Technologists' Expert Panel on Food Safety and Nutrition and the Committee on Public Information, *Diet and Hyperactivity: Any Connection?* Chicago, IL: Institute of Food Technologists, April, 1976.

Margen, S., "Why Your Child is Hyperactive," *Journal of Nutrition Education*, Vol. 7, No. 2, April-June, 1975, pp. 79-81.

National Advisory Committee on Hyperkinesis and Food Additives, *Report on Hyperkinesis and Food Additives*, New York: The Nutrition Foundation, Inc., 1977.

Obesity in Children

Huenemam R. L., "Environmental Factors Associated with Preschool Obesity, I. Obesity in Six-Month Old Children," *Journal of the American Dietetic Association*, Vol. 64: 480, May, 1974, p. 480.

Huenemann, R.L., "Environmental Factors Associated with Preschool Obesity, II. Obesity and Food Practices of Children at Successive Age Levels," *Journal of the American Dietetic Association*, Vol. 64, May, 1974, p. 488.

Winick, M. (Editor), *Childhood Obesity*, New York: John Wiley & Sons, 1975.

Wolff, J. J. and D. Lipe, *Help for the Overweight Child*, New York: Stein and Day, 1978.

Adolescents

Huenemann, R.L., M.C. Hampton, A.R. Behnke, L.R. Shaprio, B.W. Mitchell, *Teenage Nutrition and Physique*, Springfield, IL: Charles C. Thomas, 1974.

McKigney, J.J. and H.N. Munro (Editors), *Nutrient Requirements in Adolescence*, Cambridge, MA: MIT Press, 1975.

Athletes

Darden, E., *Nutrition and Athletic Performance*, Pasadena, CA: The Athletic Press, 1976.

Food and Nutrition Board, National Research Council, "Water Deprivation and Performance of Athletes," A Statement of the Food and Nutrition Board, Washington, D.C.: National Academy of Science, 1974.

Nutrition for Athletes—A Handbook for Coaches, Washington, D.C.: American Association for Health, Physical Education, and Recreation, 1971.

Smith, N.J., *Food for Sport*, Palo Alto, CA: Bull Publishing Co., 1976.

Williams, M. H., *Nutritional Aspects of Human Physical and Athletic Performance*, Springfield, IL: Charles C. Thomas, 1976.

Elderly

Rockstein, M. and M. L.Sussman, (Editors) *Nutrition, Longevity, and Aging*, New York: Academic Press Inc., 1976.

"A Study of Health Practices and Opinions, Accession No. PB 210-78," Springfield, VA: National Technical Information Service, 1972.

Winick, M., ed., *Nutrition and Aging*, Current Concepts in Nutrition, Vol. 4. New York: John Wiley & Sons, 1976.

Dietary Surveys

Center for Disease Control, U.S. Department of Health, Education, and Welfare, *Ten State Nutrition Survey, 1968-70*, V. Dietary, DHEW Publication No. (HSM) 72-8313, Washington, D.C.: U.S. Government Printing Office, 1972.

National Center for Health Statistics, *Dietary Intake Findings, United States, 1971-74*, Vital and Health Statistics Series 11, No. 202, U.S. Department of Health, Education and Welfare, Publication No. (HRH) 77-1647, Washington, D.C.: U.S. Government Printing Office, 1977.

O'Hanlon, P., and M. B. Kohrs, "Dietary Studies of Older Americans," *American Journal of Clinical Nutrition*, Vol. 31, 1978, p. 1257.

SECTION V CONTEMPORARY ISSUES IN DIET AND HEALTH

Dietary Goals

Hegsted, D.M., "U.S. Dietary Goals"; Leveille, G., "Establishing and Implementing Dietary Goals"; Peterkin, B., "The Dietary Goals and Food on the Table; (all in) *Family Economics Review*, Winter-Spring, 1978, pp. 3-24.

Short, C. J., "Dietary Goals for the United States," *Family Economics Review, Highlights,* Fall, 1978, pp. 30-32.

Coronary Heart Disease and High Blood Presurre

Advisory Panel of the British Committee on Medical Aspects of Food Policy (Nutrition), "Report on Diet in Relation to Cardiovascular and Cerebrovascular Disease," *Nutrition Today*, Vol. 12, No. 1, January-February, 1977, pp. 16-26.

Flynn, A. "The Cholesterol Controversy," *Contemporary Nutrition*, Vol. 3, No. 3, March, 1978.

"Hypertension and Weight Control," *Science News*, Vol. 113, No. 3, January 21, 1978, p. 39.

Irwin, T., *Watch Your Blood Pressure*, Public Affairs Pamphlet No. 483-A, New York: Public Affairs Committee, Inc., May, 1976.

Mann, G. V., "Medical Intelligence: Current Concepts, Diet—Heart: End of an Era," *New England Journal of Medicine*, Vol. 297, 1977, p. 644.

McGill, H. C. and G. E. Mott, "Diet and Coronary Heart Disease," in Nutrition Reviews' *Present Knowledge in Nutrition*, fourth edition, New York, Washington, D.C.: The Nutrition Foundation, Inc., 1976, pp. 376–91.

Diabetes and Hypoglycemia

Arehart-Treichel, J., "The Great Medical Debate over Low Blood Sugar," *Science News*, Vol. 103, March 17, 1973, pp. 172-73.

Malone, J. L., "Newer Aspects of Diabetes," *Advances in Pediatrics*, Vol. 24, Chicago, IL: Year Book Medical Publishers Inc., 1977, pp. 1-32.

Service, J., "Hypoglycemia," *Contemporary Nutrition*, Vol. 2, No. 7, July, 1977.

"Statement on Hypoglycemia," *Journal of the American Medical Association*, Vol. 223, No. 6, February 5, 1973.

Cancer

Barrett, V.K., *Dietary Factors in the Etiology of Cancer*, National Cancer Institute Report No. 18, Bethesda, MD: National Institutes of Health, 1975.

Gori, G. B., "Diet and Cancer," *Journal of the American Dietetic Association*, Vol. 71, October, 1977, pp. 375-78.

"Nutrition, Diet, and Cancer," *Dairy Council Digest*, Vol. 46, No. 5, September-October, 1975.

Whelan, E., *Preventing Cancer*, New York: W. W. Norton and Co., 1978.

Winick, M., (Editor) *Nutrition and Cancer*, Volume 6, Wiley Series on Current Concepts in Nutrition, New York: John Wiley & Sons, 1977.

Alcoholism

"Alcohol: A Heart Disease Preventive?" *Science News*, Vol. 112, August 13, 1977, pp. 102-3.

Halstead, C. H., "Present Knowledge in Nutritional Implications of Alcoholism, in Nutrition Reviews' *Present Knowledge in Nutrition*, fourth edition, New York, Washington, D.C.: The Nutrition Foundation, Inc., 1976, pp. 467-75.

Lieber, C. S., "Alcohol and Nutrition," *Nutrition News*, Vol. 39, No. 3, October, 1976, pp. 9, 12.

Lieber, C. S., "Alcohol-Nutrition Interaction," *Contemporary Nutrition*, Vol. 3, No. 9, September, 1978.

Roe, D. A., *Alcohol and the Diet*, Westport, CT: AVI Publishing Co., 1979.

Shaw, S. and C. S. Lieber, "Nutrition and Alcoholic Liver Disease," *Nutrition in Disease*, March, 1978.

Drugs and Diet

Committee on Nutrition of the Mother and Preschool Child, Food and Nutrition Board, National Research Council, *Oral Contraceptives and Nutrition*, Washington, D.C.: National Academy of Sciences, 1975.

"Diet-Drug Interactions," *Dairy Council Digest*, Vol. 48, No. 2, March-April, 1977.

Frankie, R. and G. Christakis, "Some Nutritional Aspects of 'Hard' Drug Addiction," *Dietetic Currents*, Vol. 2, No. 3, July-August, 1975.

King, J. C., "Nutrition during Oral Contraceptive Treatment," *Contemporary Nutrition*, Vol. 2, No. 1, January, 1976.

Lehmann, P., "Food and Drug Interactions," *FDA Consumer*, March, 1978.

Roe, D. A., "Drugs, Diet and Nutrition," *Contemporary Nutrition*, Vol. 3, No. 6, June, 1978.

Visconti, J. A., "Drug-Food Interaction," *Nutrition in Disease*, May, 1977.

Nutrients as Drugs

Anderson, T. W., "Vitamin C and the Common Cold," *Contemporary Nutrition*, Vol. 3, No. 10, October, 1978.

Anderson, T. W., R. Passmore, A. Szent-Gyorgyi, L. C. Pauling, "To Dose or Megadose—A Debate," *Nutrition Today*, Vol. 13, No. 2, March-April, 1978.

Anderson, T. W., "New Horizons for Vitamin C," *Nutrition Today*, Vol. 12, No. 1, January-February, 1977, pp.1-13.

Darby, W. J., K. W. McNutt, and E. N. Todhunter, "Niacin," in Nutrition Reviews' *Present Knowledge in Nutrition*, fourth edition, New York, Washington, D.C.: The Nutrition Foundation, Inc., 1976, pp. 162-74.

Hathcock, J. N., "Toxicity and Pharmacology," in Nutrition Reviews' *Present Knowledge in Nutrition*, fourth edition, New York, Washington, D.C.,: The Nutrition Foundation, 1976, pp. 504-15.

Herbert, V. D. "Megavitamin Therapy," *Contemporary Nutrition*, Vol. 2, No. 10, October, 1977.

Herbert V. D., "Megavitamin Therapy: Facts and Fictions," *Food and Nutrition News*, Vol. 47, No. 4, March-April, 1976, pp. 1, 4.

Hodges, R. E. "Ascorbic Acid," in Nutrition Reviews' *Present Knowledge in Nutrition*, fourth edition, New York, Washington, D.C.: The Nutrition Foundation, 1976, pp. 119-30.

Passmore, R. "How Vitamin C Deficiency Injures the Body," *Nutrition Today*,, Vol. 12, No. 2, March-April, 1977, pp. 6-ll.

Trotter, R. J., "Will Vitamins Replace the Psychiatrist's Couch?" *Science News*, Vol. 104, July 28, 1973, pp. 59-60.

U.S. Food and Drug Administration, "Vitamin and Mineral Products; Labeling and Composition Regulations," *Federal Register, 41:46156, 1976.*

SECTION VI NUTRIENTS—ARE THEY THERE WHEN WE EAT THE FOOD?

American Medical Association, *Nutrients in Processed Foods, Proteins*, Acton, MA: Publishing Sciences Group, Inc., 1974.

American Medical Association, *Nutrients in Processed Foods, Vitamins and Minerals*, Acton, MA: Publishing Sciences Group, Inc., 1974.

Committee on Nutritional Misinformation, Food and Nutrition Board, National Research Council, *Soil Fertility and the Nutritive Value of Crops*, Washington, D.C.: National Academy of Sciences, 1976.

Erdman, J. W., "Bioavailability of Nutrients from Foods," *Contemporary Nutrition*, Vol. 3, No. 11, November, 1978.

Feenema, O. "Loss of Vitamins in Fresh and Frozen Foods," *Food Technology*, Vol. 31, No. 12, December, 1977, p. 32-35, 38.

Harris, R. S. and H. V. Loesecke (Editors), *Nutritional Evaluation of Food Processing*, Westport, CN: AVI Publishing Co., 1975.

Institute of Food Technologists' Expert Panel on Food Safety and Nutrition, and the Committee on Public Information, *The Effects of Food Processing on Nutritional Values*, Chicago, IL: Institute of Food Technologists, 1974.

Bernarde, M.A., *The Chemicals We Eat*, New York: American Heritage Press, 1971.

Whelan, E. M. and F. J. Stare, *Panic in the Pantry*, _____ Atheneum, 1975.

Natural Toxicants

Committee on Food Protection, National Research Council, *Toxicants Occurring Naturally in Foods*, second edition, Washington, D.C.: National Academy of Sciences, 1973.

Hall, R. L., "Safe at the Plate," *Nutrition Today*, Vol. 12, No. 6, November-December, 1977, pp. 6-31.

Institute of Food Technologists' Expert Panel on Food Safety and Nutrition and the Committee on Public Information, *Naturally Occurring Toxicants in Foods*, Chicago, IL: Institute of Food Technologists, March, 1974.

"Microconstituents and Food Safety," *Dairy Council Digest*, Vol. 49, No. 1, January-February, 1978.

Additives

Committee on Food Protection, National Reserach Council, *How Safe is Safe? The Design of Policy on Drugs and Food Additives*, Washington, D.C.: National Academy of Sciences, 1974.

Damon, G. E., "Primer on Food Additives," *FDA Consumer*, DHEW Publication No. (FDA) 74-2002, Washington, DC: U. S. Government Printing Office, May, 1973.

Food Additives, What They Are/How They are Used, Washington, D.C.: Manufacturing Chemists' Association, Inc., 1971.

Hall, R. L., "Food Additives," *Nutrition Today*, Vol. 8, No. 4, July-August, 1973, pp. 20-28.

Hutt, P. B. and A. E. Sloan, "NAS Issues Saccharin Report," *Nutrition Policy Issues*, No. 5, March 1979.

Hutt, P. B. and A. E. Sloan, "National Academy of Sciences Issues Food Safety Report," *Nutrition Policy Issues*, No. 6, April, 1979.

Institute of Food Technologists' Expert Panel on Food Safety and Nutrition, *The Risk Benefit Concept as Applied to Food*, Chicago, IL: Institute of Food Technologists, March, 1978.

Schmidt, A. M., "The Benefit-Risk Equation," *FDA Consumer*, May, 1974, pp. 27-30.

Select Committee on GRAS Substances, Life Sciences Research Office, Federation of American Societies for Experimental Biology, "Evaluation of Health Aspects of GRAS Food Ingredients: Lessons Learned and Questions Unanswered," *Federal Proc.*, Vol 36, 1977, p. 2525.

Today's Food and Additives, Westport CN: Science Communicators, Inc. for General Foods Corp, 1976.

Contaminants

Agricultural Research Service, U.S. Department of Agriculture, *Keeping Food Safe to Eat, A Guide for Homemakers*, Home and Garden Bulletin No. 162, Washington, D.C.: U.S. Government Printing Office, Revised, 1975.

Coppack, R. H. (Editor), *Pesticides: The Issues, The Alternatives*, Berkeley, CA: University of California Division of Agricultural Sciences, 1972.

Food and Drug Administration, "Antibiotics and the Food You Eat," *FDA Consumer Memo*, DHEW Publication No. (FDA) 74-6011, Washington, D.C.: U.S. Government Printing Office, March, 1974.

Food and Drug Administration, "Safety of Cooking Utensils" *FDA Fact Sheet*, Washington, D.C.: U.S. Government Printing Office, July, 1971.

Institute of Food Technologists' Expert Panel on Food Safety and Nutrition, *Botulism*, Chicago, IL: Institute of Food Technologists, 1972.

Institute of Food Technologists' Expert Panel on Food Safety and Nutrition, *Mercury in Food*, Chicago, IL: Institute of Food Technologists, 1973.

Institute of Food Technologists' Expert Panel on Food Safety and Nutrition, *Phthalates in Food*, Chicago, IL: Institute of Food Technologists, 1973.

Institute of Food Technologists' Expert Panel on Food Safety and Nutrition, *Organic Foods*, Chicago, IL: Institute of Food Technologists, 1974.

"Toxoplasmosis: Worse than Thought," *Science News*, Vol. 113, No. 20, May 20, 1978, P. 327.

Weinberg, J. H. "Blighted Bounty: A Twist in the Staff of Life" (Aflatoxin), *Science News*, Vol 107, January 4, 1975, pp. 12-13.

SECTION VIII   MEETING THE NUTRITION CHALLENGE

Alfin-Slater, R.B. and L. Aftergood, "Misconceptions in Nutrition," *Nutrition and the M.D.*, Vol. 4, No. 14, December, 1978, pp. 1-5.

"Food Faddism," *Dairy Council Digest*, Vol. 44, No. 1, January-February, 1973.

"The Food Fad Boom," *FDA Consumer*, DHEW Publication No. (FDA) 74-2019, Washington, D.C.: U.S. Government Printing Office, December, 1973, January, 1974.

Isom, P., "Nutritive Value and Cost of Fast Food Meals," *Family Economics Review*, Highlights Fall, 1976.

Margolius, S., *Health Food Fads and Fakes*, New York: Walker & Co., 1976.

"Nutrition Misinformation and Food Faddism," *Nutrition Reviews' Supplement*, Vol. 32, 1974, pp. 1-74.

Schafer, R. and E. A. Yetley, "Social Psychology of Food Faddism," *Journal of the American Dietetic Association*, Vol. 66, February, 1975, pp. 129-33.

Tracey, M.V., "Human Nutrition (What We Don't Know)," *Nutrition Today*, Vol. 13, No. 6, November-December, 1978, pp. 17-20.

U.S. General Accounting Office, *National Nutrition Issues*, Study by the Staff of the U.S. General Accounting Office, Washington, D.C.: U.S. Government Printing Office, December 8, 1977.

Young, E. A., E. H. Brennan, G. L. Irving, "Perspectives on Fast Foods," *Dietetic Currents*, Vol. 5, No. 5, September-October, 1978.

INDEX

Absorption, of major nutrients, 122
Acid-base balance, 217–20
  and protein, 173–74
Acidophilus milk, 240
Acidosis, 367
  and fat metabolism, 162
Acne. *See* Complexion problems
Addiction. *See* Drugs, addiction; Alcoholism
Additives, to foods, 466
Adenosine diphosphate (ADP), 127, 224
Adenosine triphosphate (ATP), 126–28, 224, 253
Adipose tissue, 79, 92, 126, 160
Adolescence
  athletics in, 364–69
  malnutrition in, 355–59
  obesity, 362–63
  phases of, 352–55
  pregnancy in, 289–91, 293, 298, 360
  snacking, 518–21
  teenage growth spurt, 353–55
ADP. *See* Adenosine diphosphate
Adults
  older, 34–36, 374, 379. *See also* Aging
  single, nutritional problems of, 523–25
  young, 372
Advertising, food, 59–73
  effects on eating patterns, 40–44
Aging, 34–36, 372–81
  and BMR, 83
  drug use patterns, in older adults, 418
  effect of vitamin E on, 431
  nutrional needs and, 377–80
  snacking, patterns in older adults, 521
Alcohol, 299, 373, 414, 418, 422
  and drug addiction, 425
  effects on nutrition, 31
  metabolism, and thiamin, 260
Alcoholism, 422–25
  in pregnant women, 288–89, 291

Allergies
  to cow's milk, 317
  to food, 242–44
Aluminum, 489
American Academy of Pediatrics, 314
American College of Sports Medicine, 365
American Dental Association, 342
Amino acids, 170, 171, 176, 185
  complementary, 178, 180–81, 204
  composition, 178, 225
  essential, 36, 176, 178–79, 203, 225, 295
  infant requirements for, 309
  limiting, 177, 178
  metabolism of, 266
  nonessential, 121, 126
  and NPU, 178
Amylase, 124
Anabolism, 126
Anaerobic exercise, and glucose oxidation, 128
Anemia, 16, 356
  iron-deficiency, 227, 355
  megaloblastic, 420
  pernicious, 264–65, 378
Animal nutrition, studies of, 7
Anorexia, 50, 52, 111
  from drugs, 419
  physiologic, 330
Antacids, 420
Anthropology, cultural, food studies, 25–26
Antibiotics, 256, 421
Anti-Coronary Club, 394
Antioxidants, 481
Antivitamins, 420, 469
Appestat, 51
Appetite, 50, 419
  in preschoolers, 330
  in underweight persons, 111, 112
Arthritis, 374, 413–14
Artificial colorings and flavorings, 482
Ascorbic acid. *See* Vitamin C
Aspirin, 420, 421
Atherosclerosis, 122, 156, 379, 390, 398

Athletics, 354–55, 364–69, 435
ATP. *See* Adenosine triphosphate
Atwater, W. O., 440

Babies. *See* Infants
Baby foods, 67
Bacteria
  disease-causing, 460
  intestinal, 255
  oral, 340
Basal Metabolic Rate (BMR), 82–83, 121, 377
Basic Four, 9–14, 293, 433
  and diet for pregnancy, 297–99
Behavior modification, for weight reduction, 101
Beri-beri, 16, 424
Bile, 157, 158
Bioavailability, of nutrients, 442–43
Biotin, 225, 268
Birth control pill. *See* Oral contraceptive
Blood clotting, 221, 256
Blood pressure, 397
Blood sugar, 51, 126, 233. *See also* Glucose
  in diabetes, 404–6
  and exercise, 368
BMR. *See* Basal Metabolic Rate
Brain, critical growth period, 306
Bran. *See also* Fiber
  in preschool diet, 335
  wheat, 129, 134
Bread, 136–39
  homemade, 138
  in Indian diet, 36
Breakfast, 513–16
Breast feeding. *See* Lactation
Breast milk, nutritional value of, 309–11, 313
Brown rice, 143
Butter, 163
Buttermilk, 240
Butylated hydroxytoluene (BHT), 481
Bypass surgery, for weight control, 106

Caffeine, 336, 469
Calcium, 18, 36, 135, 147, 220–22

Calcium (Contd.)
  in childhood diet, 338
  deficiency, 16, 221
  for lactating mothers, 300–301
  need during pregnancy, 293–95
  and older adults, 378–79
  and oxalic acid, 203, 271
  percentage of weight, 216
  ratio to phosphorus, 183, 222–24
  requirements, 221
  sources, 237–38, 243
  and tooth decay, 339
  U.S. RDA, 63
  in vegetarian diet, 203
  and vitamin D, 221, 222, 253
Caloric density, 152
Calories, 81–82
  in children's diets, 329–30
  in commonly used fats, 164
  deficiency of, 16
  expended in activities, 84
  expenditure in sports, 366
  in fish, 190–91
  in fruit and vegetable group, 276–82
  for infants, 308–9
  labeling, 71–72
  for lactating mother, 300–301
  in milk and dairy products, 239, 243
  in potatoes, 278
  during pregnancy, 293
  RDA for, 7
  requirements for, 82–87
  in snacks, 518, 521
  from sugar, 147
  for teenage growth spurt, 354
  1200-calorie diet, 98
  in various bread products, 138–39
Cancer, 152, 374, 423, 474
  of the colon, 128, 183
  and fiber, 412
  and obesity, 410
  prevention of, 386
  role of diet in, 408–13
  and vitamins, 411
Canned foods, 450. See also Processing, of foods
  quality, 276
Carbohydrates, 5–6, 78, 404
  description of, 118–20
  digestion, absorption, and metabolism of, 122–28
  fiber, 128–33
  functions, 120–23
  in infant diet, 310
  low-carbohydrate diets, 104, 106–7, 121–22, 160, 182, 296

Carbohydrates (Contd.)
  needs, while dieting, 104, 121
  during pregnancy, 296
Carcinogens, 408, 475, 479
Carotene, 249, 270, 271
Cartilage, 121
Casein, 66, 238
Catabolism, 126
  of body tissue, 179
Center for Disease Control. 498
Cereal grains, 134–36
  breakfast cereals, 139–44
Chavez, Caesar, 26
Cheese, 241–44
Chemicals, in foods, 452. See also Contaminants
Chemotherapy, 419
Chewing, learning how, 320
Chicken, 194
Children
  anorexic, 111
  calcium requirements for, 221
  fluorine in diets of, 235
  and food advertising, 41–44, 60, 67
  hyperactivity in, 346–48
  iron needs of, 227
  malnutrition in, 31–32
  and obesity, 94–95
  preschool, 328–36
  serving sizes for, 332
  underweight, 110
  vegetarian diets for, 204
  zinc intake, 233
Chloride shift, in carbon dioxide transport, 220
Chlorine, 219–20
Chocolate, 241, 343, 363
Cholesterol, 63, 153, 183, 386
  controversy concerning, 395–96
  described, 157
  diet control of, 166
  and eggs, 199
  and fiber intake, 131
  formation, and saturated fats, 156
  and heart disease, 391–96
  low-carbohydrate diets and, 122
  and plant protein foods, 191–93
  in vegetarian diet, 203
Chyme, 158
Cirrhosis, of the liver, 422
Citric acid cycle, 127
Clotting, 221, 256
Coenzyme, 128, 218
  defined, 127
  folic acid as, 263
  niacin-containing, 224
Colon
  cancer of, 128, 183
  and fiber, 131

Color Additives Amendment, 473
Colostrum, 314, 315
Committee on Maternal Nutrition, 289
Complementary amino acids, 177–78, 180–81, 204
Complexion problems, 363–64
Computer, use in diet analysis, 18
Constipation
  during pregnancy, 296
  fiber intake and, 131, 296
  in older people, 379
Contaminants, 466, 486–500
Contraceptives. See Oral contraceptives
Convenience foods, 13, 472. See also Processing, of foods
Converted rice, 143
Cooking methods. See Food preparation
Copper, 188, 229, 231, 363
  function of, 127
Corn syrup, 149
Cornea, and vitamin A, 251
Coronary heart disease, 132, 156, 203, 373, 379
  causes, 396
  described, 390–96
  and diabetes, 404
  low-carbohydrate diet and, 122–23
  prevention of, 386–88
Costs
  of breakfast cereals, 141
  of breast feeding, 299
  food dollar, 512–13
  of fruits and vegetables, 273–76
  of protein foods, 194–99
  various bread products, 138–39
  of vegetarian diet, 203
Cyanide, 468

Deamination, 186
Dehydration, 121, 211
  in athletes, 364, 366–67
  of foods, 453
  in infants, 310
Delaney Clause. See Food Additives Amendment
Dental caries. See Tooth decay
Deoxyribonucleic acid (DNA), 223, 225, 233
Department of Agriculture. See United States Department of Agriculture
DES. See Diethylstilbestrol
Diabetes, 87, 126, 152, 225, 373, 404–6
  carbohydrate content in diet, 122
  and fat metabolism, 160

Diabetes (Contd.)
  and heart disease, 391
  prevention, 386
  saccharin controversy, 479
Diet aids, nonprescription, 105
Diet and Coronary Disease Study,
  394
Diet diaries, 16, 97, 101–3
  use in allergy identification,
  344
Diet recall, 16, 18
Diet therapy, 31
Dietary Goals for the United
  States, 122, 196, 386–88, 394,
  401
Dietary recommendations. See
  Recommendations, dietary
Diethylstilbestrol (DES), 491
Dieting. See Obesity; Weight control
Diets
  for babies, introduction of solid
  food, 319–24
  balanced, 9–14
  carbohydrate intake, 118
  cholesterol-control, 198
  for diabetes, 404–5
  effects on aging, 380–81
  for endurance sports, 369
  fad, 104
  Feingold, 347–48, 483
  high-fat, 410
  high-fiber, 132
  high-protein, 122, 221
  for lactation, 300–301
  liquid protein diet, 106–7, 435
  low-carbohydrate, 104, 106–7,
  121, 133, 160, 182, 296
  low-protein, 219
  for pregnant women, 110, 293–
  99
  to prevent heart disease, 393–
  96
  protein sources in, 187
  Prudent diet, 394–95
  for rheumatic diseases, 413
  and tooth decay, 339–42
  1200-calorie diet, 98
  vegetarian, 55, 104, 132, 182,
  187, 199–207, 295–96, 317,
  367
  for weight control, 97–99, 105,
  190, 360, 414
Digestion
  of carbohydrates, 125
  of fats, 157–59
  of major nutrients, 122
  of proteins, 184–85
  of starch, 310
Disaccharide, 118
Diuretics, 420
  magnesium deficiency from,
  225

Diuretics (Contd.)
  and potassium, 219, 401
DNA. See Deoxyribonucleic acid
Drugs. See also Alcoholism
  addiction to, 291, 425–26
  contamination of food by, 491
  drug–food reactions, 421
  drug-induced malnutrition,
  376, 380
  and lactation, 304
  nutrients as, 426–32
  and nutrition, 31, 373, 419–20
  during pregnancy, 298–99
  use in America, 418
  for weight loss, 105

Eating patterns, 24–55
  of children, 336, 338
  eating behavior diary, 16, 97,
  101–3
  eating out, 516–19
  of hard drug users, 425
  infant, 319–23
  and life-styles, 26–31
  nutrition education and, 44–46
  and obesity, 99–103
  physiological factors influencing, 46–52
  in preschoolers, 330–36
  for preventive nutrition, 386–
  88
  social and cultural factors affecting, 25–26
  technological changes and, 38–
  44, 59–73
  teenage, 359–60
Economic factors, and nutrition,
  31–38, 59–73. See also Costs;
  Eating patterns, technological changes
Edema, 174, 211, 401
Eggs, 188, 191
  cost, 194
  NPU, 177
  as protein source, 199
  raw, 469
Elderly. See Aging
Electron transport cycle, 127–28
Emotions, and overweight, 101,
  102
Emulsifiers, 482
Endocrine glands, regulation of
  BMR by, 82
Endurance sports, special diet
  for, 369
Energy, from food, 79–85, 377
  for athletes, 368
  metabolism, 126–28, 260
  release from fats, 79, 152, 160
  storage, 79–82, 120
Energy balance, 85–87
Enriched foods, 63

Environmental Protection Agency
  (EPA), 487, 490, 502
Enzymes, 218
  defined, 127
EPA. See Environmental Protection Agency
Essential amino acids. See Amino
  acids, essential
Essential fatty acids. See Fatty
  acids, essential
Estrogen, 468
Evaluation
  of meals, 514
  nutritional, 14, 16
Exercise, 102, 396, 435
  and aging, 377, 380
  anaerobic, 128
  and calories, 84, 87
  effect on aging, 377
  effect on children's diet, 335,
  336
  for muscle strength, 367
  for obese infants, 323
  for obese teenagers, 362–63
  weight loss and, 94–95, 97, 105
Exercise machines, 105

Fad diets, 104
Family, attitudes toward food, 5
Famine. See Hunger, world-wide
FAO. See United Nations Food
  and Agriculture Organization
Fasting, 26, 360
  effect on blood sugar, 126
  for weight control, 106–7
Fat. See Adipose tissue; Fats;
  Obesity
Fat cells, 93–94, 160
Fat-soluble vitamins. See Vitamins, fat-soluble
Fats, 5–6, 186
  in the blood, 392–93
  and cancer, 410
  daily consumption, 153
  digestion of, 157–59
  effects of cooking, 191
  energy efficiency of, 79
  in meat, 188–91
  metabolism of, 159–61
  percentage of diet, 152, 188
  in preschooler's diet, 335
  saturated fat in common foods,
  156, 244
  in vegetarian diet, 203
Fatty acids, 122, 153, 155, 267. See
  also Saturated fats; Unsaturated fats
  essential, 153
FDA. See Food and Drug Administration

Federal Trade Commission (FTC), 42, 62, 426, 434, 503
Feingold, Dr. Benjamin, 347–48, 483
Fetal alcohol syndrome, 289
Fiber, 119, 123, 128–33, 187, 221, 279
 and cancer, 412
 for constipation in pregnancy, 296
 for dental health, 340, 342
 use in breads, 138
 in vegetarian diet, 203
Flatulence, 129
Fluorine, 235, 313, 339. *See also* Tooth decay
 supplementation for infants, 309
Folacin, 13, 14, 18–19, 63, 188, 263–64, 355
 anemia in aged, 378
 supplementation during pregnancy, 293–95
Folic acid. *See* Folacin
Food Additives Amendment, 409, 473–75, 479
Food and Drug Administration (FDA), 8, 61–63, 66, 67, 72–74, 313, 478, 502
 food additives, regulation of, 473–75, 483
 food contamination, 489, 491, 499
 labels and advertisements, regulation of, 426, 433
 pesticides, 487
 saccharin ban, 479
 vitamin supplements, 427, 433
Food and Nutrition Board, 87, 249
Food composition tables, 9, 569–83
Food consumption, annual statistics, 16
Food diary. *See* Diet diary
Food dollar, 513
Food, Drug, and Cosmetic Act of 1938, 473, 476
Food guides, 9
Food industry, 38–44, 59–73, 145, 479
Food labeling, 61–72
 breakfast cereals, 140
 nutrition, 63–67, 136, 141
 regulation concerning, 61–62
Food poisoning, 460, 493–95, 498
Food preparation, 191, 457–58
Food processing, 13, 38–44, 274–75, 443–45, 448–55, 458–60
Food shortages, global, 31–38
Food Stamp Program, 34, 36
Food technology, 39, 59–73

Food value chart, 17
Fortified foods, 63
Four Food Group system. *See* Basic Four
Freeze drying, 453
Frozen food, 445, 457
Fructose, 118, 124
Fruit juice, imitation, 280
Fruits, 269
 dried, 148, 452,
 introduction into infant diet, 320–21
 juices, 279–82
FTC. *See* Federal Trade Commission
Fussy eater pattern, 54

Galactose, 118, 124
Generally Recognized as Safe (GRAS) list, 474
Genetics and nutrition, 7, 224, 267
 diabetes, 404
 and obesity, 94
Germ, of grain, 134
Global food shortages, 31–38
Glucose, 78, 118, 124–26, 233
 glucose utilization, 51
 metabolism of, 126–28
Gluten, 136
Glycogen, 79, 119, 125
Goiter, 232
Goitrogens, 468
Gout, 414, 422, 424
GRAS. *See* Generally Recognized as Safe list
Growth
 of bones, 220, 353
 in infancy, 304–6
 in preschoolers, 330
 teenage growth spurt, 353–55
Growth hormones, 491

Health foods, 503
Health professionals, as nutrition educators, 45
Heart attack, 390
Heart disease, 132, 152, 156, 203, 373, 379, 390–96
 causes, 396
 low-carbohydrate diet and, 122–23
 prevention, 386–88
Heredity, and nutrition, 7, 94, 224, 267, 404
High blood pressure. *See* Hypertension
High blood sugar. *See* Hyperglycemia
High-fiber bread, 138
High-nutrient density foods, 8, 95, 269, 380

Homemade bread, 138
Homemakers, nutrition planning by, 510–13
Honey, 148
Honey poisoning, 470
Hormones, artificial. *See* Oral contraceptives
Human nutrition, studies of, 6–7
Hunger, 50. *See also* Starvation
 in the U.S., 34–38
 world-wide, 31–34
Hydrochloric acid, 219–20
Hydrogenated oils, 155
Hydrolysis, 123, 171, 212
Hyperactivity, in children, 346–48, 419, 483
Hyperglycemia, 126, 404
Hyperkinetic behavior syndrome. *See* Hyperactivity
Hyperlipidemia. *See* Cholesterol
Hypertension, 397–404
Hypnosis, from supermarket shopping, 59
Hypoglycemia, 126, 406–8
Hypothalamus, 51

Infant formulas, 67, 309–11, 313, 314
 for premature babies, 324
Infants
 appropriate foods, by age, 320
 breast feeding, 314–19
 feeding patterns of, 319–23
 growth of, 304–6
 introduction of solid food to, 319–24
 low birth weight, 289, 323–24
 nitrogen excretion, 183
 nutritional needs of, 308–14
 obesity in, 307–8, 323
 weaning, 319–23
Ingredient list. *See* Food labeling
Insects, as food contaminants, 491–92
Insulin, 126, 225, 233, 404, 405
Insulin shock, 407
International Units, 249
Iodine, 63, 231–33
Iron, 14, 18, 133, 147, 186, 193, 220, 355
 for athletes, 367
 biologic availability, 199
 in children's diets, 328, 338
 deficiency, 16, 227
 in enriched cereals, 135
 from meat group, 187–88
 function of, 127, 226–27
 in infant diet, 311
 sources, 228–30
 supplementation, during pregnancy, 293–95
 toxicity, 227

Iron (Contd.)
U.S. RDA, 63
in vegetarian diet, 203

Jaw-wiring, for weight loss, 106
Joints, 121
Joule, 81
Juices
for athletes, 365
comparisons, 279–82
Junk foods. *See* Low-nutrient
density foods

Kelp, 232
Ketones, 182
Ketosis, 107, 121
and fat metabolism, 162
in pregnancy, 296
Key nutrients, 18
amount per dollar, 36
Kidneys, 67, 218–19, 253
babies', 309–11
and water balance, 210
Krebs cycle. *See* Citric acid cycle
Kwashiorkor, 16, 173
magnesium deficiency in, 225

La Leche League, 299–300
Labeling, food. *See* Food labeling
Lactation, 299–301
and the Basic Four, 13
diet for, 297–301
weaning, 319–23
Lactic acid, 128
Lactose, 118
Laetrile, 469
Laxatives, 420. *See also* Constipation
Lead, contamination by, 489
Lecithin, 157, 427, 482
Legumes, 13, 14, 171, 178, 186,
451
cholesterol content of, 193
enzyme inhibitors in, 469
as folacin source, 188
and mycotoxins, 499–500
Linoleic acid, 153, 310
Lipids. *See* Fats
Lipoproteins, 160
Liquid protein diet, 106–7, 435
Literacy, and food labeling, 60–61
Liver
at birth, 229
blood sugar regulation, 126
disease, 224, 422–23
drug damage, 420
in fat metabolism, 158–60
as food, 188, 191, 197
glycogen storage, 125
metabolism of vitamins, 250,
252

Liver (Contd.)
role in protein absorption, 185–
86
toxicity of alcohol to, 422–24
Longevity. *See* Aging
Low birth weight, 323–24. *See also*
Premature babies
effects on health and mortality,
289
Low blood pressure, 398
Low blood sugar. *See* Hypoglycemia
Low-nutrient-density foods, 8,
95, 281, 380, 519
alcohol, 422
in children's diets, 329–30
sugar, 147
for underweight, 112

Macroelements, 5–6, 217
Macronutrients, 5–6
Magnesium, 13, 14, 18–19, 188
deficiency, 225
functions of, 127, 224
Malnutrition, 14, 31. *See also*
Overnutrition; undernutri-
tion
from alcohol abuse, 423
in American teenagers, 355–59
in cancer patients, 409
drug-induced, 376, 380
effect on brain development,
306
Maltose, 118, 124
Manganese, 234–35
Marasmus, 16, 173
Margarine, 163–64
Meals on Wheels, 34, 36, 376
Meat analogs, 199–202
Meats, 187–91, 194–97, 320
Megadoses, of nutrients, 426–32
Memory storage, role of fats in,
153
Mercury, 488–89
Metabolism
of amino acids, 266
Basal Metabolic Rate (BMR),
82–83
of carbohydrates, 404
disorders of, 7, 14, 344–46, 408
effects of drugs, 420
energy and, 126–28, 260
of fats, 159–62
of major nutrients, 122, 128
of proteins, 185–86, 266
regulation, 82, 232
Michigan Experiment Station, 442
Microelements, 5–6, 135, 188,
217, 226–37, 442. *See also*
Copper; Fluorine; Iodine;
Iron; Manganese; Zinc
defined, 217

Microelements (Contd.)
losses, 448, 449
minor trace elements, 236–37
in vegetarian diets, 203
Micronutrients, 5–6
Microorganisms, in foods, 493–95
Milk
breast milk. *See* Lactation
and cancer, 412
comparison of cow's, human
and formula, 316–17
inability to digest, 345
in infant diet, 314–19
Milk group, 237–45
Mineral elements, 5–6. *See also*
Microelements
defined, 216
nutrient availability, 454–55
phytic acid binding, 132
during pregnancy, 293–95
requirements in infancy, 311–
13
role in metabolism, 127
supplementation, 293–95, 335,
426–34
for young children, 335
Mineral oil, 420
Mitochondria, in breakdown of
fatty acids, 160
Molasses, nutrient density of, 147
Molds, in foods, 499–500
Monosaccharides, 118
Monosodium glutamate, 517
Mormons, 409
Mycotoxins, 499

National Academy of Sciences,
479
National Heart and Diet Study,
395
National Marine Fisheries Service, 502
National Research Council, 87,
249, 289
National School Lunch Program,
34, 36, 359
Natural food diet, 55, 503
Nausea, 220
while pregnant, 297
Net protein utilization (NPU),
common sources of protein,
177
Neurotransmitters, 121
Niacin, 36, 133, 174, 188, 193,
224, 262
in enriched cereals, 135
function, 127
in megadoses, 431
sources, 262–63
U.S. RDA, 63
Nicotinic acid. *See* Niacin
Night blindness, 251

Nitrogen balance studies, 174
Nitrogen cycle, 171–72
Nitrosamines, 478
Nondairy products, 244–45
Nonessential amino acids. *See* Amino acids, nonessential
NPU. *See* Net protein utilization
Nursing. *See* Lactation
Nutrient density, 8, 69, 147. *See also* High-nutrient density foods; Low-nutrient density foods
Nutrients, 4–6
  availability, 440, 454–55
  classification of, 6
  essential, 5
  human requirements for, 7
  key, 18, 37
  losses, 448
Nutrition
  adolescent, 352
  defined, 4
  disorders of, 14–16·
  education, 44–46
  evaluation of, 14
  goals, management steps for, 510
  human, 6
  nutrition counseling, 31, 409
  prenatal. *See* Pregnancy
  preventive, 386–88
Nutritional Quality Guidelines, 72–73

Obesity, 52, 85–87, 90–107, 404, 422
  adolescent, 356, 362–63
  and cancer, 410
  in childhood, 336
  contribution to high blood pressure, 399
  eating patterns and, 99–103
  and health, 90, 123
  in infancy, 307–8, 317, 323
  and osteoarthritis, 414
  and pregnancy, 293
  prevention of, 95
  questionable reducing practices, 104–7
Obesity syndrome, 90
Oil. *See* Fats
Older American's Act, 376
Olive oil, 155
Oral contraceptives, 233, 372, 418, 419
  and milk production, 301
  nutrient depletion by, 420–21
  vitamin B₆, 266–67
  zinc, 233
Organ meats, 197. *See also* Liver, as food
Organic nutrients, 5

Organically grown foods, 503
Organoleptic qualities, of food, 48, 282–83, 472
Osmosis, 211
Osteoporosis, 183, 235, 377, 379
Overnutrition, 14
  of infants, 307
Overweight, 90. *See also* Obesity
  prevention, 95
Oxalic acid, 203, 271, 469
Oxidation, 449–50, 481

Pantothenic acid, 18–19, 267–68
  function, 127, 267
Pasta, 144
Pasteurization, described, 238, 460
PCBs. *See* Polychlorinated biphenyls
Peanut oil, 155
Pectin, in vitamin B_{12} depletion, 132
Pellagra, 16
Pennington Index Nutrients, 18
Peptide link, 171, 173
PER. *See* Protein effectiveness rating
Pesticides, contamination of foods by, 486–97
pH balance
  of the blood, 227
  of food, 452
  protein regulation of, 173–74
Phosphorus, 188, 216, 221–24
  and ATP, 127
  for lactating mothers, 300–301
  need during pregnancy, 293–95
  ratio to calcium, 183, 220–22, 313
  role in absorption of vitamin B_2, 261
  and tooth decay, 339
  and vitamin D, 253
Phthalates, 490
Phytic acid, in high-fiber diets, 132, 203
Pimples. *See* Complexion problems
Placebos, 428
Plant, Soil, and Nutrition Laboratory, 442
Plaque, dental, 340
Plaques, arterial, 390
Plastics, contamination of food by, 490
Polychlorinated biphenyls (PCBs), 490
Polysaccharide, 118
Polyunsaturated fats, 63, 155, 164–66, 396
  and heart disease, 393

Polyunsaturated Fats (Contd.)
  in protein foods, 191–93
Potassium, 121, 147, 188
  and diuretics, 219, 401
  in egg substitutes, 199, 200
  functions, sources, and requirements for, 219
  losses during sports, 365–67
  and sodium, 219
  and tooth decay, 339
Poverty. *See also* Hunger
  and diet patterns, 31–38
  in the U.S., 34
Precursors
  of essential nutrients, 7
  of niacin, 174
  of vitamin A, 249
Pregnancy
  and alcohol, 289, 424
  and the Basic Four, 13, 297–99
  calcium requirements for, 221
  dieting during 110
  drugs during, 298–99
  folacin requirements, 263
  iodine deficiency and, 232
  iron needs, 227
  megadoses of vitamin C, 432
  nutrient needs, 293–99
  and potassium, 219
  preparation for, 372
  raw meat, 493
  teenage, 289–91
  vitamin supplements, 253, 267
  zinc requirements, 233
Premature babies, developmental problems of, 323–24
Prenatal nutrition. *See* Pregnancy
Preservatives, 481
Processing, of foods, 13, 38–44, 274–75, 443–45, 448–55, 458–60
Protein, 5–6, 122, 170–74, 221, 411
  amounts in common foods, 183, 243
  for athletes, 366–67
  in bread and cereal group, 133
  complementary amino acids, 178, 180–82, 204
  complete, 178
  costs, 194–99
  digestion of, 184–85
  and growth in height, 354
  infant requirements, 309–10
  for lactating mothers, 300–301
  less complete, 178
  liquid protein diet, 106–7, 435
  metabolism of, 185–86
  needs during pregnancy, 293–95
  quality, 66
  requirements for, 174–76, 182

Protein (Contd.)
supplementation, 434–35
U.S. RDA, 63
in vegetarian diet, 204
Protein effectiveness rating (PER), 66, 177
Provitamin A. *See* Carotene
Prudent diet, 394–95
Ptyalin, 123
Pyridoxine. *See* Vitamin B₆

Questions, about nutrition, 528

RDA. *See* Recommended Dietary Allowances
Recommendations, dietary
cholesterol control, 166
Dietary Goals for the United States, 196, 386–88, 394
for fiber, 133
food preparation practices, 457
for maximization of protein availability, 187
for people living alone, 523–24
to prevent heart disease, 393–96
saturated fats, 156
for weight loss, 105
Recommended Dietary Allowance (RDA), 7
for calories, 84
for protein, 174–75
Refined foods, 135. *See also* Processing, of foods
Rehabilitation programs, nutrition counseling and diet therapy, 31
Renal solute load, and infant kidney development, 309–10, 324–25
Rheumatic diseases, 374, 413–14
Ribonucleic acid (RNA), 170, 223, 224, 233
Rice, 141–44
Rickets, 16, 222, 253
RNA. *See* Ribonucleic acid
Roughage. *See* Fiber

Saccharin, 479
Saliva, 339, 376
in carbohydrate digestion, 123
Salmonella, 460, 494–95
Salt. *See* Sodium
Salt tablets, 367
Satiety, 50
Satiety value, of diet foods, 97
Saturated fats, 63, 155, 164–66, 183
in milk and milk products, 244–45
in protein foods, 191–93
U.S. Dietary Goals, 386

Saturated Fats (Contd.)
in vegetarian diet, 203
School Lunch Program, 34, 36, 359, 516
Scurvy, 16, 256, 259
rebound, 432
Selenium, 236–37, 363
Senility, 235, 380–81
Servings
from Basic Four, 9–14
size, 196, 332
Seventh Day Adventists, 409
Shellfish poisoning, paralytic, 493
Shopping list, 511, 512
Smoking, 396, 409, 422
during pregnancy, 291
Snacking, 30, 518–22
in adolescence, 357–60
in childhood, 338
and tooth decay, 341
young children, 332
Social changes, effects on diet patterns, 26–31
Sodium, 121, 188, 387, 394, 412
in common foods, 400
during pregnancy, 288
in egg substitutes, 199, 200
functions, sources, and requirements for, 218
and high blood pressure, 399–403
in infants' food, 321
losses during sports, 367
and potassium, 219
in pregnant woman's diet, 297
Sodium nitrate, 409, 477
Sodium nitrite, 476–78
Solid food, in infant diets, 319–24
Soy products, 204, 329
as meat replacements, 200–202
Sports. *See* Athletics
Spot-reducing, 105
Staphylococcal ("staph") poisoning, 494–95
Starch, 118–19
digestion by infants, 310
Starvation, 31–38, 179–80
Storage
of energy, 79–82, 120
of foods, 448–56
of fruits and vegetables, 273
Stroke, 398–99
Sucrose. *See* Sugar
Sugar, 118, 145–49, 394, 406
and exercise, 368–69
and heart disease, 122–23
in infant diet, 316–18, 321
metabolism of, 348
percentage of common foods, 146–47
in processed fruits, 449
simple, 118

Sugar (Contd.)
and tooth decay, 341
Sulfur, 225–26
Sulfur dioxide, 452, 481
Synovial fluid, 212

Tapeworms, 493
Teenagers. *See* Adolescence
Temperature
and nutrient losses, 450–52
of refrigerator, 456
Ten-State Nutrition Survey, 355
Tetracycline, 421
Texture, food preference by, 49
Thiamin. *See* Vitamin B₁
Thyroid gland, and iodine, 232
Tooth decay, 122, 147, 148, 251, 253, 519
in children, 338–42
from drinks, 281–82
fluorine and, 235–313
in teenagers, 356
and weaning, 323
Toxemia, 288, 291
Toxicity. *See also* Contaminants
of additives, 473
of alcohol, 422–24
amino acid, 178
of drugs, 419
of fluorine, 235–36
iodine, 232
of iron, 227
naturally occurring in foods, 467–70
of nutrients, 8, 250, 295, 469
selenium, 237
Toxoplasmosis, 299, 492
Trace minerals. *See* Microelements
Transamination, 186
Tricarboxylic cycle. *See* Citric acid cycle
Trichinosis, 492
Triglycerides, 154
Tuna, mercury levels in, 489
Turbinado sugar, 148

Ulcers, 521
Undernutrition, 14, 31, 111
in children, 336
in infancy, 307
Underweight, 110–13
and health, 110
United Farm Workers, 26
United Nations Food and Agriculture Organization (FAO), 31, 34
United States Department of Agriculture (USDA), 16, 45, 66, 275, 478, 502
food composition tables, 440
grading system, 62

United States Department
of Agriculture (Contd.)
National School Lunch Program, 34, 36, 358–59
organic foods survey, 504
regulation of pesticides, 487
shopping survey, 511
United States Recommended Daily Allowances (U.S. RDA), 8, 63, 66, 73
for protein, 177–78
tables, 67–68
United States Senate Select Committee on Nutrition and Human Needs, 196, 394
Unsaturated fats, 155
for infants, 310, 314
USDA. See United States Department of Agriculture
U.S. RDA. See United States Recommended Daily Allowances

Value. See Costs
Vegetables, 269–72
flavor, 282
introduction into infant diet, 320–21
juices, 279
Vegetarian diet, 55, 104, 182, 199–207, 380
for athletes, 367
and breast milk, 317
for children, 204
Mormons and Seventh Day Adventists, 409
during pregnancy , 295–96
protein sources in, 187
risks and benefits, 203
vitamin B_{12} and, 132, 203, 265
Vinyl plastics, contamination of foods by, 490
Vitamin A, 18, 166, 188, 199, 339
and cancer, 411
deficiency, 251
sources, 249, 270, 271
toxicity, 250, 295
U.S. RDA, 63
in whole milk, 238–39
Vitamin B_1 (Thiamin), 133, 188, 193, 199, 225, 259–60
deficiency, 16, 424

Vitamin B (Thiamin) (Contd.)
in enriched cereals, 135
function, 127, 224
sources, 238, 259, 260
U.S. RDA, 63
Vitamin B_2 (Riboflavin), 188, 193, 199, 261–62
function of, 127
sources, 238
U.S. RDA, 63
Vitamin B_6 (Pyridoxine), 13, 14, 18–19, 135, 188, 266–67
Vitamin B_{12}, 13, 188, 264–66
absorption, 220, 221
anemia in aged, 378
depletion by pectin, 132
sources, 265
in vegetarian diet, 203, 265, 295–96, 317
Vitamin C, 256–59, 270, 420, 478
for colds, 430
deficiency, 16
and food processing, 459
megadoses, 432
during pregnancy, 295, 432
protection, in storage, 273
U.S. RDA, 63
Vitamin D, 153, 157, 166, 188, 251–54, 339
addition to milk, 239
in calcium absorption, 221
and cancer, 411
deficiency, 16, 222, 224, 253
for lactating mother, 300–301
need during pregnancy, 293–95
supplementation for infants, 313
Vitamin E, 13, 14, 63, 166, 254–55
in human milk, 314
megadoses, 430–31
sources, 255
in whole milk, 238–39
Vitamin K, 254–56, 314
Vitamins, 5–6
antivitamins, 420, 469
as coenzymes, 248
fat-soluble, 5–6, 153, 249–56, 310, 420, 451
heat-sensitive, 450
megadoses, 426–32
nutrient availability, 454–55

Vitamins (Contd.)
pH sensitivity, 452
for pregnant women, 293–95
requirements for infant diets, 312–14
role in metabolism, 127
supplementation, 380, 426–34
water-soluble, 5–6, 256–68, 449

Water, 5–6
binding capacity, of fiber, 131
during exercise, 364
fluoridation of, 235–36
functions of, 212
in infant nutrition, 310–11
intoxication, 468
in meats, 188
as nutrient, 210–13
in pregnancy, 293
Water balance, 210, 218–20
and carbohydrates, 121
and energy balance, 87
and protein, 173–74
Water-soluble vitamins. See Vitamins, water-soluble
Waxes, on fresh fruit and vegetables, 484
Weaning, 319–23
Weight, 85–87
average, 91
at birth. See Low birth weight
during pregnancy, 291–93, 296
excess. See Obesity
ideal, 85
of infants, 307–8
Weight control. See also Obesity; Underweight
for athletes, 369–70
during pregnancy, 291–93, 296
questionable techniques, 104–7
and snacking, 518–21
Weight Watchers, 102
Whole wheat bread, 136
Women, Infants, and Children (WIC) program, 34
World hunger, 31–38, 50

Yogurt, 240, 380

Zinc, 13, 14, 233–34, 393
in infant nutrition, 313